JOHN A. BOSWICK, Jr., M.S., M.D., F.A.C.S.

Attending Surgeon,
St. Joseph's Hospital,
Rose Medical Center,
Veterans Administration Hospital,
Denver, Colorado

Former Director of Hand Surgery Service
and Professor of Surgery,
University of Colorado Health Sciences Center

Complications in
H A N D
SURGERY

1986
W. B. SAUNDERS COMPANY
Philadelphia/London/Toronto/Mexico City
Rio de Janeiro/Sydney/Tokyo/Hong Kong

W. B. Saunders Company: West Washington Square
                            Philadelphia, PA   19105

Library of Congress Cataloging in Publication Data

Main entry under title:

Complications in hand surgery.

1. Hand—Surgery—Complications and sequelae.
   I. Boswick, John A., 1926–   . [DNLM: 1. Hand—sur-
   gery.   2. Hand Injuries—surgery.   3. Postoperative
   Complications. WE 830 C737]

RD559.C66   1986   617′.575   85–1950

ISBN 0–7216–1877–4

Designer: Karen O'Keefe
Production Manager: Laura Tarves
Illustration Coordinator: Peg Shaw
Page Layout Artist: Patti Maddaloni
Indexer: Dennis Dolan

Complications in Hand Surgery   ISBN   0–7216–1877–4

Last digit is the print number: 9   8   7   6   5   4   3   2   1

CONTRIBUTORS

JOHN A. BOSWICK, JR., M.D.
Formerly Professor of Surgery, University of Colorado School of Medicine, Denver, Colorado; Chief, Hand Surgery Service, University of Colorado Health Sciences Center, Denver, Colorado; Attending Surgeon, St. Joseph Hospital and Rose Medical Center, Denver, Colorado
Complications Following Thermal Injuries; Complications Following Electrical Injuries; Complications from Peripheral Nerve Injury; Complications Following Acute Infections of the Hand

WILLIAM H. BOWERS, M.S., M.D.
Asheville Hand Center, Asheville, North Carolina
Complications of Digital Ligament Injury

PAUL W. BRAND, M.D., F.R.C.S.
Clinical Professor of Surgery and Clinical Professor of Orthopedics, Louisiana State University School of Medicine, Shreveport, Louisiana; Chief, Rehabilitation Branch, National Hansens Disease Center, U.S. Public Health Service, Carville, Louisiana
Results of Insensitivity in Patients with Nerve Injury, Leprosy, and other Neuropathies

PAUL W. BROWN, M.D.
Clinical Professor of Orthopedic Surgery and Clinical Professor of Plastic and Reconstructive Surgery, Yale University School of Medicine, New Haven, Connecticut; Consultant in Hand Surgery, Veterans Administration Hospital, West Haven, Connecticut; Attending Surgeon, St. Vincent's Medical Center and Consultant in Hand Surgery, Bridgeport General Hospital, Bridgeport, Connecticut; Consultant in Hand Surgery, Stamford Hospital, Stamford, Connecticut
Complications Following Amputations of Parts of the Hand; Complications Following Wound Care

WILLIAM E. BURKHALTER, M.D.
Professor of Orthopaedics and Rehabilitation and Chief, Division of Hand Surgery, University of Miami/Jackson Memorial Medical Center, Miami, Florida
Complications of Tendon Transfer for Nerve Paralysis of the Hand

MACK C. CLAYTON, M.D.
Clinical Professor, University of Colorado School of Medicine, Denver, Colorado; Active Staff, St. Joseph Hospital, Denver, Colorado
Complications Following Surgery for Rheumatoid and Arthritic Conditions

WILLIAM W. EVERSMANN, JR., M.D.
Hand Surgeon, Linn County Orthopedics and Rheumatology, Cedar Rapids, Iowa; Active Staff, Mercy Hospital and St. Luke's Hospital, Cedar Rapids Iowa
Complications of Extensor Tendon Injuries; Complications of Compression or Entrapment Neuropathies

DONALD C. FERLIC, M.D.
Clinical Assistant Professor, University of Colorado School of Medicine, Denver, Colorado; Active Staff, St. Joseph Hospital, Denver, Colorado
Complications Following Surgery for Rheumatoid and Arthritic Conditions

STEWART H. HARRISON, M.D., F.R.C.S. (ENG.), F.R.C.S., L.D.S., R.C.S. (EDIN.)
Former Hunterian Professor, Royal College of Surgeons, London, England; Consultant (Plastic and Hand Surgeon), Mount Vernon Hospital and the Windsor Group of Hospitals, Northwood, England.
Juvenile Chronic Arthritis

RICHARD S. IDLER, M.D.
Clinical Assistant Professor of Orthopaedic Surgery, Indiana University School of Medicine, Indianapolis, Indiana; Associate Member, Department of Orthopaedics, St. Vincent Hospital and Health Care Center, Associate Member, Orthopaedic (Hand) Service, Methodist Hospital of Indianapolis, and Staff Physician, Orthopaedic Section, George Roudebush V.A. Medical Center, Indianapolis, Indiana
Complications in Fractures of the Phalanges and Metacarpals

MICHAEL KALISMAN, M.D.
Attending Physician, Department of Surgery, Division of Plastic Surgery, St. Luke's Roosevelt Hospital, Cabrini Medical Center, and St. Clare's Hospital, New York, New York
Complications in Flexor Tendon Injuries; Complications from Flexor Tendon Surgery

HAROLD E. KLEINERT, M.D.
Clinical Professor of Surgery, University of Louisville School of Medicine, Louisville, Kentucky, and Clinical Professor of Surgery, Indiana University School of Medicine, Indianapolis, Indiana; Director of Hand Surgery Services, University of Louisville Hospitals, Louisville, Kentucky
Complications in Flexor Tendon Injuries; Complications from Flexor Tendon Surgery

DOUGLAS LAMB, M.B., C.H.B., F.R.C.S.E.

Professor and Chairman, Department of Orthopaedic Surgery, University of Edinburgh, Edinburgh, Scotland; Consultant Orthopaedic Surgeon, Royal Infirmary and Princess Margaret Rose Hospital, Edinburgh, Scotland
Radial Agenesis

MONROE I. LEVINE, M.D.
Clinical Associate Professor of Orthopaedic Surgery, Uniformed Services

University of the Health Sciences, Bethesda, Maryland; Associate Professor of Orthopaedic Surgery, University of Missouri—Kansas City School of Medicine, Kansas City, Missouri
Complications Following Crush Injuries

ROBERT M. McFARLANE, M.D., M.Sc., F.R.C.S. (C), F.A.C.S.
Professor and Chief, Division of Plastic Surgery, University of Western Ontario, London, Ontario; Chief of Surgery, Victoria Hospital, London, Ontario
Complications of Dupuytren's Disease

HANNO MILLESI, M.D.
Professor of Surgery and Head, Department of Plastic and Reconstructive Surgery, 1st Surgical Clinic, University of Vienna Medical School, Vienna, Austria; Director, Ludwig-Boltzmann-Institute for Experimental Plastic Surgery, Vienna, Austria
Complications Following Secondary or Reconstructive Nerve Repair

ERIK MOBERG, M.D., Ph.D.
Professor Emeritus of Orthopaedic and Hand Surgery, University of Göteborg, Göteborg, Sweden
Complications and Pitfalls in Modern Upper Limb Tetraplegia Surgery

NASHAAT NAAM, M.D.
Formerly Assistant Professor of Surgery (Hand Surgery), University of Colorado School of Medicine, Denver, Colorado; Chief of Surgery and Attending Hand Surgeon, Clay County Hospital, Flora, Illinois; Attending Hand Surgeon, Richland Memorial Hospital, Olney, Illinois
Complications Following Thermal Injuries; Complications Following Electrical Injuries; Complications Following Acute Infections of the Hand

GEORGE E. OMER, JR., M.D., M.S., F.A.C.S.
Professor and Chairman, Department of Orthopaedics and Rehabilitation, University of New Mexico, Albuquerque, New Mexico; Chief of Medical Staff, Chief of Orthopaedic Surgery, and Chief of Hand Surgery, University of New Mexico Hospital, Albuquerque, New Mexico; Consultant on Upper Extremity, Carrie Tingley Hospital, Albuquerque, New Mexico
Posttraumatic Dystrophy

JOHN P. REMENSNYDER, M.D.
Associate Professor of Surgery, Harvard Medical School, Boston, Massachusetts; Visiting Surgeon, Massachusetts General Hospital and Chief of Staff, Shriners Burns Institute, Boston, Massachusetts
Radiation Injuries of the Hand

JAMES H. ROTH, M.D., F.R.C.S.(C)
Clinical Assistant Professor, University of Western Ontario, London, Ontario
Arterial Injuries of the Upper Extremity

DOUGLAS SCHREIBER, M.D.
Department of Orthopaedics, Virginia Beach General Hospital and Humana Hospital Bayside, Virginia Beach, Virginia
Complications in Fractures of Phalanges and Metacarpals

FRANK A. SCOTT, M.D., F.R.C.S.(C), F.A.C.S.
Chief, Hand and Reconstructive Surgery and Assistant Clinical Professor of Surgery, University of Colorado School of Medicine, Denver, Colorado;

Chief, Hand Surgery Service, Denver Veterans Administration Hospital and Attending Hand Surgeon, Rose Medical Center, Denver, Colorado
Complications Following Replantation and Revascularization

ALAN E. SEYFER, M.D., F.A.C.S.
Colonel, U.S. Army Medical Corps, Associate Professor of Surgery, and Chief, Division of Plastic and Reconstructive Surgery, Uniformed Services University of the Health Sciences, Bethesda, Maryland; Chief, Plastic Surgery Service and Co-Director, Hand Surgery Section, Orthopaedic Surgery Service, Walter Reed Army Medical Center, Washington, D.C.
Complications Following Crush Injuries

RICHARD J. SMITH, M.D.
Clinical Professor of Orthopaedic Surgery, Harvard Medical School, Boston, Massachusetts; Chief, Hand Surgery, Department of Orthopaedics, Massachusetts General Hospital, Boston, Massachusetts
Complications of Surgical Treatment of Tumors of the Hand

CHARLEY J. SMYTH, M.D., M.S.(Path.)
Clinical Professor of Medicine, University of Colorado School of Medicine, Denver, Colorado; Consultant, Rheumatology, St. Joseph, Mercy, St. Lukes/Presbyterian and Rose Medical Center, Denver, Colorado
Complications Following Rheumatoid and Degenerative Joint Diseases

CURTIS M. STEYERS, JR., M.D.
Assistant Professor of Orthopedic Surgery, University of Iowa Hospital and Clinics, Iowa City, Iowa
Complications in Flexor Tendon Injuries; Complications from Flexor Tendon Surgery

JAMES W. STRICKLAND, M.D.
Clinical Professor of Orthopaedic Surgery, Indiana University School of Medicine, Indianapolis, Indiana; Chief, Section of Hand Surgery, Department of Orthopaedics, St. Vincent Hospital, Director of Hand Surgical Rotation, Orthopaedic Residency, Indiana University School of Medicine, and Associate Member of the Orthopaedic (Hand) Service, Methodist Hospital, Indianapolis, Indiana
Complications in Fractures of the Phalanges and Metacarpals

ALFRED B. SWANSON, M.D., F.A.C.S.
Professor of Surgery, Michigan State University, Lansing, Michigan; Director of Orthopaedic and Hand Surgery Training Program of the Grand Rapids Hospitals and Director of Hand Fellowship and Orthopaedic Research, Blodgett Memorial Medical Center, Grand Rapids, Michigan
Cerebral Palsy

GENEVIEVE de GROOT SWANSON, M.D.
Assistant Clinical Professor of Surgery, Michigan State University, Lansing, Michigan; Coordinator of Orthopaedic Research Department, Blodgett Memorial Medical Center, Grand Rapids, Michigan
Cerebral Palsy

JULIO TALEISNIK, M.D.
Assistant Clinical Professor, University of California, Irvine, California
Complications of Fractures, Dislocations, and Ligamentous Injuries of the Wrist

KENYA TSUGE, M.D.
Professor and Chairman, Department of Orthopaedic Surgery, Hiroshima University School of Medicine, Hiroshima, Japan
Macrodactyly

JAMES R. URBANIAK, M.D.
Professor of Orthopaedic Surgery, Duke University School of Medicine, Durham, North Carolina; Chief of Orthopaedic Surgery, Duke University Medical Center, Durham, North Carolina
Arterial Injuries of the Upper Extremity

IAN WINSPUR, M.B., Ch.B., F.R.C.S.E., F.A.C.S.
Attending Surgeon (Hand Surgery and Plastic Surgery), Cottage Hospital, St. Francis Hospital, and Memorial Rehabilitation Hospital, Santa Barbara, California.
Complications Following Secondary Reconstructive Procedures of Skin and Subcutaneous Tissue; Complications Following Injury to the Skin and to the Subcutaneous Tissue

VIRCHEL E. WOOD, M.D.
Chief, Hand Surgery Service and Associate Professor, Orthopedic Surgery, Loma Linda University, School of Medicine, Loma Linda, California; Attending, Riverside General, San Bernardino County Medical Center, Jerry L. Pettis Memorial Veterans Hospital, Loma Linda Community Hospital, and Loma Linda University Medical Center, Loma Linda, California
Congenital Anomalies

PREFACE

This book was conceived during a period of intense personal involvement in the care of patients with complications arising from disease or injury of the upper extremities. Only through continuing experience was it possible to acquire the faculty of judgment so necessary in the management of these complications. As a way of broadening the knowledge base, there arose the idea of inviting expert surgeons to contribute their experiences in book form.

The soundness of the concept has perhaps been best shown by the extent to which discussions of complications have become common at meetings of hand surgeons and in the literature on the subject. To gather clinically useful expertise, published and unpublished, into a single work is the aim of this book.

Whether they are problems that make surgery of the hand more difficult or those that arise during or after an operative procedure, complications are managed by surgeons with an interest in the hand and with special training in hand surgery. It is not the intent of this volume to substitute for an appropriate development of skills and experience. Instead the book offers a detailed look at each of its topics in a way that allows readers to add the expertise of others to their own. In addition, it is hoped that all physicians who see and treat patients with injuries and disorders of the upper extremities will benefit by an understanding of the complications that can arise.

Contributors have been asked to emphasize ways to avoid pitfalls and undesirable consequences, in both surgical and nonsurgical care. Chapters stress an understanding of the indications for surgical intervention, the operative techniques employed, prevention and management of intraoperative problems, and the most practical approach to dealing with complications resulting from treatment.

I am most grateful to each of the contributing writers for sharing their experience and ideas on the often difficult subject of complications in hand surgery.

JOHN A. BOSWICK JR

CONTENTS

1

ARTERIAL INJURIES OF THE UPPER EXTREMITY

James R. Urbaniak and
James H. Roth

Arterial injuries of the upper extremity often endanger the survival of the limb, and may risk the life of the patient. The complications of treatment of these injuries may significantly affect the patient's ability to use the limb effectively. This chapter will review the vascular anatomy and its variations, the physical examination, special diagnostic tests, and acute treatment, and describe the management of complications of arterial injuries of the upper extremity.

ANATOMIC CONSIDERATIONS

A comprehensive knowledge of the arterial anatomy of the upper extremity is mandatory for all surgeons involved with arterial injury management. Hollinshead's work is an excellent reference in this regard.[20] This section is not intended to be a comprehensive study of anatomy, but rather is designed for the surgeon engaged in upper extremity vascular surgery. The anatomic structures described all have clinical relevance, and we realize the necessity of being knowledgeable about these anatomic relationships in the management of vascular problems of the upper extremity.

Normal Anatomy

The axillary artery is a direct continuation of the subclavian artery, with the change in name occurring as the vessel crosses the first rib. It becomes the brachial artery, by definition, at the lower border of the teres major muscle. At this level, the median nerve is anterolateral to the vessel, the ulnar nerve is posteromedial, and the radial nerve

is posterolateral. First, the radial nerve, then the ulnar, diverge posteriorly, and the median nerve crosses in front of the brachial artery to lie medial to it at the elbow. The artery and the median nerve then enter the antecubital fossa on the front of the brachialis muscle, and the artery ends by dividing into the radial and ulnar arteries.

Major branches of the brachial artery, which become increasingly important with compromise of brachial artery flow, provide an excellent collateral circulation to the elbow (Fig. 1–1). The first major branch of the brachial artery is the profunda brachii, which leaves the artery to pass posteriorly in company with the radial nerve. Below the profunda brachii, the brachial artery gives off muscular branches: the nutrient artery to the humerus, which enters close to the insertion of the coracobrachialis muscle, and the superior and inferior ulnar collateral arteries. The superior ulnar collateral artery arises above the middle of the arm and passes posteriorly along the medial side of the arm with the ulnar nerve, to run with the nerve behind the condyle and anastomose with the recurrent branch from the forearm. The interior ulnar collateral artery arises a short distance above the elbow, where it anastomoses with the superior ulnar collateral and with a recurrent branch ascending from the forearm.

The radial artery normally arises as the lateral terminal branch of the brachial artery in the antecubital fossae on the front of the brachialis muscle. Just below its origin, the radial artery gives off the radial recurrent artery, which supplies branches adjacent to muscles and runs upward between the brachialis muscle and the more anterior extensor muscle, following the course of the radial nerve, to anastomose with the radial collateral branch of the

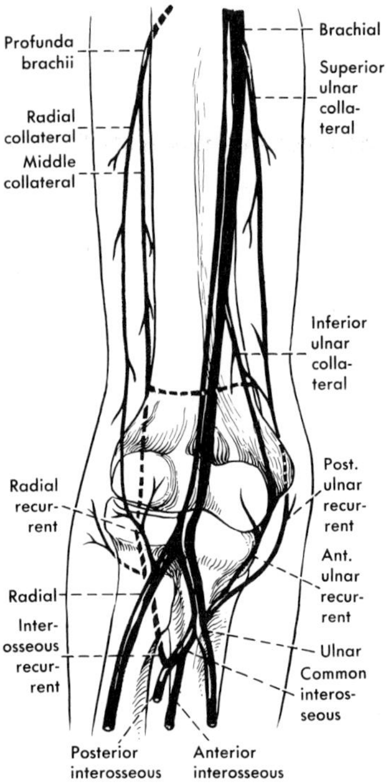

Figure 1–1. Arterial anatomy of the arm and elbow. (From Hollinshead W. H. [ed.]: Anatomy for Surgeons: Vol. 3, The Back and Limbs, New York, Harper & Row, 1969, p. 370.)

profunda brachial artery. The radial artery runs slightly laterally, under the cover of the brachioradialis muscle, anterior to the tendon of the biceps, the flexor digitorum superficialis, and the flexor pollicis longus, to appear proximal to the wrist between the tendons of the brachioradialis and the flexor carpi radialis. In the middle of the forearm, the superficial branch of the radial nerve lies just lateral to it. The radial artery leaves the anterior aspect of the thumb, arriving at the dorsum of the hand. In its further course down the arm the radial artery gives rise to unnamed muscular branches and, just before it turns dorsally, it gives off a superficial palmar branch, which enters the thenar muscle.

The ulnar artery is usually the larger terminal branch of the brachial artery. It leaves the antecubital fossae by passing posterior to the ulnar head of the pronator teres, by which it is separated from the median nerve. As it passes downward and medially, it lies medial to the median nerve between the flexor digitorum superficialis and the flexor digitorum profundus, and then descends with the ulnar nerve between the flexor carpi ulnaris and the flexor digitorum profundus. The ulnar artery emerges from behind the flexor carpi ulnaris at the wrist, crosses the anterior surface of the flexor retinaculum, and, as it enters the hand, gives off a small deep branch to the hypothenar muscles before continuing as a superficial palmar arch. While it lies behind the flexor digitorum superficialis, the ulnar artery gives off a large common interosseous artery and the small ulnar recurrent artery. The common

interosseous artery runs distally and laterally to divide after a short course into the anterior and posterior interosseous arteries. The anterior interosseous artery gives off a small median artery to the median nerve and then descends on the interosseous membrane between the flexor digitorum profundus and flexor pollicis longus, giving off muscle branches along its course. The anterior interosseous ends by passing to the pronator quadratus and dividing into anterior and posterior branches. The small anterior branch continues distally to the anterior aspect of the wrist, while the posterior branch passes through a hole in the lower part of the interosseous membrane to appear in the lower dorsal part of the forearm. In the proximal forearm, the ulnar recurrent artery divides into the anterior and posterior branches. The anterior branch passes upward between the muscle arising from the medial upper condyle and the brachialis to anastomose with the inferior ulnar collateral artery from the brachial artery. The posterior branch runs medially and upward to pass behind the medial upper condyle with the ulnar nerve, between the two heads of the flexor carpi ulnaris, and anastomose with the superior ulnar collateral artery.

The superficial palmar arterial arch, which is the continuation of the ulnar artery in the hand, gives off a digital artery to the free border of the little finger and then curves radially across the palm just deep to the palmar aponeurosis, and superficial to the nerves and tendons in the central part of the palm (Fig. 1–2). In this course it gives off three

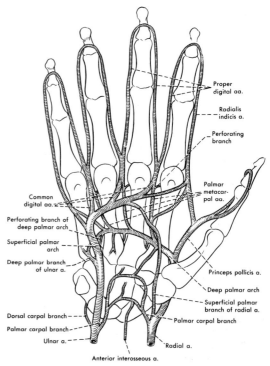

Figure 1–2. Arterial anatomy of the hand. (From Hollinshead, W. H. [ed.]: Anatomy for Surgeons: Vol. 3, The Back and Limbs, New York, Harper & Row, 1969, p. 496.)

palmar common digital arteries that run distally toward the web spaces between the little and ring, the ring and long, and the long and index fingers, where they are accompanied by common digital nerves and gradually sink into the connective tissue between the long flexor tendons. Close to the metacarpophalangeal joints, the common digital arteries are joined by palmar metacarpal arteries from the deep palmar arch. They then divide into proper digital arteries for the adjacent sides of the fingers between which they lie. The proper digital arteries course along the fingers dorsal to the proper digital nerves. The digital arteries on the ulnar side of the thumb, index, and little fingers are usually larger than the radial ones. There are transverse anastomoses that occur regularly, so that interruption of one digital artery rarely results in ischemia of the digit.

The radial artery, entering the palm from the dorsum, emerges between the two heads of the first dorsal interosseous muscle, and divides into the princeps pollicis artery and the deep palmar arch (Fig. 1–2). The princeps pollicis artery runs distally on the first dorsal interosseous between it and the adductor pollicis muscle, and usually gives off the radialis indicis artery to the radial side of the index finger. Then, as it nears the metacarpophalangeal joint of the thumb, the princeps pollicis artery divides into two proper digital arteries for either side of the thumb. The deep palmar arch runs ulnarward across interosseous muscles and metacarpals, approximately paralleling the branch of the ulnar nerve, and gives rise to the palmar metacarpal and perforating arteries. The three palmar metacarpal arteries pass directly on the interosseous muscles (close to the level of the metacarpophalangeal joints) and give off perforating branches that pass dorsally to join the dorsal metacarpal arteries. They then turn palmarward to join the common digital branches of the superficial palmar arch. The perforating branches of the deep palmar arch pass straight dorsally between the two heads of each of the second, third, and fourth dorsal interosseous muscles. These perforating branches, which carry blood to the dorsal metacarpal arteries, are frequently larger than the dorsal metacarpal arteries at their origin from the dorsal carpal rete.

The dorsal carpal arch is formed by the union of the radial and ulnar dorsal carpal arches. From this rete, the second, third, and fourth metacarpal arches arise and course distally on the surface of the dorsal interosseous muscle to the interdigital folds. They divide into two dorsal digital branches for the contiguous fingers. Distally, between the metacarpal heads, they are connected by perforating branches to a volar common digital artery of the corresponding spaces.[21]

There are three arterial sources to each finger: the common volar digital, the volar metacarpal, and the dorsal metacarpal arteries. Ultimately, two proper volar digital arteries are formed, each of which supplies adjacent sides of the digits. In most instances the main supply of the digits comes from the common volar digital arteries, but it is not

unusual for the volar metacarpal artery to supplant one of the former vessels, and, in rare instances, the chief supply may be from the dorsal metacarpal vessels. Thus, the superficial and deep volar arches can be divided, and the fingers can maintain some capillary refill through the dorsal metacarpal arteries, which have not been damaged. However, this capillary refill can be misleading, because the dorsal metacarpal arteries are often inadequate in maintaining digit viability, and, even if the digit does survive, it often becomes atrophic and painful.

Variations

A knowledge of the variations in the origin and course of the principal arteries of the upper extremity is of great practical importance in reparative and reconstructive surgery of the arm, forearm, and hand. McCormack and colleagues dissected 750 upper extremities to study the brachial and antebrachial arterial patterns. They found that 139 (19.5%) possessed major variations.[30] Of 364 cadavers, arterial variations occurred bilaterally in 23 (6.2%) and unilaterally in 89 (24.5%), for a total incidence of 112 (30.8%). The following common variations were encountered in 628 extremities: high origin of the radial artery in 15.5%, high origin and unusual course of the ulnar artery in 1.9%, and a superficial brachial artery forming a common trunk for both radial and ulnar arteries in 1.3%. Thus, the most common variations involved the radial artery.

To document the arterial patterns in the hand, Coleman and Anson studied 650 specimens.[7] In this series, 78.5% of the hands had complete superficial volar arches, implying that an anastomosis had taken place between the vessels that formed the arch (Fig. 1–3). In the absence of contribution from

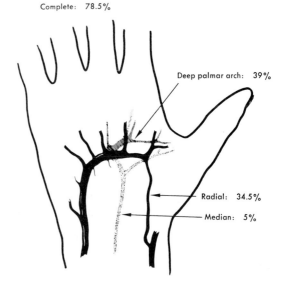

Complete: 78.5%

Deep palmar arch: 39%

Radial: 34.5%

Median: 5%

Incomplete: 21.5%

Figure 1–3. Variations of superficial palmar arch. (Adapted from Coleman, S. S., and Anson, B. J.: Surg. Gynecol. Obstet., 113:409, 1961.)

the radial or a median artery, the ulnar artery formed a complete arch by anastomosing with vessels from the deep arch in the web between the thumb and index finger. When the contributing arteries to the superficial arch do not anastomose, or when the ulnar fails to reach the thumb and index finger, the arch is incomplete. It was incomplete in a total of 140 cases (21.5%). Of 200 specimens, 97% had a complete deep arch; only 3% had an incomplete arch in which no anastomosis existed between the deep volar branches of the ulnar and radial contributions.[7] The median artery entered into the formation of the superficial volar arch in about 10% of cases. This artery always passes deep to the transverse carpal ligament. It is important to recognize patients with incomplete arches in those with arterial injuries that require arterial reconstructive surgery. Generally, an isolated radial or ulnar artery transection is "noncritical," implying that it is not associated with the signs of acute vascular insufficiency. However, in patients with incomplete arches, these injuries become critical, and demand repair or reconstruction for whole hand viability.

The upper extremity surgeon must be aware of the several variations of the first metacarpal artery and the princeps pollicis artery, as emphasized by Parks and associates.[39] The digital vessels to the thumb and radial aspect of the index finger have variations in the origin from the superficial palmar arch, deep palmar arch, and superficial palmar branch of the radial artery. Clinically, on several occasions, we have noted the capacity of the injured thumb to survive on a small dorsal artery from the dorsal carpal arch.

Nervi Vasorum

The arteries are innervated by the motor fibers that leave the branches of spinal nerves from the nervi vasorum.[21] When the nerve reaches the vessel, it usually divides into ascending and descending branches in the perivascular tissue and penetrates into the arterial wall. The distribution of the nerve endings is irregular, and the branches frequently form arches and circles. The radial part of the superficial arterial arch is supplied mostly by the medial nerve, while the ulnar part is supplied by the ulnar nerve. The deep arch is also supplied mostly by the ulnar nerve. The digital arteries receive minute twigs from the accompanying digital nerves.

Pick dissected out the nerve supply to the vasculature of the hand using the operating microscope.[42] He found that the superficial palmar arch receives nearly a dozen branches from the common digital nerves arising from the median and ulnar nerves, the deep palmar arch receives two branches from the deep branch of the ulnar nerve and one from the median nerve, and the digital arteries themselves receive anywhere from three to twelve twigs.

Pick also found that the brachial plexus does not receive its rami communicantes exclusively from the cervical thoracic sympathetic trunk.[42] Additional sympathetic fibers may reach the brachial plexus over the sinuvertebral nerve, the carotid plexus, and the nerve of Kuntz. Intermediary sympathetic ganglia, placed in spinal nerve roots or rami communicantes, bypass the sympathetic trunk. These pathways, especially in the intermediary ganglia, are often allowed to remain untouched during sympathectomy and later play an important role in residual sympathetic activity.

Osseofascial Compartments

Knowledge of the anatomy of the osseofascial compartments of the upper extremity is of great importance to the surgeon treating arterial injuries. An anatomic compartment consists of all the structures confined within a relatively closed osseofascial space. The muscles in the compartment are the functional unit, while the nerves and arteries are frequently only coinhabitants as they course through the compartment on their way to more distal destinations. Compartments of clinical importance in the upper extremity include the anterior compartment of the arm, the posterior compartment of the arm, the volar compartment of the forearm, the dorsal compartment of the forearm, and the hand compartments.

The brachial fascia covers the anterior compartment of the arm anteriorly, and firmly attaches to the medial and lateral epicondyles of the humerus distally. The medial and lateral walls are formed by the medial and lateral intermuscular septa, respectively. The septa terminate distally at the supracondylar ridges and, together with the humerus, form the posterior wall of the anterior compartment of the arm. The biceps, brachialis, and coracobrachialis muscles are contained within this compartment.

The posterior compartment of the arm contains the triceps muscle and is bounded posteriorly by the brachial fascia, medially and laterally by the respective intermuscular septa, and anteriorly by the humerus itself.

The volar compartment of the forearm is encased by the antebrachial fascia anteriorly, medially, and laterally. This fascia sends strong septal bands to the superficial border of the ulna and radius. The posterior limit consists of the ulna, radius, and intervening interosseous membrane. In the distal half of the forearm a thinner sheet of fascia extends from the medial to lateral wall, separating the three superficial muscles (palmaris longus, flexor carpi radialis, and flexor carpi ulnaris) from the deeper structures. The lacertus fibrosus proximally and the transverse carpal ligament distally are formidable barriers to volar compartment swelling. This compartment contains the flexors and pronators of the wrist and hand, and may be subdivided into superficial and deep groups. The superficial muscles include the flexor carpi ulnaris, palmaris longus, flexor carpi radialis, and pronator teres. The flexor digitorum superficialis and profundus, the flexor pollicis longus, and the pronator quadratus form the deep group muscles.

The dorsal compartment of the forearm is enveloped by the antebrachial fascia dorsally and to the sides, and by the ulna, radius, and intervening interosseous membrane anteriorly. Contained in this compartment are the wrist and finger extensors. The mobile wad consisting of the brachioradialis and extensor carpi radialis longus and brevis is separated from the rest of the dorsal compartment by fascia, and may be considered to be a separate compartment. The other muscles in this compartment include the extensor digitorum communis, the extensor indicis proprius, the extensor carpi ulnaris, the extensor digiti quinti proprius, the abductor pollicis longus, and extensor pollicis brevis and longus.

The hand can be divided into four structural compartments: the central palmar, hypothenar, thenar, and interossei compartments.[32] The central palmar compartment is bounded anteriorly by the palmar aponeurosis, radially by the thenar septum (tied posteriorly to the index metacarpal), ulnarly by the hypothenar septum (attached posteriorly to the fifth metacarpal), and distally by the palmar interosseous fascia that overlies the interossei and adductor pollicis muscle. The central palmar compartment consists primarily of the tendons of the fingers—that is, the flexor digitorum superficialis and profundus, and the lumbricals. The hypothenar compartment is bounded anteriorly and laterally by the hypothenar fascia, medially by the hypothenar septum, and posteriorly by the metacarpals. The hypothenar compartment contains the short muscles of the little finger, and the thenar compartment contains the short muscles of the thumb, except the adductor pollicis. The interosseous compartments are bounded anteriorly by the palmar interosseous fascia, and dorsally by the interosseous fascia. The metacarpals form the sides of the compartments. The interossei compartments are separate and contain the palmar and dorsal interossei of the fingers as well as the adductor pollicis of the thumb.

ARTERIAL INJURIES

General Considerations

Arterial injuries are most often the result of penetrating wounds that disrupt the wall of the artery partly or completely. Nonpenetrating injuries, usually associated with a fracture in an adjacent bone, are less frequent but often have a more serious prognosis related to extensive crushing injury of the wall of the artery and delay in diagnosis.

Most commonly the injuries are either lacerations or transections of the arterial wall. The extent of injury varies with the type of trauma. In cleanly incised wounds, injury to the arterial wall is mini-mal. In contrast, trauma from a high-velocity missile will disrupt the intima and media for a distance away from the laceration of the arterial wall. A high-velocity missile damages by virtue of its temporary cavity effect.[3] A near-miss of an artery may still be associated with intimal damage that leads to thrombosis.[27]

Arterial contusion from blunt injury may be characterized by areas of fragmentation of the arterial wall with intramural hemorrhage. The intima may become detached and prolapse into the lumen, creating an intraluminal obstruction. A serious error occurs when a contusion is misdiagnosed as a spasm. The delay in treatment as a consequence of this diagnostic error can result in gangrene. Arterial spasm is an infrequent response to injury, and intimal damage must be ruled out before making that diagnosis. The severity of ischemic response following arterial injury varies with the tolerance of different tissues for anoxia. Muscle is the most sensitive to anoxia. Skin, tendon, and bone have a greater tolerance for anoxia, and may survive an ischemic injury that has produced irreversible extensive muscle necrosis. Nerves are also sensitive to anoxia, with paralysis and anesthesia developing when blood flow is seriously decreased.

The period of tolerance of striated muscle for ischemia is in the range of 6 to 8 hours. Experimental studies by Miller and Welch have shown that successful arterial repairs in 90% of dogs resulted when the repair was performed within 6 hours after injury; the success rate decreased to 50% when the repair was delayed for 12 hours.[32] In the surviving dogs in which ischemia continued for 12 or more hours, the return of function was always delayed and incomplete. Limitation of motion and loss of strength were constant findings secondary to muscle contracture. Every effort should be made to complete arterial repair within 6 hours after injury, especially if anesthesia or paralysis are present, which indicates a severe degree of anoxia. However, a definite time limit does not exist, because the interval varies with collateral circulation. The collateral circulation, in turn, varies with the artery injured, the degree of soft tissue injury, the degree of associated shock, and the ambient temperature. In some patients in whom there is little disturbance of collateral circulation, arterial repair may be successfully performed 12 to 15 hours after injury.

Clinical Manifestations

Almost invariably patients with arterial injuries of the upper extremity are initially seen and assessed in the emergency room. Their history is that of a recent penetrating injury to the extremity or recent severe blunt trauma. Most often with a penetrating injury, the damage is isolated to the extremity. Careful assessment of the entire patient is required, however, because significant blood loss may have occurred prior to arrival in the emergency room. In patients who have sustained arterial injuries from blunt trauma, there are commonly multiple organ injuries present, including skull fractures, rib fractures, and abdominal injuries. Careful assessment of each injury and assignment of priorities are critical parts in the initial evaluation of the patient. Shock from loss of blood may occur, either as a result of hemorrhage from the injured artery or from the associated injuries. When profound shock is present, the peripheral vasoconstriction may conceal the presence of an arterial injury until the circulating volume has been restored.

Unless there is an associated fracture, patients with purely soft tissue injury do not complain of severe pain. If severe pain is present in the absence of a fracture, suspect osseofascial compartment syndrome (this entity will be discussed more fully below). Extremities with arterial injuries often have injuries of adjacent nerves and bones. A careful neurologic assessment distal to the lesion is essential in the emergency room to serve as a baseline for further examinations. If this is not documented, interpretation of a neurologic deficit that is noticed following surgery will be impossible. A careful physical examination is the most important diagnostic measure in the evaluation of extremity trauma.

In penetrating wounds, bright red bleeding, even in small amounts, immediately suggests an arterial injury. In the absence of hemorrhage, a hematoma that has evolved from extravasation of blood under significant pressure beneath the fascia may be present. However, an arterial injury can be present in the absence of bleeding or hematoma. Hence, the presence of a penetrating injury near the artery should signal the possibility of an arterial injury.

The findings of arterial insufficiency upon clinical examination include a change in the color, capillary refill, turgor, or temperature of the fingers, or a change in the pulse of the affected part. The hand should be a pale pink color. If the digits are white, this indicates arterial insufficiency, and if they are bluish, this a venous insufficiency. Capillary refill is tested by compressing the skin and watching for refill. We have found in a large number of replantations that the best location for this is the side of the fingertip between the paronychium and pulp (Fig. 1–4). Capillary refill testing by pressing on the nail and watching it refill is not as satisfactory. Capillary refill of injured digits can be compared with that of normal uninjured digits; a decrease indicates arterial insufficiency. Capillary refill that is faster than normal may indicate arterial competency but venous insufficiency. Each digit should be carefully assessed individually.

The turgor of each finger should be normal. Increased turgor suggests venous insufficiency, while decreased turgor suggests arterial insufficiency.

Skin temperature is a reliable indicator of the blood flow rate in the dermal vessels. This can be assessed by feeling with the dorsum of your fingers or hand, and comparing the temperature with that of the uninjured limb.

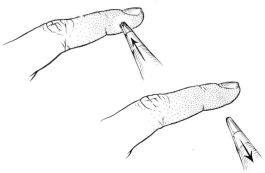

Figure 1–4. The best method of evaluating capillary refill. The tip of a blunt instrument (*e.g.,* a ballpoint pen) is used to compress the area between the nail plate and finger pulp.

A careful palpation of pulses in the injured extremity with comparison to the uninjured extremity is important. The subclavian artery is palpable in the supraclavicular fossa. The brachial artery is palpable on the medial aspect of the arm, in the groove between the biceps and triceps muscles. The radial artery is palpable on the flexor surface of the wrist, just radial to the tendon of the flexor carpi radialis. The ulnar artery is radial to the flexor carpi ulnaris tendon on the volar surface of the wrist. The ulnar artery lies deeper than the radial artery and often is not palpable, even in the normal limb. The quality and strength of the pulse should be determined in the subclavian, axillary, brachial, ulnar, radial, and even digital arteries. Auscultation may reveal a systolic bruit produced by aneurysm of an acutely angulated or partially obstructed artery. A characteristic machinery murmur is usually heard over an arteriovenous fistula.

Palpation of the peripheral pulse is the most commonly used method of screening for arterial injury, but it is not an adequate criterion of blood flow. Gelberman and co-workers reviewed 18 patients with documented complete radial or ulnar artery transections.[14] Nine of 18 had persistent palpable pulses distal to the transection: seven were due to retrograde flow, and two to transmission from the proximal artery stump or large collaterals. The Allen test was accurate in demonstrating arterial occlusions in each case.

The Allen test is a very useful clinical test for determining the patency of arteries in a double arterial supply system.[2] It can be used at the level of the wrist and in each digit individually. At the wrist, both the radial and ulnar arteries are compressed, and the hand is emptied of all blood by having the patient actively flex and extend the digits at least three times. The pressure is then removed from the radial artery and the hand is allowed to fill from the ulnar artery. The time of filling is measured. The test is then repeated, releasing the pressure on the ulnar artery and allowing the hand to fill from the radial artery. If one of the two arteries is occluded, or if the palmar arch is incomplete, the compromised circulation will then become evident, and the hand will not become fully vascularized until the occluded vessel is released. The test results should be compared with those of similar tests on the opposite hand. In the normally vascularized hand, the time of filling is generally 3 to 5 seconds, and certainly less than 7 seconds.[13] The digital Allen test can be used by selectively releasing one of the digital arteries and observing the return of vascularity to the finger.

Special Tests of Arterial Competency

Many special tests have been advocated for assessing the arterial competency of an extremity. Some are complex and involve very sophisticated instrumentation. These are usually employed in the investigation of chronic insufficiency problems, and thus may have a role in the evaluation of patients with late complications of arterial injuries. Some special tests are of great benefit in the initial assessment in the emergency department and in the inhospital monitoring of patients.

Temperature Studies. Small surface temperature probes provide reliable direct information on digital perfusion (Fig. 1–5). The efficacy of temperature monitoring in digital replantation has been demonstrated.[50] This method can also be used in the preoperative assessment of hand and finger vascular injuries. A temperature below 30° C in the digit is a very poor prognostic sign, indicating that vascular repair will likely be necessary for survival of the digit. This simple noninvasive method of monitoring the vascular status of the digit has several advantages, including the following: (1) a nurse or aide can follow the condition of these digits by reading the temperature gauge and can call the physician when significant changes are seen; (2) temperature recordings are particularly helpful when the skin color cannot be followed easily, as in dark-skinned patients, or with several traumatized or ecchymotic

digits; (3) only a small portion of the fingertip is concealed by the temperature probe, allowing adequate clinical observation of the pulp and nail bed; (4) the technique is atraumatic and does not cause damage to the digit tip; (5) in reading the temperature gauge, the fingertip is not constantly disturbed by the examiner, which is of particular benefit in children; and (6) it is inexpensive and readily available.

The Duke Diagnostic Hand Laboratory personnel have developed a technique using an environmental box for cooling (Fig. 1–6).[25] A temperature probe is placed on each of a patient's digits, and one is used to measure the ambient temperature. The subject's hands are placed into the test box and cooled to 10° C for 20 minutes. The temperatures are recorded during cooling and for 20 minutes of rewarming. A graphic computerized chart of the data is made. Simultaneous temperature and plethysmographic recording of the fingers can be obtained while altering the ambient temperature. Consistent temperature depression greater than 2.5° C, compared with that of the noninvolved digits, indicates insufficient perfusion. A rapid drop in temperature of a digit and a slow rise on rewarming also indicates relative vascular insufficiency. We have found this technique to be very useful in following our patients postoperatively, because their graphic preoperative records can be compared with their postoperative records.

Thermography. Thermography is a useful noninvasive technique that provides information similar to that obtained by the temperature probes. Absent or diminished detectable heat over an area of the hand, such as the two ulnar digits, correlates with diminished vascularities.

Doppler Recording. The Doppler is an ultrasonic flow detector that provides a noninvasive monitor of arterial (and venous) flow.[24] Ultrasound waves emitted through piezoelectric crystals are transmitted through the skin and subcutaneous tissue to the

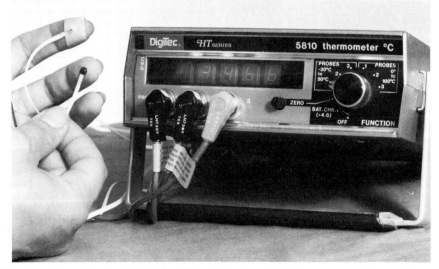

Figure 1–5. Thermister for evaluating digital blood flow. The normal digital temperature is usually between 32° and 35°C.

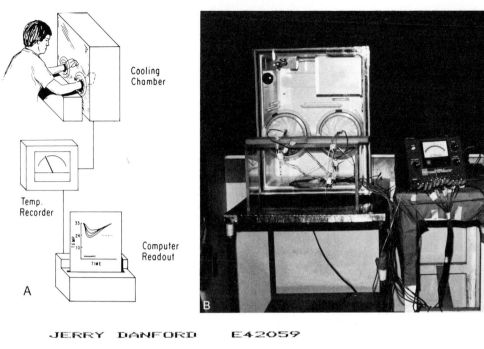

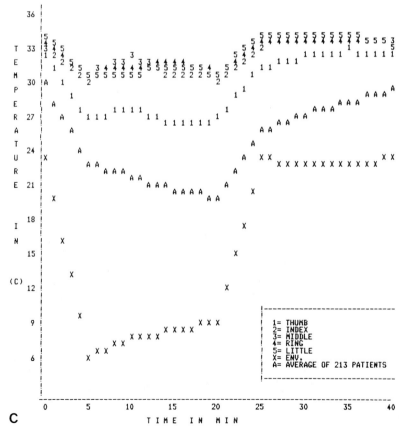

Figure 1–6. *A,* Cooling chamber of evaluation of blood flow to the hands; *B,* the hands are placed in the chamber on the left and temperature and blood flow recordings are recorded by probes on the tips of each digit and printed on a graph by a computer *(C).*

superficially located blood vessels. The radial, ulnar, superficial palmar arch, and digital vessels are accessible for monitoring with this instrument. The emitted high-frequency sound of 5 to 10 million cps strikes the soft tissues and the blood cells moving through the blood vessels. On impact, the blood cells that are in rapid motion cause an alteration in the pitch of the sound waves. These reflected waves, varying in volume and pitch according to the velocity and quantity of moving blood cells, are received by the recording part of the probe and are amplified and converted to signals in an audible range. Because digital and palmar vessels are normally audible, the Doppler is a valuable tool in the emergency room, for deciding whether or not a particular vessel has been lacerated. It is also helpful in assessing chronic vascular problems to delineate the level of thrombosis. Although Doppler mapping correlates well with arteriography, it does not allow an accurate estimate of intimal damage or of arteriosclerotic changes in these chronic problems.

Plethysmography. A plethysmograph is an instrument that measures volume. There are many types of plethysmography, including strain gauge, impedance, pneumatic, hydraulic, and inductance. Essentially all these methods utilize volume displacement attached to a recording device and amplifying system to obtain not only a quantitative but also a qualitative recording of a pulse wave, which can then be examined. The principle is the measurement of the volume increase of an organ in response to a temporary blockage of its venous outflow. In the first seconds of this blockage, the arterial inflow will be unrestricted and proportional to the volume increase. By recording the volume increase, an exact measure of the arterial blood flow can be obtained. Each normal digital pulse wave reveals a sharp systolic peak and a dicrotic notch on the down slope. Vasospasm is produced by a decreased amplitude of the wave with normal configuration. Proximal obstruction in the arterial tree, which alters normal pulsatile flow, provides a digital pulse wave with decreasing amplitude, a rounded peak, and absence of the dicrotic notch on the down slope. These pulse waves can be compared with those of other digits in the contralateral hand to obtain a percentage of normal circulation. In our experience, pulse volume recordings of less than 75% correlate with cold intolerance in patients with ulnar artery insufficiency. Intraoperative digital plethysmography can be used, and is helpful when deciding whether to ligate a particular thrombosed segment of artery or to go ahead with vein grafting. Digital plethysmography also provides a quantitative Allen test. By placing the plethysmograph on the fingertips and occluding both the radial and ulnar arteries and then releasing them sequentially, the effects on the arterial flow of the hand can be studied.

Radionuclear Scanning Techniques. Radionuclide intravenous dynamic flow studies and static profusion scans of the hand are useful. Wilgis and coworkers reported on 22 patients with various hand injuries who were examined by dynamic flow or static profusion scanning.[58] They pointed out the advantages of radionuclide angiography: (1) the technique is simple and accurate, easily reproducible, and takes only a few minutes; (2) the side effects are practically nonexistent; and (3) with a computerized image-displaying analysis system, quantitative data can be obtained. Poor resolving power and inadequate spatial resolution are the disadvantages of this method. This modality is a screening tool to visualize perfusion of the hand. We use it as a study prior to arteriography. It may make the arteriogram unnecessary, and at least it will pinpoint areas for specific study. It is also useful for repetitive monitoring of postoperative patients.

At Duke we obtained data on 50 extremities in 44 patients.[26] Of these patients, 24 were posttraumatic and 26 were diagnostic problems. Scanning was helpful in these patients but, because of the poor resolving power, anatomic errors were made that were demonstrated at arteriography. It is considerably less expensive than arteriography, and can be performed on an outpatient basis.

Wick or Slit Catheter to Measure Compartment Pressures. The Wick and more recently the slit catheters are valuable in the management of compartment syndromes.[23, 34, 47] They provide accurate and objective data, thus facilitating management decisions. The technique is particularly valuable in evaluating the critically injured, comatose, or pediatric patient in whom a reliable physical examination may not be possible. The procedure is simple and reliable but is invasive. Intracompartmental pressures higher than 30 mm Hg can produce irreversible changes, and indicate that surgical fasciotomy is probably required.

Arteriography. Contrast arteriography involves the intra-arterial injection of contrast medium and the subsequent visualization of the arterial and venous phases of circulation. This method is invaluable for the location of specific arterial defects. The femoral route is the safest puncture route. Severe complications have been reported from the transaxillary and brachial injection sites. The discomfort of this method, the requirements of special personnel and equipment, the hazards of administration of iodine, and the possible complication at the site of arterial punctures limit its application. It cannot be used routinely or repetitively. Another disadvantage is that the arteriogram is mainly an anatomic study and provides no information as to the dynamic state of the circulation. It does remain a definitive study, however, and should be performed prior to any anticipated surgery on the vasculature of the upper extremity, if time permits. It allows accurate estimation of any intimal vascular damage and allows an accurate prediction of the potential for surgical reconstruction to be made.

Opinions vary on the role of arteriography in the evaluation of vascular trauma. In most cases a thorough clinical examination will detect the presence and location of major arterial injury, and will direct surgical management correctly. When the site of arterial injury is obvious, arteriography only delays operation and does not contribute to the care of the patient. Also, arteriography occasionally will be falsely negative in the presence of an arterial injury, as demonstrated experimentally in dogs by Lain and Williams and by Mufti and colleagues.[28, 36]

Arteriography does have a role in extremity trauma, however. It is helpful in localizing the site of injury, in identifying multiple sites of injury in patients with pellet injuries or multiple fractures of the extremity, or when the track of the missile parallels a vessel. Arteriography may serve as an alternative to surgical exploration when the site of injury is close to a major artery but there are no signs or symptoms of vascular injury. In trauma management, we feel that the arteriogram should answer a specific question rather than being routinely performed. It is particularly indicated when the physical findings do not correlate with the apparent locus of the lesion.

We favor preoperative arteriograms, however, for almost all reconstructive arterial procedures, so that these procedures can be carefully planned. Special attention should be given to arteriograms of the hand. Both the deep and superficial arches should be seen; if not, a vascular defect should be strongly suspected. In the chronic situation, intraarterial vasodilators can be given following the arteriogram, and this can be both diagnostically and therapeutically helpful.

Other special investigations, including laser Doppler, intramuscular pH measurement, transcutaneous Po_2 measurement, dynamic ultrasound, and digital angiography, have been described and used. We are studying most of these in the laboratory clinically. Some of these newer tests will undoubtedly replace some of our standard techniques.

TREATMENT

Control of bleeding is the most immediate problem. This can usually be accomplished by firmly packing the wound with gauze and by applying direct pressure. A large amount of packing may be required, because the efficacy of the packing depends on the compression of the artery between the overlying skin and the underlying bone. Tourniquets are best avoided for most injuries, because they risk permanent injury to peripheral nerves. Shock, when present, should be treated by rapid infusion of fluids until the systolic blood pressure rises to 80 mm Hg, after which additional fluids can be infused more gradually. Blood is preferable but, until necessary cross matching has been done, Ringer's lactate solution, plasma, or dextran may be used. Appropriate tetanus prophylaxis should be started, as well as a wide-spectrum antibiotic.

Under no circumstances should blind clamping of vessels be attempted for control of hemorrhage in a wound that is bleeding profusely. This is dangerous because serious damage can be done to adjacent structures such as nerves and veins, or to the artery if it is clamped at a point at which it is not actually bleeding. When uncontrollable bleeding occurs in an extremity, pressure should be applied directly to the wound, and satisfactory control achieved.

An important basic attitude regarding arterial trauma is that almost all injuries can be repaired successfully with available surgical techniques. The prognosis then becomes a question of whether or not the repair was performed before irreversible muscle necrosis developed. For digital vessels, a microscope with microsurgical instruments and sutures are required.[53, 54] We prefer to perform other arterial anastomoses using the same instruments and techniques. For the brachial artery we use loupe magnification but microsurgical techniques. Surgical incisions should be placed to expose the artery proximal and distal to the site of injury, to avoid hemorrhage when clots are evacuated from the wound. High-velocity missiles frequently create such large wounds that exposure of the vessel is usually accomplished by simply extending the wound through the longitudinal incisions. However, most wounds in the civilian population are of far less destructive force, and the ideal approach is through a separate incision directly over the course of the vessel.

Most arterial injuries are best treated by excision of the injured area, followed by anastomosis. With injuries from high-velocity missiles, 2 to 4 mm of adjacent arterial wall should be excised. Repairs of lacerations are deceptive in that the suture of the laceration often results in constriction and subsequent thrombosis. Usually excision followed by direct anastomosis is preferable. Normally, 1 to 2 cm of the peripheral artery can be excised and the vessel ends can still be approximated after limited mobilization. Patman and associates found that, of 180 patients requiring repairs for civilian injuries, only 20 needed grafts.[40] Before the anastomosis is performed, the degree of back bleeding from the distal vessel should be noted, and any clots should be removed with a catheter. Also, be certain that there is good flow from the proximal cut end. This is more important the more distal the vessel. We use interrupted suture technique for all arterial repairs using 6–0 or 7–0 sutures for the brachial artery, 9–0 sutures for the forearm arteries, and 10–0 sutures for the digital arteries.

If a graft must be used to bridge a gap in the vessel because of loss of tissue, a vein graft is preferred in a patient with an open injury. If possible after arterial reconstruction, the adjacent soft tissues are approximated over the arterial repair, leaving the remaining wound open to be closed by secondary suture 4 to 7 days later. This technique will almost routinely prevent the development of infection. If a large skin defect exists, the arterial repair may be covered by the movement of a flap of muscle over the damaged artery or, if this is impossible, a meshed split-thickness skin graft may be used. We have maintained patent anastomoses with meshed split-thickness grafts over vein grafts.

Ligation of an injured artery should be performed only in minor arteries. Back bleeding is an inadequate guide to ligation of major arteries, indicating that some collateral circulation is present but not guaranteeing that collateral flow will be sufficient to prevent gangrene.

There is a lack of consensus regarding the priorities to be observed in cases of concomitant fracture and arterial injury. We agree with those who feel that bony stabilization is important prior to performing the arterial anastomosis to obviate possible disruption of the repair caused by motion.[4, 9, 29, 31] We prefer compression plating of fractures of the humerus, radius, and ulna, and pin fixation of fractures of carpus and other bones of the hand. External fixation is a good alternative if grade III wounds are present.[18, 44] To make the arterial anastomosis and also associated nerve repairs easier, we tend to shorten the bone prior to fixation. In the upper extremity length is not as important as in the lower extremity, and the shortening goes unnoticed functionally and cosmetically.

When faced with prolonged limb ischemia, a bypass shunt (silicone tubing) should be interposed between the two cut ends of the artery.[37] This allows meticulous fixation of fractures while the limb is well perfused. A shunt may also be used in the venous system. Following bone shortening and fixation, the vessels are anastomosed.

Concomitant venous injuries in the upper extremity are of less importance than in the lower extremity.[22, 46] Lacerated veins are repaired if they show evidence of hypertension after the arterial flow is resumed. Venous hypertension is visible in ligated veins that become turgid and bulge beyond the tie. The extent of damage and the location and size of the vein are all factors in determining the need for repair. Failures of arterial repairs in the upper extremity due to venous insufficiency are less common than in the lower extremity.[1]

Postoperatively, we do empirically recommend sympathetic blockade to cause vasodilation. If the procedure was performed under brachial plexus blockade, no further block is necessary. If the patient had general anesthesia, we recommend stellate ganglion blockade prior to ending the anesthetic. A useful technique for arterial repairs in the hand is to insert a fine silicone tube (number 5 ureteral stent) through a volar incision and to have the tip of the tube overlying the median nerve or ulnar nerve, or both (depending on the digits involved).[41] Postoperatively, intermittent dosages of a long-acting local anesthetic (bupivacaine) can be administered for pain relief and sympathetic blockade.

We do not recommend heparin anticoagulation as a routine. However, we do suggest aspirin, Persantine, Thorazine, and, in most cases, dextran. We reserve heparin for very distal revascularizations when venous drainage problems are anticipated.

We monitor arterial repairs postoperatively clinically by assessing capillary refill, turgor, color, and pulses, and by continuous temperature monitoring with probes. A fall below 30° C or a sudden drop of more than 1.5° C requires immediate patient assessment and problem correction.

Patients who have had major limb revascularizations or replantations must be returned to the operating room within 48 hours for wound inspection and further débridement of any necrotic tissue, if it exists. This second look will prevent many complications, especially those related to myonecrosis and infection. Of course, in more minor wounds or in digital or metacarpal revascularizations and replantations, this step is not indicated.

COMPLICATIONS OF ARTERIAL REPAIRS

Infection

The development of a postoperative infection around the site of arterial repair is a grave complication, because the anastomosis may disrupt with life-threatening hemorrhage. Infection should be treated promptly by widespread drainage and removal of necrotic tissue. If infection involves the arterial reconstruction, ligation of the artery is usually required to prevent fatal hemorrhage. Occasionally, bypass grafts may be inserted to circumvent the area of infection, with the anastomoses being performed between the artery proximal and distal to the point of injury. Prevention is the key. Leaving wounds open has dramatically decreased infection rates. Prophylactic antibiotics and tetanus prophylaxis are recommended for all arterial repairs.

Traumatic Aneurysms

A traumatic aneurysm results when a laceration is made into an artery and blood flows out of the artery into the surrounding tissue spaces (Fig. 1–7A). This may occur with unrecognized arterial injuries, or, following repair, with a breakdown of the anastomosis. Instead of clotting completely, the blood is forced out in a steady stream by arterial pressure and begins to pulsate against the soft tissues (Fig. 1–7B and C). A capsule may form around this blood, creating a cavity through which arterial flow goes out of, and then back into, the artery. The term "false aneurysm" is used for this expanding mass, because it has no true intimal lining (Fig. 1–7D). It is lined with fibrous tissue only. Rapid expansion of the false aneurysm may occur, causing severe neurologic and venous defects secondary to pressure. Continued pulsation of the false aneurysm against a nerve, even without compression, may produce serious damage. These lesions usually produce only a systolic bruit as compared with an AV fistula, which produces a continuous one. As the hematoma enlarges, the tissues are stretched and become reddened, suggesting an abscess.

Repair of a false aneurysm should be undertaken when it is diagnosed because of the inevitable outcome of enlargement and rupture. At operation, the incision should be placed to allow exposure of the uninvolved artery proximal and distal to the aneurysm. With these vessels temporarily occluded, the aneurysm can be widely incised and the origin identified. Dissection around the aneurysm before it is opened should be avoided, because it is unnec-

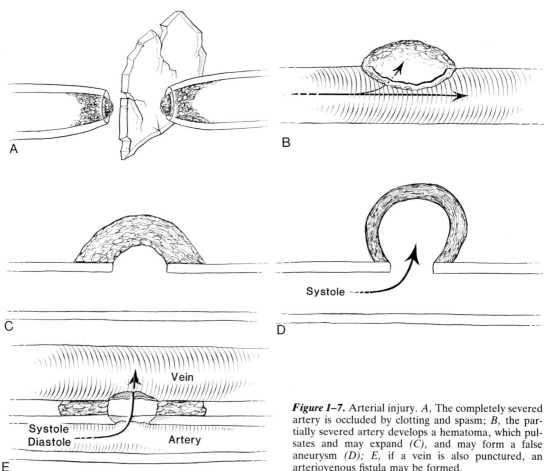

Figure 1–7. Arterial injury. *A,* The completely severed artery is occluded by clotting and spasm; *B,* the partially severed artery develops a hematoma, which pulsates and may expand *(C),* and may form a false aneurysm *(D); E,* if a vein is also punctured, an arteriovenous fistula may be formed.

essary, complicated, and often dangerous. With unusually large aneurysms it is important to remember that there is only one small opening in the arterial wall, from which the aneurysm began. Hence, if the aneurysm is inadvertently entered, the small opening can be occluded to control bleeding while further exposure is obtained. The site of communication with the parent artery can be mobilized and the injured area excised. Complete excision of the fibrous wall of the aneurysm is unnecessary and should be avoided because of the surrounding dense tissue reaction. Once the involved artery has been mobilized, arterial continuity can usually be restored by anastomosis or by insertion of a short graft. Long-term results after repair are excellent.

Traumatic Arteriovenous Fistula

An AV fistula results from a penetrating injury that simultaneously injures an artery and adjacent vein, permitting blood to flow directly from the injured artery into the vein (Fig. 1–7E). The fistula may be established immediately, in which case there is little external loss of blood, or the fistula may become apparent weeks or days following the in-

jury, in clots surrounding the artery and vein. Anatomic and physiologic changes begin to evolve when an AV fistula is produced. Immediate effects are a decrease in blood flow to tissues distal to the lesion and an increase in venous pressure. The artery, both proximal and distal to the fistula, may dilate in response to blood flow in the fistula. Venous congestion may occur and cause skin alterations. Rarely do cardiac symptoms occur with an AV fistula of the upper extremity, because the volume of blood shunted is not enough to produce heart failure.

Formerly, treatment of the AV fistula was delayed for 2 to 4 months to permit the development of collateral circulation, necessary for an extremity to survive ligation of the involved artery. Presently, most patients are treated by division of the fistula and reconstruction of the involved artery and preferably the injured vein. Most fistulas are treated at the time of the arterial injury if proper diagnosis has been made. Control of the artery and vein proximal and distal to the fistula is obtained before the fistula is dissected. Once these are temporarily occluded, the fistula can be incised and the openings isolated directly. Although a large aneurysmal sac may be present, the basic defect is usually an incomplete laceration of the arterial wall, involving only a short length of artery. Once the involved vessels have been immobilized, most of the remaining sac may be left because, as with false aneurysms, complete excision is difficult and of little benefit. Most can be repaired by anastomosis. Repair of the involved vein is indicated if the vein is a large one.

Postischemic Swelling

Compartment syndromes or Volkmann's contracture are commonly associated with arterial injuries. The necessity for fasciotomy after arterial injuries has been stressed by many authors.[8, 11, 45] A major arterial injury may produce a compartment syndrome if complete arterial occlusion has been present long enough to produce ischemic changes prior to restoration of circulation to the damaged capillary bed and muscle. This restoration of circulation may produce enough edema to initiate a compartment syndrome. With complete arterial occlusion in which the circulation is not restored, gangrene rather than a compartment syndrome will result. The total time of arterial ischemia is important. Whitesides and co-workers demonstrated that 6 hours of tourniquet-induced ischemia in dogs produced marked elevation in intracompartmental pressures after removal of the tourniquet.[57] Mubarak, in a canine tourniquet experiment, noted postischemic pressure greater than 50 mm Hg in some dogs with 4 hours of tourniquet-induced ischemia.[33] Unless fasciotomy is performed at the time of arterial repair, the resulting postischemic compartment syndrome will prolong the period of ischemia to muscles and nerves of the compartment. Fasciotomy is therefore recommended after arterial repair if the ischemic period has been longer than 6 hours.

A less common mechanism of compartment syndrome pathogenesis may result if the artery is only partially occluded, as with an intimal tear, and there is inadequate collateral circulation. The decreased perfusion and ischemia of muscle capillaries will cause an increase in the permeability of the capillary walls. The resulting edema will cause more ischemia, and the self-perpetuating formation of a compartment syndrome will be established before arterial repair. Thus, in this circumstance, both the arterial injury and the compartment syndrome are present at the same time, and both will require immediate treatment.

The early diagnosis of compartment syndrome depends on early recognition of the clinical signs and symptoms of increased intracompartmental pressure. In patients with confusing clinical findings, the diagnosis may depend on intracompartmental pressure measurements. The most important symptom of an impending compartment syndrome is pain that is greater than expected from the primary problem. This pain is usually described as deep, unrelenting, and throbbing. It is localized to the segment of the limb containing the affected compartment, and is not referred into the distribution of the traversing sensory nerve. Nerve ischemia

usually produces failure of function without pain. The pain of compartment syndromes is not relieved by immobilization. The only true objective finding is a swollen, palpably tense compartment that is the direct result of increased intracompartmental pressure. This tension is not localized to the area of injury but is perceptible in all areas of the compartment. The overlying skin is sometimes shiny and warm and this, along with the palpable tenderness, gives an impression of cellulitis. Pain with passive stretch of the muscles of the involved compartment is a common finding, and is usually attributed to muscle ischemia. However, stretch pain is not a specific sign of a compartment syndrome. If the underlying problem has caused direct muscle injury, then passive stretching of this injured muscle will in itself produce pain. Also, children often exhibit pain with passive stretching of the finger flexors following forearm and elbow injuries, even in the absence of significantly elevated intracompartmental pressures.

The first sign of nerve ischemia is alteration of sensation manifested early by subjective paresthesias in the distribution of the involved nerve, followed by hypoesthesia, and later by anesthesia. Owen has found that all his patients with intracompartmental pressure over 30 mm Hg exhibited sensory deficit.[38] He considered that, unless there is superimposed central or peripheral nerve deficit, decreased sensation to light touch or to pin prick in the distal sensory distribution is a very reliable sign of increased intracompartmental pressure. Also, the specific nerve involvement is indicative of which compartment is involved. Motor weakness secondary to nerve or neuromuscular junction ischemia and elevated intracompartmental pressure is a relatively late physical finding. It must be noted that, except in the presence of major arterial injury, peripheral pulses and capillary filling are routinely intact in compartment syndrome patients. Thus, if peripheral pulses are absent, other causes of major arterial obstruction must be sought, and arteriography is indicated. Conversely, the presence of distal pulses and capillary refill is no reassurance that a compartment syndrome does not exist. Volkmann's ischemia can develop in patients with intact pulses.[1] Uncooperative patients, unresponsive patients, and patients with peripheral nerve deficit attributable to other etiologies, such as laceration of the brachial plexus, make the clinical diagnosis of compartment syndrome confusing. It is for this

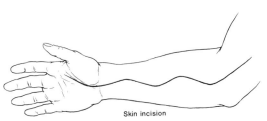

Figure 1–8. The preferred incision for a forearm fasciotomy.

reason that laboratory diagnosis using the Wick or split catheter is important.

Treatment of a compartment syndrome of the upper extremity is by fasciotomy. To release the volar forearm compartment, a single skin incision starting proximal to the antecubital fossa and extending to the midpalm is used (Fig. 1–8). The incision starts 1 cm proximal and 2 cm lateral to the medial epicondyle, and is carried obliquely across the antecubital fossa and over the volar aspect of the mobile wad. It is gently curved medially, reaching the midline at the junction of the middle and distal thirds of the forearm, and is continued straight distally to the proximal wrist crease just ulnar to the palmaris longus tendon. The incision is extended across the volar wrist crease in a curvilinear fashion, no further radially than the midaxis of the ring finger, to avoid injury to the palmar cutaneous branch of the median nerve. Termination of this incision is in the midpalm at a level even with the base of the thumb-index web. Carpal tunnel release is a standard part of forearm decompression. The lacertus fibrosus is released as part of the fasciotomy. The fascia overlying the flexor digitorum superficialis muscle belly should be divided. One must be certain that the flexor digitorum profundus, flexor pollicis longus, and pronator quadratus are adequately released. The fasciotomy is left open and dressed. Delayed primary closure at a later date is usually not possible, and split-thickness skin grafting of a portion of the defect is usually necessary.

Following the volar fasciotomy, the pressure in the dorsal compartment can be measured. If it exceeds 30 mm Hg, a dorsal fasciotomy is performed. The incision starts 2 cm lateral and 2 cm distal to the lateral condyle. It extends straight distally toward the midline of the wrist for 7 to 10 cm. The dorsal fascia is incised directly and laterally to the skin incision. The mobile wad area can be exposed easily through the volar incision. Seldom is a fasciotomy of the dorsal compartment necessary.

Compartment syndrome of the hand may present following a forearm vascular injury. Spinner and colleagues described the diagnostic triad of pain, intrinsic paralysis, and increasing pain on stretching of the involved intrinsic muscle.[49] The hand has an intrinsic minus attitude with metacarpophalangeal joint hyperextension and interphalangeal joint flexion. The hand is grossly edematous and tender. Sensation is generally normal; however, if it is diminished, carpal tunnel involvement should be suspected. The process may involve one or all intrinsic compartments, and may be acute or may persist in a subacute form for days or weeks. If untreated, an irreversible muscle necrosis occurs. The Wick catheter can be used to document an increase in pressure, and pressure greater than 30 mm Hg is an indication for fasciotomy. The most commonly involved compartments of the hand are the interossei. Dorsal decompression is performed through longitudinal incisions in the intermetacarpal spaces. The adductor is decompressed by the incision of the dorsal thumb web space.

"Crush Syndrome"

When an arterial repair is performed several hours after an injury, extensive muscle necrosis may occur and produce serious toxic manifestations. Muscle infarctions produce myoglobinemia, extracellular food loss, and acidosis-hyperkalemia. In severe cases these manifestations produce renal failure, shock, and cardiac arrhythmia.[35] This entity is known as the *crush syndrome*. Laboratory studies reflect the systemic manifestations. Muscle injury is reflected in an increase in enzyme levels, including aldolase, SGOT, LDH, and CPK. The CPK level is very elevated, usually over 10,000 IU. Myoglobin may be identified in the urine, presumptively by finding a positive benzidine test for occult blood in the absence of red blood cells on microscopic examination. The white blood count and hematocrit level may be elevated because of hemoconcentration secondary to hypovolemia. Increased creatinine and blood urea nitrogen levels reflect the severity of the renal failure. Although large amounts of potassium may be released from the injured muscle cells, normal kidneys are able to excrete the extra potassium, and hypokalemia is usually seen only in the presence of associated renal failure.

Treatment of the crush syndrome is fasciotomy and wide débridement of all necrotic muscle. The medical problems created by the muscle necrosis require aggressive medical management. Ventilatory support and dialysis may be required.[56] Successful treatment of the medical aspect of the crush syndrome is generally excellent. In contrast, however, severe limb residuals have been common.

Volkmann's Contracture

Volkmann's ischemic contracture of the upper extremity results from an irreversible necrosis of muscle tissue and subsequent fibroplastic proliferation within the muscle infarct. A variable amount of longitudinal and horizontal contraction of the resulting fibrotic mass may progress over a 6- to 12-month period following the injury. The necrotic muscle adheres to surrounding structures, fixing muscle position, reducing its mobility, and producing secondary compression of other structures in the region. The primary limitation of muscle exertion may lead to fixation of joint motion. Ischemic necrosis of the forearm muscles is most severe in the deep flexor compartment. The flexor digitorum profundus is the single most commonly and severely affected muscle. The flexor pollicis longus is the next most frequently involved muscle. In the most generalized and severe cases of Volkmann's contracture, the wrist flexors and wrist and digital extensors may also undergo varying degrees of fibrosis and contracture. The posture of the most severely involved upper extremities consists of elbow flexion, forearm pronation, and wrist flexion. The hand deformity consists of thumb flexion and adduction, and finger metacarpophalangeal joint extension and interphalangeal joint flexion, giving a claw hand appearance. Goldner noted that the muscle change caused by infarct or ischemia should be considered as a spectrum.[15]

Treatment of contractures is dependent on the severity of the deformity and on the time elapsed since injury. Mild deformity, in which hand sensibility and strength is normal but deep forearm flexors are contracted, should be managed nonoperatively with passive and dynamic extension splinting and functional training. Goldner has outlined the splinting techniques.[15] The goal of splinting is to maintain the wrist and interphalangeal joint in extension, increase the width of the thumb-index web, and augment the weakened thumb intrinsics.

The treatment of more severe contracture with evidence of nerve compression falls into four phases, as outlined by Gelberman and Blesingame: (1) release of nerve compression; (2) treatment of contracture; (3) tendon transfers for substitution reinforcement; and (4) salvage of a severely contracted or neglected forearm.[12] In the earliest stages of treatment, attention is directed toward secondary compressive neuropathies from the infarct. Neurologic return is related to the severity and duration of compression of neural tissue. Nerves may sustain compression for longer periods than muscles and still show some reversibility. If the nerves are in continuity, recovery can be expected for as long as a year and for longer periods in young patients.[48] Constriction of all three major forearm nerves may occur if fibrosis is generalized and severe. Thus, careful assessment of radial, ulnar, and median nerve function is essential early in treatment. The median nerve lies in the center of the scar, and is the most frequently and severely involved of all the nerves in Volkmann's contracture. The four major anatomic areas that may need release in the arm include the lacertus fibrosus, pronator teres, flexor digitorum superficialis, and carpal tunnel. Release of forearm neural compression should be done as soon as the condition of the extremity permits. If the nerves are in continuity, some recovery can be expected; not only will there be early return of sensibility but also marked decrease in pain in many patients.[15] Nerve grafting or repair may be required if the nerve is irreparably damaged.

At the time of nerve release or later, forearm contractures are released. The major contractures are elbow flexion, forearm pronation, wrist flexion, digital clawing, and thumb adduction. The most frequently used procedures to correct forearm contractures are excision of the infarcted muscle, flexor tendon lengthening, and flexor pronator slide. Excision of the infarcted muscle is performed by excising all muscles reduced to solid scar. This should be performed 1 to 3 or 4 months following injury.

Goldner advocates tendon lengthening proximal to the wrist, and feels that excision of the infarcted muscle may be unnecessary.[15] He recommends excision of the flexor digitorum superficialis when forearm fibrosis and digital contracture is most severe. Although flexor tendon lengthening further weakens flexor muscles, the release of contracture is more important than the maintenance of maximal strength. Tendon transfers are avoided at the time

of initial release, and are performed at a later time for reinforcement.

Tsuge uses the flexor pronator slide with and without excising the infarcted muscle, for moderate to severe deformities.[52] He does the nerve releases at the same time and tendon transfers at a later date. However, this procedure is unpredictable. There is a risk of recurrence of the deformity with growth, and the scarred necrotic muscle is not excised. There is a decrease in grip strength, especially at the distal interphalangeal joint, and there is the possibility of incomplete correction of the deformity. For these reasons we have not used this procedure at our center.

Tendon transfers are delayed until the time when some nerve recovery has occurred and the contractures have been corrected by splints or release. Goldner recommends reinforcement of tendons weakened by Z lengthening, when necessary.[15] The extensor carpi radialis longus is transferred to the flexor digitorum profundus, and the extensor carpi ulnaris is transferred to the flexor pollicis longus.

Salvage of the neglected forearm or severely contracted forearm may involve proximal or distal carpectomy, radial and ulnar shortening, wrist fusion, and digital joint fusions. In severe deformities Goldner recommends removal of the carpal bones before transfer. If the extremity is too weak for transfer, he advocates interphalangeal joint fusion, so that the extremity can function as a hook, which is generally superior to a prosthesis.

Recently, free vascularized transfers have been used in Volkmann's ischemic contracture. Taylor and Daniel used a donor nerve graft with its vascular pedicle, and transferred it to the forearm with microvascular anastomosis of the artery and vein.[51] The superficial radial nerve and its accompanying radial artery and vein were grafted to the median nerve of a Volkmann's ischemic forearm, and significant motor and sensory return were noted. Ch'en and associates first used free muscle transfer for a patient with Volkmann's ischemic contracture.[5] They transferred the lateral head of the pectoralis major to the injured forearm. Free gracilis and rectus femoris muscles have also been used to reconstruct the forearm. The ultimate role of this type of procedure is promising but must await longer follow-up to determine results.

For the severe thumb-in-palm deformity, Goldner recommends the following procedures: excision of the trapezium, metacarpophalangeal joint fusion, and adductor release. Thumb web space deepening should be considered and, in the most severely affected hands, interphalangeal joint fusions as well.

Reflex Sympathetic Dystrophy

Severe disabling pain may develop following an arterial injury of an upper extremity. Disproportionate pain after upper extremity injury should be aggressively treated so that it does not become incapacitating. The term "reflex sympathetic dystrophy" (RSD) refers to the syndrome that occurs after trauma or an exciting stimulus that causes overactivity of the sympathetic nerves and a primary or secondary vasospasm.[16] The spectrum is acute, subacute, and chronic, and the characteristics will vary according to the severity and duration of the condition. Although severe pain is always present, the separate tissues of the hand are involved to varying degrees. Drucker and co-workers have described three stages of reflex sympathetic dystrophy.[10] In stage I, the patient develops pain immediately following an injury or within a few weeks that is constant, aching, or burning in nature and disproportionate to the injury. In stage II, the edematous tissue becomes indurated and the skin cool, pale, and possibly cyanotic. Pain is continuous. In stage III, the pain spreads proximally and there are irreversible tissue changes, with fixed joint contractures and atrophic skin of the fingertips.

The chances of successful treatment diminish as the stage progresses. Our experience has demonstrated that most cases of RSD can be prevented. Tight or constrictive dressings, such as Ace wrappings, should be avoided. If undue pain is present, the dressing or cast should be immediately split to the skin. The tourniquet should be released and hemostasis obtained prior to wound closure of the hand. A bulky compressive dressing that exposes only the fingertips and postoperative elevation will diminish the incidence of RSD. Prevention is the first order of treatment for RSD.

Any treatment program for RSD should be directed toward active hand use as well as pain relief.[18] The patient must not be allowed to exclude the painful hand from daily activities. The patient is encouraged to carry a purse or similar item in the involved hand at all times, and the hand must be used for performing repetitive activities throughout the day. A supervised hand therapy program should be started to control edema, maintain joint motion, prevent contracture, and desensitize any hyperesthetic areas. Edema is reduced by active motion of the hand and by elevation. Contractures must be prevented or corrected by utilizing an active assistance exercise program. Static splinting should allow the hand to rest in the intrinsic plus position, which is least likely to lead to serious contractures. Dynamic splinting is helpful in these patients if the splints are designed to be comfortable. Passive motions by a therapist should be avoided, because this usually increases the pain and promotes further stiffness. Heat from warm packs or paraffin will increase circulation and improve the compliance of the fibrous tissue, making active exercise more effective. If possible, this program should be closely supervised by an experienced hand therapist to ensure patient compliance.

Oral medications that have proven helpful in some patients with RSD are Elavil (amitriptyline hydrochloride), Prolixin (fluphenazine hydrochloride), Haldol (haloperidol), Dilantin (phenytoin sodium), and Tegretol (carbamazepine). We have had the most success with a combination of Elavil and Prolixin. Elavil, a tricyclic antidepressant, may have an effect on the central nervous system pain receptors (endorphins).[43] Prolixin, a phenothiazine, has analgesic properties and depresses the response to peripheral stimuli. The dosage of Elavil is 25 mg each night, increased to 50 to 75 mg; that of Prolixin is 1 mg twice a day. It may take several weeks before a beneficial response is evident. Narcotics should not be used in these patients.

Reserpine administered by an intravenous block technique may be beneficial in relieving the pain of RSD. Reserpine acts as a catecholamine depletor, and inhibits adrenergic nerve endings. Using a technique similar to that used in intravenous regional anesthesia, the effect of the drug is limited to the upper extremity. The amount of reserpine is 2 mg diluted in 40 ml of 0.25% bupivacaine (Marcaine) without epinephrine. The local anesthetic in the mixture totally eliminates the arm pain, effectively breaking the pain cycle. The pain relief may last longer than the anesthetic activity of the drug. An intravenous catheter is inserted into a dorsal hand vein, and the upper extremity is exsanguinated with an Esmarch bandage. An above-elbow blood pressure cuff is inflated to 100 mm Hg above the patient's systolic pressure. The medication is administered through the intravenous catheter. The tourniquet is left inflated for 20 minutes to allow for tissue binding of the Marcaine and reserpine, and is then slowly released, and the patient is observed for a short period of time prior to discharge. The beneficial effects usually last several hours, but may last a few weeks to 3 months. The procedure may be repeated any number of times. We have found this procedure to be effective, as have others.[6] It is a safe procedure and can be done in an office setting.[55] We prefer this technique to sympathetic blockade with axillary or supraclavicular injection, because we feel that it is as effective without exposing the patient to risk. Intravenous guanethidine given by the same technique may be more effective, but its intravascular use has not been approved in this country.[17]

A nonsteroid anti-inflammatory agent should be prescribed on a long-term basis. Oral steroids may be beneficial in patients with severe discomfort. Decreasing doses for 1 week, starting with 40 mg of prednisone daily and diminishing the dose to 5 mg on the last day, is recommended. When edema is a major component, a compressive well-fitting glove may be of benefit.

The keys to treating RSD of the hand are early recognition before irreversible changes have resulted and dogmatic persistence, with a nonoperative regimen of the patient taking the active role in rehabilitation. Treatment is prolonged, and there are many peaks and valleys. Rarely is surgery indicated. Occasionally, in carefully selected patients with late stage III disease, joint releases may be indicated but beneficial results of this surgery are limited.

Late Ischemia

Symptoms of ischemia may develop as a complication of arterial injury. The most common symptoms are pain and cold intolerance. Initially the pain may be described as "tiredness," "cramping," or "general discomfort." As the ischemia persists, the pain becomes more intense.[17] Pain on exposure to cold is characteristic of ischemia.

The hand or involved digit may be pale or cyanotic, and ulcers or gangrene of the fingertips may exist. There may be a palpable difference in temperature and texture between the involved and the noninvolved digits, with the involved fingers being cooler and drier. Although claudication usually follows arterial occlusions of the leg, it is not common in the upper extremity because of less frequent prolonged use of the muscles, and because many of the lesions involve the arterial system at the wrist and hand distal to the large muscle mass. Night pain is also less common than in lesions of the lower extremity.

On examination the nail beds are often pale. Capillary refill is slow, and there is lower skin temperature when compared to that of an adjacent normal finger on the opposite hand. The Allen test may reveal diminished flow through one of the arteries at the base of the fingers.

The special tests outlined earlier are helpful in evaluating patients with finger or hand ischemia. If arteriography is performed, 1 mg of reserpine is injected intra-arterially at the end of the procedure. This results in a "medical sympathectomy," often resulting in beneficial effects that may last for months. If symptoms recur, the intra-arterial injection may be repeated. As in the treatment of RSD, reserpine by intravenous block technique may also be of value, and is probably safer than an intra-arterial injection. Systemic peripheral vasodilators, such as oral guanethidine, may be tried. We have had mixed results with systemic Ismelin (guanethidine) given orally. A starting dose of 10 mg once daily is increased by 10 mg daily each week, to a total therapeutic dose of 40 mg given in a regimen of 10 mg four times daily. While on the medication, the patient must be followed closely and monitored for development of postural hypotension.

Peripheral nerve blocks for immediate pain relief and vasodilation are often helpful. The use of a small silicone tube inserted percutaneously adjacent to a nerve allows intermittent perfusion of long-acting anesthetic agents to provide a sympathetic response for vasodilation (Fig. 1–9).[19] This effec-

tively controls vasospasm, but generally only for as long as the injections are continued.

Biofeedback techniques may decrease vasospasm in patients who have nonspecific labile syndromes. Some patients become very proficient in willing the temperature of their involved digits to rise, thereby alleviating their discomfort.

Obvious adjunctive therapy includes instructions about keeping the hands warm, wearing gloves, discontinuing smoking, and perhaps changing occupation. If gangrene progresses or symptoms persist despite nonoperative management, surgical exploration and reconstruction may be indicated. Predisposing medical conditions should be treated and stabilized prior to any surgical attempt.

References

1. Adar, R., Schramek, A., Khodadadi, J., et al.: Arterial combat injuries of the upper extremity. J. Trauma, 20:274, 1980.
2. Allen, E. V.: Thromboangiitis obliterans: Methods of diagnosis of chronic occlusive arterial lesions distal to the wrist with illustrative cases. Am. J. Med. Sci., 178:237, 1929.
3. Amato, J. J., and Rick, N. M.: Temporary cavity effects in blood vessel injury by high velocity missiles. J. Cardiovasc. Surg., 13:147, 1972.
4. Bassett, F. H., III, and Silver, D.: Arterial injury associated with fractures. Arch. Surg., 92:13, 1966.
5. Ch'en, C. S., Daniel, R. K., and Terzis, J. K.: Reconstructive microsurgery, Boston, Little, Brown & Company, 1977.
6. Chuinard, R. G., et al.: Intravenous reserpine for treatment of reflex sympathetic dystrophy. South. Med. J., 74:1481, 1981.
7. Coleman, S. S., and Anson, B. J.: Arterial patterns in the hand based upon a study of 750 extremities. Surg. Gynecol. Obstet., 113:40, 1961.
8. DeBakey, M. E., and Simeone, F. A.: Battle injuries of the arteries in World War II. An analysis of 2,471 cases. Ann. Surg., 123:534, 1946.
9. Doty, D. B., et al.: Prevention of gangrene due to fracture. Surg. Gynecol. Obstet., 125:284, 1967.
10. Drucker, W. R., et al.: Pathogenesis of post-traumatic sympathetic dystrophy. Am. J. Surg., 79:454, 1959.
11. Fowler, P. J., and Willis, R. B.: Vascular compartment syndromes. Can. J. Surg., 18:157, 1975.
12. Gelberman, R.: Volkmann's contracture of the upper extremity: Pathology and reconstruction. In Mubarak, S. J., and Hargens, A. R. (eds.): Compartment Syndromes and Volkmann's Contracture, Philadelphia, W. B. Saunders, 1981, p. 183.
13. Gelberman, R. H., and Blasingame, J. P.: The timed Allen test. J. Trauma, 21:477, 1981.
14. Gelberman, R. H., Menon, J., and Fronek, A.: The peripheral pulse following arterial injury. J. Trauma, 20:948, 1980.
15. Goldner, J. L.: Volkmann's ischemic contracture. In Flynn, J. E. (ed.): Hand Surgery, 2nd ed., Baltimore, Williams & Wilkins, 1975, p. 599.
16. Goldner, J. L.: Pain: Extremities and spine. Evaluation and differential diagnosis. In Omer, G. E., and Spinner, M. (eds.): Management of Peripheral Nerve Problems, Philadelphia, W. B. Saunders, 1980, p. 119.
17. Goldner, J. L., and Bright, D. S.: The effect of extremity blood flow on pain and cold intolerance. In Omer, G. E., and Spinner, M. (eds.): Management of Peripheral Nerve Problems, Philadelphia, W. B. Saunders, 1980, p. 176.
18. Gustilo, R. B., and Anderson, J. T.: Prevention of infection in the treatment of one thousand and twenty-five open fractures of long bones. J. Bone Joint Surg., 58A:453, 1976.
19. Hannington-Kiff, J. G.: Intravenous regional sympathetic block with guanethidine. Lancet, 1:1019, 1974.
20. Hollinshead, W. H.: Textbook of Anatomy, 3rd ed., New York, Harper & Row, 1974, p. 158.

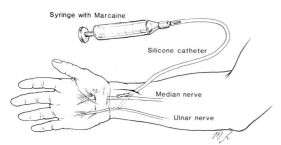

Figure 1–9. A silicone catheter is placed near the median or ulnar nerve, or near both, to infiltrate Marcaine for vasodilation of hand vessels.

21. Kaplan, E. B.: Functional and Surgical Anatomy of the Hand, 2nd ed., Philadelphia, J. B. Lippincott, 1965, p. 143.
22. Kelly, G. L., and Eisenman, B.: Civilian vascular injuries. J. Trauma, 15:507, 1975.
23. Koman, L. A., and Urbaniak, J. R.: Ulnar artery insufficiency: A guide to treatment. J. Hand Surg., 6:16, 1981.
24. Koman, L. A., Hardaker, W. T., and Goldner, J. L.: Wick catheter in evaluating and treating compartment syndromes. South. Med. J., 74:303, 1981.
25. Koman, L. A., et al.: The free vascularized scapular flap. Presented at the Annual Meeting of the Piedmont Orthopaedic Society, Colorado Springs, Colorado, May 7, 1982.
26. Koman, L. A., et al.: Upper extremity radionuclide imaging. Presented at the Annual Meeting of the American Society for Surgery of the Hand, New Orleans, Louisiana, January 18, 1982.
27. Kurchin, A., et al.: Arterial injury due to high velocity missile. Harefuah, 89:201, 1975.
28. Lain, K. C., and Williams, G. R.: Arteriography in acute peripheral arterial injuries: An experimental study. Surg. Forum, 21:179, 1970.
29. MacGowan, W.: Acute ischemia complicating limb trauma. J. Bone Joint Surg., 50B:472, 1968.
30. McCormack, L. J., Cauldwell, E. W., and Anson, B. J.: Brachial and antebrachial arterial patterns: A study of 750 extremities. Surg. Gynecol. Obstet., 96:43, 1953.
31. McNamara, J. J., et al.: Management of fractures with associated arterial injury in combat casualties. J. Trauma, 13:17, 1973.
32. Miller, H. H., and Welch, C. S.: Quantitative studies on the time factor in arterial injuries. Ann. Surg., 30:428, 1949.
33. Mubarak, S. J.: Etiologies of compartment syndromes. In Mubarak, S. J., and Hargens, A. R. (eds.): Compartment Syndromes and Volkmann's Contracture, Philadelphia, W. B. Saunders, 1981, p. 71.
34. Mubarak, S. J., et al.: The Wick technique for measurement of intramuscular pressure: A new research and clinical tool. J. Bone Joint Surg., 58A:1016, 1976.
35. Mubarak, S. J., and Owen, C. A.: Compartment syndrome and its relation to the crush syndrome: A spectrum of disease. Clin. Orthop., 113:81, 1975.
36. Mufti, M. A., et al.: Diagnostic value of hematoma in penetrating arterial wounds of the extremities. Arch. Surg., 101:562, 1970.
37. Nunley, J. A., Koman, L. A., and Urbaniak, J. R.: Arterial shunting as an adjunct to major limb revascularization. Ann. Surg., 193:271, 1981.
38. Owen, C. A.: Clinical diagnosis of acute compartment syndromes. In Mubarak, S. J., and Hargens, A. R. (eds.): Compartment Syndromes and Volkmann's Contracture, Philadelphia, W. B. Saunders, 1981, p. 98.
39. Parks, B. J., Arbelaez, J., and Horner, R. L.: Medical and surgical importance of the arterial blood supply of the thumb. J. Hand Surg., 3:383, 1978.
40. Patman, R. D., Poulos, E., and Shires, G. T.: The management of civilian arterial injuries. Surg. Gynecol. Obstet., 118:725, 1964.
41. Phelps, D. B., Rutherford, R. B., and Boswick, J. A.: Control of vasospasm following trauma and microvascular surgery. J. Hand Surg., 4:109, 1979.
42. Pick, J.: The Autonomic Nervous System. Philadelphia, J. B. Lippincott, 1970.
43. Pleasure, D. E.: The painful hand: A neurologist's perspective. Founders' Lecture, presented at the Annual Meeting of the American Society for Surgery of the Hand, New Orleans, Louisiana, January 18, 1982.
44. Rich, N. M., et al.: Internal vs. external fixation of fractures with concomitant vascular injuries in Vietnam. J. Trauma, 11:463, 1971.
45. Rich, N. M., Manion, W. C., and Hughes, C. S.: Surgical and pathological evaluation of vascular injuries in Vietnam. J. Trauma, 9:279, 1969.
46. Romanoff, H., and Goldberger, S.: Major peripheral vein injuries. Vasc. Surg., 10:157, 1976.
47. Rorabeck, C. H., et al.: The slit catheter: A new device for measuring intra-compartmental pressures. Surg. Forum, 31:513, 1980.
48. Seddon, H. J.: Volkmann's contracture: Treatment by incision of the infarct. J. Bone Joint Surg., 38B:152, 1956.
49. Spinner, M., et al.: Impending ischemic contracture of the hand. Plast. Reconstr. Surg., 50:341, 1972.
50. Stirrat, C. R., et al.: Temperature monitoring in digital replantation. J. Hand Surg., 3:342, 1978.
51. Taylor, G. I., and Daniel, R. K.: The free flap: Composite tissue transfer by vascular anastomoses. Aust. J. Surg., 43:1, 1973.
52. Tsuge, K.: Treatment of established Volkmann's contracture. J. Bone Joint Surg., 57A:925, 1975.
53. Urbaniak, J. R.: Replantation of amputated hands and digits. AAOS Instructional Course Lectures, 27:15, 1978.
54. Urbaniak, J. R.: Digit and hand replantation: Current status. Neurosurgery, 5:551, 1979.
55. Urbaniak, J. R., and Roth, J. H.: Office diagnosis and treatment of hand pain. Orthop. Clin. North Am., 13:477, 1982.
56. Weeks, S.: The crush syndrome. Surg. Gynecol. Obstet., 12:369, 1978.
57. Whitesides, T. E., Jr., Hirada, H., and Morimoto, K.: Compartment syndromes and the role of fasciotomy: Its parameters and techniques. AAOS Instructional Course Lectures, 26:179, 1977.
58. Wilgis, E. F., et al.: The evaluation of small vessel flow: A study of dynamic non-invasive techniques. J. Bone Joint Surg., 56A:1199, 1974.

2

COMPLICATIONS IN FLEXOR TENDON INJURIES

Harold E. Kleinert,
Michael Kalisman,
and Curtis M. Steyers

Of all the problems the hand surgeon is called on to treat, probably none are more prone to develop complications and consequently obtain imperfect results than flexor tendon injuries. This is especially true within the digital sheath, in which tendon injuries are one of the most problematic in hand surgery with respect to the restoration of normal function.[1-12] These undesirable situations can, however, be substantially reduced or eliminated by applying basic principles of hand surgery, which include prompt and thorough examination of the injured hand, and the appropriate choice of treatment for each condition. The treatment and complications from flexor tendon surgery will be discussed in the following chapter. To deal with these problems adequately, it is also essential to know certain facts about flexor tendon anatomy, function, and physiologic behavior.

ANATOMY

The flexor digitorum superficialis and profundus muscles originate from the medial epicondyle of the humerus, the upper part of the anterior border of the radius, the anterior and posterior surfaces of the ulna, the medial surface of the coronoid process, and the anterior interosseous membrane, respectively. Proximal to the carpal ligament the combined superficialis muscle mass forms two planes. The tendons of the most superficial plane insert to the long and ring fingers, and the deep plane tendons insert to the index and small fingers as they pass through the carpal tunnel deep to the flexor retinaculum. The profundus muscle divides into four

tendons located side by side dorsal to the superficial tendons, and pass under the flexor retinaculum with the flexor pollicis longus.

The carpal canal, approximately 4 cm in length, is formed by the flexor retinaculum, tubercles of the scaphoid and trapezium, the hook of the hamate, and the pisiform. The flexor tendons are covered with loose areolar tissue containing multiple blood vessels—that is, a vascular synovium. Only the flexor pollicis longus and the tendons of the small finger are covered with a continuous synovial sheath in the palm. The remaining tendons in the palm are covered with loose areolar tissue, called paratenon. At the level of the metacarpal neck, the flexor tendons of each finger are enveloped by a synovial sheath, which extends to the tendon's insertion. This synovial sheath is reinforced by strong fibrous pulleys: five annular pulleys and four cruciate pulleys in each finger. The annular pulleys are principally attached to the bone to ensure efficient motion and to prevent bowstringing during flexion. The cruciate pulleys lie between the annular pulleys, and are positioned over the joints to allow for movement through compression and expansion, which reduces the bulk that would limit motion. The A2 and A4 pulleys are especially critical to finger function and to the prevention of bowstringing (Fig. 2–1).

Over the proximal phalanx, each flexor superficialis tendon splits into two slips that embrace the flexor profundus tendon. After reversing their surface 180°, they reunite dorsal to the profundus tendon and then diverge to be inserted into the anterior proximal surface of the middle phalanx. The profundus tendons pass through the aperture

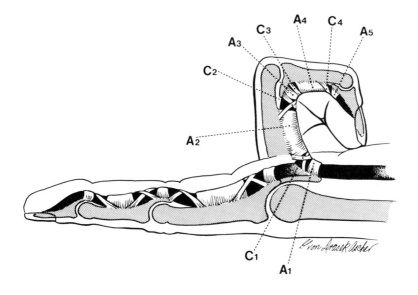

Figure 2–1. The annular pulleys remain essentially the same size in flexion and extension, whereas the cruciate pulleys expand and contract like an accordion. (From Kleinert, H.E., and Lubahn, J.: Current state of flexor tendon surgery. Ann. Chir. Main 3(1):7, 1984.)

produced by the splitting of the superficialis tendons and proceed to the base of the distal phalanx, where they terminate.

Mesotendon connects the tendons to the distal sheath. These vincula tendinum (two to the superficialis and two to the profundus tendons) are folds of synovial membranes strengthened by fibrous tissue that conduct blood vessels to the tendons. The vincula breve are located between the bone and the distal end of the tendons. The vincula longum are located between the proximal phalanx and superficialis tendons, and more distal between the proximal phalanx and the profundus tendons.

The four lumbrical muscles (one in each finger) are small cylindric muscles. The lateral two lumbricals originate just distal to the flexor retinaculum by a single head from the radial side of the flexor profundus tendon and run to the index and long fingers. The ulnar two lumbricals originate from the adjacent sides of the profundus tendons between which they lie. All four lumbricals join the radial aspect of the extensor hood at the side of the proximal phalanx.

The flexor digitorum profundus flexes the digits in slow action and the superficialis tendon assists in speed and flexion against resistance. The lumbrical muscles are important for metacarpophalangeal joint flexion. All functions of the hand—power grip, precision handling, gross motion, compression force, and power pinch—are provided by the extrinsic muscles with the assistance of the intrinsic muscles.[5, 13–18]

PHYSIOLOGIC BEHAVIOR

The vascular system of the flexor tendons within the digital sheath is markedly different from that of tendons in other regions. Outside the sheath, tendons are covered with paratenon that has a well-developed vascular network around itself. The flexor tendons within the synovial sheath region are seemingly devoid of blood vessels on their gliding volar surface. At the proximal interphalangeal joint level, the profundus tendon has a relatively avascular zone. The superficialis tendon has a similar avascular zone at its division into two slips at the base of the proximal phalanx.

Until recently it was believed that the only way to restore blood supply and tendon healing was by fibroblastic response from surrounding tissue, with ingrowth of vascular adhesions. Recent studies have demonstrated that tendons deprived of their blood supply can survive in a synovial fluid medium. Both experimental and clinical studies indicate that flexor tendons heal by a combination of intrinsic and extrinsic mechanisms whose importance depends on the level of the injured tendons. The blood supply consists of the vincula brevis and longus and on the intrinsic longitudinal vessels. The synovial fluid plays a significant role as a nutritional agent, in addition to being a lubricant. Atraumatic handling of the injured tendon, and preservation of the vincula and the synovial sheath, are mandatory for successful flexor tendon surgery.

In addition to vascular and synovial fluid nutritional supply, other important factors in tendon healing include preoperative conditions such as joint mobility, involvement of the digital nerves and arteries, fractures, suture technique, and tension. Controlled mobilization with a dynamic splint is beneficial during the postoperative period. Early unprotected active mobilization will increase tension on the suture line, with possible tendon rupture. Special care should be taken on the fifth to seventh days after repair. During this period, the tendon repair site is weaker as compared with the tendon strength immediately after the repair. Controlled mobilization of a repaired flexor tendon with dynamic rubber band traction during limited active

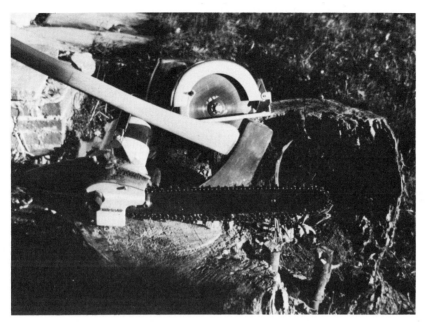

Figure 2–2. Agents that can produce injuries with multiple tissue involvement.

extension will prevent tension gap ruptures and the formation of firm adhesions.

The microcirculation of the repaired tendon is better with certain suture techniques that create less tension at the repair site and minimize adhesion and gap formation.[19–31]

There are many variations in flexor tendon injuries; the most common causes are glass, knives, saws, and farm accidents, (Fig. 2–2). Most flexor tendon injury complications can be prevented by (1) early recognition of the tendon injury, (2) early repair (primary or delayed primary if the patient's general condition is not jeopardized by such a procedure), and (3) a surgeon positively familiar with the technique of tendon repair.

For clearer understanding and simplicity of discussion of flexor tendon injuries, a zone classification was agreed on at the First Congress of the International Federation of Societies for Surgery of the Hand, held in Rotterdam in June, 1980 (Fig. 2–3; Table 2–1).

CONTRIBUTING FACTORS

Type of Injury

Tidy hand injuries are typically caused by injuries from glass or knives, and are often household injuries. Associated nerve and artery sections are common, skin edges are generally clean-cut, and skin loss or associated fractures are rare.

Untidy hand injuries result from accidents with saws and power machinery, which produce open, tearing, crushing wounds involving several tissues. This may include skin, flexor and extensor tendon,

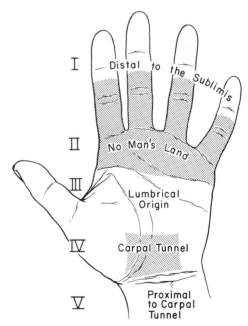

Figure 2–3. Zones of flexor tendon injury. Each influences different factors for repair. (From Kleinert, H.E., and Broudy, A.S.: Direct repair and dynamic splinting of flexor tendon lacerations. *In* Black, J., and Dumbleton, J.H. [eds.]: Clinical Biomechanics, New York, Churchill Livingstone, 1980.)

Table 2-1. CLASSIFICATION OF FLEXOR TENDON INJURIES

| | Fingers | | Thumb |
Zone	Region	Zone	Region
I	Distal to superficial insertion	I	Distal to the annular and cruciate pulleys
II	From the A1 pulley to the superficial tendon insertion	II	Annular and cruciate pulleys
III	From the distal end of the carpal tunnel to the A1 pulley	III	Thenar eminence
IV	Carpal canal	IV	Carpal canal
V	Proximal to carpal canal	V	Proximal to carpal canal

nerve, blood vessel, joint, and bone fractures, with varying amounts of tissue loss. Wound edges may not be viable. These injuries are divided into subtypes—for example, crushing, avulsion, wringer, and roller press injuries—according to the mechanism of injury (Fig. 2–4).

Associated Multiple Tissue Injury

Multiple tendon damage can occur with small stab wounds as well as with extensive trauma to the hand. The tendon may be lacerated at the level of the skin wound or some distance away, depending on the position of the fingers at the time of injury (Fig. 2–5). Associated injuries to blood vessels, nerves, bones, joints, and extensor tendons are common and are more difficult to diagnose clinically. Deep proximal wounds may have obscure injuries of the median and ulnar nerves, reflected by sensory and motor function abnormalities of the hand, whereas arterial injuries may jeopardize viability of the hand. Distal wounds involving neurovascular bundles not only cause insensitivity of the skin but also lead to the subsequent development of painful neuromas.

Unfortunately, all too frequently the diagnosis of a damaged nerve is established only after a lapse of several weeks. Recognition and primary repair of the associated neurovascular injury at the time of flexor tendon repair prevent secondary procedures, thus producing more satisfactory results.

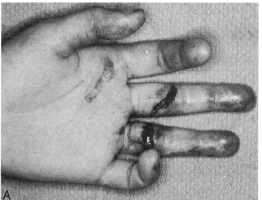
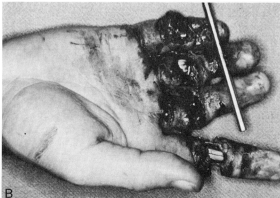
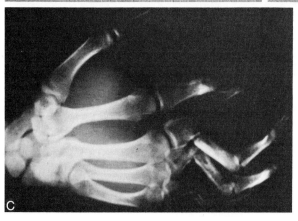

Figure 2-4. A, Tidy injury—fingers in straight position indicate flexor tendon injury; *B, C,* untidy injury (punch press), with part of flexor tendons injured and multiple tissue involvement.

Examination of the hands is usually sufficient for recognition of open fractures, whereas closed fractures are more obscure. Both types may extend into joints. The extent and severity of bone and joint injury are only accurately defined after roentgenogram examination. Anteroposterior, lateral, and oblique x-ray views should be taken whenever indicated as part of the complete hand examination.

Associated injuries of the volar plate, collateral ligaments, joint capsule, and extensor tendon are easily overlooked. Joints should be tested for stability and motion. Suspicion of injury to these structures will necessitate their exploration at the time of flexor tendon repair. Failure to recognize these injuries will result in stiff joints and in further immobility of the involved fingers.

Wound Contamination

Farm injuries, such as those caused by a cornpicker, lawnmower, or chain saw, are ordinarily heavily contaminated with foreign organic material on the surface and within tissues. Primary treatment of these injuries follows basic principles of thorough wound cleansing and irrigation, débridement of all foreign material and nonviable tissue, and tetanus immunization. Irrigation can be done with a hand irrigation syringe or a Waterpik machine, which has the advantage of controlled pressure and rapid extensive irrigation. Heavily contaminated large wounds with exposed tendons or bones, or with loss of skin, may require flap coverage. Depending on the wound condition, delayed primary or early secondary repair is advocated. In less contaminated cases with adequate skin coverage, after meticulous débridement and extensive irrigation, tendons can be repaired primarily or as a delayed procedure in 3 or 4 days. Wound and tissue cultures are obtained during initial wound management.

Skin Cover

Flexor tendon repair requires adequate skin coverage. Skin loss must be assessed in each individual case. For most wounds with no skin loss, closure is easily achieved by suture. Some wounds without skin loss, because of local tissue reaction, swelling, and hematoma, cannot be safely closed by suture without undue tension. Tension is best avoided, because it leads to tissue necrosis and potential infection. Most failures of wound closure occur in those patients with relative skin loss in whom the surgeon attempts primary suture rather than a grafting procedure. Local and occasionally distant flaps are employed to achieve closure of wounds in which underlying structures should not be left exposed. The flaps are intended to relieve tension in cases in which direct closure is impossible, to ensure the coverage of vulnerable tissue such as joints, tendons, nerves, or blood vessels by healthy skin, which will preclude heavy scar formation in this area, and

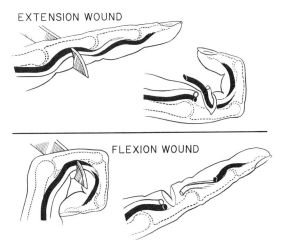

Figure 2–5. As the finger changes position, the injured profundus and superficialis tendons change in position relative to each other. (From Kutz, J.E., et al.: Evaluation of the injured hand. J. Plast. Reconstr. Surg. Nurs. 2(1):10–14, 1982.

to alter the site and direction of potential scar or tension lines. This principle can be achieved by local flaps, a Z-plasty flap or advancement, and rotation flaps. Many donor sites such as cross-finger flaps, cross-arm flaps, chest flaps, and groin flaps are available as a two-stage procedure. In extensive injuries one-stage microsurgical transfer of a flap is done as part of the emergency procedure (Fig. 2–6).

Loss of Finger Viability

The ability to replant and preserve finger or limb viability by revascularization has progressed within the last decade. At the present time, microsurgical techniques have made vascular repair possible, even at the base of the distal phalanx. With flexor tendon injuries an injury to the neurovascular bundle is common. In most cases the injury affects only one of the bundles, thus allowing for adequate blood supply through the contralateral digital artery. When both bundles are injured, the finger may be viable through collateral circulation from the dorsal skin bridge. Surgeons tend to overlook the need for vascular repair if the collateral circulation of the digit or hand is sufficient to maintain viability. Cold intolerance, claudication, and ischemic pain may result from failure to repair arterial injuries; therefore, we advocate vascular repair. Amputations, when indicated, are replanted. Tendons are repaired primarily followed by vascular microscopic repair. This may include the use of reverse vein grafts when indicated to prevent vascular repair tension. Nerves are repaired prior to skin closure.

Hematoma

Hematoma is a great danger to return of optimal functional results. Even if infection of hematoma

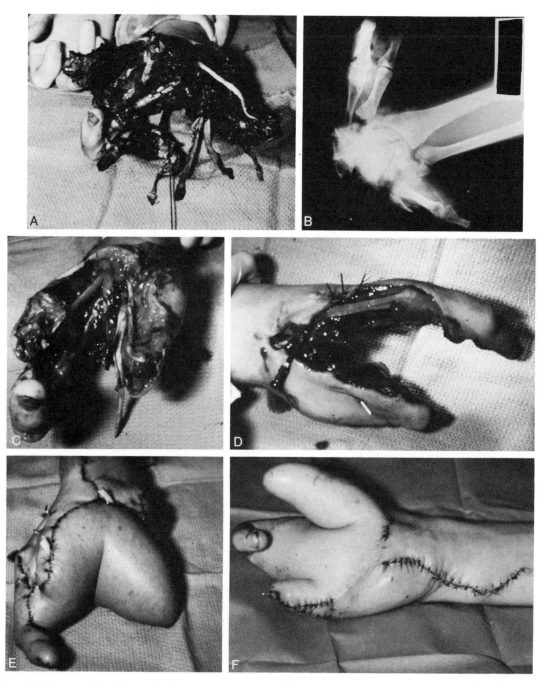

Figure 2–6. A severe blast injury necessitating microvascular reconstruction, with immediate vascularized flap skin cover. *A,* Appearance at start of emergency surgery; *B,* x-ray demonstrates finger loss and separation of remaining rays at metacarpal-carpal level; *C, D,* volar and dorsal views indicate amount of tissue cover needed after restoring bony framework and digit viability with long vein grafts to restore both arteries and veins; *E,* emergency vascularized latissimus flap for immediate coverage; *F,* appearance immediately after flexor tendolysis to improve motion.

does not occur, normal healing is delayed and tissue edges separate. Hematoma is replaced by fibrosis followed by decreased function. After flexor tendon injury, hematoma can occur from lacerated intratendinous vessels, from vincula, and from surrounding loose areolar tissue containing numerous small blood vessels. Existing hematoma must be evacu-

ated. Prevention of hematoma can be minimized by the following: (1) identification and coagulation of all bleeding vessels; (2) release of the tourniquet and attainment of hemostasis prior to wound closure; (3) elevation of the hand and extremity to reduce capillary bleeding and tissue edema; and (4) instituting wound drainage if hemostasis is doubtful.

EVALUATION OF THE INJURY

The indication for and outcome of tendon repair are influenced by several factors, including type and site of injury, time elapsed since trauma, existence of associated lesions, age, race, occupation, hobbies, associated diseases, medications, and the ability and motivation of the patient to cooperate with the intended treatment.

Clean wounds with isolated tendon injury or with associated injuries that can be treated are primarily repaired. Primary tendon repair is recommended in favorable cases up to 24 hours after injury, provided that there is no evidence of wound infection. After 24 hours delayed primary repair must be considered. Results are comparable with those of primary repair.

After 5 weeks lacerated tendons exhibit retraction, coiling, and peritendinous fibrosis. The cut muscle-tendon unit has lost tone and elasticity, and has retracted to such an extent that direct repair is probably not possible. The thickened tendon will not pass through collapsed empty pulleys, and a secondary procedure—that is, tendon graft—is indicated. Tendon grafts are further indicated in all cases with associated unstable bone or joint fracture, skin loss, or both.

Contraindications for primary, delayed primary, or early secondary flexor tendon repair include loss of significant tendon substance, inability to obtain adequate skin coverage, inadequate pulley system, multiple segmental lacerations, unstable fractures, uncooperative patient, and inexperienced surgeon. Skeletal reduction and stabilization and adequate skin cover are necessary if early motion is to be utilized. Reconstruction of severely mutilated fingers with multiple tissue injury is a salvage procedure that may require primary arthrodesis or arthroplasty and staged tendon reconstruction.

COMPLICATIONS FROM UNTREATED FLEXOR TENDON INJURIES

Partial Tendon Lacerations

In recognizing the anatomic relation of the flexor tendons and tendon sheath relative to the skin surface and skin creases, one can understand the frequent involvement of these structures in what

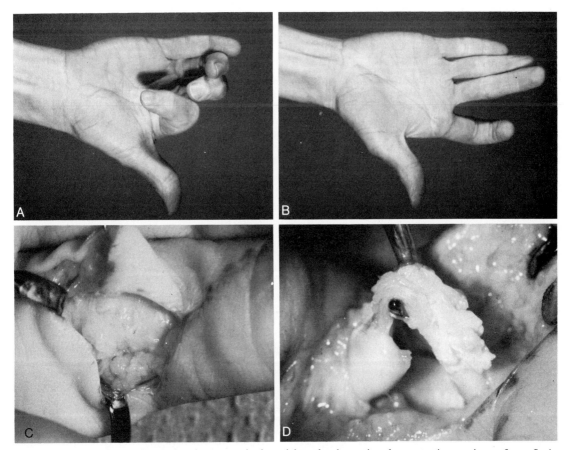

Figure 2–7. Hand of nurse 3 months after unrepaired partial tendon laceration demonstrating maximum finger flexion *(A)* and extension *(B); C,* tenosynovitis present at site of partial profundus laceration; *D,* marked fraying of tendon at site of partial profundus laceration. (From Kleinert, H.E., et al.: Complications of tendon surgery in the hand. *In* Current Management of Complications in Orthopaedics: The Hand and Wrist, S. Sandzen [ed.], Baltimore, Williams & Wilkins, in press.)

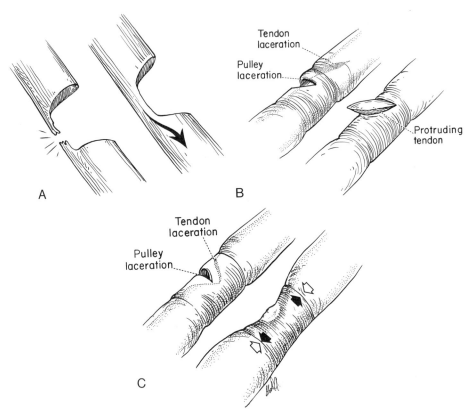

Figure 2-8. Potential complications of unrepaired and untreated flexor tendon injuries. *A*, Rupture; *B*, incomplete flexion from protruding partial laceration through aperture in sheath; trigger phenomenon and tendon adherence. (From Kleinert, H.E., et al.: Complications of tendon surgery in the hand. *In* Current Management of Complications in Orthopaedics: The Hand and Wrist, S. Sandzen [ed.], Baltimore, Williams & Wilkins, in press.)

might initially appear to be a simple, superficial skin laceration. Involvement of the tendon sheath and partial laceration of the flexor tendon are often unrecognized, ignored, or intentionally untreated (Fig. 2-7).

Three potential problems can result from not treating partial tendon lacerations: tendon rupture, decreased tendon gliding, and development of trigger finger (Fig. 2-8). Allowing a partially severed tendon to go unsutured and untreated invites the development of bulbous scar formation, producing a trigger phenomenon that causes incomplete gliding of the tendon through the pulleys. Oblique partial tendon lacerations may engage the cut tendon sheath and prevent motion. The decrease of tensile strength in the partially severed tendon illuminates the importance of treating incompletely severed tendons to prevent subsequent tendon rupture. Appropriate postoperative surgical care with splinting is similar to that of a completely severed tendon, particularly if considerable tendon substance is divided.[32, 34]

Hyperextension of the Distal Interphalangeal Joint

These injuries usually occur from a sudden dorsal hyperextension force that avulses the profundus

insertion. Most such injuries occur in athletes. The diagnosis in most cases is not made initially unless a careful history is obtained and examination for active flexion of the distal interphalangeal joint is performed. There is no flexion of the distal interphalangeal joint, which may be painful and swollen. There are three types of avulsion injuries:

1. The tendon retracts over the middle phalanx and the vinculum remains intact. A small bony fragment can pull away with the distal part of the flexor tendon. Secondary repair can be accomplished several weeks after injury, because the intact vincula prevent more proximal tendon retraction.

2. The avulsed tendon retracts into the palm, both vincula are ruptured, and a substantial portion of the blood supply is lost. There is a tender mass in the palm along with an inability to flex the distal interphalangeal joint actively. If repair is not performed within 7 to 10 days, the tendon becomes thickened and contracted, can undergo partial necrosis, and will not pass through pulleys, necessitating a tendon graft reconstruction.

3. A large bony fragment from the distal phalanx remains attached to the distal profundus tendon. The distal A4 pulley will prevent more proximal retraction. Profundus tendon lacerations in zone I are similar to types 1 and 2 avulsion injuries (above).

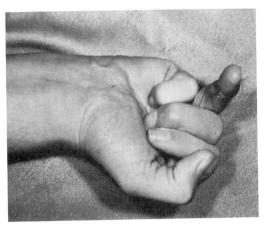

Figure 2–9. Lumbrical plus deformity.

At one time many surgeons felt that the loss of distal interphalangeal joint movement was less disabling than the operative trauma. Failure to restore active distal interphalangeal joint flexion decreases grip strength. The resulting muscle imbalance causes distal interphalangeal joint hyperextension deformity, which produces a weak pinch and pain in the joint, as well as decreased grip.[3, 33–37] The small finger may have a weak or absent superficialis tendon, resulting in minimal or weak proximal interphalangeal joint flexion.

Lumbrical Plus Deformity

Lumbrical muscles arise from the proximal profundus tendons and insert into the dorsal extensor expansion. Their main function is coordination and control of delicate movement of the fingers in flexion or extension.

When the distal insertion of the profundus tendon in the finger is disrupted or detached, the proximal end retracts, taking the origin of the lumbrical with it. This excess pull on the lumbrical insertion will limit flexion of the proximal interpha-langeal joint by the superficialis tendons. The clinical manifestation of this deformity will be "paradoxic extension" of the interphalangeal joints when the patient attempts full flexion of the finger. Lumbrical plus deformity commonly occurs in the long fingers. The ulnar three fingers' profundus tendons work in a mass action during flexion without independent function. In the long finger, when the flexor profundus tendon has lost continuity, the tendon is pulled to the ulnar side of the next lumbrical origin, thus tightening the lumbrical apparatus of the long finger. In the case of the ring and small ingers, the profundus pull is limited by the bicipital lumbrical muscle origin (Fig. 2–9).[38]

Swan-Neck Deformity

Swan-neck deformity is characterized by proximal interphalangeal joint hyperextension and by distal interphalangeal joint flexion. Isolated injury to the flexor superficialis tendon is still difficult to diagnose without careful examination, because the patient will demonstrate a full range of motion of the involved finger using the intact profundus tendon. Swan-neck deformity represents the end result of muscular imbalance from injury to the superficial flexor tendon, the volar plate, and the extensor tendon, as with mallet deformity. The significant functional disturbance with this deformity is impaired flexion of the proximal interphalangeal joint, perhaps so severe as to prevent initiating joint flexion (Fig. 2–10).[4] Restoration of the superficialis tendon function or of the volar plate check ligament will prevent such a deformity.

Retraction of the Muscle Tendon Unit

Proximal retraction of the muscle tendon unit occurs in all complete tendon lacerations. Ideally, tendon lacerations should be repaired within a few days before tissue elasticity is lost. This retraction is greatest in zones IV and V, in which the proximal

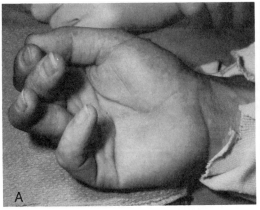
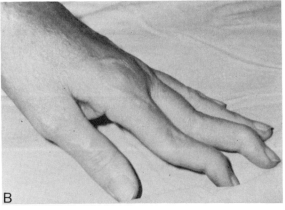

Figure 2–10. Swan-neck deformity. *A,* In single ring finger; *B,* in injured index and middle fingers.

muscle tendon unit no longer crosses a joint; hence, there is no motion to maintain muscle elasticity. The motor unit rapidly becomes fixed in this contracted position by muscular and peritendinous fibrosis, and permanent retraction of the tendon into the muscle belly will occur. Delay of tendon repair past 4 weeks in zone V usually means that the gap must be bridged by tendon grafting. Grafts to bridge the gap between tendon ends result in some loss of complete flexion, with weakness of grip.

Joint Immobility and Contractures

Joint immobility may result within a few weeks after untreated flexor tendon lacerations if the patient and physician fail to maintain passive joint motion. Untreated multiple flexor tendon lacerations are likely to produce severe joint stiffness in an extended position in all involved fingers. Loss of flexion power with subsequent extensor overpull and lumbrical plus deformity make it difficult to maintain passive joint flexion, even utilizing flexion splints. Tendon repair should be accomplished prior to the development of a fixed extension joint deformity.

Volar plate scar and adhesions, along with a lacerated tendon maintained in a flexed position, produce joint contractures. To obtain adequate tendon function joint motion must be restored in each case.

References

1. Hunter, J. W., and Salisbury, R. E.: Flexor tendon reconstruction in severely damaged hands. J. Bone Joint Surg., 53A:829, 1971.
2. Kleinert, H. E., Gropper, P. T., and Van Beek, A.: Trauma of the hand. Curr. Prob. in Surg., 15:18, 1978,
3. Kleinert, H. E., Forshew, F. C., and Cohen, M. J.: Repair of zone I flexor tendon injuries. In AAOS Symposium on Tendon Surgery in The Hand, St. Louis, C. V. Mosby, 1975, pp. 115–122.
4. Kleinert, H. E., Kutz, J. E., and Cohen, M. J.: Primary repair of zone II flexor tendon lacerations. In AAOS Symposium on Tendon Surgery in the Hand, St. Louis, C. V. Mosby, 1975, pp. 91–104.
5. Kleinert, H. E., Schepel, S., Gill, T.: Flexor tendon injuries. Surg. Clin. North Am., 61:267, 1981.
6. Kleinert, H. E., et al.: Primary repair of flexor tendons. Orthop. Clin. North Am., 4:865, 1973.
7. Lane, J. M., Block, J., and Bora, W. F.: Gliding function following flexor tendon injury. J. Bone Joint Surg., 58A:985, 1976.
8. Lister, G. L., et al.: Primary flexor tendon repair followed by immediate controlled mobilization. J. Hand Surg., 2:441, 1977.
9. Matthews, P.: The pathology of flexor tendon repair. Hand, 11:233, 1979.
10. Potenza, A. D.: Concepts of tendon healing and repair. In AAOS Symposium on Tendon Surgery in the Hand, St. Louis, C. V. Mosby, 1975, pp. 18–47.
11. Richards, J. H.: Digital flexor tendon repair and return of function. J. R. Coll. Surg., 59:25, 1977.
12. Verdan, C. E.: The decades of tendon surgery. In AAOS Symposium on Tendon Surgery in the Hand, St. Louis, C. V. Mosby, 1975, pp. 6–13.
13. Armenta, E., and Lehrman, A.: The vincula to the flexor tendons of the hand. J. Hand Surg., 5:127, 1980.
14. Doyle, J. R., and Blythe, W. F.: Anatomy of the flexor tendon sheath and pulleys of the thumb. J. Hand Surg. 2:149, 1977.
15. Leffert, R. D., Weiss, C., and Athonosoulis, C. A.: The vincula. J. Bone Joint Surg., 56A:1191, 1974.
16. Ochiai, N., et al.: Vascular anatomy of flexor tendons, I. Vincular system and blood supply of the profundus tendon in the digital sheath. J. Hand. Surg., 4:321, 1979.
17. Smith, J. W.: Blood supply of tendons. Am. J. Surg., 100:272, 1965.
18. Robb, J. E.: The termination of flexor tendon sheaths. Hand, 11:17, 1979.
19. Eiken, O., Holmberg, J., and Eikerot, L.: Restoration of the digital tendon sheath. Scand. J. Plast. Reconstr. Surg., 14:89, 1980.
20. Eiken, O., Rank, F.: Experimental restoration of the digital synovial sheath. Scand. J. Plast. Reconstr. Surg., 11:213, 1977.
21. Furlow, L. T.: The role of tendon tissue in tendon healing. Plast. Reconstr. Surg., 57:39, 1976.
22. Ketchum, L. D.: Primary tendon healing. J. Hand. Surg., 2:428, 1977.
23. Lundborg, G.: The vascularization of the human flexor pollicus longus tendon. Hand, 11:28, 1979.
24. Lundborg, G., and Frank, F.: Experimental intrinsic healing of flexor tendons based upon synovial fluid nutrition. J. Hand Surg., 3:21, 1978.
25. Lundborg, G., Holin, S., and Myrhage, R.: The role of the synovial fluids and tendon sheath for flexor tendon nutrition. Scand. J. Plast. Reconstr. Surg., 14:99, 1980.
26. Lundborg, G., Myrhage, R., and Rydevik, B.:The vascularization of human flexor tendons within the digital synovial sheath region. Structural and functional aspects. J. Hand Surg., 2:417, 1977.
27. Manske, P. R., Lesker, P. A., Bridwell, K.: Experimental studies in chickens on the initial nutrition of tendon grafts. J. Hand Surg., 4:565, 1979.
28. Matthews, P., and Richards, H.: The repair reaction of flexor tendon within the digital sheath. Hand, 7:27, 1975.
29. McDowell, C. L., and Snyder, D. M.: Tendon healing: An experimental model in the dog. J. Hand Surg., 2:122, 1977.
30. Peacock, E. E., Madden, J. W., and Trier, W. C.: Postoperative recovery of flexor tendon function. Am. J. Surg., 122:686, 1971.
31. Pennington, D. G.: The influence of tendon sheath integrity and vincular blood supply on adhesions formation following tendon repair in hens. Br. J. Plast. Surg., 32:302, 1979.
32. Jenecki, C. J.: Triggering of the finger caused by flexor tendon laceration. J. Bone Joint Surg., 58A:1174, 1976.
33. Kleinert, H. E.: Commentary on should an incompletely severed tendon be sutured. Plast. Reconstr. Surg., 57:236, 1976.
34. Schlenker, J. D., Lister, G. D., Kleinert, H. E.: Three complications of untreated partial laceration of flexor tendons. J. Hand Surg., 6:392, 1981.
35. Wray, C. R., Holtmann, B., Weeks, P. M.: Clinical treatment of partial tendon lacerations without suturing and with early motion. Plast. Reconstr. Surg., 59:231, 1977.
36. Hasham, A. I.: Closed flexor profundus injury. J. Trauma, 15:1067, 1975.
37. Leddy, J. P., and Packer, J. W.: Avulsion of the profundus tendon insertion in athletes. J. Hand Surg., 2:66, 1977.
38. Parker, A.: The "lumbrical plus" finger. J. Bone Joint Surg., 53B:236, 1971.

3

COMPLICATIONS FROM FLEXOR TENDON SURGERY

Harold E. Kleinert,
Curtis M. Steyers,
and Michael Kalisman

The results of flexor tendon repair are influenced by several factors, including not only the nature of the original wound but also the treatment method chosen (direct repair or grafting), the timing of repair (primary versus delayed primary versus secondary) and the quality of surgical technique. This chapter discusses the indications for each type of repair, recommended surgical techniques, and potential complications of each.

There are many problems associated with flexor tendon surgery, which are best avoided by eliminating their causes. Treatment modalities will vary according to the complications.

INDICATIONS AND CONTRAINDICATIONS FOR TREATMENT

Primary tendon repair is indicated for all acute flexor tendon injuries within 24 hours of injury provided there is no evidence of infection. If the suspicion of infection exists, treat the wound accordingly with cleansing, débridement, and dressing changes. Usually within 3 to 4 days the infection will have cleared, and a delayed primary repair may be accomplished. Such a *delayed primary repair* (up to approximately 2 weeks after injury) or an *early secondary repair* (2 to 5 weeks posttrauma) may also be indicated when the initial diagnosis of flexor tendon laceration has been missed, only to be discovered several days or weeks later.

Late secondary tendon repair (5 weeks postinjury) is rarely indicated. After 5 weeks the cut tendon-

muscle unit will have retracted and lost a significant degree of its elasticity, and the tendon itself will have coiled and exhibited epitenon thickening. Consequently, retrieval and direct repair may be impossible. Sheath collapse and scarring may also make direct tendon repair inappropriate at this stage.

Contraindications to primary, delayed primary, or early secondary tendon repair include the following:

1. Wounds with prolonged infection
2. Segmental tendon lacerations
3. Tendon substance loss greater than 1 cm
4. Unstable skeletal injuries requiring fixation plus immobilization
5. Destroyed critical pulleys
6. Severe tendon bed scarring from previous injury or disease
7. Insufficient skin cover

Tendon grafting procedures are indicated whenever direct tendon repair cannot be accomplished. Therefore, the indications for tendon grafting are similar to the contraindications for direct tendon repair.

Some surgeons still prefer tendon grafting to primary repair even under appropriate circumstances. It is rarely performed primarily, and is usually done several weeks or months after injury.

Tendon grafting may be performed in one or two stages. A one-stage graft is preferred over a two-stage graft. It is most often indicated in unrepaired tendon lacerations more than 5 weeks old. Two-stage tendon grafting is a salvage procedure indicated in severely traumatized fingers that require the reconstruction of a stable, mobile skeleton, or a fibro-osseous tunnel and pulley system, or both. These prerequisites are met in the first stage, after which the actual tendon graft is inserted in a separate second stage.

DIRECT FLEXOR TENDON REPAIR

Techniques

Zone I. Lacerations of the flexor digitorum sublimis in zone I (distal to flexor digitorum sublimis insertion; see Table 2–1) may be treated either by direct repair if the distal stump is at least 1.0 cm in length or by advancement of the proximal tendon to the distal bony phalanx.[3] Direct end-to-end tendon repair is accomplished utilizing a core suture of 4–0 nonreactive synthetic suture in a modified Kessler technique followed by a circumferential running 6–0 suture of the same material (Fig. 3–1).[1] The sheath is repaired whenever possible. If the proximal tendon end is difficult to retrieve, an L-shaped flap of the distal margin of the A4 pulley may be made to facilitate retrieval. Repair, however, takes priority over sheath and pulley preservation. Therefore, pulley sacrifice is preferable to tendon sacrifice. Rarely, the entire A4 pulley may have to be resected to perform a proper repair.

When insufficient distal tendon stump is available for repair (less than 1 cm), the proximal tendon may be advanced up to 1.5 cm and anchored under a distally based osteoperiosteal flap at the volar surface of the distal phalanx. A 4–0 monofilament stainless steel wire is passed through the tendon (Fig. 3–2A), through or around the distal phalanx (Fig. 3–2B), and out through the nail (Fig. 3–2C), where it is tied over a button (Fig. 3–2D). The distal tendon stump and periosteal flap are sutured with 5–0 synthetic sutures to the proximal tendon. Care must be taken to avoid damage to the volar plate and to the collateral ligaments of the distal interphalangeal joint.

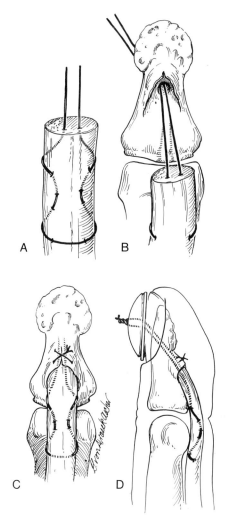

Figure 3–2. Tendon insertion utilizing a 4-0 pull-out wire. Avoid kinking the wire, which is easily removed in the direction of the repair after cutting one side and pulling on the other. (From Kleinert, H.E., Schepel, S., and Gill, T.: Flexor tendon injuries. Surg. Clin. North Am., 61:267, 1981.)

Flexor digitorum profundus avulsion from the distal phalanx (sometimes associated with a fracture) is most often encountered in the ring and middle fingers. The technique of reinsertion is virtually identical to that described above. Associated fractures are stabilized with interosseous wires, Kirschner pins, or both, where appropriate.

Flexor digitorum profundus injuries in zone I may be sutured end to end several months after injury if the vinculum brevis remains intact, because this prevents retraction of the proximal end, which is usually found distal to the A2 pulley. Reactive synovitis around the tendon ends should be excised prior to repair.

Zone II. Zone II (proximal margin A1 pulley to flexor digitorum superficialis insertion) flexor tendon lacerations present the most difficult problems of tendon surgery. The two tendons present in this zone have different excursions, and thus must move

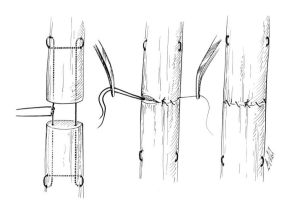

Figure 3–1. The Kessler type of tendon repair. (From Kleinert, H.E., Schepel, S., and Gill, T.: Flexor tendon injuries. Surg. Clin. North Am., 61:267, 1981.)

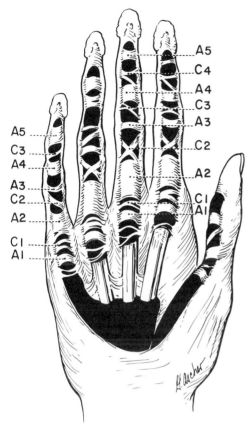

Figure 3–3. Tendon pulleys. *A,* Annular pulleys; *C,* cruciate pulleys. (From Kleinert, H.E., and Broudy, A.S.: Direct repair and dynamic splinting of flexor tendon lacerations. *In* Black, J., and Dumbleton, J.H. [eds.]: Clinical Biomechanics, New York, Churchill Livingstone, 1980.)

relative to one another as well as to their surrounding fibro-osseous tunnel. The anatomic constraints of the tunnel make tendon access difficult. However, the pulley and sheath apparatus must be preserved to maintain the normal mechanical advantage of the tendons and to provide optimal conditions for tendon nutrition and healing (Fig. 3–3).

Primary or delayed primary repair is our treatment of choice. Secondary single-stage tendon grafting, however, is still advocated by some surgeons.

Primary repair of lacerated tendons in zone II requires meticulous surgical technique. Both sheath and tendons must be handled with extreme care, because any unnecessary trauma will result in additional unwanted scarring. The tendons should never be grasped on any surface other than their cut ends.[1]

Exposure must be adequate, and is easily obtained by zigzag or midlateral extensions of the original lacerations (Fig. 3–4). Rigid skeletal stabilization is necessary. Injured periosteum and volar plate are accurately repaired to ensure a smooth tunnel floor.

The sheath is opened in an L-shaped fashion.

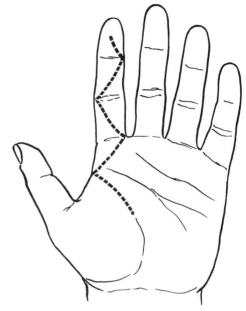

Figure 3–4. Zigzag (Bruner) incision provides maximum exposure of tendon sheath and neurovascular bundles. (From Kleinert, H.E., Schepel, S., and Gill, T.: Flexor tendon injuries. Surg. Clin. North Am., 81:267, 1981.)

Pulleys are never opened in their entirety. It is difficult to achieve a strong repair, and they must be preserved for proper tendon function.

The tendons are delivered into the sheath window. The proximal end is immobilized by a straight transfixing needle to eliminate tension during the repair (Fig. 3–5). The core suture is placed using 4–0 synthetic nonreactive suture in a manner modified from Kessler. This suture extends at least 1 cm from the cut tendon ends, and must be placed in the anterior half of the tendon to avoid damaging the blood vessels in the dorsal half (Fig. 3–6). A running circumferential 6–0 suture is then placed

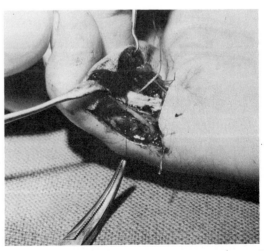

Figure 3–5. Temporary transfixion needle prevents pull on proximal cut end as the repair is accomplished.

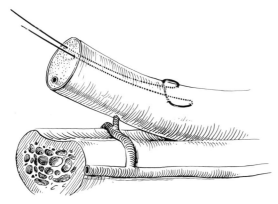

Figure 3–6. Anterior placement of suture minimizes interference with intratendinous vascular network. (From Kleinert, H.E., et al.: Complications of tendon surgery in the hand. *In* Current Management of Complications in Orthopaedics: The Hand and Wrist, S. Sandzen [ed.], Baltimore, Williams & Wilkins, in press.)

around the juncture to provide a smooth repair. Tendon ends are never everted. The digital sheath is carefully closed with 6–0 suture to provide a smooth gliding surface and to retain synovial fluid.[2, 4–8]

A closely supervised postoperative regimen is of paramount importance. A dorsal plaster slab maintains the wrist and metacarpophalangeal joints in flexion. Dynamic rubber band traction holds the injured finger in flexion in the resting state (Fig. 3–7). Active extension exercises of the interphalangeal joints against rubber band resistance are begun at 2 to 3 days postoperatively. After 3 to 3½ weeks the dorsal splint is removed. The rubber band is attached to a wrist cuff for an additional 2 to 3 weeks if the repair was less than optimal, or if the flexor digitorum superficialis was excised (Fig. 3–8). Continued supervision is necessary until optimal function has been achieved.

Zone III. Flexor tendon repair in zone III (distal edge transverse carpal ligament to proximal edge A1 pulley) may be expected to yield good results. Both tendons are provided with an excellent blood supply and are not confined within an unyielding tunnel.

Both tendons are repaired, because this provides increased strength and individual motor function. The same principles of technique are employed in zone III as were described for zone II. Palmar fascia should be left undisturbed if it has been sharply wounded; if unduly traumatized it is excised to prevent peritendinous adhesions. No attempts should be made to repair the fascia or its vertical extensions. Postoperative management is similar to that for zone III.

Zone IV. The most frequently encountered problem in zone IV (carpal tunnel) is that of laceration of flexor tendons at the distal wrist crease while the fingers are flexed. The previously described technique of tendon suture is employed, but two important points must be recognized. First, the surrounding blood-filled synovium should be excised to aid in visualization and to remove a source of increased fibrosis. Second, complete division of the transverse carpal ligament should be avoided. If completely divided, strongly reconstruct it with a woven tendon graft. Desirable postoperative management includes dynamic splinting with wrist flexion. An incompetent transverse carpal ligament leads to tendon and nerve bowstringing in a subcutaneous position.

Zone V. If early secondary repair is contemplated in zone V (proximal to carpal tunnel) it should be accomplished within 4 weeks of injury. Delays longer than 4 weeks result in permanent muscle-tendon unit shortening because the proximal end does not cross a joint. Bridge or minitendon grafts must be used to restore functional continuity. Postoperative management includes dynamic splinting, as in all other zones.

Complications From Direct Tendon Repair

Complications from direct tendon repair are determined in large part by the capability and experience of the original operating surgeon. The first surgeon to attempt the repair of a lacerated flexor tendon has the best chance of preventing complications. Complications are often due to improper surgical technique or to inadequate postoperative care.

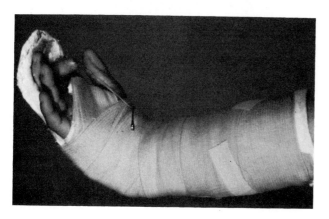

Figure 3–7. Dynamic traction on index finger with repaired flexor tendons. (From Kleinert, H.E., and Broudy, A.S.: Direct repair and dynamic splinting of flexor tendon lacerations. *In* Black, J., and Dumbleton, J.H. [eds.]: Clinical Biomechanics, New York, Churchill Livingstone, 1980.)

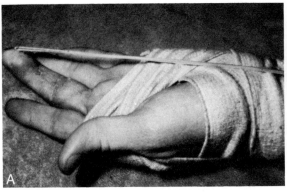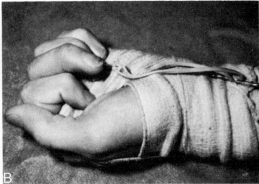

Figure 3–8. *A, B,* Rubber band traction may be continued for an extra 2 weeks by attaching to a cuff at the wrist.

Limited Tendon Excursion (Adhesions)

Adhesions between tendons or between tendons and adjacent structures limit motion and represent the most common complication. Failure to achieve adequate hemostasis will result in a peritendinous hematoma. This inevitably organizes into peritendinous fibrous tissue, which reduces tendon gliding. Traumatic handling of tendons, as in grasping the epitenon with a forceps, will also encourage fibroblastic proliferation. Tendons should be handled only by their cut ends. Likewise, the tendon pathway or tunnel should be treated with equal care. Gap formation at the repair site is also associated with increased fibrosis and scarring. It should never be allowed to occur, and may be avoided by utilizing proper suture material, proper suture placement, and proper knotting techniques. Poorly planned and supervised postoperative care leads to further tendon adhesions. Early motion facilitates better function. Utilization of a dynamic splint results in thinner, longer, and less dense adhesions.

A *bulbous repair* will not glide through the pulley system, resulting in limited tendon excursion. Such a repair is associated with an accordion effect of the tendon or with eversion of the tendon ends. Exposure of this raw tendon surface leads to tendinous-sheath scar.

A *constricted sheath* as well as an *unrepaired sheath* may restrict tendon excursion. The tunnel cross-sectional area at the edge of the unrepaired sheath decreases with attempted finger flexion. Any tendon irregularities will catch on the sheath edge (Fig. 3–9).

Limited tendon excursion should be treated initially with aggressive physical therapy. Active range-of-motion exercises isolating specific tendons and dynamic splinting are utilized. Tendolysis should not be considered until at least 6 months after repair, or until improvement with conservative therapy has plateaued. If at surgery the tendon ends are separated by more than a few (5) millimeters of scar, tendolysis will inevitably be followed by rupture. This situation requires scar excision and secondary reconstruction. Extensive scarring requires staged grafting to salvage motion. Proper postoperative exercises are mandatory following tendolysis to prevent further adhesions.

Tendon Rupture

Flexor tendon repairs are weak immediately following surgery. During the first few days following repair tensile strength is provided exclusively by the suture. The tendon ends soften during the following 10 days so that the holding ability of the suture is also diminished. Tensile strength is lowest at about day 5 and slowly increases until day 12. After day 12 tensile strength increases rapidly.

Tendon ruptures occur both *early* and *late* after repair. Strong sutures placed correctly and knotted securely aid prevention of early ruptures. Late ruptures are influenced by tendon blood supply and by nutrition. Lacerations in relatively avascular areas and those in which the sheath is not closed result in suboptimal healing conditions. Late ruptures are therefore more frequent unless appropriate precautions are taken. Both tendons are repaired whenever possible. Rupture is more likely when only one tendon is repaired. In these circumstances prolonged dynamic splinting is indicated (5 weeks).

Figure 3–9. Tendon repair site impinging on and further decreasing the diameter of the unrepaired sheath. (From Kleinert, H.E., Schepel, S., and Gill, T.: Flexor tendon injuries. Surg. Clin. North Am., 61:267, 1981.)

Treatment for ruptured tendon repair is immediate exploration and repair.

Bowstringing

Bowstringing occurs when pulleys are destroyed. Pulley destruction may occur as part of the original injury or at the time of surgery in an attempt to increase exposure. Bowstringing results in diminished tendon excursion and therefore in decreased finger flexion. If this is clinically significant, pulley reconstruction is indicated.

Joint Contracture

This complication often is secondary to severe trauma to the volar plate, or to the collateral ligaments, or to both. The surgeon may contribute to the deformity by inadvertently passing suture through the tendon into the volar plate or collateral ligaments.

Improper postoperative splinting is a frequent cause of interphalangeal joint contracture. Metacarpophalangeal joints should be splinted in flexion, allowing extension of the interphalangeal joints. Occasionally, a few degrees of flexion block is necessary in these joints to protect a neurovascular repair.

Prolonged restriction of tendon excursion results in adhesions and secondary joint contractures. If the dynamic postoperative splint is utilized, make certain that the patient extends the joints or else contracture will ensue.

Static splinting is the recommended treatment of established joint contractures. Surgical release of the contracted joint is undertaken only after conservative therapy has plateaued at an unsatisfactory level.

Infection

Infection requires immediate immobilization and administration of systemic antibiotics. Accumulated purulence is drained, and irrigation catheters are utilized for intermittent lavage. Prophylaxis against infection is initial excellent wound toilet and, for heavily contaminated or suspiciously infected wounds, delayed primary repair is indicated.

Circumstances Unique to Specific Zones

Zone I. Advancement of the flexor digitorum profundus more than 1 to 1.5 cm can restrict distal joint extension. If direct repair requires excessive advancement, alternate procedures are chosen. Tendon reconstruction is preferred, and may be achieved by lengthening at the musculotendinous junction or by tendon grafting (Fig. 3–10). In cases in which reconstruction of the tendon is impossible by grafting or by other means, there are several options: (1) tenodesis employing the flexor digitorum profundus stump, when present; (2) if suitable length is available, a dynamic tenodesis may be achieved by suturing the flexor digitorum profundus stump to the flexor digitorum superficialis insertion; (3) joint stabilization by volar capsulodesis or arthrodesis.

Pulp necrosis can occur utilizing a pull-out wire through the pulp, even in the presence of apparently sufficient padding. Avoid this complication by using correct tension or by passing the wire through the nail and securing it over a button.

Zone II. Avoid flexor digitorum superficialis excision at the proximal interphalangeal joint level. Here the superficialis tendon constitutes the tunnel floor. Its removal destroys the important gliding surface for the flexor digitorum profundus, as well as the vinculum longus to the profundus tendon. Superficialis excision enhances local scarring and has an adverse effect on profundus tendon healing and gliding. Hyperextension of the proximal interphalangeal joint frequently occurs after the distal superficialis tendon has been excised.

Zone III. Palmar fascia is not repaired. Sharply incised fascia is left unsutured. Ragged, torn fascia is cleanly excised. Failure to handle the fascia properly leads to peritendinous scarring, adhesions, and restricted motion.

Zone IV. The carpal tunnel is a large pulley. If the transverse carpal ligament is completely divided, the flexor tendons and median nerve may bowstring out of the tunnel and, with the wrist in a flexion splint, actually herniate through the skin closure.

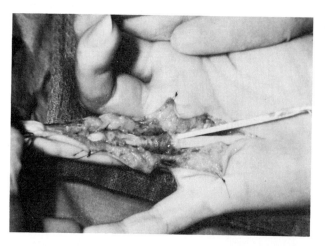

Figure 3–10. Tendon graft in the presence of an intact superficialis tendon is placed alongside rather than through the scarred or narrowed chiasm.

Avoid complete division of the ligament. If completely divided, it should be reconstructed using a woven tendon graft, which provides a strong repair.

Zone V. Motion deficits may occur if repair is done several weeks following injury because of proximal tendon retraction (see Chap. 2). Failure to repair the superficialis tendon interferes with individual finger motion, precluding return to work of those in certain professions, such as musicians, typists, and operators of small mechanical devices.

FLEXOR TENDON GRAFTING

Techniques

Flexor tendon grafting is an exacting surgical exercise requiring meticulous surgical technique. As in flexor tendon repair, skin incisions are designed so as not to cross flexor creases perpendicularly, but yet allow adequate visualization of an extensive operative field. Any scarred nonpatent fibro-osseous sheath is excised. If destroyed, the A2 and A4 pulleys must be reconstructed. If the distal superficialis tendon is intact and does not limit proximal interphalangeal joint extension, it is left in place as the posterior gliding surface. The profundus is excised, leaving a small distal stump to enhance graft attachment. A suitable motor is exposed in the palm, and surrounding scar excised. The superficialis may be chosen because of its independent motion. The little finger superficialis is frequently inadequate; thus, the profundus tendon is preferable. Should superficialis be used in preference to the profundus, the surgeon must check the lumbrical. If it is stretched from proximal migration, the lumbrical is sectioned. A suitable donor tendon is

harvested and placed through the fibro-osseous pulleys, secured to the distal phalanx in the manner described for zone I tendon reinsertions, and the proximal end is sutured using the Pulvertaft weaving technique (Fig. 3–11). The length and tension should be set so that the finger rests in slightly more flexion than its adjacent ulnar counterpart. Tendon grafts are immobilized in wrist and finger flexion for approximately 3½ to 4 weeks; nonresistant active flexion exercises are then started, along with passive joint flexion. Passive extension is started at 6 weeks, when indicated.

A two-stage tendon graft should be considered as a salvage procedure. Its use is necessary to restore motion in the scarred immobile finger; however, the procedure introduces other complications, so it is avoided unless specifically indicated. Conditions that commonly necessitate insertion of a silicone rod include a fibrotic, scarred tendon bed, destroyed critical pulleys, and joint contractures requiring surgical correction. During the first stage indicated reconstructive procedures are carried out. The silicone rod is put into place through the pulleys, where it is secured to the distal phalanx. Proximally, the rod is allowed to glide freely. Avoid large rods that stretch pulleys and contribute to bowstringing. Prior to wound closure, gliding of the rod is observed as the finger is passively flexed. The rod should glide smoothly back and forth; avoid rod buckling.[9]

In addition to restoring critical pulleys and joint motion, other indicated reconstruction procedures—for example, nerve and vascular grafts, skin scars released by Z-plasties, or by flaps, or by both—are performed. The postoperative regimen is aimed at maintaining maximal passive mobility in all joints. Passive range-of-motion exercises are

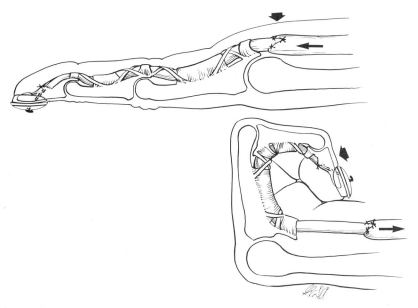

Figure 3–11. The proximal and distal attachments of the tendon graft must clear pulleys both in finger extension and flexion. (From Kleinert, H.E., and Lubahn, J.D.: Current state of flexor tendon surgery. Ann. Chir. Main, 3(1):7, 1984.)

started within a week after rod insertion. The second stage is usually performed within 3 months. Postoperative therapy following the second-stage graft is similar to that described for the single-stage procedures.

Complications

Limited Excursion

This is the most common complication, and is manifested by incomplete active digital flexion and extension. Adhesions can occur in several locations. Graft attachments must clear the distal A4 pulley and proximal A2 pulley with the finger in respective flexion and extension. Constricted scarred retinacular portions of the sheath will adhere to the graft if not excised. A traumatized tendon graft with exposed raw tendon surface will surely adhere to surrounding structures. Graft excursion limited by adhesions is treated with conservative therapy for 6 months prior to surgical intervention.

Improper Graft Length

A short graft will prevent full digital extension, while a long graft will not provide complete active flexion. Excessive graft length may produce a lumbrical plus finger by transmitting increased tension to the extensor hood via the lumbrical. Correction may necessitate lumbrical division.

Mallet deformity commonly occurs from a short graft, inadequate A4 annular pulley, improper postoperative splinting, or adhesions. Conservative measures, such as static extension splinting of the distal interphalangeal joint, which places all flexion power on the proximal interphalangeal joint, are indicated in the rehabilitation period.

Swan-neck deformity may be secondary to the mallet deformity. Other contributing factors are loss of the proximal interphalangeal joint check ligament from distal superficialis tendon excision, an inadequate or loose volar plate, tendon adhesions, and the lumbrical plus deformity. Distal interphalangeal joint extension splinting is utilized, which transfers all flexor power to the proximal interphalangeal joint and aids early correction of the deformity. It may be combined with a proximal interphalangeal joint extensor block splint. If seen late, surgical measures include proximal interphalangeal joint capsulodesis, tendolysis, and lumbrical muscle division, as indicated. Release of a mallet deformity and more proximal graft insertion may be required.

Bowstringing of the graft occurs if the pulleys are inadequate or are stretched. Flexion contracture is a frequent complication of bowstringing. Inadequate pulleys require reconstruction (Fig. 3–12).

Graft rupture occurs when active flexion or passive extension exercises are begun prior to adequate revascularization of the graft and healing of the junctural sites. Less common causes include chronic low-grade infection or protruding spicules of bone into the graft bed. Salvage can sometimes be accomplished by immediate exploration and repair.

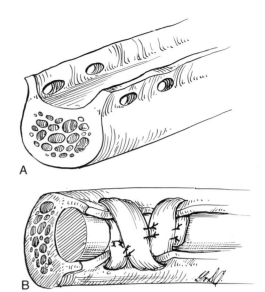

Figure 3–12. Weilby method (tendon weave) of pulley reconstruction. *A,* Openings in the fibro-osseous rim are made by scalpel point. *B,* A free tendon graft is woven through the perforations and over the tendon graft or silicone rod in 2-stage reconstruction. (From Kleinert, H.E., et al.: Complications of tendon surgery in the hand. *In* Current Management of Complications in Orthopaedics: The Hand and Wrist, S. Sandzen [ed.], Baltimore, Williams & Wilkins, in press.)

Staged Tendon Grafts

Additional complications may occur with staged tendon grafting. *Rod erosion* through the skin may occur during the period of passive mobilization (Fig. 3–13). This complication is avoided by ensuring that the rod glides smoothly and does not buckle with passive digital motion, and by providing adequate pulleys and skin cover. Mobilization should be delayed for 1 week to allow early skin healing. Rod shortening and skin closure may correct this complication.

There may be an *inflammatory reaction* around the rod. In many cases the "synovitis" is sterile. Silicone rubber rods must be handled with care, because their electrostatic charge attracts lint, talc,

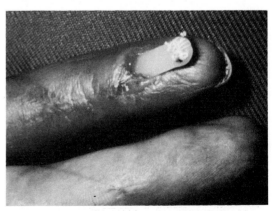

Figure 3–13. Silicone rod erosion through the skin.

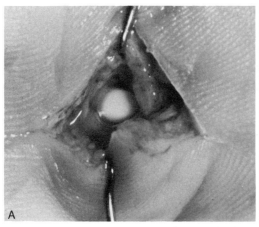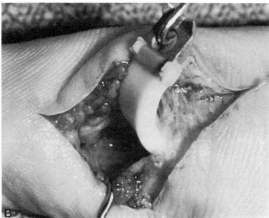

Figure 3–14. A, B, Synovitis in the presence of a rod may or may not be sterile.

wood fibers from paper drapes, and similar debris. This contamination causes the so-called "sterile synovitis." Treatment consists of immobilization and administration of anti-inflammatory medications. Once quiescent, a gradual resumption of range-of-motion exercises may be undertaken. Unfortunately, this synovitis often stretches pulleys, which contributes to bowstringing. *Infected rods* may be treated initially with decompression, antibiotic irrigation, immobilization, and systemic antibiotics. If this fails, the rod will have to be removed, and no further surgery should be contemplated for at least 6 months (Fig. 3–14).

Rod migration may occur if the distal fixation or gliding is inadequate, and this requires re-exploration and reattachment. Migration may be associated with *fracture* of the rod. Rod fracture and migration can be recognized prior to second-stage exploration by x-ray if a radiopaque rod is used (Fig. 3–15).

Bowstringing following the second-stage procedure occurs from inadequate pulleys or if an excessively large rod is used. In general, 3-mm rods are satisfactory for adults. Large rods produce larger tunnels, contributing to this bowstringing.

Late flexion contractures may follow staged graft-

ing procedures. Because the new pseudosheath is a midline longitudinal arrangement of fibrous tissue, this occurrence is understandable. Early recognition is essential, and treatment consists of static extension splinting.

Flexor tendon grafting in the presence of an intact superficialis tendon has a high complication rate. One must be very selective in choosing patients for this procedure. The patient should be motivated and have good joint mobility. The little finger may have a small and weak superficialis tendon. In this instance the profundus tendon is required for complete and strong grasp and, as such, should be reconstituted. Best results are obtained by choosing a smaller tendon graft and by passing it around the superficialis rather than through its chiasm.

References

1. Kessler, I.: The grasping technique for tendon repair. Hand, 5:253, 1973.
2. Ketchum, L. D., Martin, N. L., and Kappel, D. L.: Experimental evaluation of factors affecting the strength of tendon repairs. J. Plast. Reconstr. Surg., 59:708, 1977.
3. Kleinert, H. E., Forshew, F., and Cohen, M.: Repair of zone 1 flexor tendon injuries. *In* AAOS Symposium on Tendon Surgery in the Hand, St. Louis, C. V. Mosby, 1975, Chap. 13.
4. Kleinert, H. E., Kutz, J. E., and Cohen, M. J.: Primary repair of zone 2 flexor tendon lacerations. *In* AAOS Symposium on Tendon Surgery in the Hand, St. Louis, C. V. Mosby, 1975, Chap. 11.
5. Kleinert, H. E., Gropper, P., and Van Beek, A.: Trauma of the hand. Curr. Probl. Surg., 15:22, 1978.
6. Kleinert, H. E., and Stratoudakis, A. C.: Tendon injuries. *In* Barron, J. N., and Saad, M. N. (eds.): The Hand: Operative, Plastic, and Reconstructive Surgery, Vol. 3, New York, Churchill Livingstone, 1980, pp. 1119–1137.
7. Kleinert, H. E., Schepel, S., and Gill, T.: Flexor tendon injuries. Surg. Clin. North Am., 61:267, 1981.
8. Lindsay, W. K., Thompson, H. G., and Walker, F. G.: Digital flexor tendons: An experimental study, part 2. The significance of a gap occurring at the line of suture. Br. J. Plast. Surg. 13:1, 1961.
9. Urbaniak, J., et al.: Vascularization and the gliding mechanism of free flexor tendon grafts inserted by the silicone rod method. J. Bone Joint Surg., 56A:473, 1974.

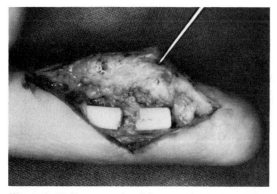

Figure 3–15. Fracture of rod just proximal to its attachment.

4

COMPLICATIONS OF EXTENSOR TENDON INJURIES

William W. Eversmann, Jr.

Although flexor tendon injuries have gained the respect of the surgical world, the extensor mechanism has not enjoyed the same careful handling and respect.[26, 30, 34, 75, 133] The extensor tendon mechanism in the fingers is thinner, more friable, and holds sutures less well than any portion of the flexor mechanism. In the area of the distal forearm and wrist, the extensor tendons are similar to the flexors because they are contained in tunnels similar but not identical to the flexor tendon sheath (Fig. 4–1).[60] As a result of their relatively exposed and superficial position, injuries to the extensor mechanism are treated daily in many practices of hand surgery. The incidence of complications from these injuries rises precipitously when the inexperienced surgeon fails to provide care necessary in the management of injuries to the extensor tendons, particularly in the fingers.[47, 54, 88, 133]

The management of complications of extensor tendon injuries is based on a sound understanding of the principles of the mechanism of this highly specialized muscle and tendon complex.[25, 66–71, 75] The wrist joint is the most important joint for the function of the fingers, and it should be remembered that finger extension and wrist flexion are synergistic.[25, 75] It follows then that muscle contraction in the extensor digitorum communis (EDC), extensor indicis proprius (EIP), and extensor digiti quinti (EDQ) will be markedly enhanced by active wrist flexion produced by the flexor carpi ulnaris, palmaris longus, or flexor carpi radialis. Inadequate active muscle contraction of the finger or thumb extensors may be largely masked if the patient learns to flex the wrist to provide finger extension, an almost natural substitution pattern. The use of wrist flexors to provide finger extension by tendon transfer, because of this synergism, provides some of the most easily retrainable tendon transfers, although they may have disadvantages when com-

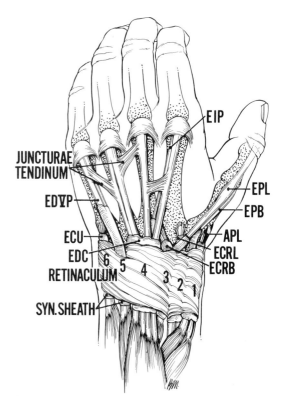

Figure 4–1. At the wrist the extensor tendons are contained in tunnels similar to but not identical to flexor tendon sheaths. The six dorsal tunnels and their associated tendons are illustrated. EIP = extensor indicis proprius; EPL = extensor pollicis proprius; EPL = extensor pollicis brevis; APL = abductor pollicis longus; EDC = extensor digitorum communis; ECU = extensor carpi ulnaris; EDVP = extensor digiti quanti proprius; ECRL = extensor carpi radialis longus; ECRR = extensor carpi radialis brevis. (Courtesy of E. Roselius. From Green, D. P. [ed.]: Operative Hand Surgery, New York-London, Churchill Livingstone, 1982.)

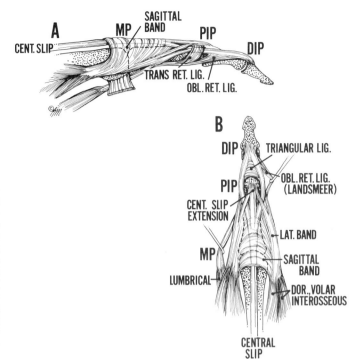

Figure 4–2. A, Lateral and *B,* dorsal views. The interosseous and lumbrical muscles form with their tendinous bands a system of interlocking functional tendons that comprise the extensor mechanism for the joints of the fingers. The sagittal band acts primarily to extend the metacarpophalangeal joint, while the more distal lateral bands coalesce and then redivide to extend the middle and distal joints of the fingers. PIP = proximal interphalangeal; DIP = distal interphalangeal; MP = intercarpophalangeal. (Courtesy of E. Roselius. From Greene, D. P. [ed.]: Operative Hand Surgery, New York-London, Churchill Livingstone, 1982.)

pared to tendon excursions of the donor and recipient muscle-tendon units.

Distal to the metacarpophalangeal joint, the extensor mechanism is composed of multiple interlocking tendon reflections whose muscles are located either extrinsic to the hand on the dorsal surface of the midportion of the forearm or intrinsic to the hand in the form of seven interosseous muscles, four lumbrical muscles, the abductor digiti quinti, and the intrinsic muscles of the thumb (Fig. 4–2).[66–71] Because of the interlocking systems of the extensor mechanism in the joints of the finger, tension in the normal extensor tendor mechanism in a joint is governed by the position of that joint as well as the adjacent joints of the fingers. Accordingly, deformities of the finger joints due to disorders in the extensor mechanisms will usually affect more than a single joint, and the prudent surgeon, in evaluating such a finger deformity, must evaluated a reciprocal relationship between the finger joints and the extensor mechanism before undertaking reconstruction of the extensor mechanism in the fingers.[25, 66–71, 75]

Boyes suggested years ago that the excursion of the extensor mechanism at the metacarpophalangeal (MP) joint varies between 11 and 13 mm from full flexion to full extension of the MP joints.[10] At the interphalangeal joints the excursion of the central slip and extensor hood varies between 2 and 3 mm, depending on the fingers studied. Accordingly, the middle and distal joints of the fingers are far more sensitive to the changes in tendinous lengths and excursions that accompany injuries to the extensor

mechanism. At the same time, the thin nature of the tendinous mechanism in the fingers, the lack of subcutaneous tissue over this mechanism, and the thinness and friability of the skin on the extensor surface of the fingers combine to stress even the most diligent surgeon in the repair and reconstruction of these interrelated tendinous units to the joints of the fingers.

MALLET DEFORMITY

Stark and associates have classified acute mallet deformities by the level and degree of extensor mechanism of distal interphalangeal joint injury.[129] When the mallet deformity is associated with loss of tendon continuity, with or without a small avulsion of bone from the distal phalanx, early treatment of the mallet deformity with an extension-producing splint at the distal interphalangeal (DIP) joint will usually result in satisfactory recovery and healing of the extensor mechanism (Fig. 4–3).[1, 27, 43, 51, 52, 72, 88, 115, 121, 129, 144] Even if a patient does not present for treatment for several weeks, an acceptable amount of extension can be gained with extension splinting for 8 to 12 weeks.[54, 58] In delayed treatment, full extension or nearly full extension will usually not be gained. In many cases, however, a loss of only 10 to 15° of extension may be acceptable to the patient and, accordingly, when a patient presents as late as 8 or 9 weeks following an acute mallet deformity secondary to loss of tendon continuity,

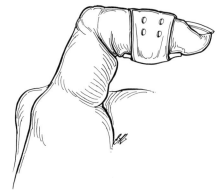

Figure 4–3. The extension-producing splint for treatment of mallet deformity of the DIP joint maintains the DIP joint in extension while allowing the free flexion and extension of the PIP joint. An adhesive bandage of adequate length prevents maceration of skin on the dorsum of the finger over the DIP joint.

extensor splinting is generally advised. Even if an acceptable amount of extension is not regained with this splinting, the additional time will allow scar tissue between the tendinous ends to be formed, which can be useful in the reconstructive procedure.

As long as compensatory swan-neck deformity or hyperextension of the proximal interphalangeal (PIP) joint does not accompany the chronic mallet deformity, it is possible to approximate the extensor tendon at the DIP joint surgically by step-cutting and overlapping the extensor tendon mechanism. By 3 to 4 months following injury, sufficient scar tissue will have bridged the gap between the ends of the tendon to hold fine suture and to shorten the tendon mechanism at the DIP joint.[26] The surgical procedure should be performed under local metacarpal block anesthesia so that, during the operative procedure, the patient can be asked to flex and extend the finger to ensure that the balance of extensor mechanism between the PIP and DIP joints is correct. Once the tension of the repair has been confirmed, internal fixation of the distal joint for healing is advisable.[26] Suturing techniques that combine a suture in the extensor tendon with suturing of the skin overlying the DIP joint are not desirable, because these techniques promote the adhesion of skin to the extensor tendon.

Chronic mallet deformities secondary to DIP joint fracture involving more than one third of the articular circumference of the dorsal distal phalanx can be satisfactorily handled, prior to 6 weeks following fracture, by open reduction and internal fixation of the small bony fragments. Although pull-out wires seem to be satisfactory in some surgeons' hands, Kirschner wires seem to be better.[44, 128, 129] With either mechanism of fixation of the fracture fragments, care should be taken to insert a transarticular Kirschner wire to prevent flexions of the distal phalanx during the early postoperative period (Fig. 4–4).

Fracture of the distal phalanx presenting more than 6 weeks after its occurrence might best be treated conservatively if the joint is stable, because operative intervention of these small fragments in porotic healing bone could produce more degeneration of the DIP joint than the volar subluxation of the joint that accompanies these injuries.

When the extensor tendon mechanism has been lost by either injury or infection over the middle phalanx, resulting in mallet deformity at the DIP joint, arthrodesis of that joint is generally preferable to an attempt at tendon grafting across the middle phalanx of the finger.

BOUTONNIÈRE DEFORMITY

The boutonnière deformity is a complication of an injury to the extensor tendon mechanism in which a laceration or avulsion of the central tendon, aggravated by subluxation of the lateral bands of the extensor mechanism, produce a flexion deformity of the PIP joint combined with an extension deformity of the DIP joint.[3, 7, 14, 24, 59, 79, 84, 85, 93, 97, 118, 120, 122, 130, 138] Harris and Rutledge, as well as Micks and Hager, observed in fresh cadaver dissections that loss of the central slip alone does not result in

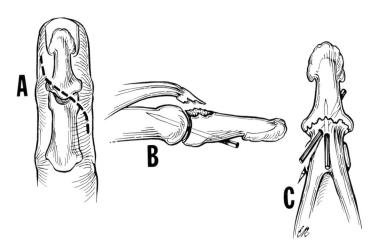

Figure 4–4. Surgery for the mallet fracture deformity requires a curvilinear incision over the DIP joint (A), and transarticulation stabilization of the joint (B). This is followed by internal fixation of the fracture fragments with small Kirschner wires (C).

boutonnière deformity, but that the deformity develops if the PIP interphalangeal joint was repeatedly flexed while tension continued to be applied to the extrinsic extensor tendon.[47, 90] With tension on the extrinsic extensor in the face of a central slip laceration, the lateral bands separated from the other fibers of the extensor hood over the PIP joint, producing the boutonnière posture. As almost no other well-defined injury of the extensor mechanism illustrates, the boutonnière deformity creates a problem of imbalance in the sequence of joints. Multiple tendinous insertions collapse the joints into an abnormal posture, creating an imbalance of the critical equilibrating forces that accomplish extension of the multiple joints in a synchronous pattern.

Most injuries to the central slip do not immediately result in a boutonnière deformity or in loss of extension of the PIP joint.[47, 90] Accordingly, following the loss of the insertion of the central slip and the continuation of the unopposed force of the flexor digitorum superficialis, stretching of the transverse retinacular ligament and triangular ligaments of the extensor hood at and just distal to the PIP joint, particularly in those areas lying between the central slips and lateral bands of the extensor mechanism, permits the lateral bands to migrate to a position volar to the axis of rotation at the PIP joint.[90] In this position the lateral bands can no longer act as extensors of the PIP joint, and simply aggravate the flexion deformity at that joint while at the same time creating an extensor posture at the distal joint of the finger. In a patient with longstanding subluxations of lateral band combined with loss of the extension thrust of the central slip, volar contracture of the PIP joint results, creating a more complex deformity from the standpoint of reconstruction with not only extensor loss but also volar contracture.

Prior to undertaking any surgical procedure for the correction of a boutonnière deformity, the involved finger must be splinted to regain passive motion of both the PIP and DIP joints, because without full passive extension of the PIP joint combined with full passive flexion of the DIP joint, the results of any surgical procedure will be severely compromised or negated by the presence of joint contracture in the finger (Fig. 4–5).[29, 73, 74, 79] Once again, the importance of the interlocking mechanisms of the extensor tendon, extensor aponeurosis, extensor hood, and central and lateral slips becomes paramount in the normal or near normal function of the finger. During the splinting of the finger, either dynamic or static splints must be used to regain full extension of the PIP joint (Fig. 4–5). Once full extension of the PIP joint has been regained, static splinting of the PIP joint combined with dynamic splinting or active flexion of the DIP joint to stretch out the oblique retinacular ligament will be necessary to complete the splinting program prior to operation (Fig. 4–5B).

Adequate splinting of the finger cannot be overemphasized as a necessary and obligatory treatment prior to operation, otherwise the oblique retinacular ligament will sustain the boutonnière deform-

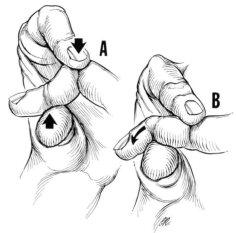

Figure 4–5. Preoperative exercises of the proximal interphalangeal joint affected with boutonnière deformity are performed by extending the middle phalanx at the PIP joint *(A)* while at the same time allowing the distal phalanx to flex *(B)*, thereby stretching the oblique retinacular ligaments. The patient can usually be instructed to perform this exercise himself.

ity because of its contracted state and its position volar to the axis of the PIP joint and dorsal to the axis of the DIP joint.

Occasionally a preliminary operation to release the volar aspect of the proximal interphalangeal joint will be necessary before correcting the boutonnière deformity itself. In these few cases I prefer the volar capsulectomy technique of Curtis, which includes, when adequate skin is available, excision of a portion of the flexor tendon sheath, tendolysis of the flexor tendons, excision of the volar plate of the PIP joint, and release of the accessory volar ligaments or fan portion of the collateral ligament on either side of the PIP joint.[19, 20] I have not found that the approach of Watson and Bowers, involving resection of the check rein ligaments of the PIP joint, to be as successful as that described by Curtis.[19] In either case, the surgical release of volar contracture of the PIP joint must necessarily lower the goals attainable after surgical reconstruction of the boutonnière deformity. Volar release of the PIP joint by operation also extends the reconstructive period for the extensor mechanism by several months, because the finger tissues must be allowed to become supple and in a state of tissue equilibrium after the volar capsulectomy release prior to undertaking a second reconstruction on the extensor mechanism. Failure to allow sufficient time between the two operations may be disastrous from the standpoint of finger function.

The multiplicity of surgical procedures that have been described for the treatment of the boutonnière deformity attests most eloquently to the complexity of this deformity and to the difficulty in its adequate surgical repair. These procedures may be divided into five major types: the anatomic repair, tendon grafting procedures, extensor tenotomy reconstructions, reconstructions using the lateral bands, and tendolysis procedures.

Mason in 1930 described the primary repair of the central tendon following acute lacerations of this tendon.[83] Kilgore and Graham applied this technique to the chronic boutonnière deformity with a technique of YV-plasty, which advances the central tendon and thereby repairs its laxity.[59, 60, 62] Elliott in 1970 resected the redundant and attenuated central tendon, performing a direct repair following the resection.[26] Internal fixation of the PIP joint is necessary for either of these procedures, allowing the joint to be stable in extension for sufficient time to allow healing of the tendinous mechanism.

Nichols in 1951 described a technique of tendon grafting of the extensor mechanism to replace the central tendon.[95] Modifications of this technique have been attributed to Fowler and described by Littler.[36, 37, 74, 79] In each of their techniques, tendinous material either from another extensor tendon or from the palmaris longus is woven into the extensor mechanism, simulating the course of the central tendon and attaching to the middle phalanx either through the previous central tendon stump or through a bone insertion. Snow in 1973 described a retrograde tendon flap in repairing the deficient extensor tendon at the PIP joint (Fig. 4–6).[117] This technique uses a portion of the proximal central tendon, reflecting it distally to its insertion in the middle phalanx to repair the deficiency of the central tendon in substance and length.[117, 119] As with other mechanisms that attempt to replace the central tendon during the repair and reconstruction of the extensor mechanism for boutonnière deformity, these tendon grafting procedures require precise tendon insertions and prolonged postoperative immobile extension, and have not achieved wide popularity in the treatment of this condition.

The third group of procedures for boutonnière deformity consists of various tenotomies of the extensor mechanism over the middle phalanx distal to the insertion of the central tendon, which release the confluence of the lateral bands that insert into the distal phalanx. Thus, the oblique retinacular ligaments for extension of the terminal phalanx are preserved, allowing the remainder of the extensor tendon to migrate proximally, tightening the central slip, and providing extension to the middle phalanx. These procedures have been described by a number of authors, including Fowler, Dolphin, Littler and Eaton, and Nalebuff and Millender.[24, 36, 37, 79, 92, 93] This procedure is generally dependable, can be performed under local anesthesia and, as long as there have been no adhesions from the extensor mechanism to the proximal phalanx or dorsal capsule of the PIP joint, which is often the case, will produce an acceptable result in a flexible boutonnière that has full passive extension preoperatively. It can be used very effectively in a select group of rheumatoid arthritic patients with boutonnière deformities if the arthritic patient has full passive extension of the PIP joint preoperatively and a minimal amount of synovitis of the PIP joint.

Reconstruction of the boutonnière deformity either by transposing the lateral bands or a portion of them, as described by Littler and Eaton, or by tendon transfer of the lateral bands to supply extension of the middle and distal phalanx, as described by Matev, can be extremely useful, particularly in those instances in which there has been considerable loss of tendinous substance over the dorsum of the PIP joint.[79, 84, 85] The procedure described by Littler and Eaton has been particularly useful in my experience for the rheumatoid boutonnière deformity, in which the dorsal tendon has been eroded and destroyed by the invasive synovium from the PIP joint.[79] This is perhaps the most satisfactory reconstruction for this difficult deformity. Once again, it is necessary to have as complete passive extension of the PIP joint as possible preoperatively. The Matev procedure, on the other hand, is difficult and demanding, and is best performed under local anesthesia during which the relative tension of the two lateral bands must be adjusted so that one may extend the PIP joint and one the DIP joint.

As with some other procedures, the patient's ability to extend the finger after insertion of the tendons, as described by Matev, permits the surgeon to evaluate the tension of the repair and, therefore, the quality of the reconstruction.[84, 85] With both the Littler and Matev procedures, the PIP joint must be maintained in extension for a sufficient period

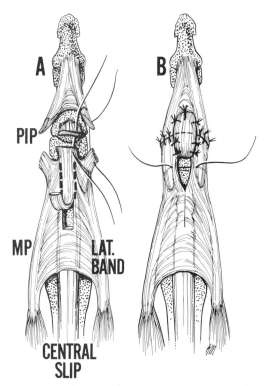

Figure 4–6. A retrograde flap method of tendon grafting of the central slip can be a simple method of repair and replacement of the central slip when it has been lost by injury or infection. (Courtesy of E. Roselius. From Greene, D. P. [ed.]: Operative Hand Surgery, New York-London, Churchill Livingston, 1982.)

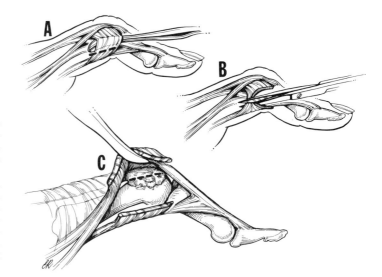

Figure 4–7. Staged tendolysis of the extensor mechanism for boutonnière deformity, beginning with division of the transverse retinacular ligaments at the lower border of the lateral bands *(A)*. Following their division, the lateral band and extensor mechanisms are elevated *(B)* to complete the tendolysis where the adhesions of the extensor tendon have fixed the extensor mechanism to the dorsal capsule of the PIP joint and to the distal portion of the proximal phalanx *(C)*.

of time to allow healing of the reconstructed tendinous mechanism prior to institution of flexion of the PIP and DIP joints.

I have used the staged tendolysis procedure described by Curtis and colleagues as my procedure of choice for the past 13 years, with excellent results for those patients with a flexible boutonnière deformity secondary to trauma.[21] During this procedure the patient, with local anesthetic infiltration of the dorsal skin of the finger, undergoes tendolysis of the extensor mechanism in a prescribed staged mechanism without altering the length-tension relationship of the extensor mechanism during the initial stages of the procedure. In many of these cases adhesions of the extensor mechanism to the proximal phalanx or to the capsule of the PIP joint have prevented direct tension from being exerted on the middle phalanx, which has resulted in the loss of PIP extension (Fig. 4–7). By tendolysis of these adhesions and usually lesser adhesions of the intrinsic tendons and the more proximal extensor mechanism, as well as division of the transverse retinacular fibers at the inferior border of the lateral band (allowing the lateral bands to reposition themselves dorsally), extension of the PIP joint can be regained. Occasionally, this procedure must be combined with an oblique tenotomy of the extensor mechanism over the middle phalanx—that is, the lateral bands distal to the central tendon insertion—which will allow the lengthened central tendon to be tightened as the extensor mechanism migrates proximally, usually no more than 1 or 2 mm.[24, 36, 37, 79, 92, 93]

One cannot overemphasize the importance of preoperative splinting in the treatment of the boutonnière deformity, because the splinting alone may in some cases regain the extension of the PIP joint. When it does not, it continues to be the necessary prerequisite for any surgical procedures that have been used to reconstruct the extensor mechanism.

COMPLICATIONS AT THE METACARPOPHALANGEAL JOINT

The area of the extensor mechanism immediately dorsal to the metacarpophalangeal (MP) joint or slightly proximal to it seems to have a unique place in our understanding of extensor tendon injuries because of its peculiar properties and unusual complications following injury to the extensor mechanism. This area of the extensor tendon is less likely to retract because of the function of the juncturae tendinum (see Fig. 4–1), which interlock the multiple extensor tendons of the fingers.[55] Accordingly, laceration of the tendon at the MP joint of the middle or ring fingers rarely results in a great deal of retraction of that tendon, and simple repair of the sharply lacerated tendon and protection of that repair for the duration of healing will result in normal or near-normal extensor function.

Because many lacerations over MP joints are the result of tooth injuries sustained in fistfights and, therefore, are really human bites, the incidence of infection on the dorsum of the hand in the extensor tendon mechanism and even into the MP joint is extremely high. When extensor tendon injuries over the MP joints are the result of human bite or tooth-type lacerations, repair of the tendon is contraindicated until the wound is cleansed, irrigated, débrided, and closed by a delayed primary or secondary technique. The repair of the lacerated extensor tendon, when the laceration is due to a human bite, is contraindicated as a primary repair. If, however, the wound or human bite are treated by careful débridement, irrigation, exploration of the wound and then a later delayed primary closure, repair of the tendon can be accomplished at the time of delayed primary closure of the skin in an otherwise clean uninfected wound that has been treated by staged management technique.

Adhesions of the capsule, extensor tendon, and

MP joint following extensor tendon injury are extremely common, and require careful surgical intervention if conservative measures to gain MP joint flexion fail. In those cases in which there has been fracture of the metacarpal head and resultant adhesions to the metacarpal or capsule, capsulectomy of the MP joint and possibly even arthroplasty of the joint surfaces may be necessary at the time of tendolysis of the extensor mechanism. Ordinarily, only excision of the dorsal capsule of the MP joint is necessary, unless long-standing extension contracture of the MP joint has resulted in contractures of the collateral ligaments and adhesions of those collateral ligaments to the metacarpal head. If a rigid extension contracture of the MP joints exists together with extensor tendon adhesions to the capsule and metacarpal head, the method of capsulectomy as described by Howard seems to be preferable to regain motion of the MP joint.[10]

Subluxation of the extensor tendon following injuries to the extensor mechanism at the MP joint produces a disabling snapping of the finger in addition to asynchronous motion during flexion of the fingers at the MP joint. In most cases, the subluxation is due to tearing of the sagittal bands on the radial side of the extensor tendon at the MP joint. If the incompetence of these fibers secondary to acute injury is recognized at the time of the injury, their repair by direct suture, as advocated by Kettelkamp and co-workers, is often sufficient to restore the stability of the extensor tendon, maintaining its position in a middorsal area.[57] Following chronic subluxation of the extensor tendon, reconstruction seems to be much more difficult, and methods of stabilizing the extensor tendon using either the juncturae tendinum or a transposed slip or extensor tendon tissue looped around the lumbrical, may have some benefit in stabilization of the tendon.[86]

Whether using the juncturae tendinum repair, as described by Wheeldon, or the tendon slip repair, as described by McCoy and Winsky, the procedure should be done under local anesthesia so that the patient can flex and extend the MP joint during the surgery, applying the usual and normal tendon forces and, accordingly, the operating surgeon can adjust the tension of the repair to the needs of the patient.[86, 143] Many surgeons dealing with this difficult deformity have entertained the concept that those patients susceptible to it may have a configuration of the metacarpal head that predisposes to subluxation of the extensor tendon and conversely makes stabilization of the extensor tendon dorsal to the metacarpal head difficult or impossible.

In a few selected cases, I have undertaken repair of the subluxation of the extensor tendon deformity by tenodesis of the extensor tendon to the proximal phalanx of the involved finger, after a method initially described by Kaplan and others in the treatment of the deformities of rheumatoid arthritis.[53] When this method is used, the tenodesis to the proximal phalanx should be performed with the PIP and DIP joints in full flexion, because the tendon of the extensor digitorum communis is balanced in its normal tension when the wrist and MP joints are straight. If the patient has normal intrinsic extensors of the PIP and DIP joints, a chevron cut just distal to the tenodesis site at the most proximal portion of the proximal phalanx will dissociate the extrinsic from the intrinsic extensors of the finger, ensuring by early motion of the PIP and DIP joints in the postoperative period that there will be no extension contracture of the PIP joint by the tenodesis to the proximal phalanx of the extensor digitorum communis tendon.

Loss of extensor tendon material at the MP joint, when there is adequate skin for coverage of this joint, requires an intercalated tendon graft from the distal stump of the extensor digitorum communis on the dorsum of the hand, either to the proximal phalanx of the digit or to the stump of the extensor hood on the dorsum of the proximal phalanx.[42, 45] Once again, if there is adequate intrinsic extension of the PIP and DIP joints, the surgeon need not anastomose the tendon graft to the dorsal hood, because tenodesis of the extensor digitorum communis to the proximal phalanx will be sufficient to gain full extension of the MP joint, allowing the intrinsic extensors of the PIP and DIP joints to maintain extension of those joints.

When the extensor tendon graft of the extensor digitorum communis across the MP joint, because of a deficiency of intrinsic extensors, must be attached to the dorsal hood of the extensor mechanism over the proximal phalanx, or even as far as the central slip of the extensor mechanism at the PIP joint, the delicate balance between the flexion and extension of the MP and PIP joints will be affected. In such cases, tension on the graft must be adjusted carefully, often with the patient under a local anesthesia and awake to ensure the best possible outcome of extensor tendon grafting.

COMPLICATIONS ON THE DORSUM OF THE HAND

Extensor tendon injuries on the dorsum of the hand proximal to the attachment of the juncturae tedinum (see Fig. 4–1), when the tendon is completely divided, result in immediate retraction of the proximal stump of the tendon by contraction of the more proximal muscle in the forearm. If the magnitude of these injuries is realized within a few days of the injury, retrieval of the proximal stump of the extensor tendon and primary or delayed primary repair of the tendon provide the best functional result following the necessary healing and rehabilitation of the patient. If, however, these injuries are recognized several weeks following the acute injury, a more complex reconstruction of the extensor mechanism will generally be necessary, because retrieval of the proximal stump of the tendon and primary suture of that tendon to the

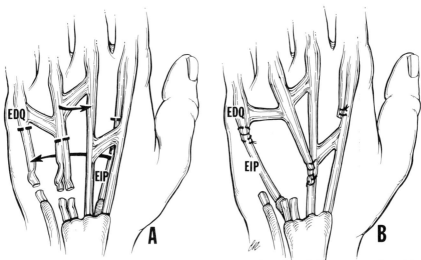

Figure 4–8. Cross-tendon transfer of the extensor tendons to replace function of the extensors lost either by attritional rupture or trauma can be accomplished in various ways, such as the one illustrated. *EDQ,* extensor digiti quinti; *EIP,* extensor indicis proprius.

distal stump result in a fixed extension contracture of the finger at the MP joint. Accordingly, alternative methods of reconstruction will be necessary.

Tendon transfer, often using the extensor indicis proprius, offers the most satisfactory alternative for restoring function of the extensor mechanism.[10] The use of the extensor indicis proprius to replace the extensor pollicis longus is a time-honored and excellent procedure that can be depended on to restore normal extension to the distal joint of the thumb. When one or even two extensor tendons are lost in the fingers, the extensor indicis proprius again can be used in a tendon transfer to restore extension to one or more fingers. Particularly in the rheumatoid arthritic with multiple tendon ruptures at approximately the radiocarpal joint, side-to-side suturing of multiple extensors—suturing the distal stumps of ruptured tendons to the distal segment of intact tendons and the proximal stumps of ruptured tendons to the proximal portions of intact tendons—provides an excellent reconstruction and will restore the best possible extension in most cases (Fig. 4–8). The combination of a tendon transfer of the extensor indicis proprius, possibly with a side-to-side repair as just described for another tendon or two, is probably a better alternative than producing a single massive anastomosis of tendinous tissue on the dorsum of the hand, particularly in rheumatoid arthritis patients.[34]

Tendon graft is the third choice for restoration of extensor tendon function in the delayed treatment of extensor tendon lacerations on the dorsum of the hand. In such cases, multiple intercalated tendon grafts, which bridge the distance between the proximal stump of the extensor digitorum communis and its corresponding fellow distally, can provide excellent functional results if the tension on the tendon graft at the time of insertion is adjusted meticulously and is checked by passive flexion and extension of

the wrist to judge the relative tension of the several fingers. These intercalated tendon grafts often require tendolysis, which probably should not be performed for at least 6 months following the tendon graft insertion.

When the extensor tendon graft is routed from the proximal stump of the extensor digitorum communis to the MP joint, the insertion of that graft as a tenodesis into the proximal phalanx, combined with dissociation of the normal extrinsic from the intrinsic extensors, seems to be the most desirable method for providing extension of the MP joint and

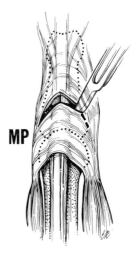

Figure 4–9. Dissociation of the extrinsic from the intrinsic extensor mechanisms of the fingers can be accomplished with a chevron incision just distal to the MP joint, which will effectively isolate the extensor force from the extensor digitorum communis to the MP joint alone. The intrinsic extensors will then be the sole extensors for the middle and distal joints of the fingers.

for retaining normal independent extension of the middle and distal joints of the fingers.[25, 74, 75] Dissociation of the extrinsic and intrinsic extensors by a chevron cut on the dorsal hood of the extensor mechanism distal to the insertion of the tendon graft at the base of the proximal phalanx, and the early active motion of the PIP and DIP joints in both flexion and extension while the MP joint is immobilized in extension, provide the best possible result from the standpoint of finger function (Fig. 4–9). With this technique, the tendon graft functions only at the MP joint and is prevented from contributing to the delicate interlocking tendinous mechanisms between the three finger joints on the extensor surface. This technique can only be used when there is normal intrinsic extension of the middle and distal finger joints.

POSTOPERATIVE CARE

Following either primary repair, tendon transfer, or extensor tendon grafting, the extremity should be immobilized with the wrist extended, and with the MP and PIP joints of the involved fingers and thumb similarly extended. This extension should not be forced but should be comfortable and maximal. The DIP joints can be allowed to flex over the end of the cast or splint that maintains the wrist in comfortable extension and the MP joints and PIP joints in an extended position.

Three weeks following surgery to restore the extensor mechanism, the PIP joints can be released and their early flexion begun while the wrist and MP joints continue to be held in the extended position. At 4 weeks following the replacement procedure, the MP joints can be released, but the wrist should be maintained in a comfortable position of extension until 6 weeks postsurgery.

The wrist can be released for active motion in flexion 6 weeks after extensor restoration to the fingers and thumb. If, however, the wrist extensors themselves were repaired, grafted, or had a tendon transfer from, for example, the pronator teres to the extensor carpi radialis longus or brevis, an additional period of wrist splinting may be desirable to allow further strengthening of these large and important tendons.

TECHNIQUE OF TENDOLYSIS OF EXTENSOR TENDONS

Although the technique of tendolysis of the extensor tendons on the dorsum of the hand, wrist, or distal forearm is similar to that for the flexor surface—that is, careful dissection of scar from the tendon itself, which frees the tendon along its entire length—little attention has been directed to the problem of tendolysis of the extensor mechanism within the digit itself. When the extensor tendon is tenodesed by adhesions proximal to the MP joint,

flexion of the MP joint results in an extension contracture at the PIP joint. Accordingly, if the patient manifests signs of adhesions proximal to the MP joint, tendolysis must be started on the dorsum of the hand or even more proximally. When the extensor tendon adhesions are at or distal to the MP joint, usually overlying the proximal phalanx of the finger, the tendolysis procedure becomes much more complex, and parallels very closely the procedure described by Curtis for capsulectomy of the interphalangeal joints.[20]

On opening the finger through a middorsal incision or through an incision modified either by previous incisions or by trauma on the dorsum of the finger, the extensor tendon mechanism is exposed by dissection in the plane between the subcutaneous tissue and the tendinous mechanism. The entire extensor tendon and hood must be tendolysed from the skin. Using a small flat elevator inserted beneath the extensor tendon between the extensor tendon and the periosteum of the proximal phalanx, the extensor tendon can be gently elevated from the bone to which it may be adherent. By inserting the elevator beneath the extensor hood in the distal half of the proximal phalanx, this elevator can be advanced both proximally and distally to free the dorsal hood structure from the phalanx. Working on either side of the phalanx, the elevator is used to free the intrinsic tendons from any adhesions to capsule or bone in the proximal half of the proximal phalanx. This maneuver may require additional sharp dissection, and care should be taken to separate the lumbrical from the interosseous tendon on the radial side.

Having exposed the dorsal and lateral aspects of the PIP joint, the transverse retinacular fibers of Landsmeer are separated from the deep collateral ligaments of the PIP joints, usually with a pair of sharp curved scissors with a relatively fine point, taking care to preserve the transverse retinacular fibers. If this area is deeply scarred, these fibers can be divided at the lower border of the lateral band at each side of the PIP joint. This maneuver is generally facilitated by tracing the lateral band from a point just distal to the PIP joint proximally, and then dividing the transverse retinacular fibers at the PIP joint while tracing the lower border of the lateral band. If the transverse retinacular fibers are divided, care must be taken to preserve the collateral ligaments of the PIP joints to ensure stability of that joint.

By elevation of the extensor tendon after division of the transverse retinacular fibers, the dorsal capsule of the PIP joint can be visualized. Careful dissection will separate the dorsal tendon and central slip from the dorsal capsule to ensure the freedom of this small but important section of the extensor mechanism (see Fig. 4–7). In some cases, excision of the dorsal capsule of the PIP joint will facilitate flexion of that joint during extensor tendon tendolysis of the finger.

If the PIP joint is stiff in extension and capsulectomy of the joint is necessary, the procedure of extensor tendon tendolysis must be modified to preserve the transverse retinacular fibers and their attachments to the extensor tendon at the PIP joint so they can maintain the PIP joint's stability after excision of the collateral ligaments, as described by Curtis.[20] Accordingly, after separating the transverse retinacular fibers of Landsmeer from the capsule and collateral ligaments of the PIP joints, they are protected and elevated so that the cord portion of the collateral ligament beneath them can be excised carefully.

Tendolysis of the extensor mechanism distal to the PIP joint is even more difficult because of the friability of the small lateral bands, the dense scar that often envelops these bands and the so-called triangular ligament, and the difficulty in maintaining freedom of this section of tendon following the tendolysis procedure. Once again, a flat elevator is used. It is introduced beneath the lateral edge of the lateral bands along their entire expanse across the middle phalanx to their insertion in the distal phalanx of the digit. This simple maneuver, when completed from both sides of the extensor tendon, freeing both lateral bands, and combined with a capsulectomy or capsulotomy of the dorsal capsule of the DIP joint, usually provides sufficient excursion of the DIP joint.

As with any tendolysis operation, early postoperative motion of the digit is necessary to preserve the freedom of the tendon. Careful attention to maintenance of the tendolysis postoperatively is at least as important as the surgical procedure itself.

Rarely, insertion of thin portions of Silastic sheet between the tendolysed extensor tendon and either the skin dorsally or the bone volarly seems to be helpful in the maintenance of a sliding mechanism for the freshly tendolysed extensor tendon. In these cases the Silastic sheet is generally sutured at several points to maintain its position as a flat interface between the several tissue layers. In all cases in which I have used this technique, an additional surgical procedure has been necessary to remove the Silastic sheeting following the tendolysis.

References

1. Abouna, J. M., and Brown, H.: The treatment of mallet finger. The results in a series of 148 consecutive cases and a review of the literature. Br. J. Surg., 55:653, 1968.
2. Adams, J. P.: Correction of chronic dorsal subluxation of the proximal interphalangeal joint by means of a criss-cross volar graft. J. Bone Joint Surg., 41A:111, 1959.
3. Aiche, A., Barsky, A. J., and Weiner, D. L.: Prevention of boutonnière deformity. Plast. Reconstr. Surg., 46:164, 1979.
4. Ambrose, J., and Goldstone, R.: Anomalous extensor digiti minimi proprius causing tunnel syndrome in the dorsal compartment. Report of a case. J. Bone Joint Surg., 57A:706, 1975.
5. Bate, J. T.: An operation for the correction of locking of the proximal interphalangeal joint of the finger in hyperextension. J. Bone Joint Surg., 27:142, 1945.
6. Bevin, A. G., and Hothem, A. L.: The use of silicone rods
under split-thickness skin grafts for reconstruction of extensor tendon injuries. Hand, 10:254, 1978.
7. Bingham, D. L. C., and Jack, E. Q.: Buttonholed extensor expansion. Br. Med. J., 2:701, 1937.
8. Blue, A. I., Spira, M., and Hardy, S. B.: Repair of extensor tendon injuries of the hand. Am. J. Surg., 132:128, 1976.
9. Bowers, W. H., and Hurst, L. C.: Chronic mallet finger: The use of Fowlers' central slip release. J. Hand Surg., 3:373, 1978.
10. Boyes, J. H.: Bunnell's Surgery of the Hand, 5th ed., Philadelphia, J. B. Lippincott, 1970, pp. 439–442, 616–618.
11. Boyes, J. H.: Boutonnière deformity (discussion). In Cramer, L. M., and Chase, R. A. (eds.): Symposium on the Hand, Vol. 3, St. Louis, C. V. Mosby, 1971, p. 56.
12. Bruner, J. M.: The zigzag volar digital incision for flexor tendon surgery. Plast. Reconstr. Surg., 40:571, 1967.
13. Bunnell, S., Doherty, E. W., and Curtis, R. M.: Ischemic contracture, local, in the hand. Plast. Reconstr. Surg., 3:424, 1948.
14. Burkhalter, W. E., and Carneiro, R. S.: Correction of the attritional boutonnière deformity in high ulnar nerve paralysis. J. Bone Joint Surg., 61A:131, 1979.
15. Burton, R. I., and Eaton, R. G.: Common hand injuries in the athlete. Orthop. Clin. North Am., 4:809, 1973.
16. Casscells, S. W., and Strange, T. B.: Intramedullary wire fixation of mallet-finger. J. Bone Joint Surg., 39A:521, 526, 1957.
17. Casscells, S. W., and Strange, T. B.: Intramedullary-wire fixation of mallet finger. J. Bone Joint Surg., 51A:1018, 1969.
18. Cleland, J.: On the cutaneous ligament of the phalanges. J. Anat. Physiol., 12:526, 1978.
19. Curtis, R. M.: Treatment of injuries of proximal interphalangeal joints of fingers. In Adams, J. P. (ed.): Current Practice in Orthopaedic Surgery, St. Louis, C. V. Mosby, 1964, p. 1410.
20. Curtis, R. M.: Capsulectomy of the interphalangeal joints of the fingers. J. Bone Joint Surg., 36A:1219, 1954.
21. Curtis, R. M., Reid, R. L., and Provost, J. M.: A staged technique for repair of the traumatic boutonnière deformity. J. Hand Surg., 8:167, 1983.
22. Dargan, E. L.: Management of extensor tendon injuries of the hand. Surg. Gynecol. Obstet., 128:1269, 1969.
23. Devos, R.: Conservative treatment of mallet finger. Acta Orthop. Belg., 43:203, 1977.
24. Dolphin, J. A.: Extensor tenotomy for chronic boutonnière deformity of the finger. Report of two cases. J. Bone Joint Surg., 47A:161, 1965.
25. Eaton, R. G.: The extensor mechanism of the fingers. Bull. Hosp. Joint Dis., 30:39, 1969.
26. Elliott, R. A.: Injuries to the extensor mechanism of the hand. Orthop. Clin. North Am., 1:335, 1970.
27. Elliott, R. A.: Splints for mallet and boutonnière deformities. Plast. Reconstr. Surg., 52:282, 1973.
28. Elson, R. A.: Dislocation of the extensor tendons of the hand. Report of a case. J. Bone Joint Surg., 49B:324, 326, 1967.
29. Engelbrecht, J. A.: A method for repair of extensor tendons. S. Afr. Med. J., 40:623, 1966.
30. Entin, M. A.: Repair of the extensor mechanism of the hand. Surg. Clin. North Am., 40:275, 1960.
31. Eversmann, W. W.: Extensor tendon injuries of the digits. In Boswick, J. A. (eds.): Current Concepts in Hand Surgery, Philadelphia, Lea & Febiger, 1983.
32. Eyler, D. L., and Markee, J. E.: The anatomy and function of the intrinsic muscles of the fingers. J. Bone Joint Surg., 36A:1, 1954.
33. Finochietto, R.: Retraction de Volkmann de los musculos intrinsecos de la mano. De la Sociedad de Cirugía de Buenos Aires, 1920, Tomo IV.
34. Flatt, A. E.: The Care of Minor Hand Injuries, 4th ed., St. Louis, C. V. Mosby, 1979.
35. Flinchum, D.: Mallet finger. J. Med. Assoc. Ga., 48:601, 1959.
36. Fowler, S. B.: Extensor apparatus of the digits. Proceedings of the British Orthopaedic Association. J. Bone Joint Surg., 31B:477, 1949.
37. Fowler, S. B.: The management of tendon injuries. J. Bone Joint Surg., 41A:579, 1959.
38. Furnas, D. W., and Spinner, M.: The sign of "horns" in the

diagnosis of injury or disease of the extensor digitorum communis of the hand. J. Plast. Surg., 31:263, 1978.

39. Gama, C.: Results of the Matev operation for correction of boutonnière deformity. Plast. Reconstr. Surg., 64:319, 1979.

40. Goldner, J. A.: Deformities of the hand incidental to pathological changes of the extensor and intrinsic muscle mechanisms. J. Bone Joint Surg., 35A:115, 1953.

41. Haines, R. Q.: The extensor apparatus of the fingers. J. Anat., 85:251, 1951.

42. Hakstian, R. W., and Tubiana, R.: Ulnar deviation of the fingers. The role of joint structure and function. J. Bone Joint Surg., 49A:299, 1967.

43. Hallberg, D., and Lindholm, A.: Subcutaneous rupture of the extensor tendon of the distal phalanx of the finger; "mallet finger." Acta Chir. Scand., 119:260, 1960.

44. Hamas, R. S., Horrell, E. D., and Pierret, G. P.: Treatment of mallet finger due to intra-articular fracture of the distal phalanx. J. Hand Surg., 3:261, 1978.

45. Hamlin, C., and Littler, J. W.: Restoration of the extensor pollicis longus tendon by an intercalated graft. J. Bone Joint Surg., 59A:412, 1977.

46. Harris, C., Jr., and Riordan, D. C.: Intrinsic contracture in the hand and its surgical treatment. J. Bone Joint Surg., 36A:10, 1954.

47. Harris, C., and Rutledge, G. L., Jr.: The functional anatomy of the extensor mechanism of the finger. J. Bone Joint Surg., 54A:713, 1972.

48. Hauck, G.: Die Ruptur der Dorsal Aponeurose am ersten Interphalangeal Gelenk, zugleich eim Beitrag zur Anatomic and Physiologic der Dorsal Aponeurose. Arch. Klin. Chir., 123:197, 1923.

49. Heywood, A. W. B.: Correction of the rheumatoid boutonnière deformity. J. Bone Joint Surg., 51A:1309, 1969.

50. Hillman, F. E.: New technique for treatment of mallet fingers and fractures of the distal phalanx. J.A.M.A., 161:1135, 1956.

51. Howie, H.: The treatment of mallet finger: A modified plaster technique. N. Z. Med. J., 46:513, 1947.

52. Hunter, J. M., et al.: Rehabilitation of the Hand, St. Louis, C. V. Mosby, 1978.

53. Kaplan, E. B.: Extension deformities of the proximal interphalangeal joint of the fingers. An anatomical study. J. Bone Joint Surg., 18:781, 1936.

54. Kaplan, E. B.: Anatomy, injuries and treatment of the extensor apparatus of the hand and fingers. Clin. Orthop., 13:24, 1959.

55. Kaplan, E. B.: Functional and Surgical Anatomy of the Hand, 2nd ed., Philadelphia, J. B. Lippincott, 1965.

56. Ketchum, L. D., et al.: A clinical study of forces generated by the intrinsic muscles of the index finger and the extrinsic flexor and extensor muscles of the hand. J. Hand Surg., 3:571, 1978.

57. Kettlekamp, D. B., Flatt, A. E., and Moulds, R.: Traumatic dislocation of the long finger extensor tendon. A clinical, anatomical, and biomechanical study. J. Bone Joint Surg., 53A:229, 1971.

58. Kilgore, E. S., Jr., and Graham, W. P.: Operative treatment of swan-neck deformity. Plast. Reconstr. Surg., 39:468, 1967.

59. Kilgore, E. S., Jr., and Graham, W. P.: Operative treatment of boutonnière deformity. Surgery, 64:999, 1968.

60. Kilgore, E. S., Jr., and Graham, W. P.: The Hand: Surgical and Nonsurgical Management, Philadelphia, Lea & Febiger, 1977.

61. Kilgore, E. S., Jr., et al.: Correction of ulnar subluxation of the extensor communis. Hand, 7:272, 1975.

62. Kilgore, E. S., Jr., et al.: The extensor plus finger. Hand, 7:159, 1975.

63. King, T.: Injuries of the dorsal extensor mechanism of the fingers. Med. J. Aust., 2:213, 1970.

64. Kleinert, H. E., and Kasdan, M. L.: Reconstruction of chronically subluxated proximal interphalangeal finger joint. J. Bone Joint Surg., 47A:958, 1965.

65. Laine, V. A. I., Sairanen, E., and Vainio, K.: Finger deformities caused by rheumatoid arthritis. J. Bone Joint Surg., 39A:527, 1957.

66. Landsmeer, J. M. F.: Anatomy of the dorsal aponeurosis of the human finger and its functional significance. Anat. Rec., 104:31, 1949.

67. Landsmeer, J. M. F.: A report on the coordination of the interphalangeal joints of the human finger and its disturbances. Acta Morphol. Neerl. Scand., 2:59, 1953.

68. Landsmeer, J. M. F.: Anatomical and functional investigation on the articulation of the human fingers. Acta Anat. (Suppl. 24), 25:1, 1955.

69. Landsmeer, J. M. F.: Report on the coordination of the interphalangeal joints of the human finger and its disturbances. Acta Morphol. Neerl. Scand., 2:59, 1958.

70. Landsmeer, J. M. F.: The coordination of finger-joint motions. J. Bone Joint Surg., 45A:1654, 1963.

71. Landsmeer, J. M. F.: Atlas of Anatomy of the Hand, New York, Churchill Livingstone, 1976.

72. Lewin, P.: A simple splint for baseball finger. J.A.M.A., 85:1059, 1925.

73. Littler, J. W.: Principles of reconstructive surgery of the hand. Am. J. Surg., 92:88, 1956.

74. Littler, J. W.: Principles of reconstructive surgery of the hand. In Converse, J. M. (ed.): Reconstructive Plastic Surgery: Principles and Procedures in Correction, Reconstruction, and Transplantation, 2nd ed., Vol. VI, Philadelphia, W. B. Saunders, 1964, pp. 1612–1632.

75. Littler, J. W.: The finger extensor mechanism. Surg. Clin. North Am., 47:415, 1967.

76. Littler, J. W.: On the adaptability of man's hand, with reference to the equiangular curve. Hand, 5:187, 1973.

77. Littler, J. W.: The digital extensor-flexor system. In Converse, J. M. (ed.): Reconstructive Plastic Surgery: Principles and Procedures in Correction, Reconstruction, and Transplantation, 2nd ed., Vol. VI, Philadelphia, W. B. Saunders, 1977, pp. 3166–3214.

78. Littler, J. W., and Colley, S. G. E.: Restoration of the retinacular system in hyperextension deformity of the interphalangeal joint. Proceedings of the American Society for Surgery of the Hand. J. Bone Joint Surg., 47A:637, 1965.

79. Littler, J. W., and Eaton, R. G.: Redistribution of forces in correction of boutonnière deformity. J. Bone Joint Surg., 49A:1267, 1967.

80. Long, C., and Brown, M. E.: Electromyographic kinesiology of the hand. Muscles moving the long finger. J. Bone Joint Surg., 46A:1683, 1964.

81. Mann, R. J., Hoffeld, T. A., and Farmer, C. B.: Human bites of the hand: Twenty years experience. J. Hand Surg., 2:97, 1977.

82. Mason, M. D., and Allen, H. S.: The rate of healing of tendons—an experimental study of tensile strength. Ann. Surg., 113:424, 1941.

83. Mason, M. L.: Rupture of the tendons of the hand. Surg. Gynecol. Obstet., 50:611, 1930.

84. Matev, I.: Transposition of the lateral slips of the aponeurosis in treatment of long-standing "boutonnière deformity" of the fingers. Br. J. Plast. Surg., 17:281, 1964.

85. Matev, I.: The boutonnière deformity. Hand, 1:90, 1969.

86. McCoy, F. J., and Winsky, A. J.: Lumbrical loop operation for luxation of the extensor tendons of the hand. Plast. Reconstr. Surg., 44:142, 1969.

87. McFarlane, R. M.: Observations on the functional anatomy of the intrinsic muscles of the thumb. J. Bone Joint Surg., 44A:1073, 1962.

88. McFarlane, R. M., and Hampole, M. D.: Treatment of extensor tendon injuries of the hand. Can. J. Surg., 16:366, 1973.

89. McMurtry, R. Y., and Jochims, J. L.: Congenital deficiency of the extrinsic extensor mechanism of the hand. Clin. Orthop., 125:36, 1977.

90. Micks, J. E., and Hager, D.: Role of the controversial parts of the extensor of the finger. J. Bone Joint Surg., 55A:884, 1973.

91. Milford, L. W., Jr.: Retaining Ligaments of the Digits of the Hand. Gross and Microscopic Anatomic Study. Philadelphia, W. B. Saunders, 1968.

92. Nalebuff, E. A., and Millender, L. H.: Surgical treatment of the swan-neck deformity in rheumatoid arthritis. Orthop. Clin. North Am., 6:733, 1975.

93. Nalebuff, E. A., and Millender, L. H.: Surgical treatment of the boutonnière deformity in rheumatoid arthritis. Orthop. Clin. North Am., 6:753, 1975.
94. Newmeyer, W. L.: Primary Care of Hand Injuries, Philadelphia, Lea & Febiger, 1979.
95. Nichols, H. M.: Repair of extensor tendon insertions in the fingers. J. Bone Joint Surg., 33A:836, 1951.
96. Nichols, H. M.: Manual of Hand Injuries, 2nd ed., Chicago, Year Book Medical Publishers, 1960, pp. 180–181, 191.
97. Pardini, A. G., Costa, R. D., and Morais, M. S.: Surgical repair of the boutonnière deformity of the fingers. Hand, 11:87, 1979.
98. Parkes, A.: The lumbrical plus finger. Hand, 2:164, 1970.
99. Parkes, A. R.: Traumatic ischaemia of peripheral nerves, with some observations on Volkmann's ischaemic contracture. Br. J. Surg., 32:403, 1945.
100. Peacock, E. E., Jr.: The dynamic splinting for the prevention and correction of hand deformities. A simple and inexpensive method. J. Bone Joint Surg., 34A:789, 1952.
101. Portis, R. B.: Hyperextensibility of the proximal interphalangeal joint of the finger following trauma. J. Bone Joint Surg., 36A:1141, 1954.
102. Pratt, D. R.: Internal splint for closed and open treatment of injuries of the extensor tendon at the distal joint of the finger. J. Bone Joint Surg., 34A:785, 1952.
103. Pratt, D. R., Bunnell, S., and Howard, L. D., Jr.: Mallet finger classification and methods of treatment. Am. J. Surg., 93:573, 1957.
104. Rabischong, P.: L'innervation proprioceptive des muscles lombricaux de la main chez l'homme. Rev. Chir. Orthop., 48:234, 1962.
105. Ramsay, R. A.: Mallet finger (letters). Lancet, 2:1244, 1968.
106. Reef, T. C., and Brestin, S. G.: The extensor digitorum manus and its clinical significance. J. Bone Joint Surg., 57A:704, 1975.
107. Riddell, D. M.: Spontaneous rupture of the extensor pollicis longus; the results of tendon transfers. J. Bone Joint Surg., 45B:506, 1963.
108. Riordan, D. C., and Stokes, H. M.: Synovitis of the extensors of the fingers associated with extensor digitorum brevis manus muscle. A case report. Clin. Orthop., 95:278, 1973.
109. Rosenzweig, N.: Management of the mallet finger. S. Afr. Med. J., 24:831, 1950.
110. Sakellarides, H. T.: The extensor tendon injuries and the treatment. R. I. Med. J., 61:307, 1978.
111. Sarrafian, S. K., et al.: Strain variation in the components of the extensor apparatus of the finger during flexion and extension. A biomechanical study. J. Bone Joint Surg., 52A:980, 1964.
112. Schenck, R. R.: Variations of the extensor tendons of the fingers—surgical significance. J. Bone Joint Surg., 46A:103, 1964.
113. Schultz, R. J., and Furlong, J. P.: Observations on the fiber pattern of the extensor mechanism of the finger at the level of the proximal interphalangeal joint. Bull. Hosp. Joint Dis., 39:100, 1978.
114. Shrewsbury, M. M., and Johnson, R. K.: A systemic study of the oblique retinacular ligament of the human finger: Its structure and function. J. Hand Surg., 2:194, 1977.
115. Smillie, I. S.: Mallet finger. Br. J. Surg., 24:439, 1937.
116. Smith, R. J.: Non-ischemic contractures of the intrinsic muscles of the hand. J. Bone Joint Surg., 53A:1313, 1971.
117. Snow, J. W.: Use of a retrograde tendon flap in repairing a severed extensor tendon in the PIP joint area. Plast. Reconstr. Surg., 51:555, 1973.
118. Snow, J. W.: A method for reconstruction of the central slip of the extensor tendon of a finger. Plast. Reconstr. Surg., 57:455, 1976.
119. Snow, J. W., and Switzer, H.: Method of studying the

relationships between the finger joints and the flexor and extensor mechanism. Plast. Reconstr. Surg., 55:242, 1975.
120. Souter, W. A.: The boutonnière deformity. A review of 101 patients with division of the central slip of the extensor expansion of the fingers. J. Bone Joint Surg., 49B:710, 1967.
121. Spigelman, L.: New splint for management of mallet finger. J.A.M.A., 153:1362, 1953.
122. Spinner, M., and Choi, B. Y.: Anterior dislocation of the proximal interphalangeal joint, a cause of rupture of the central slip of the extensor mechanism. J. Bone Joint Surg., 52A:1329, 1970.
123. Spoor, C. W., and Landsmeer, J. M.: Analysis of the zigzag movement of the human finger under influence of the extensor digitorum tendon and the deep flexor tendon. J. Biomech., 9:561, 1976.
124. Stack, H. G.: Muscle function in the fingers. J. Bone Joint Surg., 44B:899, 1962.
125. Stack, H. G.: Mallet finger. Hand, 1:83, 1969.
126. Stack, H. G.: Buttonhole deformity. Hand, 3:152, 1971.
127. Stack, H. G.: The anatomy of the muscles and tendons of the hand. In Proceedings of the Second Hand Club. Copenhagen, 1961. London, British Society of Surgery of the Hand, 1975, p.95.
128. Stark, H. H.: Troublesome fractures and dislocations of the hand. In AAOS Instructional Course Lectures, Vol. 19. St. Louis, C. V. Mosby, 1970, pp. 130–149.
129. Stark, H. H., Boyes, J. H., and Wilson, J. N.:Mallet finger. J. Bone Joint Surg., 44A:1061, 1962.
130. Stewart, I. M.: Boutonnière finger. Clin. Orthop., 23:220, 1962.
131. Swanson, A. B.: Surgery of the hand in cerebral palsy and the swan-neck deformity. J. Bone Joint Surg., 42A:951, 1960.
132. Thompson, J. S., Littler, J. W., and Upton, J.: The spiral oblique retinacular ligament: S.O.R.L. J. Hand Surg., 3:482, 1978.
133. Tubiana, R.: Surgical repair of the extensor apparatus of the fingers. Surg. Clin. North Am., 48:1015, 1968.
134. Tubiana, R., and Valentin, P.: Anatomy of the extensor apparatus and the physiology of the finger extension. Surg. Clin. North Am., 44:897, 1964.
135. Tubiana, R., and Valentin, P.: The physiology of the extension of the fingers. Part 2. Surg. Clin. North Am., 44:907, 1964.
136. Vainio, K., and Oka, M.: Ulnar deviation of the fingers. Ann. Rheum. Dis., 12:122, 1953.
137. Van Denmark, R. E.: A simple method of treatment for recent mallet finger. Milit. Surg., 106:385, 1950.
138. Van der Meulen, J. C.: The treatment of prolapse and collapse of the proximal interphalangeal joint. Hand, 4:154, 1972.
139. Varian, J. W., and Pennington, D. G.: Extensor digitorum brevis manus used to restore function to a ruptured extensor pollicis longus. Br. J. Plast. Surg., 30:313, 1977.
140. Verdan, C. E.: Primary and secondary repair of flexor and extensor tendon injuries. In Flynn, J. E. (ed.): Hand Surgery, 2nd ed., Baltimore, Williams & Wilkins, 1975, p. 149.
141. Weeks, P. M., and Wray, R. C.: Management of Acute Hand Injuries. A Biologic Approach, 2nd ed., St. Louis, C. V. Mosby, 1978, p. 314.
142. Weinberg, H., Stein, H. C., and Wexler, M. R.: A new method for treatment of mallet finger. Plast. Reconstr. Surg., 58:347, 1976.
143. Wheeldon, F. T.: Recurrent dislocation of extensor tendons. J. Bone Joint Surg., 36B:612, 1954.
144. Williams, E. G.: Treatment of mallet finger. Can. Med. Assoc. J., 57:582, 1947.
145. Zancolli, E.: Structural and Dynamic Bases of Hand Surgery, Philadelphia, J. B. Lippincott, 1968, pp. 105–106.

5

COMPLICATIONS OF TENDON TRANSFER FOR NERVE PARALYSIS OF THE HAND

William E. Burkhalter

MEDIAN NERVE PARALYSIS

Certainly the major sources of complications or failure of any tendon transfer rest in the surgeon's failure to adhere to the precepts of Steindler and Mayer.[14, 20] These have been stated in many different articles, but in any chapter on complications of tendon transfer they must be restated. The bed is bad, the motor is weak, a contracture persists, or we forget that a single muscle tendon unit primarily performs only a single function. The excursion of the motor is too limited. These are all causes for tendon transfer failures.

Although these may result in the failure of the operative procedure, a new set of circumstances should not arise. This is what I mean by complications. An example of this is an opposition transfer using the flexor digitorum superficialis of the ring finger in which a normal motor is used, the pulley is fixed in the area of the pisiform with a loop of the flexor carpi ulnaris, the bed is normal, the thumb is free of contractures, the attachment is perfect, and the tension is correct. Postoperatively, opposition of the thumb is perfectly restored but the patient has difficulty with hand function secondary to either a swan-neck deformity of the ring finger or a flexion contracture of the proximal interphalangeal (PIP) joint. This is then a complication, even though the operative procedure was completely successful and excellent opposition was restored. Obviously, we may have the same complication with an unsuccessful operative procedure.

In the case of the operative procedure bringing about opposition of the thumb, the complications may involve the area from which the motor has been removed, the course of the muscle tendon unit through nerves, vessels, and other tendons to the

thumb, secondary deformities along the course of the transfer, including the thumb itself, or the donor finger. Because the flexor digitorum superficialis to the ring finger is the most commonly used motor for opposition transfer, complications of the motor should be seen relatively frequently.

Jacobs and Thompson say that some type of PIP joint deformity occurs in 8% of cases in which the flexor digitorum superficialis has been utilized as a motor.[8] One is the swan-neck deformity in the supple hand, in which the flexor digitorum superficialis is cut over the midphalanx or certainly at the level of the PIP joint. However, to blame this deformity completely on the suppleness of the patient's tissues would be incorrect. Even in this type of patient with long tails on the distal flexor digitorum superficialis, a flexion contracture or swan neck of the PIP joint may be seen. The key seems to be the PIP joint area. What we need to do is avoid this area when removing the flexor digitorum superficialis. If we do not, the result may be a swan-neck or flexion contracture of this joint postoperatively.

In the case of opposition transfers, we do not need full length of the flexor digitorum superficialis to reach the thumb. Avoiding the area of the PIP joint when removing the superficialis by making the incision between the A1 and A2 pulley areas would avoid the area of the PIP joint (Fig. 5–1). Here, the superficialis is divided on both sides of the flexor digitorum profundus. The two slips may be divided proximal to Camper's chiasm to avoid the PIP joint area completely. Because the division is proximal to Camper's chiasm, there is no difficulty in removing the flexor digitorum superficialis from the finger.[15] No "hang-up" occurs on the flexor digitorum profundus similar to that in the more distal division,

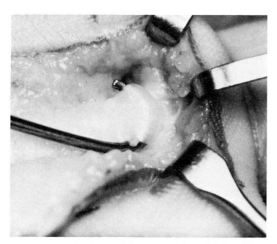

Figure 5–1. The interval between A1 and A2 pulleys at the base of the finger is a good area to remove the superficialis for tendon transfer. There is no hang-up on the profundus and the area around the PIP joint is avoided, with its attendant complications.

when the chiasm must be divided to free the superficialis from the profundus. A slip, however, remains proximal to the PIP joint if the division of the superficialis is made in the area between the A1 and A2 pulleys.[15]

Postoperatively, when the patient is in a cast holding the thumb in opposition and perhaps the wrist in slight flexion, we should not forget the PIP joint of the donor finger. If, postoperatively, we exercise the same care as during the operative procedure, we will be rewarded with no contracture of the donor finger. Elastic extension splintage, if there is a tendency toward flexion contracture, is important. Do not let a lag become a contracture. Avoid the hyperextension problem because a 10° flexion contracture of the digit is certainly preferable to a swan-neck deformity with or without associated locking.

Classically, the ring finger flexor digitorum superficialis has been used as a primary muscle tendon unit for an opposition transfer. The use of the superficialis of the long finger has been advocated as an alternative if there has been damage to the ring finger. The long flexor superficialis should not be used for opposition of the thumb. This motor has excellent control, and is probably the most powerful individual muscle in the hand. Removal of this motor severely affects power grip and control. Alternative transfers are usually available and should be utilized in the low median nerve injury, rather than sacrificing this extreme powerful and well-coordinated individual muscle tendon unit. I have had many patients in whom this has been used for adductor transfers to the thumb as well as for opposition transfers, and the patients' complaints have generally been lack of control and loss of ultimate function in the hand, in spite of improved thumb function.

Until recently, extensor proprius transfers were

rarely utilized.[5, 6, 18] The limited excursion, long course, and relative weakness as compared with the flexor digitorum superficialis has made them definitely a second choice. However, because most opposition transfers are now performed for the residuals of trauma as opposed to paralytic disease, these transfers are much more valuable. Rarely with median nerve laceration in the forearm is any flexor digitorum superficialis (FDS) undamaged, and certainly in the high lesion it is not available for use. The major complication of using either proprius motors is loss of extension of the donor finger through the metacarpophalangeal joint. In the case of the extensor indicis proprius (EIP), careful repair of the extensor mechanism after removal of the tendon will obviate this problem.[2] Failure to do this may result in a lag or, in extreme cases, in subluxation of the hood radially, with resultant failure of extension due to radial displacement of the remaining extensor tendon.[5]

In the case of the extensor digiti minimi being used as an opposition transfer, it must be remembered that both the extensor digiti minimi and extensor digitorum communis (EDC) to the small finger may have a common muscle belly, proximally, or the EDC may be completely absent to the small finger. These problems must be recognized at the time of surgery and treated appropriately, or a small finger extensor lag will result. If a single muscle belly proximally controls both tendons distally, the tendon must be separated so that the extensor digit quinti (EDQ) proximally will be asked to only bring about opposition of the thumb. No muscle tendon unit can bring about two dissimilar functions. In this case, the distal portion of the EDC of the small finger may be sutured to the ring EDC at the time of transfer for opposition. This transfer should be protected during immobilization of the EDQ opponensplasty, which may, however, pose a problem. Utilizing a relatively short excursion propius tendon for the opposition means that the wrist should be in some flexion during the postoperative immobilization.

Full flexion of all metacarpophalangeal joints drags the entire EDC system distally, thereby reducing tension on the repair even in the presence of wrist flexion.

Most, if not all, opposition transfers that utilize a motor other than the FDS exhibit difficulty with full extension of the thumb. Opposition may be full and effective but, with a proprius transfer either from the small or the index finger, full extension in maximal abduction is usually not possible. That is, it is not possible to lay the hand completely flat on a table unless the thumb is somewhat adducted. This is not true on all occasions but, when performing either an EIP or an extensor digiti minimi opponensplasty, the surgeon must be prepared to accept less than the flat hand position as well as full opposition. The true or potential excursion is usually not adequate when compared with the FDS to bring about full extension.

I feel that the excessive concern regarding exten-

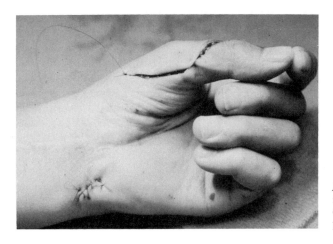

Figure 5–2. Using short excursion opponensplasty motors the thumb, at the conclusion of the procedure, should rest in full opposition, or else incomplete thumb function could result.

sion of the thumb may jeopardize a satisfactory opponensplasty secondary to putting up the tendon transfer under low tension. For a proprius opponens transfer, the thumb must be in full opposition with the wrist in neutral both in flexion-extension and in radioulnar deviation (Fig. 5–2). Failure to recognize the problem with radial and ulnar deviation makes tension assessment and postoperative immobilization a problem. With any opposition transfer that utilizes the ulnar border of the wrist as a pulley, the hand tends toward ulnar deviation. Obviously, ulnar deviation of the hand reduces tension on the transfer in the postoperative dressing. If the hand tends to deviate ulnarly thumb position may be lost. If a postoperative cast is applied and the wrist

remains in ulnar deviation, rehabilitation of the wrist and transfer may be difficult postoperatively. At the time of operation, in the immediate postoperative dressing, and in the postoperative immobilization, the wrist should be volar-flexed 30°, and the thumb placed in full opposition, and the wrist should be in neutral regarding radial and ulnar deviation.

The so-called Camitz transfer for thumb opposition is valuable for improving thumb position (Fig. 5–3).[1, 13] This transfer utilizes the palmaris longus as a muscle tendon unit. Extending the length with a strip of palmar fascia means that this transfer is usually performed at the time of carpal tunnel release. The motor is weak and there is limited

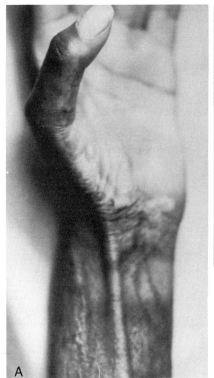

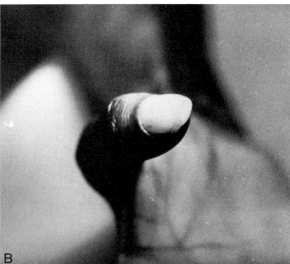

Figure 5–3. A, B, The Camitz transfer gives excellent abduction but, unless positioning of the transfer in the abductor pollicis brevis tendon is exact, flexion of the metacarpal phalangeal joint and lack of extension of the interphalangeal joint will result, in addition to inadequate rotation.

excursion, but the palmaris longus can position the thumb in abduction. The palmaris longus lengthened by the palmar fascia subcutaneously tunneled to the abductor pollicis brevis tendon in the metacarpophalangeal (MP) joint area, however, does not bring about appreciable pronation of the thumb.

At the present time in the United States longstanding median nerve compression at the wrist is certainly a prime indication for this tendon transfer. Release of the carpal tunnel at the time of opposition transfer, coupled with postoperative maintenance of the wrist and flexion, may create some problems. With short excursion motors such as the palmaris longus some flexion is obviously going to be required at the wrist in the postoperative immobilization. If the flexor tendons of the fingers subluxate volarly from the wrist joint during the postoperative period of immobilization, this greater distance from the wrist joint increases the moment arm of the flexor tendons of the fingers for wrist flexion. This combined finger flexor mass may make restoration of normal motion in the wrist during rehabilitation a real problem. A flexon contracture may result postoperatively that is quite resistant to treatment. Wrist flexion to reduce tension on any opposition transfer is certainly appropriate. Its use, however, when coupled with a carpal tunnel release, should be limited to the absolute minimum in terms of degrees of flexion.

The abductor digiti minimi opposition transfer popularized by Littler and Cooley (described initially by Huber and Nicholayson) utilizes an intrinsic muscle to replace an intrinsic muscle.[12] The ulnarinnervated abductor digiti minimi is used to substitute for an absent or denervated abductor pollicis brevis. The transfer assumes that the abductor digiti minimi can remain viable and can function with almost all of its origin divided. The muscle must survive and function on a neurovascular pedicle.

The procedure as described by Littler and Cooley is the most technically demanding opponensplasty. The abductor digiti minimi must be released from all of its bony attachments, and remains anchored only to the flexor carpi ulnaris (FCU). The muscle is then rotated on its long axis like the leaf of a book into the thumb position. Only by this complete release will the abductor digiti minimi transfer function as a true opposition transfer (Fig. 5–4A). Without this extreme release proximally, the muscle acts only as a flexor pollicis brevis.[21]

The point of this is that denervation or an infarction of the muscle must constantly be kept in mind during the procedure. The chance of neurovascular loss is not as great with minimal release of the origin, but only short flexor function results. This may be ideal in the completely intrinsically minus thumb, but it is not true opposition.

In addition to possible loss of the muscle from technical failure still another complication should be considered, especially in the patient with a high median nerve paralysis. In this situation, although the ulnar three fingers close completely, the long finger is usually quite weak as far as the flexor is concerned, because it is really being flexed by the

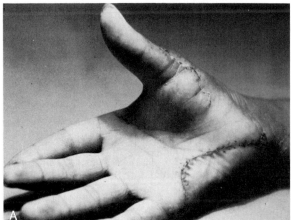

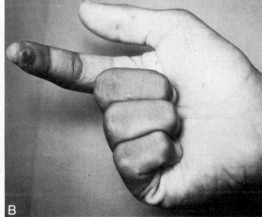

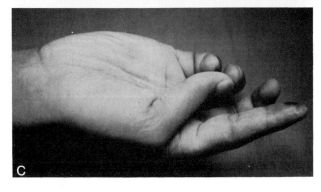

Figure 5–4. *A*, An aductor digiti quinti opposition transfer, in which true opposition is brought about. This muscle, in order to be a true opposition transfer, must be attached proximally only by its artery, nerve, vein, and a small attachment to the flexor carpi ulnaris. Otherwise, only short flexor action will result. *C*, Removing the intrinsic flexor from the only normal digit in the hand in the case of a high median nerve injury probably creates additional weakness volarly, and I feel that other transfers can better substitute for the lack of opposition in this case.

more ulnar-innervated musculature of the flexor digitorum profoundus. Certainly, the radial side of the hand is weak as far as power and precision grip are concerned. True powerful flexion exists only in the ulnar two digits, and then only through the flexor digitorum profundus (Fig. 5–4B). In this situation, to weaken the only normal or near normal finger in the hand is hardly justified (Fig. 5–4C). To remove the abductor digiti minimi in this situation consequently reduces the strength and dexterity of the only normal digit in the hand, and I don't feel that it should be done. Other transfers can be used to bring about positioning of the thumb without damaging the small digit.

The next area of concern is the pulley. Although opposition transfers can become adherent in the area of constructed pulleys, with reasonable care adherence is usually not a problem. However benign the subcutaneous ulnar border of the hand seems to be as a pulley, it may be a problem if the suture line of the opposition transfer fails in this area. The two transfers that have a suture line on the ulnar border of the hand are the combined extensor carpi ulnaris (ECU) motor with a distal attachment by the extensor pollicis brevis tendon, and the ECU to the extensor pollicis longus (EPL). In addition, the ECU may be prolonged with a tendon graft with similar results. Both of these transfers may not function because of failure of gliding on the ulnar border of the wrist.[8, 10, 11]

A Bunnell transfer utilizing a fixed pulley in the area of the pisiform constructed from a slip of FCU is standard in opposition transfers. However, when doing the FDS ring opposition, the first few times one notices how easily the FDS loops around the FCU from radial and deep to the ulnar and superficial, and from there to the thumb. No fixed pulley is constructed. The loop of the FDS around the FCU acts as a pulley. Opinions are varied on the loop pulley. It is said that if the FCU is completely normal proximal migration of this dynamic pulley will not occur, and the FDS opposition transfer will function normally. However, I have seen the dynamic pulley fail with a normal FCU, and would suggest continuing to use a fixed pulley for the FDS opposition transfer. Certainly, if the FCU is partially or completely denervated, it will rapidly become ineffective as a dynamic pulley. Remember that pulleys and suture lines do not mix, and that to try to mix these will result in adherence of the transfer.

Problems With The Thumb

There are three major problems of thumb motion following opposition transfer. Using short excursion motor units such as wrist motors or proprius tendon, extension of the thumb is usually incomplete. This lack of extension may be minimal and of no functional consequence, which is usually the case with a normal functioning EPL. However, in the absence of a functioning EPL, a lack of extension may sometimes be significant. In such a case there is no

antagonist to the opposition transfer. Only the abductor pollicis longus and extensor pollicis brevis can move the thumb away from the fingers so that the fingers can close, as into a tight fist. If the thumb cannot be moved away from the fingers, as the fingers try to close they will constantly hit the opposed thumb. If the transfer to restore opposition is not too tight, the abductor pollicis longus and extensor pollicis brevis will be able to clear the thumb from the fingers during power grip. If not, however, the thumb will be constantly interfering with power grip activities. Riley and colleagues have described an opponensplasty utilizing the EPL muscle tendon unit around the ulnar border of the forearm.[17] They again make the point that here tension is very important, and too high a tension will result in a thumb constantly held in opposition.

The high median nerve lesion at the elbow or proximal has been a good indication for an early opposition transfer. The transfer allows maximal use of the hand without external splintage, and avoids the development of contractures of the thumb web space area. Since the work of Riordan and Brand, the method of distal attachment of most opposition transfers to the thumb has been to the intrinsic mechanism, to the EPL over the proximal phalanx, or to both. Previously, a bony attachment to the ulnar border of the proximal phalanx had been suggested by Bunnell.[3] Motoring the lateral bands over the extensor pollicis longus has been felt to be important to increase interphalangeal extension. Littler and Cooley, however, feel that motoring the tendon of the abductor pollicis brevis reproduces the motion of true opposition.[12, 13] Motoring the two lateral bands or the EPL over the proximal phalanx with the opposition transfer increases considerably the interphalangeal joint extension of the thumb. In the cases of high median nerve lesions with no functioning flexor pollicis longus, an unbalanced situation is created. Without careful attention to detail in the management of the interphalangeal joint, hyperextension will result. With this the condyles of the proximal phalanx are presented to the finger for prehension.

This is not to say that lack of normal flexion of the interphalangeal (IP) joint is not extremely disabling. It certainly is not, and arthrodesis of the IP joint in full extension is sometimes performed in ulnar nerve paralysis to obviate hyperflexion of the IP joint and to shift the excursion of the flexor pollicis longus to the more proximal joints. Full extension, however, and hyperextension of the IP joints are not synonymous. Arthrodesis in full extension presents the largest pulp surface of the thumb to the fingers for prehension. Hyperextension presents only the skin covering the condyles to the fingers for pinch. In addition, the imbalance created usually results in ankylosis of the joint in hyperextension. Even with return of flexor pollicis longus function following neurorrhaphy or a transfer, IP joint motion will not be regained.

It seems, therefore, in the patient with a high median nerve lesion, care should be exercised in doing an opponensplasty. In general, attachment to

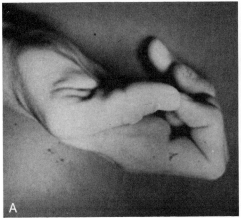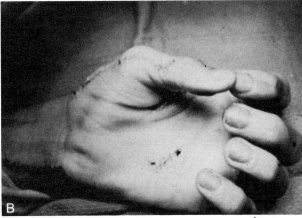

Figure 5–5. *A,* A completely intrinsically minus thumb *(A)* with a satisfactory opposition transfer but with persisting metacarpal phalangeal joint flexion *(B).* Note the crank handle effect that the index finger will exert on this intrinsically minus thumb. An additional surgical procedure will be necessary to make the thumb functional; opposition is really only a positioning maneuver. (From Green, D. P.: Operative Hand Surgery. New York, Churchill Livingstone Inc., 1982, with permission.)

the EPL over the proximal phalanx should be discouraged unless something is done simultaneously to motor the flexor pollicis longus by tendon transfer. An alternative to this is arthrodesis of the IP joint in extension at the time of opponensplasty. However, being careful about increasing the tension on the extensor pollicis longus would seem to be preferable. This can be accomplished by utilizing only the tendon of the abductor pollicis brevis and MP joint capsule as an attachment or the more distal attachment to the bone, as pointed out by Bunnell.[3] Opposition involves abduction and rotation of the MP joint, in addition to basilar joint motion. Failure to maintain the tendons of the transfer radial to the MP joint will reduce overall effectiveness of the transfer. Placement volarly will result in flexion of the MP joint, and excessive dorsal placement will result in hyperextension of the MP joint.

In general, the presence of some adduction and short flexor function will protect against the hyperextension deformity. The extensor pollicis brevis is not strong enough to overcome a volarly placed opposition transfer. With the abductor pollicis brevis tendon capsule and EPL over the proximal phalanx method of attachment, an excess volar or dorsal course of the tendon across the MP joint should not occur. The Bunnell method of bony attachment on the ulnar aspect of the proximal phalanx is more likely to unbalance the MP joint by excessive volar or dorsal migration.

Since Bunnell's article on opponensplasty, various methods of distal attachment have been used.[3] One that has been pointed out and widely used is utilization of the extensor pollicis brevis tendon.[11] This tendon is cut free from its muscle belly in the area of the first dorsal compartment and is drawn into the incision in the area of the MP joint of the thumb. With this persisting bony attachment to the proximal phalanx, the proximal tendon can be tunneled across the thenar eminence to attach to any motor for thumb opposition. This obviously wastes one muscle tendon unit. The attachment of the

extensor pollicis brevis distally, however, may migrate further distally with function of the transfer. This is obviously due to some attritional changes in the hood system. The result is that the opposition transfer gradually ceases to function and gradually becomes a flexor of the MP joints, where previously muscle tendon unit acted as an extensor. Proponents of this procedure have said that looping the extensor pollicis brevis around the EPL immediately proximal to the MP joint will mitigate this distal migration of the tendon of the EPL.

In the usual isolated low median nerve lesion with functioning ulnar-innervated thumb intrinsics, opposition should be restored well by opponensplasty (Fig. 5–5). However, in a combined lesion with no intrinsic thumb musculature, the problem is quite different. Even in the absence of contractures and with normal thumb extrinsic extensor muscles, maximum thumb function will probably require an opposition transfer and a short flexor replacement, or the so-called adductorplasty. Even

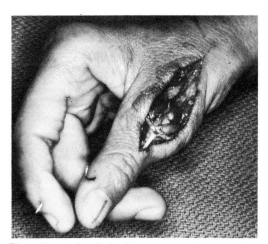

Figure 5–6. Arthrodesis of the metacarpal phalangeal joint in the case of an intrinsically minus thumb increases the stability and usefulness of the thumb tremendously, even without adductorplasty.

with these two transfers, thumb function may be improved by arthrodesis of the MP joint and extension, slight adduction, and slight pronation (Fig. 5–6). The increased stability with normal joint proximally and distally greatly improves the overall usefulness of the thumb.[7]

Development of Nerve Problems Secondary to the Course of the Tendon

In addition to structural complications involving the thumb or donor finger or tendon adherence, the development of nerve problems, usually secondary to the course of the tendon, can be seen. In the area of the thumb at the site of bony attachment, the nerve most likely to be in jeopardy is a continuation of the radial nerve that gives sensibility to the radial aspect of the thumb. When attaching an opposition transfer in this area, especially if one is going to use the method of Riordan, in which the transfer is attached to the EPL over the proximal phalanx, this nerve is very definitely encountered. In the median nerve paralysis patient it may offer a significant amount of sensibility to the patient, and may be quite useful. Its damage may reduce sensibility in the thumb but, in addition, may bring about signs and symptoms of a neuroma in this area. If one is doing an opposition transfer, I feel that this nerve should be found and protected during the final attachment of the tendon transfer (Fig. 5–7). Spinner has pointed out that, if this is not done, occasionally there is a tendency to run the transfer superficial to this nerve branch, in which case signs and symptoms of a sensory neuritis may occur.[19] In addition, Wood has pointed out that, in various types of pulleys in the area of the pisiform, it might be possible to develop entrapment of the ulnar nerve. This is especially obvious, and must be guarded against if using the so-called Brand pulley, in which a portion of the tunnel of Guyon may be used as the pulley for the transfer of the FDS, or

in the Pallazi pulley, in which the deep part of the abductor of the small finger is used as a pulley. In such a situation, Wood noted that an intrinsic paralysis ensued because of compression of the ulnar nerve by this tendon transfer.[22]

In general, I think it best to maintain the tendon transfer away from direct access to the major nerves in the extremity, and certainly in a superficial situation to make certain that the transfer passes deep to the sensory nerves in question. This is most commonly a problem in the area of the dorsal cutaneous branch of the ulnar nerve when performing either of the proprius transfers from the dorsum—the EIP or the extensor digiti minimi transfers—which use the ulnar border of the wrist as a pulley. In general, however, the compression neuropathies, either motor or sensory or both, have not been a major problem in tendon transfer, in spite of the fact that a significant portion of the transfer is done by subcutaneous tunneling within the palm, wrist, and distal forearm. However, when using tunneling techniques for the first time, it is best to think in anatomic rather than in surgical terms.

Complications of Extrinsic Replacement

There are a series of transfers that may be done to bring about extrinsic flexor power to the fingers via two different modes. In the high median nerve paralysis, in which all superficialis tendons are paralyzed, as well as the profundus to the index and long fingers and the flexor pollicis longus, power grip needs to be restored to the hand in some way. Powerful flexion exists in the ring and small fingers, and the long finger is somewhat "dragged along" with the profundus to the ring finger and usually demonstrates full motion but is quite weak when tested against resistance. To bring about index flexion, the index profundus tendon can be joined to the profundus of the long or ring finger, or both, to bring about simultaneous flexion of all fingers.

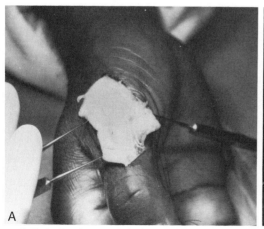
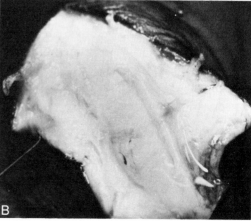

A   B

Figure 5–7. A, B, The superficial branch of the radial nerve on the dorsal radial aspect of the thumb must be protected during a tendon transfer both from the standpoint of developing neuroma at the site of injury, and because in many patients with median nerve injuries this is a useful area of sensibility.

Although this results in simultaneous flexion of all fingers, it does not individualize the motions, nor does it add essential power to that activity. If it is felt that power is necessary, one must use the extensor carpi radialis longus (ECRL) to bring about powerful finger flexion on the radial side of the hand. Here the problem is one of a difference in excursion between a wrist extensor such as the ECRL and the flexor digitorum profundus tendon. The tension on this transfer must be adjusted using the dynamic tenodesis principle; otherwise, satisfactory flexion or extension, or both, will not be obtained.[5, 16]

The method involves bringing the wrist into full extension and ensuring that the finger is capable of flexing. If at that point the power is brought from the ECRL through its transfer, reasonably good terminal power may be obtained. However, the hand can only be opened completely by considerable volar flexion of the wrist to release the tension on the ECRL.

A major complication of tendon transfer for median nerve paralysis in using the ECRL is setting the tension too high so that the patient ends up with a hooked index finger, which can't be extended out of the way except by extreme volar flexion of the wrist. If this occurs the transfer must be lengthened, because the flexed index finger constantly in the way prevents the patient from getting a mobile thumb if there has been an opposition transfer to the more sensible fingers on the ulnar border of the hand. This hooked index finger is a definite complication of the use of short excursion motors to bring about digital flexion. This can only be obviated by essentially full wrist motion and by ensuring that the tension is set up using the dynamic tenodesis principle.

The same situation exists regarding transfer of the brachioradialis to the flexor pollicis longus to bring about IP joint flexion. Significant amounts of IP joint flexion are probably not required: what is more important than a high degree of IP joint flexion is stability to the IP joint plus power to bring the thumb across the palm. Thus, when the transfer is set up, it must be set up again using the dynamic tenodesis principle. Full passive extension of the thumb should be possible in the operating room with the wrist in 20 to 30° of volar wrist flexion. Dorsiflexion of the wrist should passively bring about terminal joint flexion. The resulting power will then be related to the effective excursion of the brachioradialis.

To obtain satisfactory excursion of the brachioradialis, the brachioradialis tendon must be freed far proximally to get the 2 to 3 cm of excursion necessary to make the flexor pollicis longus function. The tendon unit must be carved out of the investing fascia of the forearm, at least as far as the muscle belly and slightly further. Also, note that when using the brachioradialis for this, the effectiveness of the brachioradialis is related to elbow position. With the elbow flexed, for instance, the brachioradialis with its short excursion motor will be able to do very little in regard to powerful tip

flexion. With the elbow in full extension there will be much more tone to the flexor policis longus transfer via the brachioradialis, and greater power can be exerted with this transfer. This amounts to a considerable difference between full extension of the elbow and flexion to 90°.

Technique of Transfers in High Median Nerve Paralysis

A few points need to be made regarding technique in tendon transfers for high median nerve paralysis, which are basically attempts to replace the function of six finger flexors by transfer for digital flexion. I don't feel that simply joining or side-to-side suturing of the flexor digitorum profundus of the index to the flexor digitorum profundus of the long finger will suffice. Certainly, both these rwo radial flexor digitorum profundi should be sutured to the ring finger, unless the flexor digitorum profundus to the long finger is extremely strong, and usually it is not. Patients who undergo side-to-side suturing techniques in the distal forearm have good photographs but poor strength on the radial side of the hand.

Thus, unless strength is of no concern, I would transfer the ECRL to the flexor digitorum profundus of the index and long fingers. The ECRL is tenotomized immediately distal to the muscle bellies of the extensor pollicis brevis and abductor pollicis longis, and withdrawn proximal to these muscles. The fascia in the forearm is excised over a large segment, so that the tendon will pull in a straight line from its dorsal radial aspect to the volar side of the wrist. The direct route should be subcutaneous; it will be if the brachioradialis is also going to be used for the flexor pollicis longus. Considerable fascial excision is necessary if the brachioradialis is going to obtain useful excursion so it may act as a flexor pollicis longus.

Following this extensive freeing from fascial attachment, the ECRL is interwoven into the musculotendinous junction of the flexor digitorum profundus of the index and long fingers. Avoid the tendency to make the suture line too distal, where the possibility of adhesions is greater than more proximally. The course of this transfer is in relationship to the radial artery. Initially, I felt that this tendon should be passed deep to the radial artery, so that when tension developed in the musculotendinous unit there would be no compromise of arterial flow. However, I have not seen this as a problem in other patients, even if the transfer had been placed superficial to the radial artery.

These same comments apply to the use of the brachioradialis for the flexor pollicis longus. There should be concern for tension, the need for extensive freeing of the tendon from the investing fascia of the forearm, and the straight line pull.

Finally, in regard to tendon transfers for extrinsic replacement in median nerve paralysis, the most frequent complication is related to incorrect tension. Use the dynamic tenodesis principle at the time of surgery to adjust the tension correctly. If minimal excursion is obtained postoperatively after a rehabilitation effort, use tenolysis, especially for the ECRL to the index and long profundi.

RADIAL NERVE PARALYSIS

Complications in this group of transfers are generally related to the wrist, with radial deviation, inadequate extension of the fingers, or a combination of these two, in which the functional problem is related to power grip. In the initial case, the most commonly performed operative procedure to regain wrist extension in a radial nerve paralysis is transfer of the pronator teres to the wrist extensors to gain dorsiflexor stability of the wrist. An extensive incision, generally on the volar side of the wrist, is required to mobilize the pronator from its extensive osseous attachment. The osseous attachment may be easily identified by elevating the volar surface of the brachioradialis and noting the radial artery and the radial nerve as it exits from beneath the brachioradialis.

Once the pronator teres is removed from the radius and is freed proximally to obtain adequate excursion, there is usually a great tendency on the surgeon's part to continue beneath the brachioradialis to reach the wrist extensors immediately to the dorsum. This, however, should not be done, and the transfer should pass subcutaneous to the brachioradialis so that the periosteum, which has been elevated from the radius with the tendinous portion of the pronator teres, will not interfere with the gliding of this tendon transfer.

The transfer of the pronator teres should be passed superficial to the brachioradialis, and the brachioradialis allowed to fall down onto the raw surface of the radius. The fleshy dorsum of the brachioradialis allows a smooth sliding plane for the pronator teres muscle tendon unit. Failure to do this may result in limitation of excursion of the pronator teres and limitation of motion of the wrist, both dorsiflexion and volar flexion.

It must be remembered that the transfer will be attached to the wrist extensors proximal to the dorsal retinaculum, so that the function that is carried out by the transfer will be directly related to the tendon to which it is attached. Both the extensor carpi radialis brevis (ECRB) and ECRL should be motored by the pronator teres, but the ECRL is primarily a radial deviator of the wrist; thus, the problem is not so much radial deviation as it is dorsiflexion and radial deviation. In this case it is important to motor primarily the ECRB, and to avoid carefully motoring the ECRL. Previous attempts to avoid any sort of radial deviation of the wrist by trying to "tether" the ECU and the ECRB together as a single tendon transfer, so that the wrist comes up in neutral, have not been effective.[30]

The tendon that has the least excursion for wrist dorsiflexion is the one that will limit the action of the tendon transfer. Because the ECRB is a radial deviator, in addition to being a dorsiflexor, the only way to avoid radial deviation is to insert the pronator teres in a dual fashion. If this is done, the ECU must be cut and brought out of its pulley and run subcutaneously from the metacarpal base to the ERCB.[24, 25] Unless the ECU is removed from its dorsal compartment, dorsiflexion of the wrist will be limited. The moment for dorsiflexion of the ECU is smaller than that of the ECRB, so the ECU will effectively tether the ECRB. However, generally only one tendon should be motored, and this can be the ECRB; no attempt should be made to motor the combination of the ECRB and ECU or of the ECRB and ECRL.

Assuming that the transfer of the pronator teres and other transfers have been carried out and are functioning satisfactorily, but the dorsiflexion of the wrist may not be strong. If the FDS to the ring or long finger has not been previously utilized to bring about extension of the fingers or thumb, or of all of these, they are available to transfer dorsally, either through the interosseous membrane to the dorsum or around the radial or ulnar side of the wrist to bring about more powerful extension of the wrist. The more direct route would involve using the long finger superficialis to the radial side of the interosseous artery and nerve, on the radial side of the profundus to the index, and then putting it through a large opening in the interosseous membrane and attaching it directly to the wrist extensor proximally.

The use of the sublimi for unstable or weakened wrists is quite rewarding, and patients gain considerable use of their hand with the stable wrist. An alternative to this, which has often been said not to be indicated in radial nerve paralysis, is an arthrodesis of the wrist. If an arthrodesis is done to stabilize a wrist, it should not be done primarily. Initially a standard set of transfers should be done to gain wrist, finger, and thumb extension. If, after rehabilitation, the patient has good use of the hand and good extension of the fingers, but continues to complain of an unstable or weak wrist, stabilizing the wrist in some type of splint for a period of time may indicate the exact position in which the wrist should be arthrodesed to have maximum function of the fingers, both for flexion and extension. If arthrodesis of the wrist is to be used in lieu of a tendon transfer for wrist stability, it should not be used as an alternative until the patient has regained satisfactory finger and thumb extension. Even then it should be only used if it is felt that hand function is markedly improved with the wrist control splint in varying degrees of flexion or extension.

Thus, by having the patient completely rehabilitate the finger extensors and thumb extensor-abductor prior to arthrodesis of the wrist, one can get a general feeling that the transfer is going to be successful, even after solid wrist arthrodesis. Formerly, when arthrodesis was combined with tendon transfer for the finger, the tendon transfer often did not function well when done in conjunction with the arthrodesis, and extension and flexion of the fingers were compromised by carrying out two procedures at the same time.

Although the use of the FDS and pronator teres tendon transfer has been widely used for wrist extension, a controversy has evolved about what should be done to regain finger extension. In the classic case of isolated radial nerve paralysis, there are essentially three structures that are usable for finger or thumb extension. The motoring of the EDC can be performed by the FCU, which is transferred around the ulnar border of the wrist and sewn by an interweaving technique into the EDC dorsally. Another method is the use of the flexor carpi radialis passed through the interosseous membrane and sutured to the EDC on the dorsum. Alternatively, the FDS of the ring or long finger, or of both, may be passed again through the interosseous membrane. The ring finger FDS is passed to the ulnar side of the profundus wad, and that of the long finger is passed to the radial side of the profundus wad to motor the EDC, the abductor of the thumb, or both.[1, 5]

Generally it has been felt that removing the FCU eliminates a very powerful ulnar and volar flexor of the wrist, which should be preserved to maximize wrist flexion activities.[23, 26] Thus, use of the FDS has been advocated by Boyes and others.[23] However, the problem with retraining or with adhesions of the FDS musculotendinous unit as it passes through the interosseous membrane has been a major problem, and Riordan has pointed out that often prolonged retraining of the transfer is necessary to get satisfactory finger extension.[29] Most authorities would agree that use of a wrist flexor to gain finger extension is more synergistic and more easily learned by the patient than use of a finger flexor to become a finger extensor, in spite of the fact that it has been frequently pointed out that synergy is unimportant.

The flexor carpi radialis transfer does use a wrist flexor to work for a finger extensor, has a rather direct course through the interosseous membrane, does not remove the FCU, and thus seems to be in many respects an ideal transfer. The only real deterrent to its use is that it does have relatively limited excursion when compared with an FDS musculotendinous unit. This limited excursion, though, is not a major problem as long as the wrist has some mobility. It can easily be seen that the only tendon transfers in which the patient can dorsiflex the wrist completely and still extend the fingers completely are those using the relatively long excursion FDS tendons. Whether or not this is important is questionable. Nevertheless, the problem of adherence to the interosseous membrane and retraining must be remembered when this tendon is used for a motor (Fig. 5–8).[28, 31]

Some thought should be given to motoring the thumb. There are two traditional ways of motoring the two short muscles and the one long muscle of the thumb. It is debatable whether or not a single tendon transfer should be used to bring about extension or abduction of the thumb. Often the use of the palmaris to motor a translocated EPL gives an excellent functional result. Certainly, EPL function is not particularly needed in the patient. Basically the thumb requires EPL function pulling in the general direction of the abductor pollicis longus. However, if two sublimi are going to be removed from the fingers to bring about extension, one of these could easily be used to bring about extension of the fingers and one to aid in double motoring the thumb. That is, the palmaris longus plus the FDS could be used, one to act as an abductor pollicis longus and the other to act as an EPL.

The major problem with this, however, is that if both sublimi are removed, one for the extensor EDC and the other for double motoring the thumb and perhaps the index finger, there may very well be a requirement (as pointed out above) for additional power to stabilize the wrist in dorsiflexion. With two sublimi removed for thumb and finger extension they obviously cannot be used to strengthen the wrist. Some type of wrist flexor is required to compensate for this wrist dorsiflexor weakness, which brings back the same problem of trying to retrain essentially nonphase muscles. Generally, it is unnecessary to double motor the thumb, and usually a subluxated radially EPL motor by a palmaris longus gives satisfactory extension and true abduction to all three thumb joints.

One major complication in radial nerve tendon transfers occurs in the following example. The classic group of tendon transfers has been used: the

Figure 5–8. When using short excursion motors such as the flexor carpi ulnaris or the flexor carpi radialis, finger extension is usually incomplete with the wrist in dorsiflexion. This, however, is usually of little functional significance.

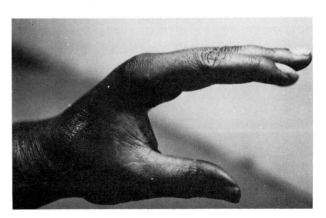

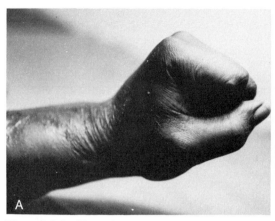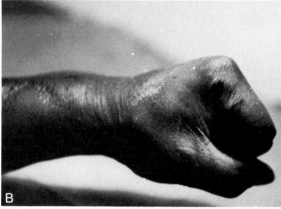

Figure 5–9. In this particular patient with a radial nerve tendon transfer, the tension on the extensor digitorum communis has been adjusted properly. The patient is able to dorsiflex the wrist with the pronater teres transfer *(A),* and the tension is not so high that the hand opens by dorsal tenodesis if the wrist comes to neutral *(B).* This is proper tension for radial nerve transfers to the extensor digitorum communis.

pronator has been used to motor the wrist, the palmaris longus has been used to motor the thumb, and the translocated EPL and either the FCR or the FCU have been used to motor the finger extensors. If the tendon transfer for finger extension is slightly tighter than normal, tighter than it should have been, or if the suture line has been placed so far distal that as the fingers come into flexion there is a tendency for the suture line to hang up on the dorsal retinaculum, an interesting series of events ensues. In a movie the patient may be able to show excellent function of the tendon transfer. However, when trying to use the hand for power grip activities, there may be complaints of extreme weakness. This is not merely isolated dorsiflexor weakness of the wrist but represents limited excursion or too high tension on the tendon transfer for function of the EDC.

As the patient attempts to make a tight fist the wrist comes out of full dorsiflexion because of this enormous flexor power working against the pronator teres muscle, and the patient loses power grip. This occurs because, if there are a few tendon adhesions that don't allow full motion and full gliding of this tendon transfer to the EDC then, as the wrist drops into a little flexion, the fingers are actually brought open by a tenodesis effect, which essentially forces the patient to lose the grip. Thus, in general, the grip or power grip may be weak because the patient's wrist cannot be stabilized in maximum dorsiflexion.

If the wrist can be stabilized in maximum dorsiflexion this sequence of events does not occur. However, if there is a tendency for the wrist to drop slightly into flexion, the fingers will tend to open by tenodesis function. This is especially the case when short excursion motors have been used for finger extension. The freely moving FDS obviously have plenty of excursion to compensate for any portion of the wrist, as far as finger extension or flexion are concerned. If short excursion motors are used, or the suture line is too distal, as the hand comes out of full dorsiflexion with power grip the

fingers will have a tendency to open by a dorsal tenodesis action.

This must be constantly guarded against when the transfer tension is adjusted at surgery. When the tendon transfer tension is adjusted, the patient's fingers should be able to be closed passively with the wrist in only slight dorsiflexion. If this cannot be done, the transfer tension on the EDC will be too high, resulting in a dorsal tenodesis of the EDC. The obvious treatment for this is either tenolysis—depending on whether there is adherence of the transfer dorsally—strengthening of the wrist dorsiflexors by transfer of an FDS to the wrist extensor, or opening of the retinaculum if the transfer suture line has been made too distal. This fine balance between tension on the wrist extensor and tension on the finger extensor must always be remembered when doing radial nerve palsy transfers (Fig. 5–9). It constitutes one of the reasons for unsatisfactory tendon transfers for radial palsy. Much of this has been attributed to a weak dorsiflexor of the wrist, but this may be only part of the problem, and the high tension or adherence of the EDC transfer must also be considered.

ULNAR NERVE PARALYSIS

Intrinsic Replacement

When attempting to replace intrinsic function in the fingers, we generally plan on not trying to replace all function of the intrinsic muscles. Our concern is in regard to the claw deformity, with lack of full PIP joint extension. The functions of abduction and adduction of the fingers are not taken into consideration, and these are almost never replaced. Many procedures have been advocated for the control of the claw hand, as well as for improving the pattern of grasp. In addition, since the work of Mannerfelt, some concern regarding a loss of power and its restoration has been mentioned.[46]

Many procedures to replace intrinsic function

include the observation that the EDC is capable of full PIP joint extension in the absence of intrinsic function if the MP joints are prevented from hyperextension. This is the so-called "Fowler" test. Some patients may lack full extension of the PIP joints during this test, either because of a contracture or an extensor lag. In the case of the contracture, either static or dynamic splints are necessary to regain full passive extension. Once the contracture has been relieved, there may be a persisting lag of full extension. At this point an MP joint block to full extension with a PIP extensor elastic outrigger should be applied to all the fingers. This splint should be comfortable enough to be worn almost constantly. In certain cases with this mode of treatment continued for several weeks, the extensor lag will be completely eliminated and the patient will pass the Fowler's test. The lag is caused by prolonged flexion of the PIP joints with attritional elongation of the central slip over the PIP joint, the so-called attritional boutonnière deformity.[40]

If prolonged splinting does not relieve the problem and a lag continues, some operative procedure will be necessary to shorten or tighten the extensor system, thereby increasing the tension to the PIP joint extension. The intrinsic tendon replacement will need to be prolonged to the central slip of the extensor system at the PIP joint rather than sutured to the lateral band, bone, or pulley over the proximal phalanx. An alternative is to increase the tension by doing a Littler-type boutonnière repair.[45] This repair, however, in the absence of functioning intrinsic muscles, must be carried far enough proximally so that hyperextension of the MP joint is prevented. With this increased tension the EDC can then bring about full PIP extension.

Certain points should be made regarding the timing and selection of transfers for intrinsic paralysis.[36, 39, 48] In the case of the recently repaired nerve laceration in the midforearm or wrist, at least some intrinsic return should be expected in the hand. The internal splint should then control the claw and improve the pattern of grasp, but power should not be added to PIP extension, and probably no attempt should be made to improve the strength of grasp by

tendon transfer. If significant nerve return occurs, secondary deformities will not be seen if these guidelines are followed. In such a case a Zancolli volar capsulorrhaphy or a Zancolli lasso procedure fulfills these criteria.[50] In addition, the split FDS of the ring finger may be transferred to the A1 pulley, as described by Brooks and Jones, or to the bone of the proximal phalanx, as described by Burkhalter and Strait.[35, 39]

All these procedures control the claw, improve the pattern of grasp, and do not increase power grip or tension in the extensor system. In the more proximal lesions with repairs above the elbow or still more proximally, for instance, or in certain disease states in which minimal to no intrinsic return is likely, any intrinsic replacement selected should be based on available motors and on the functional requirements of the patient. It is in this group of patients that PIP flexion contractures and extensor lags in the PIP joint are seen, because usually the transfers are carried out much later. In addition, these patients develop a flexor habitus of the wrist (Fig. 5–10).

Although most patients utilize their hand from 30° volar flexion to 30° dorsiflexion of the wrist, the patient with a long-standing intrinsic paralysis does not. It is rare to have these patients bring their wrist into more dorsiflexion than 30° volar flexion for any activity. Some may have a contracture of the wrist but many do not, and they develop this habitus in an attempt to increase the strength of extension and, hopefully, to improve PIP extension. Obviously, this never occurs, so it is not beneficial for the patient and results in a difficult rehabilitation problem, which must be considered when doing intrinsic replacements.

In all intrinsic replacements the motors cross the wrist either volar or dorsal to the axis of motion (Fig. 5–11). If the transfer tendon passes volar to the wrist joint, and the tension of the transfer is adjusted with the wrist in neutral during surgery, the flexor habitus of the wrist will render the transfer ineffective. In addition to concern about contractures and lags in the fingers, therefore, the flexor habitus of the wrist should be noted and treated, if

Figure 5–10. This patient with a combined median and ulnar nerve palsy shows a wrist flexor habitus, but does not have any true contracture.

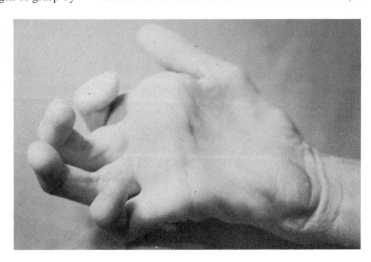

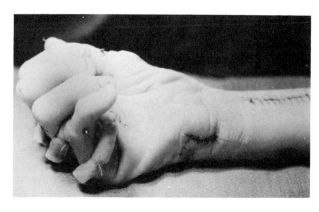

Figure 5–11. This transfer for intrinsic function and opposition was done at the same time, with the transfers passing volar to the wrist joint.

possible prior to the tendon transfer if the intrinsic replacement is to pass volar to the axis of the wrist joint. This type of retraining prior to actual tendon transfer is extremely important, and cannot be overemphasized (Fig. 5–12). The flexor habitus, although a major problem if the transfer passes volar to the wrist, is not as important if the motor is passed dorsal to the axis of wrist motion. Wrist flexion in this case will increase tension on the intrinsic transfer, and it will become more and not less effective.

In certain patients with supple hands, and in some others without but with an increase of strength of PIP extension, a swan-neck deformity may result following intrinsic replacement. Certainly, if two, three, or four FDS tendons are removed from the flexor surface of the finger and transferred to the lateral bands of all digits, a swan-neck deformity would be expected to develop. The combination of increased extensor force and loss of PIP joint flexor power makes the deformity obvious. This deformity will occur without a flexion contracture of the MP joints.

Brand felt that even using only one FDS puts the PIP joint in enough jeopardy that all sublimus tendons should be left in place to protect the PIP joint.[33] His alternative method was not to weaken the PIP joint flexor system but simply to increase PIP joint extension via a transfer to the lateral bands. This transfer utilizes a dorsal motor, a four-

tailed tendon graft, and the intermetacarpal route volar to the axis of the deep intermetacarpal ligament to the lateral bands.[34] With this transfer, Brand could correct the intrinsic minus problem and largely avoid the swan-neck deformity seen with the Stiles-Bunnell sublimus interosseous transfer.[33] This transfer, in addition, obviated the flexor habitus of the wrist problem; with the motor crossing dorsal to the wrist joint, wrist flexion increases MP joint flexion and IP extension, and the transfer becomes more effective.

Although wing tendon or lateral band attachments have been traditionally used in intrinsic replacements, postoperative splintage is a problem. The maintenance of MP joint flexion and simultaneous PIP extension by external means is difficult. Allowing the PIP joints to drop into flexion in the postoperative period will compromise tendon tension and result in less than an optimum result. K-wire fixation across the PIP joints has been utilized to maintain full extension in this joint postoperatively. However, with or without K-wire fixation, loss of PIP flexion is seen in about 5 to 10% of patients that have had this Brand-type intrinsic replacement.[34]

Because of the problem with the PIP joints, several authors have felt that if the patient is capable of PIP joint extension via the EDC with the MP joints blocked in less than full extension, lateral band attachment is unnecessary. The pulley over

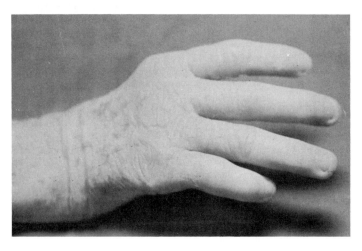

Figure 5–12. This patient had a very difficult rehabilitation problem because of the persisting flexor habitus of the wrist but, once the patient was able to relearn wrist extension with finger extension, the transfers became effective and the claw was completely controlled.

the proximal phalanx or the bone of the proximal phalanx has been used for distal attachment for intrinsic replacements. This is not true intrinsic replacement, but rather is a substitution of MP joint flexion for the intrinsic mechanism. The transfer acts as a prime MP joint flexor, so that in finger flexion all joints close simultaneously, and the pattern of flexion is improved. The transfer stabilizes the MP joint so that the patient, by control of the transfer, can overcome the EDC and avoid hyperextension of the MP joint. If MP joint hyperextension is avoided, PIP extension is then achieved by the EDC. The pulley or bony attachment does not increase the power of PIP joint extension directly.

Generally, as a result, fewer posttransfer swanneck deformities should be seen. The real advantage, however, is that postoperatively PIP joint immobilization is unnecessary. Only the wrist needs positioning, either into volar flexion or dorsiflexion, depending on the course of the motor used and on the MP joints that need to be maintained in flexion. The PIP joints can be moved throughout the period of postoperative immobilization.

It would be advantageous here to indicate the differences between a stable MP joint secondary to a pulley or a bony attachment of an intrinsic replacement and an MP joint flexion contracture (Fig. 5–13A). Most patients with pulley or bony attachments to the proximal phalanx will be able to demonstrate active MP joint flexion and extension.

Hyperextension will be prevented by normal muscle tone of the transfer, and perhaps by a mild contracture. The transfer never gives a severe contracture and, in most patients, amounts to no more than 10 to 15°, if present at all. Some patients with a long excursion FDS transfer can even demonstrate an active claw deformity by relaxing the transfer and overusing the EDC.

A severe contracture—for instance, 30 to 45° in the small finger MP joint—is quite another story. If this contracture results from an excessively tight volar capsulorrhaphy or from an adherent intrinsic replacement, a different set of circumstances is seen (Fig. 5–13B and C). The patient will be annoyed by the contracture and will constantly push against it—not, however, on the proximal phalanx, but on the tips of the fingers, thereby increasing tremendously the pressure of the PIP joint on the volar plates. In addition, the EDC will be attempting to overcome the contracture. Most of its power will go to the PIP joint, because the EDC will be unable to overcome the MP joint flexion deformity. It has been shown by some unpublished studies that the power of PIP joint extension can be increased as much as 30% by blocking the MP joint in flexion. These short-term studies of normal hands showed that considerable EDC power can be made to go one joint distal. Thus, with significant MP joint flexion contracture, swan-neck deformities may occur even in the absence of intrinsic function. In

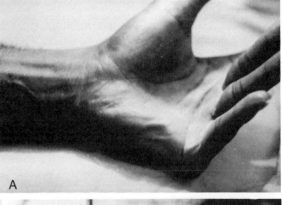

Figure 5–13. A, Severe flexion contracture of the metacarpal phalangeal joints may bring about the swan-neck deformity, even in the presence of functioning superficial tendons. A contracture of this degree needs early treatment to avoid secondary deformities. *B, C,* The flexion contracture of the hand may be secondary to adherence because the suture line of motor to graft was on the dorsum of the hand rather than in the proximal forearm.

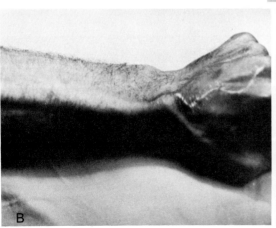

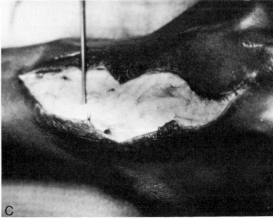

general, then, dynamic control of the MP joint by transfer is preferable to the development of a contracture.

Another potential problem arises with the Zancolli loop procedure, when using the FDS of each finger to act as a prime MP joint flexor of that finger. Will swan-neck deformity result? It usually will not, except in the most supple hands. Use of the long excursion FDS will not produce a significant contracture of the MP joints of any of the fingers. Control is dynamic, not static, and there is no increase in PIP extensor force except that mentioned previously as coming from the EDC.

Swan-neck deformity has been seen, however, and if this loop operation is used, some preparations should be made for its control in the extreme supple hand. One slip of the FDS in these patients should be sutured across the volar plate of the PIP joint to the opposite side, to where the pulley attaches to the bone. This reinforces the volar plate and should protect against hyperextension of the PIP joint.

Flexion contracture of the MP joints may occur with or without swan-neck deformity of the finger, and may be secondary to two particular problems. As might be expected, they more often occur with the Brand-type of intrinsic transfer rather than with the sublimus interosseous transfer, as described by Bunnell.[33] The course of the Brand transfer, coming as it does from the dorsum of the hand between the metacarpals to the individual fingers, sets up a possibility of two contractures: (1) there may be adherence of the tendon graft as it passes through the intermetacarpal fascia overlying the intrinsic muscles; (2) the four-tailed grafts may be sutured so distally to the ECRL or to the brachioradialis that the division of the graft may actually bind on the shaft of the metacarpal, which could result in a rather severe flexion contracture that cannot be treated except by lengthening the divisions of the graft. This is rarely seen, though, because the graft is usually sutured to the tendon motor in the distal third of the forearm proximal to the wrist joint, and certainly should never be sutured on the dorsum of the hand. Here adherence is possible in the area of the intermetacarpal fascia.

Regardless of the causes of a severe flexion contracture of 30 to 45°, it should not be allowed to persist. Many secondary changes will occur if it goes on as long as several months, in addition to the problems with swan-neck deformity of the PIP joint. Surgical release of this MP contracture will improve overall hand function, and should be done as soon as it seems that the problem will not correct itself spontaneously after the tendon transfer.

In a small group of patients it has been noted that, in addition to hyperflexion of the MP joints or the development of a flexion contracture postoperatively, some do not seem to have such a flexion contracture but end up with deviation of the finger and failure to control MP joint hyperextension (Fig. 5–14). In these situations the problem is obvious. During transfer of the tendon from the dorsum of the hand into the base of the proximal phalanx or

into a lateral band area, the proper course of the transfer was not followed. Instead of going volar to the deep intermetacarpal ligament, the transfer basically was found to pass dorsal to it, so it will not control MP joint hyperextension and will act only as a deviator of the finger. If this is seen the patient should be reoperated on and the tendon graft repositioned more volar to the axis of MP joint flexion. When the transfer is placed too dorsal, only further deviation of the finger will result, and there will be failure to control the claw, which will not improve with time.

Another complication analogous to the wrist flexor habitus seen in intrinsic paralysis is wrist extension contracture. This complication follows tendon transfers for intrinsic replacement. The tendon course is dorsal to the axis of the wrist joint. The so-called Brand transfer or its modifications cause this to occur.

Classically, the ECRL motor is prolonged with a tendon graft through the intermetacarpal spaces to the fingers after passing volar to the deep intermetacarpal ligament. The ECRL is primarily a radial deviator in its anatomic location. Its transfer dorsally, plus its removal from the dorsal retinaculum, increase the moment arm for wrist dorsiflexion and also add a new dorsiflexor motor. Use of the brachioradialis prolonged with tendon grafts similarly adds a new motor to wrist dorsiflexion, and its subcutaneous location also gives this tendon a large

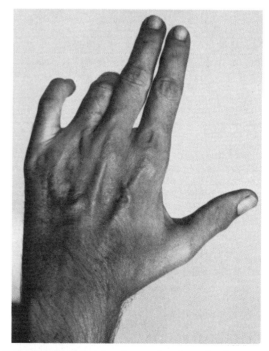

Figure 5–14. If the transfer coming from the dorsum of the wrist does not pass volar to the deep intermetacarpal ligament, deviation of the digits without control of the claw will be the result. (From Burkhalter, W. E.: Restoration of power grip in ulnar nerve paralysis. Orthop. Clin. North Am., 5:302, 1974.)

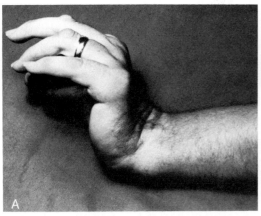 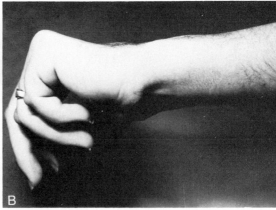

Figure 5–15. This patient is years postintrinsic replacement. The ECRL was prolonged with a tendon graft passed to the proximal phalanx of all fingers. There is good power grip, good pattern of flexion, and good control of claw *(A),* but limited wrist flexion *(B),*

moment arm (Fig. 5–15). Utilizing the flexor carpi radialis prolonged with a graft around the radial aspect of the wrist to its dorsum adds similar power but weakens wrist flexion.

Almost all long-term patients with these transfers develop a fixed extension deformity of the wrist, and seem to use the hand with the wrist in a position of 60° to 25° dorsiflexion. The wrist never flexes. In spite of the patient's satisfaction with the procedure, the complication is a biomechanical certainty.

A final complication of attempts to restore intrinsic action to the fingers is balance, or rather the inability to balance MP joint flexors and extensors. If the surgical plan involves replacement of MP joint flexion only, either by a pulley or a bony attachment, the antagonist of the transfer is the EDC. We are really trying to balance the forces of the transfer against those of the EDC, which hopefully is normal. One would think that the wrist extensor or brachioradialis would certainly be stronger than the combined EDC of all fingers, but this is not always true, and the MP joint flexor sometimes seems to be too weak, with the claw deformity recurring gradually in the postoperative period. This apparent weakness may mean that a poor motor has been selected, but more probably it indicates that adhesions about the transfer are limiting the excursion and power of the motor. In tendon transfers in peripheral nerve injury adhesions are the most frequent cause of weakness.

Another cause for failure in regard to recurring claw deformity following tendon transfer is residual adherence, or limited excursion of the flexor tendons volarly. This is most frequently seen in the combined ulnar nerve and tendon injury at the wrist level. Using the Brand transfer, or the Brand route at least, the aim is to have the transfer tighten passively by wrist flexion—that is, the MP joints flex with wrist flexion. This is directly antagonistic to the EDC, which passively extends the MP joints with wrist flexion. With some adherence of the

flexor tendons volarly the fingers will straighten only passively: through the MP and PIP joints simultaneously with wrist flexion.

Consider the following situation. A patient has an intrinsic paralysis secondary to nerve and tendon injury at the wrist. There is residual volar adherence of mild or perhaps moderate degree. The EDC is extremely strong secondary to the use of a lumbrical bar, with the EDC extending the PIP joints well. A Brand route transfer with the tendon graft is performed. (Surgery probably should have been postponed to overcome completely the flexor tendon adherence volarly, but it was done nevertheless.) Postoperatively, immobilization is in wrist dorsiflexion and MP joint flexion. During the period of immobilization there is full PIP joint motion.

Following removal of the immobilization in 4 to 6 weeks, initial work should be aimed toward flexion of the MP joints. *First, obtain isolated function and control of the tendon transfer. In this situation wrist flexion must be avoided for a long time, probably several months. Wrist flexion puts passive stretch on the tendon graft and suture lines dorsally.* In addition, the tension on the EDC is increased by wrist flexion and, because the motor is strong, all these factors tend to attenuate the transfer and the tendon graft. Because of the flexor tendon adherence volarly, though, the fingers can only be extended through the PIP joints by wrist flexion.

This hypothetical situation is difficult, and should be avoided when doing intrinsic replacement surgery for local injury at the wrist. Remember that the dorsal route was devised for intrinsic muscle paralysis secondary to a disease process, not for direct injury volarly with adherent flexor tendons. There has not been much work done in regard to intrinsic replacement in patients with combined low ulnar nerve and tendon injuries. Obviously, some patients regain intrinsic function, but not all. In the United States I am sure that trauma is the major etiology in patients needing intrinsic substitution.

Thus, one should make absolutely certain that the wrist and all three finger joints can be brought into full passive extension prior to doing any transfer utilizing the dorsal route.

Tendon Transfers for Pinch

The weakened or unstable pinch is usually secondary to loss of intrinsic muscles supplied by the ulnar or median and ulnar nerves. Occasionally direct injury to the thumb index web with loss of muscle tissue results in a similar problem. Operative procedures to improve precision grip have been variously called pinch transfers, adductorplasties, and short flexor plasties, and all concentrate on improving thumb function.

In addition to the thumb, some thought must be given to the index or index and long fingers.[47] These fingers, in the classic ulnar nerve lesions, are extremely weak even though there is no claw deformity. The absence of claw in these two radial fingers is secondary to median innervated lumbricals, which are weak but still can prevent claw deformity. Because of the relatively good control, lack of claw deformity, and normal sensibility, there is a tendency to attribute much greater power and dexterity to these fingers than they really possess. This deficit is most obvious when the patient attempts to use these fingers against a strong thumb. The fingers collapse into MP extension, hyperflexion of the PIP joint, and hyperextension of the DIP joint. Tendon transfers in ulnar nerve paralysis have concentrated on controlling the ulnar two fingers and their claw deformity. Certain operative procedures have, in addition, sought to improve the pattern of closure of the two ulnar fingers, and little attention has been given to the radial two fingers.

It is our feeling now that, even in an isolated ulnar nerve lesion, intrinsic function should be replaced to all four fingers. The additional strength and stability to the index and long fingers will make the pinch function between the thumb and the radial digits more stable and powerful. This improvement is secondary to two separate but interrelated situations. When one observes pinch in ulnar nerve paralysis between the thumb and index fingers, there is much concentration on the thumb. The thumb hyperflexes at the DIP joint and extends or hyperextends at the MP joint (Froment's or Jeanne's sign). The index finger, however, flexes at only one of its three joints (Fig. 5–16).

Why are the MP and DIP joints in extension or in hyperextension? Hyperextension at the MP joint occurs because there is no prime MP joint flexor, except the lumbrical. In the case of the DIP joint it appears as if the flexor digitorum profundus is not functional, in spite of the fact that the musculotendinous unit is normal. This is a valid observation. I have done EMGs of the flexor digitorum profundus to the index finger during pinch in cases of ulnar palsy, and have found it to be electrically silent, in spite of a normal EMG with isolated flexion of the finger. If the flexor digitorum profun-

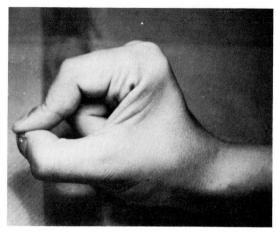

Figure 5–16. In ulnar nerve paralysis there is no action of the flexor digitorum profundus to the index during pinch. In this patient the only motor flexing the index finger is the superficialis in addition to a weak lumbrical.

dus were firing in addition to the flexor digitorum superficialis, the index finger would present the fingernail to the thumb for prehension, not the pulp of the digit, and obviously this is not functional. With hyperflexion of the PIP joint and MP joint extension, the only way a stable pulp can be presented to the thumb is by hyperextension of the distal joint, with electrical silence of the profundus tendon. With stabilization of the MP joint in flexion, either with hand pressure dorsally over the proximal phalanx or with the MP joint flexor replacement, the flexor digitorum profundus becomes active, the pinch strength improves with the use of the MP flexor replacement, and the patient can now utilize the flexor digitorum profundus in pinch activities.

Assuming that our concern for the thumb has now spread to the index finger, it should continue to the long finger. The long finger supports the MP joint of the index finger from either rotational collapse, ulnar deviation, or both during pinch, even in a normal hand. In the weakened situation, I feel that we should also motor the long finger.

Thus, to repeat, in the intrinsic paralysis of the ulnar nerve–injured patient all four fingers should undergo intrinsic replacement to control the claw and improve the strength of the ulnar two fingers. On the radial two fingers only strength is improved, because claw does not exist on the radial side and the closing pattern is normal.

It may be that one elects to improve pinch or precision grip without a procedure to control claw ulnarly, or uses only a static or semidynamic procedure ulnarly. In this case both index and long fingers should be motored with the same transfer, and something should be done to improve the thumb as well (Figs. 5–17 and 5–18). Obviously, if all four fingers have intrinsic replacements, then only the thumb requires additional procedures to improve pinch.

Results from operative procedures to improve pinch have generally been successful. Reports by Brown, Hamlin and Littler, and Goldner reveal

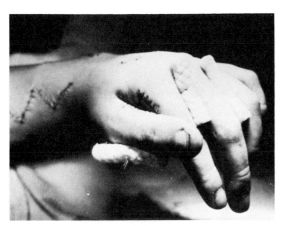

Figure 5–17. Improvement of pinch in this patient was achieved by transfer of the flexor digitorum superficialis across the palm deep to the index flexor tendon to the thumb and brachial radialis to the proximal phalanx of the index and long fingers.

improvement in strength, up to 65 to 85% of the normal side, when only a tendon transfer is used to the thumb.[37, 42, 43] Smith has given us yet another motor with the ECRB musculotendinous unit prolonged with a tendon graft to the thumb through the intermetacarpal route.[49]

What is one really trying to restore by the pinch transfer, the adductoplasty, or the short flexor plasty? Clearly, it is short flexor function—that is, MP joint and carpometacarpal joint flexor action. Rotation into supination is not desirable, certainly not with a combined median and ulnar nerve lesion with weakness of the abductor pollicis brevis function. As far as the thumb is concerned, pronation is acceptable but not supination.

The Boyes transfer of the brachioradialis, prolonged with a tendon graft running between the

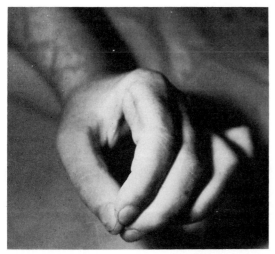

Figure 5–18. Note the position of the thumb and index and long fingers now during power pinch, with good power in the profundus tendons.

third and fourth metacarpals to the adductor tendon, and also the Smith ECRB transfer, prolonged with a graft to the adductor area, give good adduction to the thumb.[32] The EIP adductorplasty has a similar course, running beneath the index flexors to the adductor tubercle. This transfer requires no graft, as do the other two, but is considerably weaker than they are. As pointed out by Littler, the FDS of the ring finger transferred beneath the index flexors to the adductor tendon does not require a graft, and has a great excursion of motion.[44] These transfers all run beneath the flexor digitorum superficialis and profundus to the index finger, and actually use these tendons as a pulley. If the transfer runs superficial to the tendon, adductor function is satisfactory, but this bowstring is uncomfortable when picking up hard objects in the palm.[37]

All these transfers are best placed beneath the flexor digitorum superficialis and profundus to the index finger. With the exception of the FDS of the ring finger, all these motors have relatively short excursions. An adduction contracture of the thumb is one of the most common and annoying complications of adductorplasty. Thus, when using short excursion motors, great care must be taken so as not to create an opposite deformity. This complication is most often seen in the presence of a median and ulnar nerve injury, when weakness of the opposition function of the thumb exists. A strong adductorplasty, with its tendency toward thumb supination, may very well compromise an excellent opposition transfer. All these transfers bring the thumb toward the fingers (i.e., those with an intermetacarpal palmar route or both). The Goldner adductorplasty, on the other hand, brings the thumb to the side of the hand and supinates the thumb excessively.[42] This transfer reinforces the function of the EPL, which is already an adductor of the thumb and is excessively active in the median and ulnar nerve–injured patient, or even in the patient with an isolated ulnar nerve injury. Secondary contractures were common with Goldner's procedure and presently, if I were to use the FDS to the ringfinger, I would utilize the Littler course through the palm of the hand rather than the Goldner course across the dorsum.

In the combined median and ulnar nerve injury, in which the patient has had an opposition transfer for a maximal thumb position, selection of an adductorplasty is extremely important.[41] At the time of the opponensplasty I feel that the patient needs an arthrodesis of the MP joint of the thumb (Fig. 5–19). The arthrodesis position is quite important because of the existing pronation weakness, in spite of excellent thumb opposition. The position of hyperpronation and extension through the MP joints is good, with minimal abduction of the thumb through this MP joint. Thumb hyperpronation neutralizes the supinatory effect of the fingers as they strike the thumb in power pinch. Full extension arthrodesis of the MP joint has the same effect by reducing the "crank handle" effect of the MP joint in flexion. Consequently, only short flexor action is

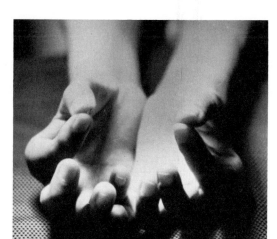

Figure 5–19. The hand on the right shows hyperpronation of an arthrodesis of the metacarpal phalangeal joint performed on a combined median and ulnar nerve injury patient. Not that this hyperpronation with extension of the metacarpal phalangeal joint reduces considerably the rotational component to the thumb created by the flexing index finger. This helps to obviate the Brand crank effect, which the powerful index finger may exert against the weak thumb. On the left is an arthrodesis without hyperpronation. (From Green, D. P.: Operative Hand Surgery. New York, Churchill Livingstone, 1982.)

needed. That is, in the patient with a combined median and ulnar nerve palsy, there is no need for supination of the thumb.

Some thought should be given to attaching the pinch transfer radial to the flexor pollicis longus in the thumb in the area of the attachment of the radial head of the flexor pollicis brevis. This will bring about thumb pronation with short flexor action instead of supination with short flexor action. Excessive pronation is not a problem with the power of the EPL still in position. Although pinch between the thumb and index finger or index and long fingers can be improved by almost any of the procedures mentioned, rotational abnormalities in the combined lesion, in which the pronatory effect has been replaced by a transfer, should be prevented. Utilizing short excursion motors such as the EIP, brachioradialis, and ECRB, tension is extremely important. In the more severely damaged hands there is a tendency for a secondary contracture to develop in the thumb if there is weakness of abductor pollicis brevis function.

References

Median Nerve Paralysis

1. Braun, R. M.: Palmaris longus tendon transfer for augmentation of thenar musculature in low median nerve palsy. J Hand Surg., 3:5, 488, 1978.
2. Brown, E., Teague, M., and Snyder, C.: Prevention of extensor lag after indicis proprius tendon transfer. J Hand Surg., 4:168, 1979.
3. Bunnell, S.: Opposition of the thumb. J. Bone Joint Surg., 20:269, 1938.
4. Burkhalter, W.: Tendon transfer in median nerve palsy. Orthop. Clin. North Am., 5:271, 1974.
5. Burkhalter, W., Christenson, R., and Brown, P.: The extensor indicis proprius opponensplasty. J. Bone Joint Surg., 55:725, 1973.
6. Chouhy-Aguirre, S., and Coplan, S.: Sobre secuelas de lesion alta e irriparable di nervio mediano y cubital y su tratamiento. Prem. Med. Argentina 43:2341, 1956.
7. Edgerton, M., and Brand, P.: Restoration of abduction and adduction to the unstable thumb in median and ulnar nerve paralysis. Plast. Reconstr. Surg., 36:150, 1965.
8. Henderson, E. D.: Transfer of wrist extensor and brachioradialis to restore opposition of the thumb. J. Bone Joint Surg., 44A:513, 1962.
9. Jacobs, B., and Thompson, T. C.: Opposition of the thumb and its restoration. J. Bone Joint Surg., 42A:1015, 1960.
10. Kaplan, I., Dinner, M., and Chait, L.: Use of extensor pollicis longus as a distal extension for an opponens transfer. Plast. Reconstr. Surg., 57:186, 1976.
11. Kessler, I.: Transfer of extensor carpi ulnaris to tendon of extensor pollicis brevis for opponensplasty. J. Bone Joint Surg., 45A:1389, 1963.
12. Littler, J., and Cooley, S.: Opposition of the thumb and its restoration by adductor digiti minimi transfer. J. Bone Joint Surg., 45A:1389, 1963.
13. Littler, J., and Cooley, S.: Primary restoration of thumb opposition with median nerve decompression. Plast. Reconstr. Surg., 39:74, 1967.
14. Mayer, L.: The physiologic method of tendon transplantation. Surg. Gynecol. Obstet., 22:182, 1977.
15. North, E., and Littler, J. W.: Transferring the flexor superficialis tendon: Technical considerations in the prevention of proximal interphalangeal joint disability. J. Hand Surg., 5:498, 1980.
16. Phalen, G., and Miller, R.: The transfer of wrist extensor muscles to restore or reinforce flexion power of the fingers and opposition of the thumb. J. Bone Joint Surg., 29A:993, 1947.
17. Riley, W., Burkhalter, W., and Mann, R.: Extensor pollicis longus opponensplasty. J. Hand Surg., 5:217, 1980.
18. Schneider, L.: Opponensplasty using the extensor digiti minimi. J. Bone Joint Surg., 51A:1297, 1969.
19. Spinner, M. D.: American Society for Surgery of the Hand, Correspondence Newsletter 1980–36, May 30, 1980.
20. Steindler, A.: Tendon transplantation in the upper extremity. Am. J. Surg., 44:260, 1939.
21. Weissinger, H., and Singsen, E.: Abductor digiti quinti opponensplasty. J. Bone Joint Surg., 59A:895, 1977.
22. Wood, V.: Nerve compression following opponensplasty as a result of wrist anomalies. J. Hand Surg., 5:279, 1980.

Radial Nerve Paralysis

23. Boyes, J.: Tendon transfer for radial palsy. Bull. Hosp. Joint Dis., 21: 1960.
24. Brand, P.: Tendon transfer in the forearm. In Flynn, J. E. (ed.): Hand Surgery. Baltimore, Williams & Wilkins, 1966, pp. 331–342.
25. Brand, P.: Biomechanics of tendon transfer. Orthop. Clin. North Am., 5:203, 1974.
26. Chuinard, R., et al.: Tendon transfer for radial nerve palsy. J. Hand Surg., 3:560, 1978.
27. Jones, R.: Tendon transplantation in cases of musculospinal injuries not amenable to suture. Am. J. Surg., 35:333, 1921.
28. Moberg, E., and Nachemson, A.: Tendon transfer for defective long extension of the wrist and finger. Acta Chir. Scand., 133:31, 1967.
29. Riordan, D.: Radial nerve paralysis. Orthop. Clin. North Am., 5:283, 1974.
30. Said, G.: A modified tendon transfer for radial nerve paralysis. J. Bone Joint Surg., 56B:320, 1974.
31. Thomson, M., and Rassmussen, K.: Tendon transfer for defective long extension of the wrist and fingers. Scand. J. Plast. Reconstr. Surg., 3:71, 1969.

Ulnar Nerve Paralysis

32. Boyes, J.: Bunnell's Surgery of the Hand, 5th ed., Philadelphia, J. B. Lippincott, 1970.

33. Brand, P.: Paralytic claw hand with special reference to paralysis in leprosy and treatment by the sublimus transfer of stiles-bunnell. J. Bone Joint Surg., 40B:618, 1958.
34. Brand, P.: Tendon grafting illustrated by a new operation for intrinsic paralysis of the finger. J. Bone Joint Surg., 43B:444, 1961.
35. Brooks, A., and Jones, D.: A new intrinsic tendon transfer. Presented at the Annual Meeting of the American Society for Surgery of the Hand, San Francisco, 1975.
36. Brown, P.: The time factor in surgery of upper extremity peripheral nerve injury. Clin. Orthop., 68:14, 1970.
37. Brown, P.: Reconstruction for pinch in ulnar intrinsic palsy. Orthop. Clin. North Am., 5:323, 1974.
38. Burkhalter, W. E.: Early tendon transfer in upper extremity peripheral nerve injury. Clin. Orthop., 104:68, 1974.
39. Burkhalter, W. E., and Strait, L.: Metacarpal phalangeal flexor replacement for intrinsic muscle paralysis. J. Bone Joint Surg., 55A:1667, 1973.
40. Burkhalter, W. E., and Carneiro, R.: Correction of the attritional boutonnière deformity in high ulnar nerve paralysis. J. Bone Joint Surg., 61A:131, 1979.
41. Edgerton, M., and Brand, P.: Restoration of abduction and adduction to the unstable thumb in median and ulnar paralysis. Plas. Reconstr. Surg., 36:150, 1965.
42. Goldner, J.: Replacement of the function of the paralyzed adductor pollicis with flexor digitorum sublimus—a ten-year review. J. Bone Joint Surg., 49A:583, 1967.
43. Hamlin, C., and Littler, J. W.: Restoration of power pinch. J. Hand Surg., 5:396, 1980.
44. Littler, J. W.: Tendon transfers and arthrodesis in combined median and ulnar nerve paralysis. J. Bone Joint Surg., 24A:225, 1949.
45. Littler, J. W., and Eaton, R.: Redistribution of forces in the correction of the boutonnière deformity. J. Bone Joint Surg., 49A:1267, 1967.
46. Mannerfelt, L.: Structure of the hand in ulnar nerve paralysis: A clinical experimental investigation in normal and anomalies of innervation. Acta Orthop. Scand. (Suppl)., 87:91, 1966.
47. Neviaser, R., Wilson, J., and Gardner, M.: Abductor pollicis longus transfer for replacement of first dorsal interosseous. J. Hand Surg., 5:53, 1980.
48. Omer, G.: The technique and timing of tendon transfers. Orthop. Clin. North Am., 5:243, 1974.
49. Smith, R.: ECRB adductorplasty, presented at the Annual Meeting of the American Society for Surgery of the Hand, Las Vegas, 1981.
50. Zancolli, E.: Structural and Dynamic Bases of Hand Surgery, 2nd ed., Philadelphia, J. B. Lippincott, 1978, p. 174.

RADIATION INJURIES OF THE HAND

John P. Remensnyder

Radiation injuries to the hand constitute some of the most difficult and subtle injuries in hand surgery. Fortunately they are not common injuries, but occur sporadically, frequently under unusual circumstances. Radiation injuries and thermal burns are not to be equated therapeutically: successful treatment of thermal burns requires a careful appraisal of the visible injury (see Chap. 7); for radiation injuries, success follows an appreciation of the unseen and future effects specific to this group of injuries, as well as a detailed knowledge of the mode and physics of the accident.

The purpose of this chapter is to discuss the therapy of two different forms of complications: the treatment of the complications of the radiation injury itself, and the management of complications peculiar to the surgical therapy of radiation injuries to the hand.

HISTORICAL NOTE

From the vantage point of the present atomic age, the beginning days of x-ray tubes and radium experiments appear dim and confused. However, the early workers seem to have perceived promptly both the beneficial and harmful effects of the mysterious rays. Physicians and scientists rapidly became aware of radiation damage to skin and other tissues, literally within months after the discovery and recognition of x-rays.

On November 8, 1895, Wilhelm Roentgen, during his experiments in Wurzburg, Germany, recognized the existence and character of x-rays, and published his findings on January 5, 1896.[1] Of ironic interest to the present discussion is the fact that the first published x-ray was the famous picture of the bones of Frau Roentgen's hand.

The first published description of radiation skin damage appeared early in 1896, when H. D. Hawks, a fourth-year medical student at Columbia Univer-

sity, described a severe inflammation dermatitis of his hands after intense exposure to his experimental apparatus.[2] He postulated that the skin damage was due to a secondary rather than primary effect of the irradiation. Daniel and Marcuse, early in the same year, described epilation as a result of exposure to x-rays, correctly concluding the effect to be a direct one.[3, 4] In October 1896, Elihu Thompson, a physicist at the General Electric Company in Lynn, Massachusetts, deliberately exposed the little finger of his left hand to the rays from his experimental tube to determine the skin effects. In a fascinating article and series of published correspondence with Dr. E. A. Codman, he described a long-lasting inflammation and the appearance of a very painful and indolent ulceration of his finger.[5] The importance of his experience is that he appears to be the first investigator to conclude rightly that the damage was caused directly by x-rays, and was not a secondary effect.

In the summer of 1897, Walter Dodd, the first roentgenologist at the Massachusetts General Hospital, had suffered severe radiation damage to both hands as a result of experiments conducted during the preceding year. He suggested to Dr. Charles Allen Porter that he remove the painful ulcerated areas of radiation injury to his forefinger. Porter did so, and covered this defect immediately with a split-thickness skin graft, which brought about prompt relief of the unremitting pain and secure healing. Dodd's case represents the earliest reported instance of surgical treatment of a radiation ulceration.[6]

Thus, radiation damage was identified and its surgical treatment accomplished within 18 months following Roentgen's discovery, and by 1909, Porter was able to report the surgical treatment of 47 patients.[7] The identity of the worker who suffered the first malignancy induced by x-ray exposure is not known but, in 1902, Frieben in Hamburg reported a case of irradiation carcinoma.[8] Dodd himself had the first of two amputations of his fingers for squamous cell carcinoma in the autumn of 1902, just 6 years after his initial exposure.[6] Dr. Percy Brown, a victim of early x-ray usage, compiled a series of short biographies of the early radiation workers and their ultimate fates.[9] He noted that average time between exposure and development of their first radiation malignancies was between 5 and 7 years, and most of the 28 individuals reported died with disseminated disease.

RADIATION PHYSICS

Radiation damages tissue either by a direct ionizing effect from particulate radiation or by secondary ionization within cells from electromagnetic wave sources. Irradiation produces varying levels of damage depending on several factors, including the dose delivered, the time course of delivery, the tissue involved, and the age of the patient. All cellular elements, especially the nucleus and cell membrane, are affected by high-energy ionization, which produces various immediate and remote metabolic, biochemical, and physiologic changes.

Clinically, radiation from both electromagnetic and particulate sources can result in problems (Tables 6–1 and 6–2). X-rays are part of the electromagnetic spectrum produced by high-energy activation of appropriate targets and, in the higher energy ranges, cause well-known biologic changes. Gamma rays are essentially the same as X-rays but emanate from radioactive nuclei. Direct ionizing effects on tissue occur also with particulate radiation from beams of various atomic particles. Alpha particles have heavy mass but naturally low energy levels, which are inadequate to penetrate tissues to any significant degree. Beta rays, or high-energy electrons, have sufficient energy to penetrate skin and subcutaneous tissues, and cause major damage at these levels. Neutrons having a high linear energy cause either direct damage or secondary particle emission within cells as a result of neutron capture.

In a civilian practice, patients usually present with radiation damage due to x-rays and beta radiation. Occasionally, patients are seen with damage resulting from high-energy accelerator accidents, which show the effects of highly activated heavy particles. Accidents in atomic energy laboratories and installations may produce a combination of electromagnetic and particulate radiation effects; there is even the occasional patient who has had radioactive material accidentally injected into the clean tissues.[10]

Table 6–1. ELECTROMAGNETIC WAVE TYPES AND SOURCES

Wave Type	Sources
Hertzian (radio waves and microwaves)	Radio Transmitters
Infrared	Hot materials
Visible	Hot materials—activated molecules
Ultraviolet	Hot materials—activated gases
X-rays and gamma rays*	Atoms struck by high-energy particles; radioactive materials; cosmic sources

*Similar to x-rays, but from radioactive nuclei.

Table 6–2. PARTICULATE RADIATION TYPES AND SOURCES

Particle Type	Sources
Alpha (He nuclei)	Radioactive material and cosmic rays
Beta (electrons)*	Accelerators; radioactive materials
Neutron	Nuclear reactors; cosmic rays; accelerators
Proton (H nuclei)	Accelerators; cosmic rays

*Same as cathode rays.

PATHOLOGIC EFFECTS OF RADIATION

The acute effects of ionizing radiation, regardless of the source, show up as a peculiar three-phase inflammatory response, the severity of which depends on the intensity of exposure and on several other variables.[11] The first change noted is an *early erythema,* which occurs as a pale pink itchy change that usually disappears by the third day after exposure. The *main (second) erythema* begins in the affected area about the eighth or tenth day, gradually becoming a deep violaceous color by the end of the second week, when the reaction is at its height. As it subsides, a deep brawny pigmentation supervenes, frequently making it difficult to decide when the second stage has ended. The *late (third) erythema* begins during the fifth to sixth week, and may last several weeks. Because of residual pigmentation from the second stage, the third phase may not always be noted. The early changes seem to be due to the release of vasoactive amines, while the latter two stages are the result of direct destructive changes in the capillary walls and of altered vascular reactivity.

If a very high dose is given over a short period of time, the acute picture may include an intense inflammatory exudative dermatitis, blister formation, and even acute ulceration of the skin and subcutaneous tissues. Pain and itching are intense, and healing may be slow and quite delayed.

The chronic effects of radiation damage to the skin and superficial tissues were beautifully described by Wolbach in 1909, and have hardly been improved on since.[12] He pointed to four major changes: (1) loss of skin appendages; (2) collagen changes in the dermis; (3) dermal necrosis and thinning; and (4) progressive vascular obliteration. Sweat glands, hair follicles, and sebaceous glands are all destroyed at moderate levels of radiation (1200 to 2400 R), producing the typically hairless dry cracked skin of chronic radiation damage. Alteration of fibroblast function reduces collagen production, and the matrix organization of collagen is markedly disturbed. Both factors lead to characteristic thinning and atrophy of radiated skin, which has reduced resistance to superficial trauma and infection.

Perhaps the most important pathologic change is that of progressive vascular obliteration. This is the prime factor that makes radiation damage an advancing destructive lesion, characterized by progressive shutdown of the local blood supply and development of ischemic tissue changes. The atrophic ischemic skin is especially prone to develop necrosis and ulceration. Pain is the outstanding characteristic of the chronic radiation ulcer and may be due to radioneuritis, pH changes, micro- or macroinfections, or compression of the nerves by fibrosis.[13]

The clinical picture of fully developed chronic radiation dermatitis of the hand has been graphically described by Urbach (Fig. 6–1):

". . . the earliest changes are flattening of the epidermal ridges of the fingers, followed by diffuse drying of the skin, thickening of the creases, scantiness of hair, atrophy of sebaceous and sweat glands and the appearance of numerous hyperkeratotic warty lesions. The nails become cracked and brittle. The general appearance of the skin is that of premature aging. Eventually, there are interference with motion and pain. Persistent ulcers appear which are exquisitely painful."[11]

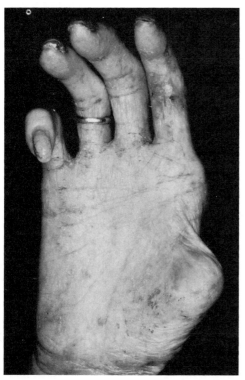

Figure 6–1. Chronic radiation dermatitis and superficial ulceration. Hand was radiated as treatment for eczema 40 years previously; thumb was amputated 3 years previously for squamous cell carcinoma.

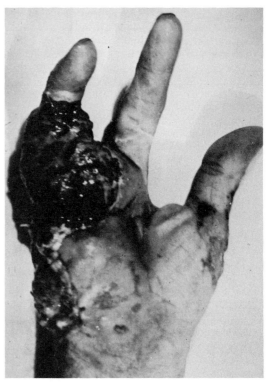

Figure 6–2. Fungating squamous cell carcinoma in hand of radiology technician who inadvertently received multiple doses of radiation while holding cassettes in the early days of clinical radiology. Note previous two amputations for chronic painful ulceration of fingers and healed skin graft proximal to lesion. (Courtesy of History of Radiology Archives, Department of Radiology, Massachusetts General Hospital.)

The final and disastrous end stage of chronic radiation damage occurs with the appearance of malignant degeneration (Fig. 6–2). I have already mentioned the development of malignancies in the early physicians and scientists who were inadvertently exposed to high cumulative doses of radiation. Malignancies usually appear in association with the characteristic hyperkeratotic lesions of the skin, and always occur in skin with some degree of radiation damage.

Exactly what percentage of patients will develop cancer following low-level exposure remains uncertain, but figures from several series indicate that from 11 to 36% of these at-risk patients will develop carcinoma, either squamous cell or basal cell (Table 6–3). The interval from insult to onset of malignancy varies from 7 to 28 years, averaging 17.4 years.[13]

TREATMENT OF RADIATION COMPLICATIONS

The treatment of complications of radiation injury to the hand requires the surgeon to deal with three quite different types of problems: (1) superficial skin reactions, both acute and chronic, which involve no tissue loss; (2) tissue loss, either early or

Table 6–3. INCIDENCE OF DEVELOPMENT OF POSTRADIATION SKIN CANCER (ALL CELL TYPES)

References	Year	Total of Patients Irradiated	Patients Who Developed Cancer Total	%
Saunders and Montgomery[14]	1938	226	26	11
Teloh et al.[15]	1950	112	34	30
Cannon et al.[16]	1959	165	36	22
Robinson and Masters[17]	1960	105	31	30
Hartwell et al.[18]	1964	39	12	31
Conway and Hugo[19]	1966	63	23	36
Rintala[13]	1967	198	37	19
Holmstrom and Johanson[20]	1972	170	37	22

late, requiring replacement; and (3) malignancies developing in areas of chronic radiation damage.

Radiation Dermatitis. *Acute radiation dermatitis* usually requires no operative treatment, and therapy is directed toward the control of both pain and inflammation as well as preventing infection. With respect to pain, the acute injury comes in three peaks, and usually the patient suffers with minor irritation and itching during the first 10 to 12 days. In the second week the inflammatory response becomes intense and pain may become severe and unremitting, requiring narcotics for control. During this time, analgesic agents help during active and passive manipulation to maintain joint mobility. Because acute radiation injury produces a partial thickness skin injury, it is imperative during this time to prevent the hand from becoming infected, which would convert the partial thickness damage into a full-thickness injury that would require tissue replacement. Various topical antiseptic agents are available for this purpose, including 0.5% silver nitrate solution, silver sulfadiazine, and Sulfamylon. The skin of the hand, other than being a bit dry, resumes a relatively normal character following healing.

Chronic radiation dermatitis slowly advances as a result of progressive vascular shutdown and the effects of chronic tissue ischemia. The skin becomes fragile, dry, cracked, and fissured due to dermal thinning and loss of sebaceous and sweat glands. Emollient creams help to maintain skin softness and keep cracking at a minimum. Mild escharotic agents (e.g., 3% sulfur and salicylic acid ointment) prevent build-up of hyperkeratotic material. Particular attention should be paid to the nails that, due to nail bed damage, become distorted and raised from the bed, presenting a ragged, fragmented appearance. Chronic paronychia occurs and if poor hygiene, repeated infection, and snagging become a problem, consideration should be given to excision of the entire nail and to replacement with a full-thickness skin graft. Regular periodic examinations of the hand are critical to detect any changes suggestive of malignant degeneration. Areas of unstable tissue such as premalignant keratoses should be removed for pathologic examination and closed, either primarily or with a graft.

Tissue Loss in Acute Radiation Injury. This is uncommon unless the insult has been massive.

Krizek and Ariyan reported such an injury in 1973, in which there had been massive accidental exposure of the hands to 19,500 rads.[21] Despite conservative measures, excision and grafting were necessary to gain initial wound closure. A similar instance was reported by Caldwell and McCormack, with nonhealing following uncontrolled therapeutic exposure of the patient's hands to radiation.[22] The hands of patients in both of these cases responded to grafting because the damage was superficial. With even more severe damage, two courses are possible: if tendons and joints are exposed, pedicle flap coverage will be necessary; in some instances, no repair is possible, and amputation is the only recourse.[21, 23]

Chronic radiation ulceration occurs in the setting of established dermatitis and presents as an extremely painful nonhealing ulceration, with low-grade sepsis. Treatment is surgical and temporizing measures, such as topical therapy and dressings, cannot be expected to heal tissues ulcerated from long-standing ischemia. Again, because the radiation ulcer is an ischemic lesion, preliminary débridement is contraindicated because it leads to enlargement of the ulcer as a result of dieback at the débrided margins. Successful treatment of radiation ulceration consists of the prompt and wide excision of all involved tissue and repair with either a free graft or pedicle flap. The accurate assessment of the depth of damage is essential in the choice of graft or flap. If, following excision of the ulcer and adjacent tissues, the bed shows good vascularity and reasonably healthy tissue, then *immediate grafting* is indicated (Fig. 6–3). Wide excision is essential to prevent secondary breakdown at the edge of the graft, and immediate graft application prevents deterioration of the partially ischemic bed, which occurs if delayed grafting is attempted. If, after ulcer excision, the damage is obviously very deep, exposing tendons and joints, then a blood-bearing pedicle flap is essential to ensure proper healing. Brown and colleagues emphasized the use of flaps to bring in new blood supply to the area of radiation damage as a necessity for healing deeply damaged tissues.[24] Again, adequate and wide excision and immediate flap application are critical to successful repair.

Radiation-Induced Malignancies. Successful treatment of radiation-induced carcinoma of the hand requires early diagnosis and prompt aggressive

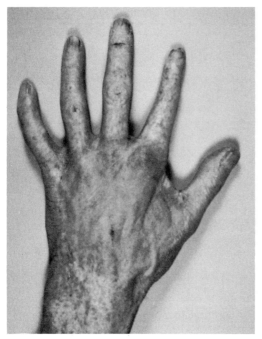

Figure 6–3. Well-healed skin graft 6 years after excision and immediate grafting of chronic radiation ulcer dorsum of the hand of an early demonstrator of x-ray machines. (Courtesy of Dr. B. Cannon.)

therapy. Constant surveillance of patients with radiation dermatitis helps to detect early degenerative changes, and any suspicious hyperkeratotic areas should be biopsied. All tissues removed in the course of treatment of either chronic radiation dermatitis or ulceration should be subjected to pathologic examination to eliminate the possibility of occult cancer.

The most common malignancy to appear in a radiation-damaged hand is squamous cell carcinoma, and its treatment is surgical; radiation therapy plays no role. The principle of wide local removal guides therapy, which should be either amputation or wide excision and grafting, depending on the location of the tumor. Amputation should include one normal proximal joint to avoid possible intramedullary spread. Regional node dissection is indicated when the primary lesion is extensive or deeply invasive, or if there are palpable nodes. Metastasis in some series have run as high as 25%.[13]

TREATMENT OF THERAPEUTIC COMPLICATIONS

Virtually all complications that appear following the surgical treatment of radiation ulceration may be thought of as being caused by inadequate excision of the ulcer and surrounding damaged ischemic tissue. Such complications include infection, hemorrhage, graft loss, separation of flap edges, continued pain, development of carcinoma, and continued progressive necrosis. Given an accurate knowledge

of the pathology of radiation dermatitis and ulceration and its intrinsic progressive ischemic nature, development of all these complications becomes understandable. Unfortunately, as difficult as the complications of radiation are to treat, the complications of such treatment are even more difficult to remedy.

Infection. This is one of the major complications following surgical treatment of radiation ulceration. It is frequently unclear whether the appearance of infection in the setting is primary or appears secondarily in areas that were inadequately excised and hence are still undergoing necrosis. Preoperative measures should be taken to attempt to reduce the incidence of postoperative infection. Following culture and sensitivity determinations of the bacterial flora, a radiation ulcer should be treated to make it mechanically clean and to reduce the bacterial level as much as possible. Appropriate measures include repeated dressing changes, use of local antibiotics, and the use of specific systemic antibiotics. Débridement should be avoided except when there is obviously loose and separated necrotic tissue; sharp débridement into bleeding tissue simply invites further necrosis. Local antibiotics may be more effective than systemic agents because of the reduced blood supply in the neighborhood of a radiation ulcer.

If, despite appropriate preoperative precautions and accurate surgical treatment, one encounters a postoperative infection, the general principles of treatment for any postsurgical infection should be followed, but more intensively and for a longer period of time: culture and determination of sensitivity of the predominating organism; intensive use of appropriate systemic antibiotics and, if possible, local antiseptics; establishment of drainage; and use of proper dressing schedules. Application of local heat should be used sparingly for fear of adding damage to already compromised tissue. Not uncommonly, severe local infection will induce necrosis of either wound edge or repair tissue, and a secondary ulceration may remain following the successful treatment of postsurgical infection.

Hemorrhage and Hematoma. These are real dangers following excision of radiation-damaged tissue. Not only have small vessels lost a good deal of their intrinsic contractility due to damage to the media, but also they are rigidly encased in dense fibrotic tissue. Both factors serve to keep the cut vessels open and bleeding after excision. Careful hemostasis with thorough coagulation of all bleeding points is essential to forestall hematoma formation. Adequate stenting of skin grafts may prevent a certain amount of postoperative ooze, but undue reliance should not be put on "stent pressure" to offset inadequate hemostasis. Although delayed grafting following excision of thermal burns to allow for hemostasis is useful, delay in the application of a graft to an excised radiation ulcer invites secondary infection and ischemic edge loss, leading to graft failure. Hemostasis must be careful and complete, permitting immediate repair.

Graft Loss and Separation of Pedicle Flap Edges. These occur regularly if the initial excision does not encompass all the compromised tissue. Application of a graft or flap to an inadequately excised bed with essentially no circulation and no proliferative ability of the few remaining vessels guarantees loss. When a skin graft has been lost, prompt regrafting is essential. If the loss occurs because of motion, mechanical factors, or hematoma, yet the bed is healthy, then prompt regrafting is indicated. If the bed simply cannot support the graft due to inadequate blood supply, re-excision down to healthy tissue will be necessary with application of either a graft or flap. If, following every effort to excise all damaged tissue, some clearly compromised areas must remain, a pedicle flap bringing in its own blood supply should be used. Pedicle flaps confer another potential benefit to the excised bed—that is, normal wound-healing mechanisms. Radiated tissue loses much of its intrinsic ability for wound contraction, epithelialization, and blood vessel proliferation. Small defects due to separation of flaps from wound edges can be treated conservatively and expected to heal, because the normal flap tissue side of the wound will provide wound contraction and epithelialization; the radiated side will not.

Other Complications. The three remaining complications are logical and tragic outcomes of inadequate excision. *Continued pain* occurs if substantial ischemic tissue remains, secondary necrosis occurs, or repair tissue breaks down. The remaining severely injured tissue is still prone to the long-term *development of radiation-induced carcinoma,* as well as *continued progressive tissue necrosis.* All are preventable by wide, adequate initial excision, and accurate and appropriate repair.

References

1. Roentgen, W. C.: On a new kind of ray. Erst. Mitt. Sitzgrber., Physik-Med. Ges. Wurzburg, 137: Dec., 1895. (Translated by Stanton, A.: Nature, 53:274, 1896.

2. Hawks, H. D.: The physiologic effects of x-rays. Elect. Eng., 22:276, 1896.
3. Daniel, J.: The x-rays. Science, 3:562, 1896.
4. Marcuse, W.: Nachtrag zu dem Fall von Dermatitis and Alopecie nach Durchleuchtungeversuchen unit Roentgen Strahlen. Dtsch. Med. Wochenschr., 22:681, 1896.
5. Codman, E. A., and Thompson, E.: The cause of burns from x-rays. Boston Med. Surg. J., 135:610, 1896.
6. Porter, C. A., and White, C. J.: Multiple carcinomata following chronic x-ray dermatitis. Ann. Surg., 46:649, 1907.
7. Porter, C. A.: The surgical treatment of x-ray carcinoma and other severe x-ray lesions. J. Med. Res., 21:357, 1909.
8. Frieben, A.: Cancroid nach laugdauernder Einwirkung von Roentgenstrahlen. Fortschr. Roentgenstr., 6:106, 1902.
9. Brown, P.: American Martyrs to Science through the Roentgen Rays. Springfield, IL, Charles C Thomas, 1936.
10. Schofield, G. B., et al.: Assessment and management of a plutonium-contaminated wound case. Health Phys., 26:541, 1974.
11. Urbach, F.: Pathologic effects of ionizing radiation. In Fitzpatrick, T. B. (ed.): Dermatology in General Medicine, New York, McGraw-Hill, Inc. 1971. pp. 1036–1043.
12. Wolbach, S. B.: Summary of effects of repeated roentgen-ray exposure on human skin antecedent to formation of carcinoma. Am. J. Roentgenol., 13:139, 1925.
13. Rintala, A.: Local radiation burns: a clinical study of 198 burns with special reference to treatment by plastic surgery. Acta Chir. Scand. (Suppl):376, 1967.
14. Saunders, T. S., and Montgomery, H.: Chronic roentgen and radium dermatitis. J.A.M.A., 110:23, 1938.
15. Teloh, H. A., et al.: A histopathologic study of radiation injuries of the skin. Sugery, Gynecology and Obstetrics, 90:335, 1950.
16. Cannon, B., et al.: Malignant irradiation for benign conditions. N. Engl. J. Med., 260:197, 1959.
17. Robinson, D. W., and Masters, F. W.: Surgery for radiation injury. Arch. Surg., 80:946, 1960.
18. Hartwell, S., et al.: Radiation dermatitis and radiogenic neoplasms of the hand. Ann. Surg., 160:828, 1964.
19. Conway, H., and Hugo, N. E.: Radiation dermatitis and malignancy. Plast. Reconstr. Surg., 38:255, 1966.
20. Holmstrom, H., and Johanson, B.: Local radiation injury and its surgical treatment. Scand. J. Plast. Reconstr. Surg., 6:156, 1972.
21. Krizek, T. J., and Ariyan, S.: Severe acute radiation injuries of the hands. Plast. Reconstr. Surg., 51:14, 1973.
22. Caldwell, E., and McCormack, R. M.: Acute radiation injury of the hands. Report of a case with a 21-year follow-up. J. Hand Surg., 5:568, 1980.
23. Lanzl, L. H., Rosenfield, M. L., and Tarlov, A.: Injury due to accidental high dose exposure to 10-meV electrons. Health Phys., 13:241, 1967.
24. Brown, J. B., et al.: Application of permanent pedicle blood-carrying flaps. Plast. Reconstr. Surg., 8:335, 1951.

7

COMPLICATIONS FOLLOWING THERMAL INJURIES

John A. Boswick, Jr.
Nashaat Naam

Severe burns of the hands often result in marked impairment of function, severe deformities and, consequently, severe emotional problems. The definitive treatment of burned hands is sometimes delayed because of concentrating on the acute resuscitation of the patient, a delay that could lead to serious complications. In recent years, more attention has been directed toward an early and aggressive treatment regimen to salvage more burned hands. Several factors contribute to the outcome of treatment and occurrence of complications in severe burns of the hands, such as the nature of the burn, location, extent, and depth of the burn, patient's age, type of treatment, and patient cooperation.[1, 2]

INCREASED INTRACOMPARTMENTAL PRESSURE

Circumferential burns of the extremity have the potential of compromising blood flow to the distal part, producing varying degrees of ischemic necrosis. The progressive accumulation of edematous fluid in the unyielding fibromuscular compartment gradually obstructs lymphatic and venous drainage, capillary flow and, ultimately, arterial flow. The presence of rigid burn eschar and the massive fluid therapy used in burn resuscitation contribute significantly to the increase in compartmental pressure in burned extremities.[3] The fingers are particularly at risk of ischemia because of their thin skin, minimal soft tissue protection, and scanty collateral circulation.

The presence of pallor, cyanosis, impaired capillary filling, or impairment of neurologic function should alert the physician to the possibility of compromised blood flow. All distal pulses should be monitored periodically using Doppler ultrasound. However, relying only on Doppler pulses may sometimes delay the performance of escharotomies.[3, 4] Many studies have confirmed the inaccuracies of Doppler pulses in assessing the state of limb perfusion. Clayton found absent or significantly decreased muscle blood flow in burned extremities, despite the presence of distal pulses.[4]

Direct measurement of intramuscular compartment pressure using the wick catheter can help in defining the indications for escharotomy more accurately, without reliance on inconsistent clinical signs.[9] The catheter is inserted percutaneously into the underlying muscle. The position of the catheter tip can be confirmed by the appearance of a pressure spike when the muscle contracts. The site of catheter placement is usually the volar aspect of the forearm, midway between the elbow and the wrist. Sometimes another catheter is placed in the dorsum of the hand in the second interosseous muscle.[5] An intramuscular pressure of 30 mm Hg is considered to be the upper limit of normal, and any increase above that limit means a significant increase in intracompartmental pressure.

It has been found that patients who have greater than 30% of total body surface area burn, greater than 10% total body surface area full-thickness burn, or circumferential burns of the arms have a significantly higher incidence of elevated intramuscular pressure measurement.[3] Direct measurement of the intercompartmental pressure is generally recommended in all patients with extensive extremity burns.

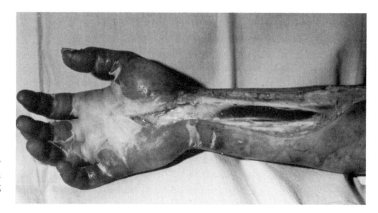

Figure 7–1. Fasciotomy in severely burned upper extremity. The incision should be extended to the palm, opening the transverse carpal ligament.

Decompressive escharotomy should be performed immediately if distal pulses are absent by Doppler, or if the intramuscular pressure is greater than 30 mm Hg.[3, 6] Escharotomy or fasciotomy is done on the volar aspect of the forearm, extending to the palm and dividing the transverse carpal ligament (Fig. 7–1). The interosseous muscles are decompressed by vertical incisions between the metacarpals, which open the fascial sheath surrounding the muscle. Digital escharotomy is performed through unilateral or preferably bilateral incisions, which are placed more toward the dorsum of the digit to avoid injury to the neurovascular bundles. The incision is carried down to the fat. Hemostasis is achieved with direct pressure and electrocautery.[7, 8] Effective decompressive escharotomy restores distal lymph perfusion. The return of pulses in the superficial palmar arch is an indication of adequate perfusion of the hand, but not necessarily of the fingers. Using Doppler ultrasound, Moylan and colleagues found that it took up to 24 hours to detect a return of digital blood flow in patients who had upper extremity escharotomy.[9] Thus, the absence of digital Doppler pulses in the early postescharotomy period does not necessarily indicate irreversible ischemia of the fingers.

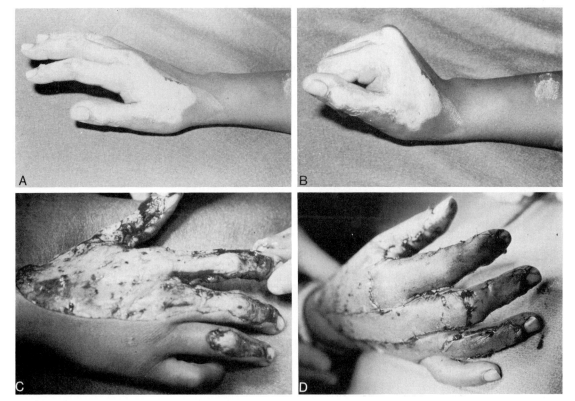

Figure 7–2. A through D, A full-thickness burn of the dorsum of the hand treated by early excision and grafting.

POSTBURN CONTRACTURES

Improper treatment of burned hands will result in different types of contractures, extensive scarring, and severe impairment of hand function. Early tangential excision and immediate autografting of deep burns of the hand have contributed significantly to improvement in functional results of treating burned hands. Early excision and grafting have the advantage of removing the necrotic tissue and converting open wounds into closed ones. This decreases wound edema, reduces the incidence of infection, reduces pain, enhances early mobilization of the hand and fingers and, consequently, helps to obtain maximal functional return (Fig. 7–2).[10-19]

Hand deformities secondary to burns are not due to contracture of collagen fibers per se, but to the fact that these fibers form around joints that are not optimally positioned. When collagen fibers mature, they will hold these joints in abnormal positions. This explains why the hand should be kept in functional position, and why careful attention should be directed toward keeping each joint in the hand in maximal functional position, using either external or internal splinting.[1, 20] Internal splinting is achieved by pinning the joint using K-wires. The wrist joint should be maintained in dorsiflexion. The metacarpophalangeal joints are kept in 70 to 90° flexion, the interphalangeal joints are kept extended, the thumb is kept in the position of grasp (abducted and anteposed), and the fingers are separated from each other.

Contractures of the Dorsum of the Hand. Severe burns of the dorsum of the hand frequently result in hypertrophic dorsal scarring, even in cases treated by early excision and skin grafting.[21] This dorsal scarring may cause hyperextension of the metacarpophalangeal joints and clawing of the fingers, with contracture of web spaces. The resulting impairment of function is especially important in the first web space. Boutonnière deformity or swan-neck deformity may result from destruction of the extensor mechanism of the fingers.

Contractures of Web Spaces. Several techniques have been described to correct these deformities. Z-plasty or YV advancement is usually sufficient to widen the web space. Cases with severe contractures may need excision or division of the scarred area

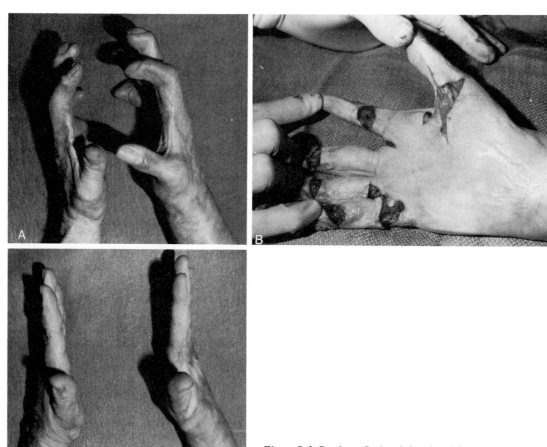

Figure 7–3. Postburn flexion deformity of fingers of both hands (A) treated by scar division (B) and skin grafting, with good functional result (C).

and coverage of the resulting raw area by split- or full-thickness skin grafts, or by regional or distant flaps.[21, 23]

Volar Scars. Mild contractures of the volar aspects of the fingers can be corrected by simple or multiple Z-plasty. Extensive scarring needs excision of the scar, taking care not to injure the neurovascular bundles; the gap is then grafted with a thick split-thickness or full-thickness skin graft. Deep burns of the volar aspect of the fingers result in contracture of deep structures. Therefore, release of the contracted volar plate may be necessary to correct deformities of the finger. The tourniquet should be deflated before any attempt to straighten the finger is done. Otherwise, vascular compromise and ischemia may develop secondary to stretching the shortened neurovascular bundles. The finger is straightened gradually after deflating the tourniquet while the circulation of the finger is carefully watched. The joints are pinned in the maximally correct position with K-wires (Fig. 7–3).[21, 24]

Contractures of the Wrist, Elbow, and Axilla. Volar contractures of the wrist, elbow, and axilla should be treated surgically if they cause significant impairment of functional activity. The contracture is treated by division or excision of the hypertrophic scar, followed by grafting or flap reconstruction.

HYPERTROPHIC SCARS

Hypertrophic scars may complicate burns of the hand and upper extremity. Apart from the disfiguring effect, they cause other problems such as itching, blistering, and discomfort. Serious joint contractures and deformities may develop if the scarring occurs around joints.[25] Hypertrophic scars usually soften and become flattened in 1 to 2 years, but sometimes it takes longer or persists permanently. Robitaille and co-workers have shown that the presence of edematous fluid inside the scar is a very important factor in formation and persistence of hypertrophic scars.[26] Various methods of treatment have been used, such as surgical excision, local steroid injection, and radiotherapy. The recurrence of the scarring frequently follows surgical excision, and it may even be larger than before the excision. Steroid injection is associated with a low response rate. Radiotherapy has the potential of inducing skin cancer.

In recent years, pressure garments have been used in treating hypertrophic scars, with excellent results. Control of local edema by the pressure garment may be the major factor in that type of treatment.

Using the electron microscope, Kischer found that external pressure could induce an internal rearrangement of the collagen fibers within the hypertrophic scar.[27] Biochemical changes related to collagen metabolism have been noticed in hypertrophic scars after local steroid injections and external pressure application.[28] The pressure garments are supposed to exert a uniform pressure on the desired area, and should maintain even pressure on the scar. The patient is supplied with two sets of garments, so that one set is worn while the other is being washed. The garments should be checked regularly, making sure that they fit snugly and that they exert firm pressure on the scarred area. Treatment should continue for not less than 6 months, and the condition is then reassessed to determine if further treatment is necessary.

HETEROTOPIC PERIARTICULAR OSSIFICATION

Heterotopic periarticular ossification is an uncommon complication of thermal injury. The injury site of this periarticular ossification is the posterior aspect of the elbow joint, but it may affect other joints. It has also been reported in the interosseous membrane between the radius and the ulna at the wrist or elbow level.[6, 29] Spontaneous resolution has been reported to occur in this type of calcification.[24] The incidence of heterotopic calcification varies in different reports. Jackson found an incidence of 0.1% in the patients treated at the Birmingham Accident Hospital Burn Unit.[30] However, Munster and associates noted that, in 160 burned upper limbs, 18 (11.3%) developed heterotopic calcification, but 13 of them (8.1%) showed spontaneous resolution with return to normal range of motion. The remaining five limbs (3.1%) required surgical intervention.[31]

The true etiology and pathogenesis of this calcification are unknown, but it seems that it is unrelated to intra-articular bony ankylosis that sometimes complicates burns.[29, 31, 32] There is no correlation between the area of the body surface burned or the immobilization of the patient and the periarticular calcification. However, there is a significant correlation between the severity and depth of upper extremity burns and the development of heterotopic calcification.

The relationship between disturbance in calcium metabolism, which is often seen in burn patients, and heterotopic calcification is not fully known. November-Dusansky and colleagues found that a high protein intake, in excess of 150 g/day, increases calcium mobilization and negative calcium balance, thereby leading to extraosseous calcium deposits and the formation of renal stones.[33] Postburn heterotopic calcification that is associated with normal alkaline phosphatase levels is not similar to ossification in paraplegic patients, in whom the serum alkaline phosphatase level is usually elevated.[34] Local injury and formation of hematoma between the triceps and humerus may be the initiating factor leading to calcium deposition and later ossification of the area.[31]

Clinically, the earliest sign is slight loss of active range of motion, which progresses gradually to partial or complete limitation of joint movement. Heterotopic calcifications appear on radiographs as a fluffy shadow posterior to the elbow joint and anterior to the triceps insertion. The calcification gradually spreads to the medial epicondyle, and sometimes to the lateral epicondyle. The calcifica-

tion may resolve spontaneously or progress into ossification with formation of mature bone.

Surgical excision of the heterotopic ossification should be delayed until the heterotopic bone is

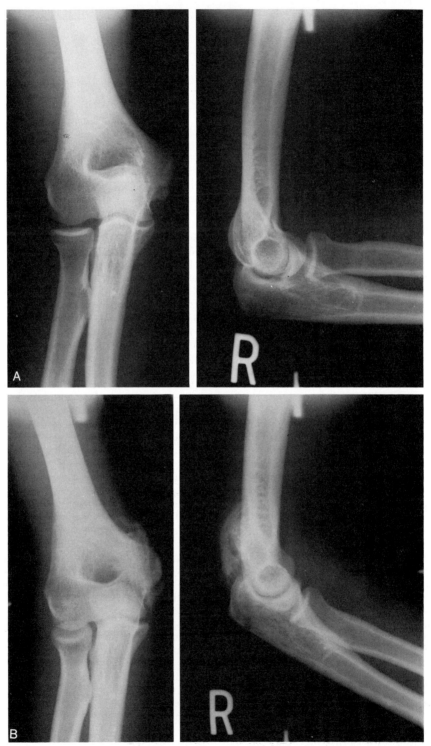

Figure 7–4. *A,* Periarticular heterotopic ossification of the right elbow extending toward the medial side; *B,* the same elbow after surgical excision of the heterotopic bone. The patient regained full range of motion.

mature to prevent recurrence. The results of surgical treatment are generally very good, with return of excellent range of motion (Fig. 7–4).

DISORDERS OF BONY GROWTH

Occasionally in children, premature fusion of epiphyseal plates of the hand bones occurs following burns. This leads to growth arrest or progressive angulation if growth in one part of the plate is arrested while it continues in the rest.[22, 30] Recently, a new surgical technique has been described to correct this problem by removal of the bony bridge caused by the premature fusion and replacement of a free graft. This will result in healing of the epiphyseal plate with cartilage, and the deformity will be corrected spontaneously over 2 to 3 years by normal growth, avoiding the need for multiple osteotomies.[35]

AMPUTATIONS

The indications for amputations following burns are diminishing. Severe ischemia leading to limb necrosis, severe postburn infection, or clostridial myonecrosis that threaten the patient's life are probably the only indications for amputation.

References

1. Boswick, J. A.: Thermal burns of the upper extremity. *In* Flynn, J. E. (ed.): Hand Surgery, 3rd ed., Baltimore, Williams & Wilkins, 1982, p. 586.
2. Boswick, J. A.: The management of fresh burns of the hand and deformities resulting from burn injuries. Clin. Plast. Surg., 1:621, 1974.
3. Saffle, J. R., Zeluff, G. R., and Warden, G. D.: Intramuscular pressure in the burned arm: Measurement and response to escharotomy. Am. J. Surg., 140:825, 1980.
4. Clayton, J. M., et al.: Sequential circulatory changes in the circumferentially burned extremity. Ann. Surg., 185:391, 1977.
5. Mubarak, S. J., et al.: The wick catheter technique for measurement of intramuscular pressure. J. Bone Joint Surg., 58A:1016, 1976.
6. Pruitt, B. A.: Complications of thermal injury. Clin. Plast. Surg., 1:667, 1974.
7. Salisbury, R. E., Taylor, J. W., and Levine, N. S.: Evaluation of digital escharotomy in burned hands. Plast. Reconstr. Surg., 58:440, 1976.
8. Boswick, J.A.: Management of the burned hand. Orthop. Clin. North Am., 1:311, 1970.
9. Moylan, J. A., Inge, W. W., and Pruitt, B. A.: Circulatory changes following circumferential extremity burn evaluated by the ultrasonic flowmeter. J. Trauma, 11:763, 1971.
10. Janzekovic, Z.: A new concept in the early excision and immediate grafting of burns. J. Trauma, 10:1103, 1970.
11. Hunt, J. L., Sato, R., and Baxter, C. R.: Early tangential excision and immediate mesh autografting of deep dermal hand burns. Ann. Surg., 189:147, 1979.
12. Monafo, W. M.: Tangential excision. Clin. Plast. Surg., 1:591, 1974.
13. Hunt, J. L., Sato, R. M.: Early excision of full-thickness hand and digit burns: Factors affecting morbidity. J. Trauma, 22:414, 1982.
14. Levine, B. A., et al.: Efficacy of tangential excision and immediate autografting of deep second-degree burns of the hand. J. Trauma, 19:670, 1979.
15. Salisbury, R. E., and Wright, P.: Evaluation of early excision of dorsal burns of the hand. Plast. Reconstr. Surg., 65:670, 1982.
16. Magliacani, G., Bormioli, M., and Cerutti, V.: Late result following treatment of deep burns of the hand. Scand. J. Plast. Reconstr. Surg., 13:137, 1979.
17. Habal, M. G.: The burned hand: A planned treatment program. J. Trauma, 18:587, 1978.
18. Corlett, R. J.: The treatment of deep burns of the hand. Aust. N.Z. J. Surg., 49:567, 1979.
19. Wexler, M. R., and Rousso, M.: The immediate treatment of the burned hand. Prog. Surg., 16:165, 1978.
20. Mehrotra, O. N.: Salvage procedures for mutilated burnt hands. Aust. N.Z. J. Surg., 50:278, 1980.
21. Rousso, M., and Wexler, M. R.: Secondary reconstruction of the burned hand. Prog. Surg., 16:182, 1978.
22. Craven, R. E., and Duran, R. J.: Management of burn deformities of a hand. Am. J. Surg., 100:802, 1960.
23. Leung, P. C., and Chow, Y. Y. N.: Treatment of burned hand. Burns, 8:338, 1981.
24. Salisbury, R. E., and Dingeldein, G. P.: The burned hand and upper extremity. *In* Green, D. P. (ed.): Operative Hand Surgery, New York, Churchill Livingstone, 1982, p. 1523.
25. Leung, P. C., and Ng, M.: Pressure treatment of hypertrophic scars resulting from burns. Burns, 6:244, 1979.
26. Robitaille, A., Halpern, D., and Kottke, F. J.: Correction of keloids and finger contractures in burn patients. Arch. Phys. Med. Rehab., 54:515, 1973.
27. Kischer, C. W.: Predictability of resolution of hypertrophic scars by scanning electron microscopy. J. Trauma, 15:205, 1975.
28. Michael, J. C., Mulleken, J. B., and Hoopes, J. E.: Effect of intralesional injection of triamcinolone on G-6-PD and alanine aminotransferase activity in keloids. Plast. Reconstr. Surg., 56:660, 1975.
29. Heslop, J.H.: Heterotopic periarticular ossification in burns. Burns, 8:436, 1982.
30. Jackson, D. M.: Destructive burns: Some orthopedic complications. Burns, 7:105, 1980.
31. Munster, A. M., et al.: Heterotopic calcification following burns: A prospective study. J. Trauma, 12:1071, 1973.
32. Boyd, B. M., Roberts, W. M., and Miller, G. R.: Periarticular ossification following burns. South. Med. J., 52:1048, 1959.
33. November-Dusansky, A., Moylan, J. A., and Linkswiler, H.: Calciuretic response to protein loading in burn patients. Burns, 6:198, 1980.
34. Furman, R., Nicholas, J. J., and Jivoff, L.: Elevation of the serum alkaline phosphates coincident with ectopic bone formation in paraplegic patients. J. Bone Joint Surg., 52A:1131, 1970.
35. Langenskiold, A.: An operation for partial closure of an epiphysial plate in children and its experimental basis. J. Bone Joint Surg., 57B:325, 1975.

COMPLICATIONS FOLLOWING ELECTRICAL INJURIES

John A. Boswick, Jr.
Nashaat Naam

Electrical injuries may have three major types of effects: (1) those that occur distant to the site of entrance and exit of the current (e.g., the heart, central nervous system, eyes); (2) those that occur as a direct effect of the current as it travels from the point of entrance to exit; and (3) those caused by flashes and flames, such as burning clothing, which result from the current igniting a fire or from the arcing effect of electrical energy as it passes from one area to another. In this chapter we will discuss the complications that occur from the direct effect of electrical energy on the tissues of the upper extremity. To understand the complications and problems that occur as a result of electrical energy passsing through living tissue, it is necessary to remember that electrical energy is converted to heat when it meets a resistance—that is, Joule's law. Therefore, the greater the resistance of a tissue, the greater the heat and presumably the amount of damage to the involved structures.[1-3] In the extremities, tissue resistance to electrical current, in order of diminishing resistance, is bone, cartilage, tendon, skin, muscles, vessels, and nerves.

An excellent example of this phenomenon is the electrical injury that occurs when a hand is the point of entrance of the current and the other hand or another anatomic area is the exit. As the current moves into the forearm, the muscles that flex the wrist and fingers contract, causing the fingers and wrists to flex. This results in the offending object being grasped more firmly and when the wrist flexes, there is an arcing effect from the flexed fingers that are holding the electrically charged object to the volar surface of the wrist, causing a concentration of the current at the wrist area. A full-thickness skin injury usually occurs. The skeletal muscles are damaged by the generated heat and by the ischemic

effect resulting from thrombosis of their blood vessels. The muscle damage may be remote from the site of skin injury and out of proportion to the skin damage.[4]

Peripheral nerves may show a refractory period while keeping their anatomic integrity, unless the generated heat is sufficient to cause tissue death.[5, 6] Microscopically, there is perivascular hemorrhage, edema, and demyelination associated with neuronal death. Delayed neurologic injury has been described to occur as late as 1½ to 2 years following the injury.

Vascular damage from electrical injury may occur secondary to three different mechanisms:

1. Direct effect of electric current. The intensity of an electric current has sufficient heat to burn the vessel wall. The extent of vascular wall damage is more manifest in the inner layer of the vessel wall. The endothelial cells become necrotic and, in some areas, may show severe edema with degeneration of the internal elastic membrane and of the internal layer of smooth muscles. These changes may be found at a distance from the site of injury.

2. Effect of heat transmitted from the surrounding tissues. This causes full-thickness degeneration or necrosis, as seen in thermal burns.

3. Liquefaction necrosis of the blood vessels. Infection may cause this at a later stage. The resulting vascular injury may lead to thrombosis or delayed hemorrhage.[7-9]

INCREASED COMPARTMENTAL PRESSURE

A major problem in patients with electrical injuries is the increase in muscle compartmental pressure that, if left to progress, may lead to permanent

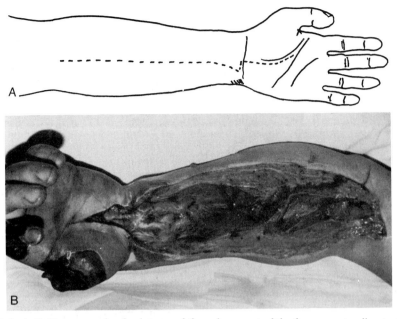

Figure 8–1. A, B, Decompressing fasciotomy of the volar aspect of the forearm extending to the palm.

tissue damage from inadequate perfusion. The increase in compartmental pressure is mainly due to capillary damage and the resultant interstitial edema, which occur even before the fluid resuscitation. Decompressive fasciotomy should be done as early as possible to prevent further compromise of tissue perfusion and to allow direct inspection of these tissues to assess their viability. Direct measurement of compartmental pressure using the wick catheter may be helpful in deciding early fasciotomies.

The decompressing incision should start in the palm, including opening the transverse carpal ligament and the fascia over the flexor muscles well into the proximal forearm (Fig. 8–1). Occasionally,

neurolysis of median and ulnar nerves may be necessary if they are swollen and severely edematous.[5] Digital escharotomy and intrinsic fasciotomy may be indicated in cases with marked swelling of the hand and fingers (Fig. 8–2).

Clinical assessment of muscle viability is often inaccurate. The initial appearance of the muscle may be deceiving, because residual hemoglobin gives the muscle a normal red color when exposed to air.[4, 10] Use of arteriography is also not helpful in assessing muscle viability because it fails to visualize the small muscular branches. Muscle biopsies are accurate but not practical because of the time factor and the necessity of obtaining a large number of biopsies.

Figure 8–2. Fasciotomy of the dorsum of the hand in electrical injury.

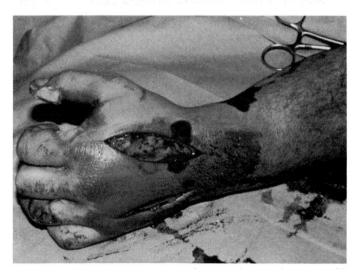

The technetium-99m (^{99m}Tc) pyrophosphate scan has emerged as a reliable and sensitive diagnostic adjunct in determining the degree and extent of muscle damage. It has been very helpful in guiding subsequent débridement following initial fasciotomy.[4, 11, 12] The necrotic or irreversibly nonvascularized tissues appear as "cold" (i.e., nonperfused) areas on the scan. Areas with increased uptake that appear "hot" on the scan correspond to muscles with 20 to 80% necrotic muscle fibers.[11, 12] Those areas with partially damaged muscle fibers should be observed frequently to determine the necessity of débridement.

The débridement is better done in the operating room using the Bovie to minimize blood loss. If more than one limb needs to be débrided, it is preferable to use a two-team approach. Débridement should be conservative, removing only the obviously necrotic areas and repeating the débridement at 48-hour intervals.

Wound care after fasciotomy is of the utmost importance in preserving the exposed tissues, which should be kept moist. Saline wet dressings, topical agents such as silver sulfadiazine or Sulfamylon, or biologic dressings such as homografts or heterografts have been used successfully in wound management. Primary closure of the fasciotomy wound can be done if tissue edema subsides rapidly. Otherwise, some form of skin coverage using grafts or flaps may be necessary for wound coverage.

NEUROLOGIC INJURY

As stated above, nerve tissue has the least resistance to electric current. It is also very susceptible to thermal injury. Neurologic injury can be immediate or delayed, and may even appear after up to 2 years.[13] Early fasciotomy is extremely important to prevent further ischemic injury of the nerve and to permit return of function. It is very difficult clinically to assess nerve viability or the possibility of return of function. The nerves may be grossly anatomically intact, but they may lose their function either temporarily or permanently. The exposed nerve should be covered, perferably by the patient's own skin through local or distant flaps, to preserve viability.[4]

ARTERIAL INJURY

Apart from the extensive soft tissue damage caused by the electrical injury, major blood vessels of the upper extremity may be also segmentally damaged, leading to impairment of the blood supply of the distal part of the extremity. As a result the limb becomes necrosed, and amputation may become necessary. If residual circulation is maintained and collateral circulation is established the limb may survive, but ischemic contractures may render the limb functionally useless.[8]

Manifestations

In the early stages the hand appears swollen and cyanotic, with low temperature. Fasciotomy provides only slight improvement. Gradually, the hand color becomes dark and the temperature progressively drops. Ischemia may progress into frank gangrene. Pulses at the radial, ulnar, and digital levels should be monitored periodically. Disappearance of pulsations is an indication of arterial obstruction. The presence of pulse at the early stage cannot, however, rule out arterial injury, because thrombosis secondary to intimal injury may take a few days to occur.

Treatment

Arteriography may show filling defects, beady appearance, thrombosed segments, or nonvisualization of the distal part of the ulnar or radial artery, or of both. The involved arteries should be explored, and the damaged segment excised. The excision should be done sequentially until adequate pulsatile flow is obtained. Frozen section biopsies should be taken from the cut ends of the vessel wall to make sure that the resection of the damaged vessel is adequate and that the remaining vessel is normal. Following adequate resection, a transposition vein graft is used to bridge the defect in the resected vessel.[8] In patients with injury to the deep or superficial palmar arch, vascular grafts using microvascular techniques may prove valuable in restoring the blood supply of the hand.

WOUND COVERAGE

Following fasciotomy and repeated débridement, the wound should be covered with a biologic dressing, either a homograft or heterograft. Such a dressing is bacteriostatic, promotes healthy granulation tissue, and prevents tissue dessication.[6] Maintenance of tissue integrity of nerves is often difficult with a homograft. Therefore, definite wound closure with an autograft or flaps should be achieved as early as possible.

Split-thickness skin grafts are very useful for definitive closure because of their simplicity, good chance of success, low risk, and relatively good endurance in contact with prosthesis.[5, 14, 15] Local or distant skin flaps may be necessary for covering the vital structures and areas in which secondary reconstruction is to be performed. In recent years, with advanced microvascular techniques, free skin flaps have been used for wound coverage.[16] However, because of the associated arterial injury, it may not be suitable in some cases.

SEPTIC COMPLICATIONS

Wound infection and clostridial myonecrosis may complicate electrical injuries. Early débridement

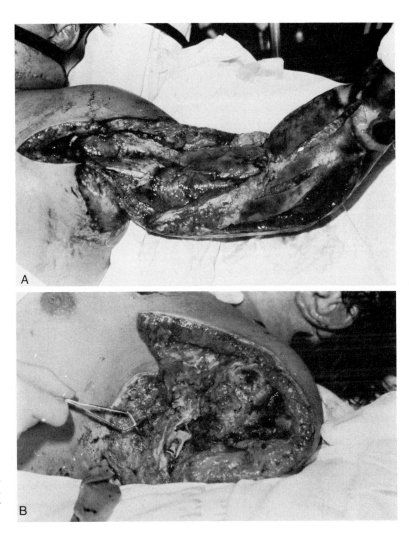

Figure 8–3. Severe electrical injury with massive soft tissue necrosis *(A)* resulting in shoulder disarticulation*(B)*.

and wound coverage are very important in preventing wound infection. Osteomyelitis, septic arthritis, and infection of amputation stumps are other infrequent septic complications.

AMPUTATION

The overall incidence of amputation following electrical injury remains high. The United States Army Institute of Surgical Research treated 85 patients with electrical injury to the upper extremities between 1950 and 1974, and 43% of these patients required limb amputation.[17] In another series, 65% of the patients needed some type of amputation.[5]

Amputation is indicated to save the patient's life if extensive muscle necrosis or infection threatens the patient's life (Fig. 8–3). It is also indicated in cases of severe irreparable vascular injury. If amputation is necessary, the maximal possible length of limb should be kept for adequate prosthetic fitting and function.

MAINTENANCE OF FUNCTION

Active motion of all joints should be encouraged as early and as much as possible to avoid joint stiffness and wound contracture. The involved extremity should be elevated above the level of the heart for 24 hours to minimize edema formation. The use of splints may be helpful in preventing deformities and in maintaining appropriate positioning. The wrist should be kept in the dorsiflexion position to provide a better balance for the extensor muscles over the powerful flexors and to improve the flexion of the metacarpophalangeal joints. The metacarpophalangeal joints should be kept in flexion to keep the collateral ligaments stretched and to prevent joint stiffness. Extension of the interphalangeal joints is important to avoid disruption of the center slip and boutonnière deformity. If deformities develop later in spite of all the precautionary measures, and they do not respond to splinting, surgical correction is indicated.

References

1. Hunt, J. L., and Pruitt, B. A.: Vascular lesions in acute electrical injuries. J. Trauma, 14:461, 1974.
2. Hunt, J. L., and Pruitt, B. A.: The pathophysiology of acute electrical injuries. J. Trauma, 17:487, 1977.
3. Ponten, B., Erikson, U., and Olding, L.: New observations on tissue changes along the pathway of the current in an electrical injury. Scand. J. Plast. Reconstr. Surg., 4:75, 1970.
4. Holliman, C. J., et al.: Early surgical decompression in the management of electrical injuries. Am. J. Surg., 144:733, 1982.
5. Butler, E. D., and Grant, T. D.: Electrical injuries with special reference to the upper extremities: A review of 182 cases. Am. J. Surg., 134:385, 1977.
6. Solem, L., and Strate, R. G.: The natural history of electrical injuries. J. Trauma, 17:487, 1977.
7. Hunt, J. L., and Pruitt, B. A.: Vascular lesions in acute electrical injuries. J. Trauma, 14:461, 1974.
8. Wang, X., et al.: Early vascular grafting to prevent upper extremity necrosis after electrical burns. Burns, 8:303, 1982.
9. Wang, X., and Xoh, W.: Arterial injuries in electrically burned upper limbs and effect of early reconstruction of blood circulation to the wrist. Burns, 8:379, 1982.
10. Burke, J. F., et al.: Pattern of high-tension electrical injury in children and adolescents and their management. Am. J. Surg., 133:492, 1977.
11. Hunt, J., et al .: The use of technetium-99^m stannous pyrophosphate scintigraphy to identify muscle damage in acute electrical burns. J. Trauma, 19:409, 1979.
12. Hunt, J. L., Sato, R. M., and Baxter, C. R.: Acute electric burns. Arch. Surg., 115:434, 1980.
13. Christensen, J. A., et al.: Delayed neurologic injury secondary to high-voltage current with recovery. J. Trauma, 20:166, 1980.
14. Salisbury, R. E., and Pruitt, B. A.: Management of electrical burns of the upper extremities. J. Plast. Reconstr. Surg., 51:648, 1973.
15. Peterson, R. A.: Electrical burns of the hand: Treatment by early excision. J. Bone Joint Surg., 48A:407, 1966.
16. Sharzer, L. R., and O'Brien, M. C.: Clinical application of free flap transfer in the burn patient. J. Trauma, 15:767, 1975.
17. Salisbury, R. E., and Pruitt, B. A.: Burns of the Upper Extremity, Philadelphia, W. B. Saunders, 1976, pp. 72–83.

9

POSTTRAUMATIC DYSTROPHY

George E. Omer

Pain is an intensely personal perceptual behavior state. Reflex sympathetic dystrophy is a neurovascular process involving severe pain, swelling, discoloration, stiffness, and dysfunction of a peripheral nerve containing many sympathetic axons. The most significant description of this process following gunshot wounds was reported by Mitchell, and he initiated use of the word "causalgia" (from the Greek words meaning burning pain).[28] Later, similar symptoms were recorded following minor trauma, such as the "acute bone atrophy" described by Sudeck.[12] Reflex sympathetic dystrophy is not the only cause of pain, but it is well known as a group of disastrous symptoms following trauma or a surgical procedure in what may seem to have been a normal extremity.

NEUROPHYSIOLOGY

The sympathetic nervous system of the upper extremity is concentrated in the thoracic portion of the spinal cord. Myelinated sympathetic axons exit the cord via the anterior nerve root and then separate to form the white rami that enter the thoracic ganglia. A synapse occurs, and the postganglionic unmyelinated axons exit from the thoracic ganglia and enter the peripheral nerve. Because preganglionic axons form plexuses and synapse with many different postganglionic axons, a sympathetic discharge may affect several different target organs represented in more than one dermatome. Activation of a sympathetic discharge may elicit either an excitatory or an inhibitory response in different target organs, based on the relative potencies of the various catecholamines released at the neuroeffector junction. During an abnormal process, such as reflex sympathetic dystrophy, there may be great variations in the extremity, such as vasodilation or vasoconstriction, increased redness or pallor, sweating or dryness, and coolness or heat, depending on the severity or stage of involvement of different target organs.

Pain is related to free nerve endings termed nociceptors. In the peripheral nervous system, ap-

proximately 25% of the small myelinated axons ("A-delta"; class III), and approximately 50% of the smaller unmyelinated axons ("C-delta"; class IV) are nociceptors. The action potential produced by stimulation of the nociceptors passes to a synapse in the dorsal horn of the spinal cord, which has six laminae of cell networks that process as well as transmit the impulses.[26] The convergence of visceral and cutaneous axons into the dorsal horn may represent the basic mechanism of referred pain. Nociceptive impulses are transmitted from the dorsal horn to all levels of the central nervous system through specific tracts such as the spinothalamic system or multisynaptic afferent systems such as the spinoreticular system. Supraspinal descending neural systems modify the nociceptive impulses and affect transmission in the thalamus, reticular formation, dorsal column of the spinal cord, and other relay systems.[8, 27]

There is a relationship between humoral mediators and pain. All injured cells release prostaglandins and thromboxanes. These mediators are also liberated by mechanical, electrical, radiation, or thermal injury. They induce pain by lowering the threshold to pain transmission and by increasing the intensity of the stimulus.[30] Injured nerve axons are excited by norepinephrine, which is the substance released at the neuroeffector junction by efferent impulses in the sympathetic nervous system.[35] In the normal intact sensory nerve, sympathetic transmitters do not evoke obvious injury signals, although they may modulate sensitivity. Partially damaged nerve membrane and the unmyelinated axons (sprouts) within a neuroma are highly sensitive to norepinephrine. Stimulation of myelinated axons releases local endorphins, which dampen or stop the oversensitive spontaneous activity of these unmyelinated axons at the spinal cord level. When tissue is injured, the nociceptors are influenced by sympathetic efferents, the chemical environment, the vasculature, the temperature, and high-frequency antidromic impulses.[36]

Peripheral nerve irritation, abnormal sympathetic function, and psychological factors all contribute to reflex sympathetic dystrophy. The treatment program for every patient afflicted with this difficult neurovascular process must be approached on an individual basis.

TREATMENT

There are only two principles in the treatment of an established pain syndrome involving an extremity—relieve the pain, and institute active use of the involved extremity.[20-23] The pain process related to reflex sympathetic dystrophy may be divided into three categories: "trigger-point" excitation; diffuse burning pain; and referred or systemic response.

The surgeon should avoid unnecessary tissue trauma and accidental nerve injury, such as laceration of the superficial radial nerve, during an elective procedure. Meticulous hemostasis will decrease the potential for edema. Prevention of pain before and after elective surgery minimizes the risk of persistent postoperative pain. Aspirin is effective to block the metabolic pathway from injured cells to prostaglandins and thromboxanes.[37] A number of patients will develop gastritis with aspirin. The prescription should be changed to a buffered preparation, such as Ascriptin. Other oral medications, such as vitamin C, which can increase gastric activity, should be discontinued. A mild tranquilizer, such as hydroxyzine pamoate, reduces the incidence of analgesic side effects, including nausea and vomiting, and promotes the inhibition of anxiety.[15] These medications are most effective during the first 24 to 72 hours after surgery. Precarious preservation of all possible segments of an injured extremity may result in prolonged pain. Poor skin coverage and diminished sensation complicate functional retraining and increase cold sensitivity. Postoperative elevation of the extremity will decrease intracellular edema and accumulation of pain mediators.

Every patient who suppresses voluntary movement of an injured extremity because it is painful should be placed on a supervised program of gentle but active mobilization. Early motion is essential to prevent joint contractures and muscle atrophy, and will eliminate pain in many patients. The best management anticipates the problem, and active motion is begun before pain has become an established neurovascular process.

"Trigger-Point" Pain

A distorted quality of sensation, or of altered sensibility, is a transient experience in almost all injuries involving peripheral nerves, and may be related to the preponderance of unmyelinated fibers during regeneration. Injured nerve axons are excited by the norepinephrine released by sympathetic activity. A neuroma can become the trigger point for prolonged spontaneous pain, leading to narcotic addiction and emotional deterioration in a susceptible individual.

Transcutaneous electrical stimulation attempts to stimulate the larger myelinated axons selectively and to control pain by activating antidromic inhibitory mechanisms. The intensity should be varied by the patient because stimuli that are too intense overcome the inhibition mechanism and produce additional pain. Loeser and coworkers reported 198 patients in whom 68% obtained short-term relief and 12.5% used the stimulator for long-term pain control.[13] Long studied 400 patients with pain; 33% found the stimulating device to be of sufficient value to use it as the only method of pain therapy, while an additional 44% found stimulation to be a beneficial adjunct in their overall treatment program, which included behavior modification, drug withdrawal, and physical activity.[14] The best results are obtained when electrical stimulation is given within 3 months of the onset of pain. In my patients with

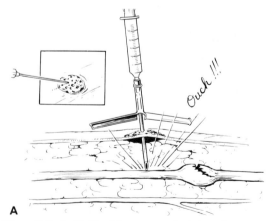 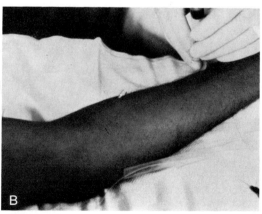

Figure 9–1. A, B, The 16-gauge needle is introduced near the "trigger point" of pain after local cutaneous anesthetic block. Usually the needle should be proximal to the "trigger point." Continuous pain after insertion would suggest penetration of the epineurium, and the needle should be withdrawn slightly. (*A* from Omer, G. E., Jr.: Continuous peripheral epineural infusion for the treatment of acute pain. *In* Omer, G. E., Jr., and Spinner, M. (eds.): Management of Peripheral Nerve Problems, Philadelphia, W. B. Saunders, 1980.)

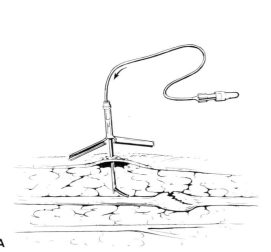

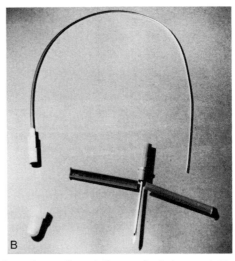

A

B

Figure 9–2. The 18-gauge intravenous catheter *(A)* is inserted down the needle and close to the "trigger point" of pain *(B)*. *(A* from Omer, G. E., Jr.: Continuous peripheral epineural infusion for the treatment of acute pain. *In* Omer, G. E., Jr., and Spinner, M. (eds.): Management of Peripheral Nerve Problems, Philadelphia, W. B. Saunders, 1980.)

chronic well-established pain, the percutaneous stimulator has produced consistent improvement only if operated continuously.

At Massachusetts General Hospital, operative placement of the electrodes directly on involved peripheral nerves for prolonged stimulation resulted in lasting relief of pain in only 30% of 44 patients followed for at least 6 months.[38] A similar study at Duke University reported lasting relief of pain in 36% of 20 patients followed for 30 months.[17, 18]

A peripheral chemical sympathetic block may be performed on the ward.[20, 24, 25] A 16-gauge needle is inserted into the trigger point (Fig. 9–1), and a flexible 18-gauge polyethylene intravenous catheter is inserted through the needle (Fig. 9–2). The needle is removed, leaving the catheter in place, and a solution of 0.5 ml of lidocaine hydrochloride 0.5% is injected (Fig. 9–3). If the pain is relieved,

the catheter is capped and taped into place, allowing exercise activity (Fig. 9–4). Additional periodic injections of lidocaine solution are based on the time of pain-free activity. The periodic infusion has been continued for a few days up to 2 weeks. If there is more than one trigger point, separate catheters should be used. This method is not effective in those patients in whom chronic pain has been untreated for 3 or more months.

Percutaneous injection of triamcinolone acetonide about the neuroma after a cutaneous block with lidocaine hydrochloride 2% has been reported to relieve pain symptoms in 50% of patients after one injection and in 80% of patients after multiple injections.[31] It was surmised that the steroid softens the fibrous tissue about the neuroma.

Percussion or massage of painful neuromas has been a clinical procedure in amputees since World

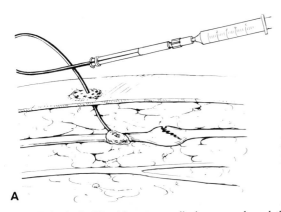

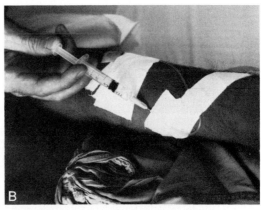

A

B

Figure 9–3. *A, B,* The 16-gauge needle is removed, and the local anesthetic agent is injected to obtain a peripheral chemical sympathetic block. Additional injections are given to provide pain-free activity. *(A* from Omer, G. E., Jr.: Continuous peripheral epineural infusion for the treatment of acute pain. *In* Omer, G. E., Jr., and Spinner, M. (eds.): Management of Peripheral Nerve Problems, Philadelphia, W. B. Saunders, 1980.)

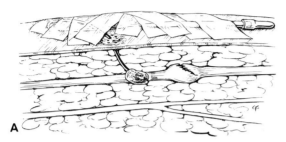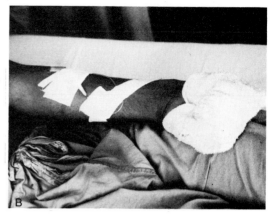

Figure 9–4. A, B, The intravenous catheter is capped and taped in place for physical medicine therapy. If the block cannot sustain relief after 2 or 3 days, the catheter is replaced to obtain an effective block. (*A* from Omer, G. E. Jr.: Continuous peripheral epineural infusion for the treatment of acute pain. *In* Omer, G. E., Jr., and Spinner, M. (eds.): Management of Peripheral Nerve Problems, Philadelphia, W. B. Saunders, 1980.)

War I. Controlled clinical studies have indicated that the technique is useful in selected cases.[7] Rubber mallets, mechanical vibrators, or ultrasonic treatments will provide the repetitious percussion. Anesthesia may be necessary over the trigger area at the onset of treatment, but percussion or massage may be done later without local anesthesia.

The best surgical procedure for a painful neuroma is transfer of the neuroma, attached to the proximal nerve stump, to a new site at which compression is unlikely and traction is minimal. The neuroma should be placed in an area of good circulation with a thick subcutaneous layer that is free of scar.

Success has been reported in 82% of patients treated with this technique.[4, 9] Only one repeat procedure is indicated in those patients with continued pain.[34] One should check for potential external pressure, such as a ligament or traction scar, on the neuroma in the healing wound.

Diffuse Burning Pain

This neurovascular process most often results from an injury to the median nerve or the brachial plexus. There is usually incomplete severance of the

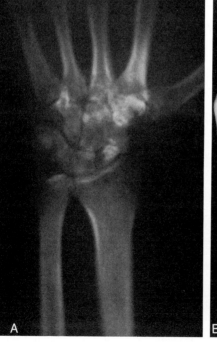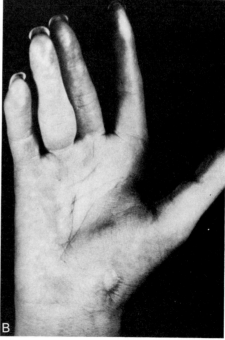

Figure 9–5. A and *B,* Sudeck's atrophy of the carpus following a fracture of the scaphoid. The proximal portion of the scaphoid is avacular, and retains normal density. The hand has trophic changes.

injured nerve, with retention of partial sensory and motor function. There has been an associated injury to a major artery in more than one third of my cases, in which burning pain was the immediate and dominant feature.[21] Half of my patients had characteristic symptoms on the day of injury and two thirds of the patients had them by the end of the first week after injury.[19, 22]

The loss of vascular, sudomotor, pilomotor, and muscle tone controls will result in profound nutritional (trophic) changes. There is atrophy of subcutaneous tissue, skin, muscle, and bone (Fig. 9–5). In the early stages the residual limb is markedly swollen and warm. There is hyperesthesia to light touch and sensitivity to cold. After 2 to 3 months there is fibrotic brawny edema. Contractures become fixed due to lack of active motion. Roentgenograms of the distal bones show patchy osteopenia. A bone scan (^{99m}Tc-etidronate disodium) will be positive before the bone resorption is visible on plain films.[29] Six to 9 months after onset of pain, the extremity becomes pale and cool, with either hyperhidrosis or dryness.

Initial treatment is interruption of the abnormal sympathetic reflex, and chemical central sympathetic block should be performed as a diagnostic test as well as a therapeutic procedure. I use solutions of either lidocaine hydrochloride 1% or mepivacaine hydrochloride 1% to produce peripheral warming and loss of sweating, as well as relief of pain. A series of four or five blocks should be given on consecutive days; one placebo of normal saline solution given during the series will confirm the value of the sympathetic block. Prognosis can be related to the effect of the sympathetic block: (1) one block may provide total relief; (2) one block may provide tolerable relief; (3) the duration of the first block may exceed that expected, and subsequent blocks may provide progressively longer relief; (4) the duration of the first block may exceed that expected, but subsequent blocks provide progressively shorter relief; and (5) the block may provide relief only for the duration expected from the anesthetic agent used.[20] For responses 1 through 3, a series of chemical central sympathetic blocks should lead to resolution of the pain syndrome and further treatment, other than physical medicine procedures, may be unnecessary.

Chemical blocks may be complicated by accidental penetration of the peripheral nerve. This potential problem is related to all injection therapy.

For responses 4 or 5, permanent improvement by sympathetic block should not be expected. Transcutaneous electric nerve stimulation should be considered for those patients whose pain persists after chemical central sympathetic block. Stilz and associates have shown an increase in cutaneous skin temperature of 1.5 to 2.5° C with this technique.[33] Some researchers have implanted electrodes to stimulate cells in the periaqueductal periventricular gray matter to release β-endorphin and obtain analgesia.[10]

In those patients with pain and associated is-chemia, various drugs that decrease sympathetic activity may be beneficial, including α-receptor blocking agents such as tolazoline hydrochloride and phenoxybenzamine hydrochloride, the β-adrenergic receptor blocking drug propranolol hydrochloride, and the neuronal norepinephrine depletors such as reserpine, methyldopa, or guanethidine. Chuinard and colleagues injected 1 mg of reserpine diluted in 50 ml of normal saline solution intravenously in the same technique as that used for intravenous regional anesthesia block.[3] Wynn-Parry used the same technique to inject 20 mg of guanethidine in 20 ml of normal saline solution. The tourniquet is released after 20 minutes.

Surgical sympathectomy should be performed when the burning pain responds to central chemical sympathectomy but requires as repeated series of blocks for long-term relief. Surgical sympathectomy will relieve only burning pain; associated painful neuromata or arthritic pain will not be altered. I prefer the transaxillary approach with removal of the sympathetic chain from the fourth thoracic level distal to the stellate ganglion.[11] Horner's syndrome often is not present after the transaxillary approach, which permits removal of only half of the stellate ganglion, but is more often present following the supraclavicular approach and can be most annoying to the patient. For a satisfactory result, postoperative precise sudomotor function tests should demonstrate complete sympathetic denervation of the involved extremity.

Patients with distal injuries such as frostbite or local crush have been treated with a digital artery surgical sympathectomy by Flatt.[5] Spinner has explored neuromas-in-continuity to reattach disrupted axon bundles or to release isolated compression.[25]

Attempts to interrupt the sensory pathways of the spinal cord and brain have led to various ineffective procedures with disappointing long-term results. White and Sweet have recorded that postcordotomy analgesia cannot be expected to last longer than 3 months, with somewhat better results in cases involving the lower extremity rather than the upper extremity. Rhizotomy, posterior column tractotomy, postcentral gyrectomy of the sensory cortex, and frontal leukotomy have all been ineffective for sustained relief of pain.[6] Most of the procedures interrupt the spinothalamic tract, which projects pain to the ventroposterolateral nucleus of the thalamus and to the parietal cortex. The return of pain after surgery is related to the increased activity of polysynaptic systems (paleospinothalamic or spinoreticulothalamic) that are widespread in the brain stem and thalamus. These polysynaptic systems are infinitely complex and diffuse, and eventually frustrate any ablation procedure.

Referred or Systemic Response Pain

The shoulder-hand sydrome is associated with heart attacks and strokes.[32] Cervical disc disease and osteoarthritis may refer pain to the upper extremity. Rheumatoid arthritis, diabetes, and other systemic conditions may result in a massive episode of stiffness and pain. Corticosteroids are useful for the patient trapped in a massive episode of painful inflammatory stiffness.[23] Benson has used a mixture of 40 to 80 mg of methylprednisolone sodium succinate with 50 ml of 0.5% lidocaine hydrochloride as an intravenous regional anesthesia block.[1] After 15 minutes, one can gently manipulate stiff joints and stretch contracted soft tissue webs. The tourniquet can be lowered in 30 to 45 minutes, utilizing oxygen and intravenous diazepam for disorientation reaction. The procedure may be repeated in 3 days, if necessary. Salicylates should be used to abort ongoing inflammatory metabolic pathways.

Hypnosis and Personality Dysfunction

Pain may be relieved by hypnosis or distraction conditioning. In the latter part of the eighteenth century, the German physician Franz Anton Mesmer developed modern techniques for hypnosis. Experiments in hypnosis have shown that subjects can distort perception as well as motor movements, and through hypnosis partial to total anesthesia can be produced. Acupuncture has become popular in the United States, and seems to be effective in the susceptible individual. However, there is minimal scientific evidence, anatomic or physiologic, that acupuncture points or meridians exist.[2] Successful acupuncture and hypnosis both require the cerebral cortex to activate complex conditioned reflexes that raise pain thresholds, remove anxiety and tension, and relieve depression.[16]

It is worthwhile to relieve the patient's anxiety while pain is unrelieved. Trifluoperazine, 1 to 2 mg twice daily, is effective, or diazepam and chlordiazepoxide hydrochloride may be used in younger patients. Narcotics are extremely dangerous for these problems, and should be withheld. A battery of psychometric tests, such as the Minnesota Multiphasic Personality Inventory, may be valuable in evaluating depression, hypochondriasis, and other personality disorders.

FUNCTIONAL ACTIVITY

The second principle in the treatment program of an established pain syndrome is functional activity. Passive modalities will improve circulation, decrease edema, and prepare the patient for voluntary participation in active modalities such as athletics.

Passive modalities include massage, vibrators, stump wrapping, faradic muscle stimulation, ice packs, hot packs, paraffin packs, microwaves, ultrasound, and inflatable splints with positive-negative pressure. In the apprehensive patient, use of these methods may have to be preceded by very delicate techniques, such as stroking the skin with a feather. Some passive modalities may be contraindicated, such as the whirlpool bath, because it is dependent heat and may increase edema.

The more important phase is voluntary functional activity. Special care should be directed to warming up key areas of circulation, such as the rotator cuff muscles in a shoulder-arm-hand syndrome. Total body conditioning is important, and the patient should be ambulatory if possible. Function can be developed with diversional games, athletics, assigned work, and activities of daily living. It is important that the health-care team be compassionate and yet obtain maximum effort from the patient. The best functional activity occurs when the patient returns to work as usual.

I have followed several patients for years beyond their acute onset of pain. Medications and surgical procedures were not entirely effective in all these patients but, in time, almost all used their involved extremities, and a high percentage of them returned to work. Under emotional stress, their pain seems as severe as it was during active treatment. Most can vividly recall their "pain state." Life goes on, though, and many patients adapt and inhibit their response to the pain. Appropriate treatment will assist the patient to shorten the interval between overwhelming pain and tolerance. Ultimately, patients "cure" themselves.

References

1. Benson, W. F.: Treatment of the Painful Extremity (booklet). Personal communication, 1978.
2. Cantrell, J. R.: Acupuncture: A form of psychological healing. Southwest Med., 63:14, 1975.
3. Chuinard, R. G., et al.: Intravenous reserpine for treatment of reflex sympathetic dystrophy. J. Hand Surg., 5:289, 1980.
4. Eaton, R. G.: Painful neuromas. In Omer, G. E., Jr., and Spinner, M. (eds.): Management of Peripheral Nerve Problems, Philadelphia, W. B. Saunders, 1980.
5. Flatt, A. E.: Digital artery sympathectomy. J. Hand Surg., 5:282, 1980.
6. Glidenberg, P. L.: Central surgical procedures for pain of peripheral nerve origin. In Omer, G. E., Jr., and Spinner, M. (eds.): Management of Peripheral Nerve Problems, Philadelphia, W. B. Saunders, 1980.
7. Grant, G. H.: Methods of treatment of neuromata of the hand. J. Bone Joint Surg., 33A:841, 1951.
8. Hagbarth, K. E., and Kerr, D. I. B.: Central influences on spinal afferent conduction. J. Neurophysiol., 17:295, 1954.
9. Herndon, J. H., et al.: Management of painful neuromas in the hand. J. Bone Joint Surg., 58A:369, 1976.
10. Hosobuchi, Y., et al.: Stimulation of human periaqueductal grey matter for pain relief increases immunoreactive beta-endorphin in ventricular fluid. Science, 203:279, 1979.
11. Kleinert, H. E., et al.: Surgical sympathectomy—upper and lower extremity. In Omer, G. E., Jr., and Spinner, M. (eds.): Management of Peripheral Nerve Problems, Philadelphia, W. B. Saunders, 1980.
12. Lankford, L. L.: Reflex sympathetic dystrophy. In Omer, G. E., Jr., and Spinner, M. (eds.): Management of Peripheral Nerve Problems, Philadelphia, W. B. Saunders, 1980.
13. Loeser, J. D., et al.: Relief of pain by transcutaneous stimulation. J. Neurosurg., 42:308, 1975.
14. Long, D. M.: Electrical stimulation for the control of pain. Arch. Surg., 112:884, 1977.
15. Momose, T.: Potentiation of postoperative analgesic agents by hydroxyzine. Bonica, J. J. (ed.): Considerations in Management of Acute Pain, New York, Hospital Practice Publishing, 1977.

16. Murphy, T. M., and Bonica, J. J.: Acupuncture analgesia and anesthesia. Arch. Surg., 112:896, 1977.
17. Nashold, B. S., Jr., et al: Direct electrical stimulation of the peripheral nerves for relief of intractable pain. J. Bone Joint Surg., 57A:729, 1975.
18. Nashold, B. S., Jr., et al.: Electrical stimulation of peripheral nerves with micro-electrical implants for pain relief. *In* Omer, G. E., Jr., and Spinner, M. (eds.): Management of Peripheral Nerve Problems, Philadelphia, W. B. Saunders, 1980.
19. Omer, G. E., and Thomas, S. T.: Treatment of causalgia, Review of 70 cases at Brooke General Hospital. Tex. Med., 67:93, 1971.
20. Omer, G. E., and Thomas, S. T.: The management of chronic pain syndromes in the upper extremity. Clin. Orthop., 104:37, 1974.
21. Omer, G. E., Jr.: Management of pain syndromes in the upper extremity. *In* Hunter, J. M., et al. (eds.): Rehabilitation of the Hand, St. Louis, C. V. Mosby, 1978.
22. Omer, G. E., Jr.: The reflex sympathetic dystrophies and other pain syndromes. *In* Fredricks, S., and Brody, G. S. (eds.): Symposium on the Neurologic Aspects of Plastic Surgery, Vol. 17, St. Louis, C. V. Mosby, 1978.
23. Omer, G. E., Jr.: Management of the painful extremity. Curr. Pract. Orthop. Surg., 8:86, 1979.
24. Omer, G. E., Jr.: Continuous peripheral epineural infusion for the treatment of acute pain. *In* Omer, G. E., Jr., and Spinner, M. (eds.): Management of Peripheral Nerve Problems, Philadelphia, W. B. Saunders, 1980.
25. Omer, G. E., Jr.: Nerve, neuroma, and pain problems related to upper limb amputations. Orthop. Clin. North Am., 12:751, 1981.
26. Rexed, B.: The cytoarchitecture organization of the spinal cord of the cat. J. Comp. Neurol., 96:415, 1952.
27. Reynolds, D. V.: Surgery in the rat during electrical analgesia induced by focal brain stimulation. Science, 164:444, 1969.
28. Richards, R. L.: Causalgia, a centennial review. Arch. Neurol., 16:339, 1967.
29. Schnell, M. D., and Bunch, W. H.: Management of pain in the amputee. *In* The Committee on Prosthetics and Orthotics and N. C. McCollough, III (eds.): Atlas of Limb Prosthetics, Surgical and Prosthetic Principles, St. Louis, C. V. Mosby, 1981, pp. 464–482.
30. Singer, S. J.: Architecture and topography of biologic membranes. *In* Weissman, G., and Claiborne, R. (eds.): Cell Membranes: Biochemistry, Cell Biology and Pathology, New York, Hospital Practice Publishing, 1975.
31. Smith, J. R., and Gomez, N. H.: Local injection therapy of neuromata of the hand with triamcinolone acetonide: A preliminary study of 22 patients. J. Bone Joint Surg., 52A:71, 1970.
32. Steinbrocker, O.: The shoulder-hand syndrome: Associated painful homolateral disability of the shoulder and hand with swelling and atrophy of the hand. Am. J. Med., 3:402, 1947.
33. Stilz, R. J., et al.: Reflex sympathetic dystrophy in a 6-year-old: Successful treatment by transcutaneous nerve stimulation. Anesth. Analg. (Cleve.) 56:438, 1977.
34. Tupper, J. W., and Booth, D. M.: Treatment of painful neuromas of sensory nerves in the hand: A comparison of traditional and newer methods. J. Hand Surg., 1:144, 1976.
35. Wall, P. D., and Gutnick, M.: Ongoing activity in peripheral nerves: The physiology and pharmacology of impulses originating from the neuron. Exp. Neurol., 43:580, 1974.
36. Wall, P. D.: Modulation of pain by nonpainful events. *In* Bonica, J. J., and Albe-Fessard, D. G. (eds.): Advances in Pain Research and Therapy, Vol. 1, New York, Raven Press, 1976.
37. Weissman, G.: Pain mediators and pain receptors. *In* Bonica, J. J. (ed.): Considerations in Management of Acute Pain, New York, Hospital Practice Publishing, 1977.
38. White, J. C., and Sweet, W. H.: Pain and the Neurosurgeon: A Forty-Year Experience, Springfield, IL, Charles C Thomas, 1969.
39. Wynn-Parry, C. B.: Correspondence Newsletter 1981–2, American Society for Surgery of the Hand.

10

COMPLICATIONS FROM PERIPHERAL NERVE INJURY

John A. Boswick, Jr.

Loss of motor function and decreased sensibility to heat, cold, and other modalities are often considered to be the major complications resulting from injury to the peripheral nerves in the upper extremity. This decrease in motor and sensory function is serious. However, in reviewing the detailed histories and carefully examining a large number of patients with injuries to one or more of the major peripheral nerves in the upper extremity, it becomes quite obvious that various problems and complications arise following these injuries. They are not the same in all patients, although the patterns are somewhat consistent.[1]

RADIAL NERVE INJURY

The radial nerve can be injured in any location after separating from the brachial plexus. The more common locations are in the middle and distal thirds of the humerus after it becomes exposed on the lateral side of the arm and at the level of the wrist, at which the superficial sensory branch is vulnerable to operative and accidental trauma.

When injury occurs to the radial nerve in the arm, there is a loss of wrist, finger, and thumb extension, a significant decrease in thumb abduction, and a decrease in wrist supination. The loss of these actions severely impairs hand function. Without wrist extension, the hand cannot be placed in the optimal position for grasp. It is the wrist extensors, especially the extensor carpi radialis longus and brevis, which provide the action that brings the wrist into dorsiflexion and stabilizes it in the appropriate position for grasp. This position will vary from an almost neutral position to one of essentially full dorsiflexion. After the wrist has been positioned for grasp by the wrist extensors, further stabilization is maintained by the counterbalancing effects of the

wrist flexors. When the extensor mass is paralyzed by loss of radial nerve function, not only is the ability to extend the wrist lost, but also the potential for stabilizing the wrist in grasping. The powerful wrist flexor remains unchecked and the ability to position the wrist in extension or a neutral position is lost, with the grasp severely compromised.[2]

When a radial nerve injury occurs at a more distal level, and the wrist extensors maintain their action, hand function is not as severely compromised. The ability to extend the fingers and thumb is lost, as well as some degree of thumb abduction (Fig. 10–1). These actions are partially compensated by the action of the intrinsic muscles, which can extend the digits at the interphalangeal joint as well as abduct and rotate the thumb. Although these actions of the intrinsic muscles allow some hand function (and in some patients the function is quite adequate), loss of full extension of the fingers and thumb and full abduction of the thumb significantly compromises the ability to open the hand for grasping large objects and the performance of other tasks that require full digital extension and complete thumb abduction.

With injury to the radial nerve in the arm and forearm, there is also loss of sensibility over the dorsal surface of the thumb, index finger, some of the long finger, and most noticeably in the web space between the thumb and index finger. This decrease in sensibility from radial nerve injury in the arm and forearm is noticed by most patients with this type of injury, but rarely presents a functional problem.

Injury to the sensory branch of the radial nerve after it surfaces from beneath the wrist is one of the more common injuries to the radial nerve in the upper extremity. This injury occurs from accidental wounds that may involve other structures, such as the extensor tendons. On occasion, only the sensory

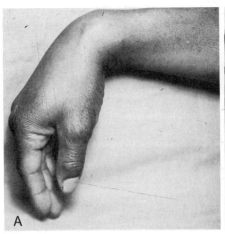
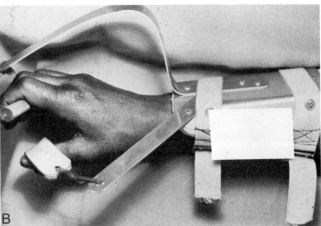

Figure 10–1. Loss of active extension of the wrist and of the metacarpophalangeal joint of the fingers in a patient with radial nerve injury. There is loss of abduction of the thumb. *B,* Dynamic splinting in the recovery period of radial nerve injury. Note that the metacarpophalangeal joints are maintained in extension and the thumb in abduction.

branch of the nerve is involved. Injury to the sensory branch of the radial nerve at the distal forearm may occur during surgery for various procedures. These include operations for release of the tendon sheath of the first dorsal compartment, procedures on the extensor tendon on the radial side of the wrist, and operations on the wrist joint or the base of the thumb.[3]

The incidence of injury to the sensory branch of the radial nerve in the distal forearm is unknown, because the symptoms are insignificant in many patients. They may be detected only on suspicion from an accidental wound or an operative procedure in the area. The decreased sensibility that may occur often goes unnoticed, unless checked for by pin prick or two-point discrimination. However, in some patients with injury to the sensory branch of the radial nerve, a painful neuroma may develop that is often extremely uncomfortable and disabling. It is not known why neuromas of sensory nerves are a problem in some patients and not in others, but it appears to be related to scar formation in the area of the injury. This is not always the situation, however, because many patients with extremely sensitive neuromas in the sensory branch of the radial nerve do not have noticeable scar formation in the area of the neuroma. In such patients, the relocation of the painful neuroma often fails to relieve the discomfort; therefore, scar formation alone is not the only factor contributing to the discomfort. The modalities of pressures and massage have been used to treat the discomfort of neuromas, often with very effective results. The earlier these techniques are applied, the more effective they appear to be. Based on meticulous observations and examination in a large number of patients, the early and extensive use of the hands after nerve injury tends to reduce or eliminate the problem of the painful neuroma.[1] Depending on the type of work the patient performs, pressure and massage therapy may be added to ensure adequate

stimulation of the area in which the neuroma is likely to develop.

MEDIAN NERVE INJURY

Interruption of median nerve function results in an interesting decrease in sensibility and motor function of the hand. The most common location of injury to the median nerve is at the level of the wrist. However, injury in the arm (*i.e.,* above the elbow) is not unusual. When injury occurs at the more proximal level, the muscles that contribute to pronation of the wrist are impaired, as well as the radial wrist flexor, the superficial flexors of the fingers, the long flexor of the thumb, the deep flexor (profundus) of the index finger, some components of the thenar mass, and digital intrinsic muscles. The component of thenar intrinsic loss that occurs will determine the ensuing pattern of motion performed by the fingers and thumb. In studies of patients with isolated injury to the median nerve above the elbow, all have been found to have a decreased ability to pronate the forearm and to flex the wrist, and a complete loss of the capacity for flexion of the interphalangeal joint of the thumb, and of both interphalangeal joints of the index finger (both interphalangeal joints of the long, ring, and little fingers would actively flex; Fig. 10–2). In 65% of the patients there was a slightly decreased ability to rotate the thumb to a position of grasp, and in the remaining 35% there was a marked and often complete ability to rotate the thumb to a position perpendicular to the index finger (Fig. 10–3). This variation in the ability to rotate the thumb is accounted for by the variation in the contribution of the median nerve to the muscles of the thenar mass, and by the ability of the long abductor of the thumb to abduct and rotate the thumb metacarpal.

Patients with injury to the median nerve above

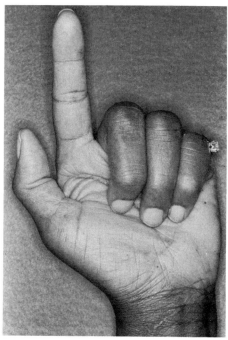

Figure 10–2. Patient with high median nerve injury showing the inability to flex the distal interphalangeal joints of the little, ring, and long fingers fully, and with no flexion of the interphalangeal joints of the thumb or index finger.

the elbow always have loss of the forearm flexion mass and obvious atrophy of the thenar intrinsic muscles (Fig. 10–4). This loss of muscle tissue is noticeable and measurable; the denervation of the muscles can be detected by electrical studies (electromyography) within 4 weeks. Repair of the median nerve above the elbow using appropriate suture techniques always provides a return of axon regeneration to the denervated forearm and thenar muscles and an improvement in the end-organs of sensibility in the palm and digits. The return of electrical activity as detected electromyographically varies from 4 to 6 months for the forearm muscles

and from 12 to 18 months for the thenar area. The rate of return of muscle innervation depends on the location of the injury, age of the patient, and extent of scarring (if this is a problem). Active flexion of the thumb and index finger returns in 3 to 6 weeks after electrical activity returns to the superficial and deep flexors of the digits. In the adult patient with a median nerve injury above the elbow, in whom there is significant loss of thumb rotation, this function seldom if ever returns following nerve suture. Tendon transfer is required to restore this action. It is felt that the small delicate fibers of the thenar intrinsics undergo atrophy to the extent they can no longer function satisfactorily. In addition to atrophy precluding sufficient action to accomplish thumb rotation, the possibility of a conduction defect from the motor end-plate to the muscle fibers may account for some loss of active motion.[4]

The impairment of function of the sensory component of the median nerve results in decreased sensibility of the radial side of the palm, the volar surface of the thumb, and index, and long fingers, and the radial half of the ring finger. There is some variation in this pattern of decreased sensibility, explained by the crossover of fibers from the median and ulnar nerves in the forearm, and by the actual anatomic variation of the ulnar nerve supplying the radial side of the ring and ulnar side of the long fingers. A rare occurrence is the ulnar nerve's providing the sensory distribution of the radial side of the long finger and the ulnar side of the index finger. These variations in anatomic pattern also occur in the motor distribution, and explain the variation in the ability to rotate the thumb with injury to the median nerve.

In about 35% of patients, the problem that occurs with injury to the median nerve above the elbow is a decrease in grip strength that never fully returns (although there is a return of full active motion of the digits), injury to the hands due to decreased sensibility, decreased pinch strength between thumb and index finger, and loss of the ability to rotate the thumb to a position of grasp.

With injury to the medial nerve at the level of

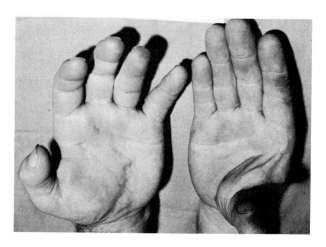

Figure 10–3. Patient with high median nerve injury showing the inability to rotate the thumb of the injured hand to a position of grasp.

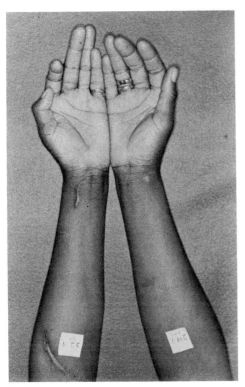

Figure 10–4. Forearm atrophy is shown in this patient with a median nerve and brachial artery laceration approximately 2 cm proximal to the median condyle of the humerus.

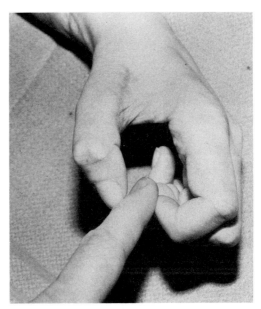

Figure 10–5. Froment's sign. Note flexion of the interphalangeal joint of the thumb.

the wrist the problems are the same as in the more proximal injuries, except for the loss of flexion of the thumb and index finger, and of the independent flexion of the long, ring, and little fingers at the proximal joint due to denervation of the sublimis muscle group.

ULNAR NERVE INJURY

The ulnar nerve, like the median nerve, is most commonly injured at the level of the wrist. Isolated injuries occur in the arm and proximal forearm that do not cause impairment significantly greater than the injuries at the more distal level.

With injury to the ulnar nerve in the distal forearm, there is a loss of sensibility over the ulnar side of the palm, the volar surface of the little finger, and the ulnar half of the ring finger. The hypothenar, interosseous, thumb adductor, some of the thenar, and the little and ring finger lumbrical muscles are denervated.

This denervation of the hypothenar mass results in loss of the ability to cup the hand for grasp and a subsequent decrease in grip strength. Denervation of the thumb adductor produces in some patients a marked decrease in pinch strength between the thumb and index finger. The loss of the adductor in aiding pinch forces the flexor pollicis longus to

become a major contributor to thumb adduction and a contributor to pinch. Due to the forceful action of the long flexor of the thumb in contributing to pinch, the interphalangeal joint flexes, a sign described by Froment (Fig. 10–5).[5]

When the ulnar nerve is injured, all the interosseous muscles and the muscles of the little and ring fingers are usually denervated. This causes an imbalance of action at the metacarpophalangeal joint. Without the action of the interosseous, the long extensors that have an insertion into the proximal phalanges of the fingers will extend their influence almost unchecked, and cause the metacarpophalangeal joint to hyperextend. When the metacarpophalangeal joint hyperextends, the flexor sublimis and profundus extend their action at the proximal and distal interphalangeal joints, with a resulting flexion of approximately 90° at each location. The deformity of metacarpophalangeal hyperextension and flexion of the interphalangeal joints is known as claw hand (Fig. 10–6). This deformity creates a function problem, because the involved fingers cannot extend to grasp objects, and the patient with this deformity will often knock objects off tables when attempting to grasp a glass or bottle. In a few patients, the long finger is involved in an ulnar nerve injury; that is, it hyperextends at the metacarpophalangeal and flexes at the interphalangeal joints. I have seen two patients in whom all four fingers were involved. Some of the thenar muscles become denervated following injury to the ulnar nerve. However, this presents only a minor (if any) problem regarding thumb flexion and adduction.

The decreased sensibility on the ulnar side of the hand from an ulnar nerve injury allows these areas to become easily injured by heat and sharp objects.

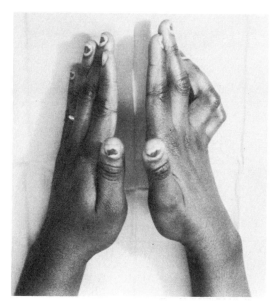

Figure 10–6. Atrophy of the interossei associated with hyperextension of metacarpophalangeal joints and with flexion of proximal interphalangeal joints in a patient with right ulnar nerve injury.

Until sensibility returns following nerve suture, or if the nerve injury is irreversible, patients should be taught to be careful when using their hands to prevent such accidents.

In addition to the claw deformity that occurs following ulnar nerve injury, muscle atrophy is also characteristic. Interosseous wasting is noticed between the metacarpal, especially on the first dorsal interosseous muscle when viewed from the dorsal surface to the radial side of the index finger. On the palmar surface, wasting of the hypothenar area is most noticeable, along with flattening of the area of the adductor and following the effect in the thenar area from the atrophy of the ulnar-innervated thenar muscles.

When injury to the ulnar nerve occurs above the elbow, the effect is basically the same as in below-elbow injuries, except that there is less tendency for the interphalangeal joints of the little and ring fingers to flex because the ulnar profundus mass is denervated.

Thus, the complications that occur on the distal upper extremity as a result of nerve injury are predictable but somewhat variable. Decreased sensibility, loss of motion, and positional deformities are the primary problems. Decreased sensibility may result in injuries, especially burns; however, all types of accidents may result. Loss of motion from nerve injury results in decreased use and resultant loss of strength. The positional deformities that occur due to muscle denervation (*e.g.,* claw deformities, wrist drop, loss of thumb rotation) cause problems of use ranging from minimal to almost complete disability. Many complications and problems that occur from nerve injury in the upper extremity can be corrected by appropriate nerve suture and prevented by instruction and care in using the hands.[6]

References

1. Boswick, J. A., Jr.: Consequences of peripheral nerve injuries in the upper extremity. *In* Boswick, J. A. Jr., (ed.): Current Concepts in Hand Surgery, Philadelphia, Lea & Febiger, 1983, pp. 83–86.
2. Boswick, J. A., Jr.: The hand. *In* Committee on Trauma, American College of Surgeons: Early Care of the Injured Patient, 3rd ed., Philadelphia W. B. Saunders, 1982, pp. 248–264.
3. Omer, G. E.: The results of untreated traumatic injuries. *In* Omer, G. E., and Spinner, M. (eds.): Management of Peripheral Nerve Problems, Philadelphia, W. B. Saunders, 1980, p. 502.
4. Boswick, J. A., Jr., and Stromberg, W. B., Jr.: Isolated injury to the median nerve above the elbow. J. Bone Joint Surg. 49A:653, 1967.
5. Boswick, J. A., Jr., and Scott, F. A.: Repair of peripheral nerves (upper extremity). *In* Eiseman, B. (ed.): Prognosis of Surgical Disease, Philadelphia, W. B. Saunders, 1980.
6. Fisher, G. T., and Boswick, J. A., Jr.: Neuroma formation following digital amputation. J. Trauma, 23:136, 1983.

11

COMPLICATIONS OF COMPRESSION OR ENTRAPMENT NEUROPATHIES

William W. Eversmann, Jr.

Entrapment neuropathies are nerve injuries that result from intermittent or prolonged ischemia of segments of the peripheral nerve trunk in predictable areas.[43, 44] Unless the entrapment neuropathy involves all or nearly all of the motor function of the peripheral nerve in addition to complete sensory loss, or is extremely longstanding in its presence, recovery of the function of the peripheral nerve is anticipated by both the patient and the surgeon following decompression of the peripheral nerve segment.[43] Following surgical decompression, failure of the nerve to recover will often call both the patient and the surgeon's attention to a possible complication of the entrapment neuropathy.

One cannot emphasize too greatly the absolute necessity of complete preoperative evaluation of the patient with a nerve compression syndrome and its value in assessing the recovery of the patient following surgical decompression.[43, 170] Without an accurate preoperative detailed evaluation of the patient's neurologic function, both motor and sensory, the presence of a postoperative complication cannot be assessed to determine the need for further treatment, whether surgical or nonsurgical. Muscle testing and sensory evaluation including two-point discrimination testing, tactile ognosis, and testing of pinch and grip, in addition to the evaluation of a trained observer on the patient's hand use, are essential for evaluation of the patient's postoperative circumstances. Ideally, this examination should be performed prior to the initial surgery but, in its absence, it is mandatory to determine the presence of complications of entrapment neuropathies.

Because entrapment and compression neuropathies are nerve injuries, the basic principles surrounding the degree of nerve injury must of necessity apply to these neuropathies. Accordingly, the classification of nerve injuries by Seddon—neurapractic, axonotmetic or neurotmetic—or that of Sunderland—loss of conduction in the axons, loss of continuity of the axons with an intact endoneurial sheath, loss of continuity of the nerve fibers, loss of continuity of the nerve fibers perineurium and fasciculi, and loss of continuity of the nerve trunk—applies to these nerve lesions.[170, 180]

Following decompression of a compression neuropathy, if the degree of nerve injury has been neurapractic, the patient will note recovery of function within the sphere of the nerve trunk in the first 3 to 6 weeks, and the recovery will affect the entire field innervated by that peripheral nerve, both motor and sensory, at about the same time.[180] Following decompression of the nerve trunk, if recovery begins by progressive migration of Tinel's sign distally along the nerve axis, with linear reinnervation of muscle and sensory receptors, the diagnosis of an axonotmetic response would be appropriate. Finally, following decompression of the nerve trunk, if no advancement in percussion sensitivity and no recovery of the nerve function is noted, then a neurotmetic injury to the nerve would have occurred.

In the postoperative evaluation of a patient whose response to surgical decompression of an entrapment neuropathy has been compromised, one of three clinical syndromes is observed. First, the patient experiences no relief of pain nor of dysesthesia and no recovery of peripheral nerve function following the decompression. In the second, the patient might experience relief of pain and dysesthesia but continues to have a lack of motor or sensory nerve function. The third syndrome occurs when the pain and dysesthesia were initially relieved but then recur several weeks after the surgical procedure. The third syndrome may or may not be accompanied by recovery of the nerve function.

The first syndrome, that of no relief of pain nor of dysesthesia and no recovery of the nerve trunk, must be regarded as the most ominous in the prognosis of nerve function. Such a response normally suggests that the original diagnosis was incorrect, the decompression was insufficient, or insufficient time has been allowed to pass for the observation of any recovery of the nerve.

The second syndrome, that of pain and dysesthesia relief but no observable recovery of the nerve, normally suggests that there was an axonotmetic lesion and that the decompression was properly diagnosed and decompressed, and that insufficient time has transpired to allow the axons to progress in their migration toward the sensory and motor receptors. Accordingly, this circumstance is best handled by continued observation, allowing sufficient time for the axons to regenerate toward areas in which, receptors having been reinnervated, changes in clinical signs would indicate nerve regeneration. When pain and dysesthesia are initially relieved only to recur several weeks after the decompression, with or without evidence of nerve regeneration and reinnervation, one must draw the conclusion that the rest, lack of motion, or even immobilization generated by the surgical decompression and postoperative care have been sufficient to relieve the severity of the compression neuropathy temporarily, but that the compression neuropathy has been inadequately relieved and completion of the surgical decompression may be necessary.

The onset of a reflex sympathetic dystrophy after decompression of a compression or entrapment neuropathy can be a devastating complication that requires the same thoughtful, decisive, and expert care that will accompany this syndrome regardless of its cause. Those stages and classifications common to reflex sympathetic dystrophy from other causes are no less likely to be associated following surgery for a compression or entrapment neuropathy. Accordingly, the description by a patient of a burning sensation, a cutting, searing, pressure, or tearing pain, and the findings of painful paresthesias to light touch and painful stiffness of the proximal interphalangeal (PIP) joints following surgery for a compression neuropathy, often in conjunction with hyperhidrosis and redness or a mottled red appearance of the palm, must be a cause of extreme concern for the surgeon dealing with such a patient. The use of stellate ganglion blocks, somatic nerve blocks, periodic perineural infusions, sympatholytic medication, or even sympathectomy combined with aggressive hand therapy may be necessary for this patient.

ENTRAPMENT NEUROPATHIES

In addition to the complications that may affect any of the entrapment neuropathies, each specific entrapment has a group of complications or potential complications that must be addressed at the time of surgical decompression to ensure their avoidance, or dealt with postoperatively if the patient fails to respond to the surgical decompression of that compression syndrome. Each complication is most properly considered by reviewing the particular compression syndromes.

Pronator Syndrome

Failure of the median nerve to recover motor and sensory function following decompression for a pronator syndrome requires the surgeon to evaluate first whether the diagnosis of a pronator syndrome was correct.[7, 9, 51, 85, 91, 94, 160] Although the anterior interosseous syndrome will occasionally mimic signs of a pronator syndrome, exploration and decompression of the median nerve for pronator syndrome most often will also include decompression of the anterior interosseous nerve.[174] A detailed review of the diagnostic studies, both physical examination and sensory evaluation of the median nerve in the hand, and electrodiagnostic studies will ordinarily differentiate the pronator syndrome, which involves the median nerve above the anterior interosseous nerve, from the anterior interosseous syndrome, which involves the anterior interosseous nerve and deep volar compartment of the forearm exclusively.

Symptoms of pronator syndrome can be caused by anomalies in and about the brachial plexus, particularly when the contribution to the median nerve from the lateral cord of the brachial plexus is involved in either a fascial or vascular compression.[170] If a vascular compression is involved, arteriography of the axillary artery and its tributaries, particularly the posterior humeral circumflex artery, will be necessary in varying positions of abduction of the shoulder to diagnose a vascular compression of the brachial plexus. Fascial bands lying within the lateral cord of the brachial plexus, or the contribution of the lateral cord to the median nerve, which can certainly produce symptoms similar to a pronator syndrome, will only be able to be diagnosed at surgical exploration.

During the evaluation of a patient with continuing symptoms from a pronator syndrome after surgical decompression, the surgeon must evaluate the patient for the adequacy of the decompression.[94] Ordinarily, surgeons will be more reluctant to evaluate their own surgical decompression than that of someone else.

The most common surgical error in a decompression of pronator syndrome is failure to carry the dissection sufficiently proximal to decompress the ligament of Struthers.[7, 85, 130, 177–179] It is well known that the ligament of Struthers may arise from a supracondylar process, beneath which the median nerve, brachial artery, or both may suffer compression. The ligament of Struthers, arising from the osseous process, blends with the fascia of the humeral head of the pronator teres to form a compressive band across the median nerve.[177-179] Less well known is that a ligament of Struthers arising from the diaphysis of the humerus without a supracondylar process of bone may also compress the median nerve, brachial artery, or both within the distal 5 cm of the humerus (Fig. 11–1). Accordingly, adequate surgical decompression for pronator syndrome must include a dissection of the distal 5 cm of the humerus to ensure adequate decompression of the proximal portion of the median nerve. Failure to decompress the median nerve in the distal 5 cm of the humerus may only be reflected in the position of a previous surgical scar and, therefore, a surgical scar that begins at the elbow flexion crease must alert the surgeon to the possibility that the exploration for a ligament of Struthers compression may have been neglected (Fig. 11–2).

Before undertaking re-exploration for a pronator syndrome, the surgeon must be very sure that the patient is continuing to have symptoms of a compression of the median nerve. (This evaluation can be aided by electrodiagnostic studies.) Cutaneous nerve dysesthesia attendant to a previous operative procedure could well be confused by the patient with a continuing syndrome of deep nerve

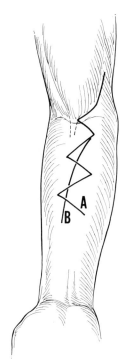

Figure 11–2. The surgical incision for the pronator syndrome should begin above the elbow (as in *A*). An incision that begins at or distal to the elbow crease may not afford the surgeon sufficient exposure to explore for the ligament of Struthers, or possibly even to divide the lacertus fibrosis completely. (Courtesy of E. Roselius. From Greene, D. P. (ed.): Operative Hand Surgery, New York-London, Churchill Livingstone, 1982.)

compression. If the patient's symptoms are largely dysesthetic on the volar cutaneous skin of the proximal forearm, a series of diagnostic, subcutaneous infiltrations of local anesthetic should be performed as diagnostic blocks to assess the relief from symptoms that the patient may obtain with this relatively simple diagnostic procedure. If the patient obtains relief by simple subcutaneous infiltrations of local anesthetics in the distal third of the brachium, it is usually unlikely that a continuing compression of the median nerve exists.

Because the median nerve may undergo compression in the proximal forearm as well as the carpal tunnel, the failure to resolve symptoms within the median nerve following release of a pronator syndrome must logically call attention to the possibility of a more distal compression neuropathy of the median nerve at the carpal tunnel. Percussion testing of the median nerve is not a useful sign of localization of compression at the carpal tunnel following decompression of a pronator syndrome, because an advancing Tinel's sign may become sensitive at the wrist during the examination. Phalen's test, however, continues to be useful, as are electrodiagnostic nerve conduction velocity tests across the carpal tunnel. If there is any question of a concomitant carpal tunnel syndrome following

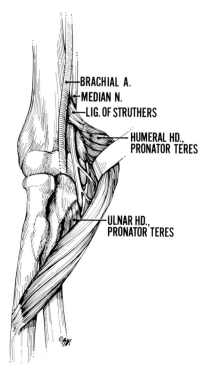

BRACHIAL A.
MEDIAN N.
LIG. OF STRUTHERS
HUMERAL HD., PRONATOR TERES
ULNAR HD., PRONATOR TERES

Figure 11–1. The ligament of Struthers may arise from the humerus directly or from the supracondyloid process of the humerus, and may entrap either the median nerve alone (as shown) or the median nerve and brachial artery together. The ligament of Struthers becomes confluent with the fascia of the humeral head of the pronator teres distal to its origin from the humerus. (Courtesy of E. Roselius. From Greene, D. P. (ed.): Operative Hand Surgery, New York-London, Churchill Livingstone, 1982.)

release of a pronator syndrome, re-examination of the patient 4 to 6 weeks following initial evaluation will usually resolve the confusion between a pronator syndrome that is resolving with distal regeneration of axons from an additional compression syndrome at the carpal tunnel.

Anterior Interosseous Syndrome

When surgical decompression of the anterior interosseous syndrome fails to produce the desired neurologic recovery, the surgeon is faced with a complex problem that is difficult to evaluate and requires detailed re-evaluation. Initially, the surgeon must be certain that the patient does not have an occult deep volar compartment syndrome, in which there is no longer any viable muscle tissue to respond favorably to the decompression. Second, it is important to be certain that there is not a rupture of the flexor pollicis longus tendon, with or without a concomitant rupture of the flexor digitorum profundus tendon of the index finger. Osteophyte formation, particularly in the rheumatoid arthritic, or a history of trauma, such as a small laceration at the wrist leading to loss of continuity of the flexor pollicis longus and index profundus tendon, might very well simulate the anterior interosseous syndrome. In some cases a carpal tunnel view radiograph of the distal forearm and wrist reveals an osteophyte that might be responsible for the spontaneous rupture of these tendons.

Even when surgeons perform the exploration and release of the anterior interosseous nerve themselves, there is still the question of whether adequate exploration has been performed on the patient's previous decompression.[19, 45, 46, 87, 96, 113, 132, 134, 157, 161, 165, 168, 173, 174, 185, 199] Review of the previous operation report is certainly desirable but, when unavailable, the size of the surgical incision may provide some indication of the extent of the exposure and decompression (see Fig. 11–2).

Evaluation of the complicated interosseous syndrome will necessarily require an electromyogram of the deep volar compartment, particularly including the pronator quadratus and flexor pollicis longus.[43, 170] This electromyogram should effectively rule out a deep compartment syndrome, in which there would be limited electrical response of the muscles, and a rupture of the flexor pollicis longus or index profundus tendons, in which the response of the muscles should be normal or nearly normal. A persistence of denervation potentials and fibrillations within these muscles would seem to indicate a continuing neurologic cause for the denervation. Accordingly, one must begin to search the multitude of anatomic variations that could be responsible for the anterior interosseous syndrome.[170] These would include an accessory head of the flexor pollicis longus (Gantser's muscle), the so-called palmaris profundus, and the flexor carpi radialis brevis.[115, 146, 170] Complete release of the anterior interosseous syndrome usually includes elevation of the radial head of the flexor digitorum superficialis arch (Fig. 11–3).

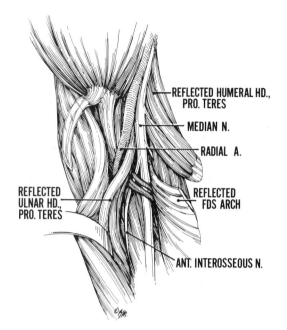

Figure 11–3. The completed release of the anterior interosseous syndrome and anterior interosseous nerve usually includes elevation of the radial origin of the flexor digitorum superficialis *(FDS)* and reflection of the superficial or humeral head of the pronator teres to expose the median nerve and anterior interosseous nerves completely. (Courtesy of E. Roselius. From Greene, D. P. (ed.): Operative Hand Surgery, New York-London, Churchill Livingstone, 1982.)

If this arch has not been elevated, it will be difficult or impossible to visualize these anatomic variations and, therefore, to decompress the anterior interosseous nerve completely.[43]

Persistent anterior interosseous syndrome after decompression may also be caused by anatomic variations at the brachial plexus, particularly those involving the posterior humeral circumflex artery as it crosses the contribution from the medial cord to the median nerve.[43, 170] This anatomic variation can be diagnosed by angiography of the axillary artery, taking care to observe the filling of the posterior humeral circumflex artery in varying degrees of abduction and external rotation of the shoulder. A loss of filling of the posterior humeral circumflex artery on axillary angiography in an abducted position, especially if this position is associated with symptoms of anterior interosseous syndrome and pain in the shoulder, may indicate the medial cord of the brachial plexus as the site of compression. Surgical exploration of the contribution of the medial cord of the brachial plexus to the median nerve will be necessary to rule out this lesion further.

Carpal Tunnel Syndrome

Carpal tunnel syndrome is the most common compression neuropathy of the upper extremity. Nearly all major series of patients with this syn-

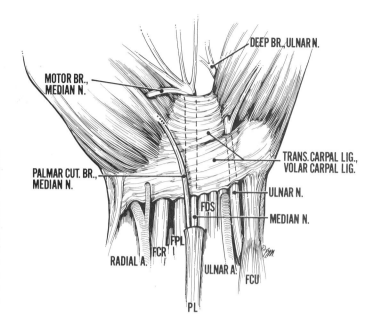

Figure 11–4. Exploration of the motor branch of the median nerve is an important part of the release of the transverse carpal ligament and of decompression of the median nerve for carpal tunnel syndrome. Various anomalies of the motor branch have been described and must be searched for so that the surgeon can be certain that no continuing entrapment of the motor branch exists following decompression. (Courtesy of E. Roselius. From Greene, D. P. (ed.).: Operative Hand Surgery, New York-London, Churchill Livingstone, 1982.)

drome contain a small group of patients, varying from a few percent to as high as 20%, who fail to respond to decompression of the median nerve.[24, 44, 48, 63, 90, 92, 142, 207] A few of these patients have such advanced injury to the median nerve that they must be considered as neurotmetic and, therefore, will be unresponsive to simple decompression of the median nerve. As with other compression neuropathies, the complications of carpal tunnel syndrome should be avoided whenever possible. The evaluation of these complications must necessarily include a review of the previous surgical procedure. If the surgical decompression does not divide the fascia of the distal forearm at the proximal wrist crease, a transverse band of forearm fascia may very well perpetuate the compression of the median nerve at the proximal flexion crease of the wrist.[43] Thus, adequate decompression might logically include fasciotomy of the distal several inches of the forearm in addition to release of the transverse carpal ligament.

Exploration of the motor branch of the median nerve will be an important element of the original operation (Fig. 11–4).[94] If the motor branch of the median nerve has a transligamentous course to the thenar muscles, it will be necessary to relieve the nerve as it passes through the deep transverse carpal ligament so that continuing compression of the motor branch does not exist postoperatively.[80] The presence of more than one motor branch, or the paralysis of a portion of the thenar muscles, might well herald the presence of multiple or anomalous motor branches, one or more of which may be transligamentous.[56, 66, 80, 116, 136, 140] Postoperative neuropathy of the palmar cutaneous branch of the median nerve, secondary either to poor positioning of the operative incision or to continuing neuropathy of the palmar cutaneous branch as it pierces the palmar fascia, will be a cause of persistent

disagreeable symptoms that may require exploration of the palmar cutaneous branch of the median nerve.[172] When the palmar cutaneous branch is compressed, the compression is usually located at the base of the palm just distal to the wrist crease as the nerve pierces the palmar fascia and assumes its subcutaneous position to innervate the skin on the thenar eminence (Fig. 11–5).

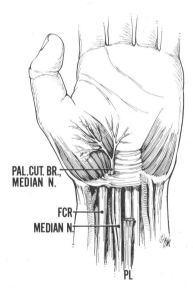

Figure 11–5. An entrapment of the palmar cutaneous branch of the median nerve as it passes through the volar carpal ligament and palmar fascia at the base of the palm may cause continuing paresthesias and dysesthesias in the base of the palm, suggestive of continuing neuropathy of the median nerve. (Courtesy of E. Roselius. From Greene, D. P. (ed.): Operative Hand Surgery, New York-London, Churchill-Livingstone, 1982).

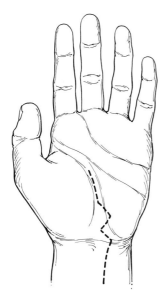

Figure 11–6. An incision for carpal tunnel syndrome should lie ulnar to the long axis of the ring finger at the base of the palm to avoid the branches of the palmar cutaneous branch of the median nerve. (Courtesy of E. Roselius. From Greene, D. P. (ed.): Operative Hand Surgery, New York-London, Churchill Livingstone, 1982.)

If an ulnar incision for release of the transverse carpal ligament, as advocated by Taleisnik, is used for decompression of the carpal ligament, the canal of Guyon is likely to be opened or partially opened during the course of deep transverse carpal ligament division (Fig. 11–6).[183] When Guyon's canal is partially opened ulnar nerve neuropathy may result, and the patient will complain of ulnar nerve neuropathic symptoms following carpal tunnel surgery. If the surgeon performing a release of the deep transverse carpal ligament recognizes that Guyon's canal has been partially decompressed at the time of the surgery on the carpal tunnel, the decompression of Guyon's canal should be completed, freeing the ulnar nerve and vascular bundle from the distal third of the forearm to the distal extent of Guyon's canal. If, following decompression of the carpal tunnel, the patient begins to complain of ulnar neuropathic symptoms, it is likely that this is the result of incomplete decompression of Guyon's canal, and completion of this decompression may be necessary to relieve the patient's ulnar tunnel syndrome.

The patient being evaluated for complications of carpal tunnel syndrome will require a radiograph of the carpal tunnel as part of the evaluation to search for osteophytes or osseous deformity, which could perpetuate the disagreeable symptoms of median neuropathy and neuritis. The patient with rheumatoid arthritis who has undergone release of the deep transverse carpal ligament but whose surgery has not included a synovectomy of the flexor tendons, or who has continuing deformity at the border of the distal radius, may well require further surgical decompression and débridement.

A patient with a history of previous laceration of the wrist must also be suspect in that such a laceration might have caused previous injury to the median nerve, an injury that existed prior to carpal tunnel release. Most such patients will have had a partial laceration of the median nerve, which will further confuse the motor and sensory evaluation, both prior to the initial carpal tunnel decompression and following that decompression.

Tumorous conditions of the median nerve are a particular problem from the standpoint of evaluation. Fibrofatty degeneration of the median nerve, one of the more common tumorous or tumorlike conditions that affect the area of the carpal tunnel, will be difficult to manage, because the patient, as the median nerve increases in size, will develop progressive and increasing neuropathy that will be largely unresponsive to surgical care.

Following a detailed re-evaluation of the median nerve—motor and sensory evaluation, as well as electrodiagnostic studies that include nerve conduction velocity tests across the wrist and electromyograms of median- and ulnar-innervated muscles of the hand—a few patients will have continuing severe neuropathy for which there is little or no explanation, and for whom surgical re-exploration of the median nerve will be selected.[20, 48, 73, 84, 109, 110, 112, 128, 149, 186, 187] At the time of re-exploration, epineurotomy of the median nerve or even internal neurolysis of the median nerve across the carpal tunnel may be indicated.[34, 57] If either of these procedures are chosen, magnification and fine instruments will be necessary to preserve the interfascicular plexus of nerves and the microcirculation of the median nerve during the course of the incision of the epineurium and the treatment of the interfascicular fibrosis.[34, 43]

Various systemic diseases have been described as presenting with carpal tunnel syndrome.[3, 11, 25, 38, 52, 53, 63, 65, 67–69, 83, 86, 90, 92, 93, 99, 104, 105, 120, 121, 123, 129, 135, 137, 143, 145, 153, 155, 164, 176, 185, 196, 203] In most cases the usual operation for decompression of the median nerve at the carpal tunnel will be sufficient to relieve the patient of neuropathic symptoms.[15, 142] Certain of these systemic diseases, however, will retard or delay the usual response to decompression of the median nerve.[25, 52, 135, 196] Nearly any major peripheral neuropathy will delay the response of decompression of the median nerve.[203] Apparently, these neuropathies have an additive effect with the compression of the fascicles from the transverse carpal ligament, and result in a slowed response to decompression and a considerably slowed recovery of the nerve. Patients with multiple compression neuropathies are particularly suspect for an underlying peripheral neuropathy of this nature. A congenital sensitivity to compression has been described in some patients who present with multiple compression neuropathies. Diabetes mellitus, probably because of its effect on the microcirculation of the nerve, enhances the symptoms of carpal tunnel syndrome and delays the response of decompression of the median nerve.[135] In patients whom I have treated who had both diabetes mellitus and a compression neuropathy, the delay in recovery of the nerve, if it recovered at all, was prolonged two to three times.[44]

Another cause of delay in recovery of the median nerve would be a "double crush" syndrome, in which another compression neuropathy of the median nerve proximal to the carpal tunnel exists.[43] A pronator syndrome in the proximal forearm, or a more proximal lesion of the median nerve even at the brachial plexus level, would be the second portion of a "double crush." Thus, detailed examination for a pronator syndrome or for a vascular or fascial anomaly of the distal brachial plexus may be required to complete the evaluation of a carpal tunnel syndrome unresponsive to surgical decompression.

Cubital Tunnel Syndrome

The cubital tunnel syndrome is a compression neuropathy of the ulnar nerve near the elbow; it is unique among the compression neuropathies because of the difficulty that many surgeons have experienced regaining normal or near normal function in its surgical treatment.[28, 29, 41, 78] Many surgical procedures have been developed in attempts to treat this neuropathy.[43]

Because the neuropathy occurs at a level of the ulnar nerve that makes the diagnosis difficult until the degree of nerve injury is advanced, many patients seem to be too long neglected, either by their own lack of concern or by that of their physician, to the relatively less severe symptoms of numbness of the little and a portion of the ring finger. In many patients attention to the diagnosis of this severe compression neuropathy is ignored until such time as severe atrophy of the intrinsic muscles of the hand, and consequently an axonotmesis or neurotmesis, have developed in the ulnar nerve.[41, 47, 49, 60, 141, 194]

In defense of the physicians who see these patients, the early diagnosis of this neuropathy is difficult, and may commonly be confused with a nerve root lesion of the eighth cervical root, a thoracic outlet syndrome, or even a "double crush" injury of the ulnar nerve, with concomitant and lesser compressions at either the thoracic outlet, nerve root, or ulnar tunnel.[1, 14, 16, 27, 36, 62, 75, 95, 200, 206] Thus, it is easy to see that the most common complication of the cubital tunnel syndrome may very well be the late diagnosis or incorrect diagnosis of this compression neuropathy.

Each operation for cubital tunnel syndrome seems to have its unique complications. The simple decompression procedure, during which the surgeon sections the aponeurosis of the flexor carpi ulnaris and, therefore, decompresses the ulnar nerve from the ulnar notch distally into the forearm, has gained considerable popularity because of its dependability in those patients in whom the compression can be localized at the aponeurosis of the flexor carpi ulnaris.[188, 202] This aponeurosis, which has also been referred to as the medial retinaculum of the elbow,

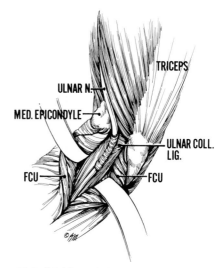

Figure 11–7. Division of the aponeurosis of the flexor carpi ulnaris *(FCU)* to decompress the ulnar nerve as it passes distal to the medial epicondyle maintains both the intrinsic and extrinsic blood supplies of the nerve. (Courtesy of E. Roselius. From Greene, D. P. (ed.): Operative Hand Surgery, New York-London, Churchill Livingstone, 1982.)

can be safely divided and the ulnar nerve decompressed. An advantage of this operation is its simplicity, because the aponeurosis is simply divided over the ulnar nerve and into the proximal third of the forearm. This operation is generally quite safe, because the ulnar nerve is not disturbed and, therefore, is not robbed of either its extrinsic or intrinsic blood supply (Fig. 11–7).

The most serious complication of this procedure is the onset of subluxation of the ulnar nerve to or across the medial epicondyle after simple decompression of the nerve.[28, 29, 78] This can be avoided by limiting the decompression to an area distal to a line drawn from the medial epicondyle to the olecranon. Once this subluxation begins, there is little short of either epicondylectomy or transposition of the ulnar nerve that will relieve the symptoms experienced by the patient.

Over 35 years ago King and Morgan published their experience with medial epicondylectomy for the treatment of traumatic ulnar neuritis at the elbow.[88] The removal of the medial epicondyle, permitting the nerve to seek its own optimal position without disturbing its intrinsic or extrinsic vascular supply, seemed popular for its simplicity, advantageous because the nerve was not excessively manipulated, and desirable because damage to any branches of the ulnar nerve was avoided (Fig. 11–8).[31, 54, 81, 88, 133] Several reports on this operation have continued to find favor with this procedure through the advantage of early postoperative motion, which allows the patient to return to the usual activities in the shortest possible interval.[33, 54, 81]

The most important disadvantage of medial epicondylectomy continues to be the loss of the pro-

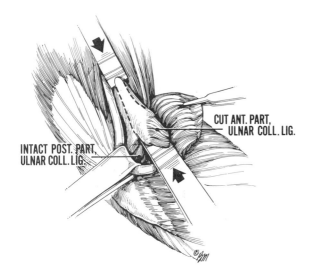

CUT ANT. PART,
ULNAR COLL. LIG.

INTACT POST. PART,
ULNAR COLL. LIG.

Figure 11–8. By retracting the ulnar nerve posteriorly during medial epicondylectomy, the branches of the ulnar nerve and its blood supply are left undisturbed. The origin of the flexor muscle mass is replaced beneath the nerve following epicondylectomy. (Courtesy of E. Roselius. From Greene, D. P. (ed.): Operative Hand Surgery, New York-London, Churchill Livingstone, 1982.)

tecting prominence of the medial epicondyle, which may subject the nerve to repeated direct external trauma following epicondylectomy. Because the nerve is not explored during medial epicondylectomy the surgeon usually cannot identify the site or degree of compression, and as a result the possibility of partial or total lack of relief of symptoms may be more than just theoretically unacceptable. Subluxation of the ulnar nerve, with secondary compression at the medial intermuscular septum, has been identified as a postoperative complication of this procedure.

Anterior transposition of the ulnar nerve, although certainly popular with many surgeons, is a most demanding operation.[18, 23, 33, 101, 108, 126, 147] It has been accompanied by a number of variations since its description by Learmonth in 1942.[101] Many authors favor this approach in the surgical treatment

of the cubital tunnel syndrome, reserving it for the more severe and difficult compression neuropathies of the ulnar nerve at the elbow.[126]

The potential complications of this procedure are related to the extensive exposure of the ulnar nerve, which not only places the branches of the nerve at some risk, especially those of the flexor carpi ulnaris, but also may increase the scar in the new bed to which the ulnar nerve has been transposed. During the transposition the ulnar nerve may be separated from its blood supply, causing further injury to the nerve and an increase in neuropathy. Commonly, anterior transposition of the nerve, either subcutaneous or submuscular, could create a new site of compression if the surgeon fails to adhere to the details of the dissection and transposition.

The most proximal site of creation of a secondary

Figure 11–9. Following transposition of the ulnar nerve anteriorly, care must be taken that a secondary site of entrapment is not created at the arcade of Struthers or the medial intermuscular septum, or beneath the flexor muscle mass. (Courtesy of E. Roselius. From Greene, D. P. (ed.): Operative Hand Surgery, New York-London, Churchill Livingstone, 1982.)

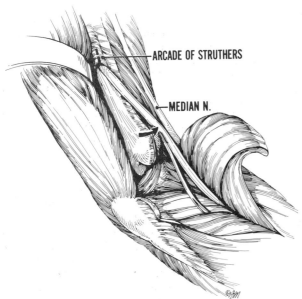

ARCADE OF STRUTHERS

MEDIAN N.

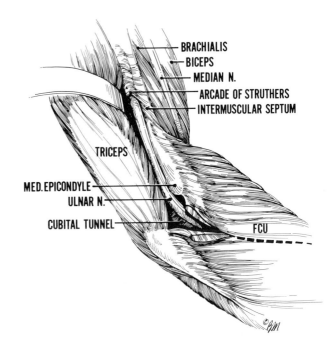

BRACHIALIS
BICEPS
MEDIAN N.
ARCADE OF STRUTHERS
INTERMUSCULAR SEPTUM
TRICEPS
MED. EPICONDYLE
ULNAR N.
CUBITAL TUNNEL
FCU

Figure 11–10. The medial intermuscular septum must be excised prior to transposition of the ulnar nerve anteriorly with either subcutaneous or submuscular transposition technique. *FCU,* flexor carpi ulnaris. (Courtesy of E. Roselius. From Greene, D. P. (ed.): Operative Hand Surgery, New York-London, Churchill Livingstone, 1982.)

compression neuropathy after anterior transposition occurs at the arcade of Struthers, approximately 10 cm proximal from the medial epicondyle of the humerus.[177–179] At this position, a fascial reflection of the triceps muscle adjacent to the intermuscular septum may create a site of secondary neuropathy across the ulnar nerve, which has been transposed anteriorly from the posterior compartment of the brachium (Fig. 11–9).[152] This fascial reflection must be released by the surgeon transposing the nerve or it will create a new site of compression.

The second potential site of a secondary neuropathy following anterior transposition is at the medial intermuscular septum, which will lie directly beneath the ulnar nerve following transposition anteriorly (Fig. 11–10). The medial intermuscular septum compression will produce a positive percussion test 3 to 5 cm proximal to the medial epicondyle along the medial intermuscular septum. The medial intermuscular septum should be excised at the time of anterior transposition or, if causing a secondary compression, should be excised at re-exploration of the ulnar nerve.

If a submuscular transposition has been selected for the patient, a tight fascial band lying between the flexor carpi ulnaris and the flexor carpi radialis, as the medial muscle mass is elevated for submuscular transposition, may be a source of compression on replacement of the flexor muscle mass and its reattachment to the medial epicondyle. At the time of anterior transposition, therefore, this aponeurotic band lying within the flexor muscle mass will require removal over a sufficient distance to allow an unobstructed passage of the ulnar nerve. Failure to excise the aponeurotic band may create a secondary site of compression neuropathy in the transposed ulnar nerve, with a positive percussion test over the flexor

muscle mass just distal to the medial epicondyle.[43] If examination of the patient elicits a positive percussion test in the flexor muscle mass of the anteriorly transposed ulnar nerve, re-exploration of the nerve and relief of the nerve in this area are indicated.

A similar band may be created when the surgeon has selected a subcutaneous transposition for the ulnar nerve, in which case the band will be a reflection of the flexor carpi ulnaris as the nerve *re-enters* the flexor compartment of the forearm between the two heads of this muscle. Once again, a sensitivity of the nerve to percussion over the flexor muscle mass may dictate re-exploration and relief of the nerve at the point of sensitivity.

Obviously, re-exploration of the ulnar nerve following anterior transposition should not be undertaken if there has been significant improvement of function of the nerve until the surgeon and patient are convinced that recovery has been unsatisfactory or has not occurred, or that recovery has deteriorated postoperatively. In all cases, a simple neuritis or neuroma of the superficial skin nerves, which may be divided by the surgical incisions on the medial side of the elbow, should be carefully ruled out, usually using diagnostic blocks. Specifically, neuromas of the medial antebrachial or medial brachial cutaneous nerve can be disturbing to the patient, suggesting that the desired improvement to have been obtained by decompression of the cubital tunnel was limited or nonexistent and may, following treatment, relieve the patient sufficiently that the ulnar nerve may not need re-exploration or surgical manipulation.

The systematic evaluation of the patient who has undergone a previous operation for cubital tunnel syndrome requires at least three distinct methods of examination. The first is a detailed and probably repeated elbow flexion test, which seems to be particularly useful in those patients who have undergone simple decompression of the ulnar nerve. With these patients a positive elbow flexion test will usually underscore the necessity for a more aggressive surgical approach to cubital tunnel syndrome, either by medial epicondylectomy or by anterior transposition of the ulnar nerve.

The subcutaneous blocking of the sensory nerves on the medial side of the arm and forearm with local anesthetic is absolutely essential in the evaluation of the postoperative patient who continues to have symptoms of cubital tunnel syndrome. Whenever possible, this block should be performed using a long-acting local anesthetic to evaluate the presence of dysesthesia, paresthesia, or neuroma formation in one or more branches of the medial antebrachial and medial brachial cutaneous nerves. On several occasions I have found that the postoperative symptoms that disturb patients the most have nothing to do with the ulnar nerve itself but are, instead, related to these superficial cutaneous nerves, branches of which are all too commonly divided by the usual surgical incisions at the medial epicondyle.

Third, and probably most important, a period of immobilization of the elbow either in a surgical orthosis, a plaster splint, or a cast, relieved along the course of the ulnar nerve so that no pressure is exerted along the ulnar nerve, will usually provide valuable information concerning the patient's symptoms. If, for instance, the patient experiences relief of the dysesthetic or paresthetic symptoms with simple immobilization of the elbow, there is a possibility of benefit from surgical re-exploration as long as the preoperative criteria of lack of improvement following surgery, insufficient improvement following surgery, or deterioration following improvement after surgery have been met. That is, if a patient has either signs or symptoms of lack of improvement or deterioration following an initial surgical procedure for cubital syndrome, and if that patient has dysesthetic or paresthetic symptoms in the ulnar nerve distribution that are relieved by simple immobilization, the likelihood that the patient will benefit from re-exploration of the nerve with or without a more aggressive surgical approach is extremely high. If the previous operative procedure was a simple decompression of the ulnar nerve, anterior transposition—removing the nerve from its bed—will probably be most satisfactory. If, however, the previous surgical procedure was a subcutaneous transposition, it might be advisable to proceed to a submuscular transposition, combined with re-exploration of the ulnar nerve proximal to the elbow.

Ulnar Tunnel Syndrome

Because many patients have symptoms of ulnar tunnel syndrome as a direct result of misuse of the

hand, most commonly using the hypothenar eminence in a hammerlike fashion, a detailed work history and change of work routine will often relieve the symptoms of what may be considered an occupational neuritis of the ulnar nerve.[39, 70, 89, 125, 154, 156, 162, 182, 184, 190, 208] Complications of this syndrome are thus relatively infrequent.[79, 114, 124, 150, 159, 189] Thrombosis or aneurysm of the ulnar artery associated with or as the result of this syndrome, however, is common.[89] Accordingly, the surgeon undertaking decompression of the ulnar tunnel should be aware of the occasional problem of having to deal with either an aneurysm or a thrombosis of the ulnar artery, even with resection and end-to-end anastomosis or vein grafting of the ulnar artery if the thrombosis is over a significant segment.

At the time of decompression of the ulnar tunnel, it is important to carry the decompression into the distal third of the forearm so that a band of forearm fascia does not complement the flexion of the wrist at the proximal wrist crease to perpetuate the compression syndrome of the ulnar nerve at the crease (Fig. 11–11).[6, 12, 30, 43, 64, 74, 144, 191, 192, 204, 205] A surgeon who confines decompression to the canal of Guyon, without continuing into the distal third of the forearm, will usually leave a compressive band at the proximal wrist crease, with symptoms of percussion sensitivity at the wrist crease and a positive wrist flexion test for the ulnar nerve if the decompression is incomplete.

Although a neuroma of the palmar cutaneous branch of the ulnar nerve is theoretically possible,

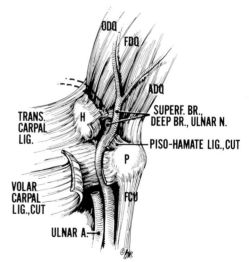

Figure 11–11. Decompression of the ulnar tunnel syndrome must be accompanied by fasciotomy of the distal 2 or 3 inches of the forearm proximal to the wrist creases, exposing the ulnar artery and nerve so that a compressive band does not remain at the proximal wrist crease. *FCU,* flexor carpi ulnaris, *ODQ,* opponens digiti quinti; *FDQ,* flexor digiti quinti; *ADQ,* abductor digiti quinti, *P,* pisiform bone. (Courtesy of E. Roselius. From Greene, D. P. (ed.): Operative Hand Surgery, New York-London, Churchill Livingstone, 1982.)

it is extremely rare, and does not seem to cause an extended period of discomfort or disability for the patient.[42] If a neuroma of the palmar cutaneous branch of the ulnar nerve is suspected by dysesthesias over the hypothenar eminence, conservative measures such as desensitization, with progressively increasing severity of percussion of the neuroma, would ordinarily be sufficient to provide relief for the patient.

A neuritis of the medial antebrachial cutaneous nerve, unlike that of the palmar cutaneous branch of the ulnar nerve, may produce disabling and disagreeable symptoms that can be annoying and affect a worker's performance. The diagnosis of neuritis of the medial antebrachial cutaneous nerve is usually confirmed by a subcutaneous injection of a local anesthetic at the midforearm level, which would relieve the neuritic pain at the distal forearm, wrist, or hypothenar eminence but at the same time would not produce a complete motor and sensory block of the ulnar nerve. Medial antebrachial cutaneous nerve neuritis that does not respond to desensitization procedures in the area of the neuroma is probably best treated by resection of the brachial portion of the medial antebrachial cutaneous nerve, which would render a large portion of the medial side of the forearm anesthetic.

COMPRESSION NEUROPATHIES

Dorsal Branch of the Ulnar Nerve

Compression neuropathy of the dorsal branch of the ulnar nerve is relatively infrequent. However, following decompression, persistent neuroma of the dorsal branch with or without dysesthesia in its distribution on the dorsal surface of the ring and little fingers may persist as an annoying and even disabling symptom. In the presence of continuing symptoms after decompression, as long as the decompression has been complete and extends from the ulnar nerve to the dorsum of the hand, the surgeon must only be certain that the patient's symptoms are due to the dorsal branch. A series of diagnostic blocks injected subcutaneously 2 to 4 cm proximal to the ulnar styloid, on the dorsoulnar aspect of the distal forearm, should provide temporary relief of the dysesthesia if it is caused by persistent neuroma of the dorsal branch of the ulnar nerve.

It is important to differentiate this pain syndrome from other conditions that could cause pain in the same area—specifically, tear of the triangular cartilage lying between the distal ulna and the triquetrum of the wrist, with or without chondromalacia of the triquetrum, extensor carpi ulnaris tendinitis, neuritis of the antebrachial cutaneous nerve, and neuritis of an aberrant branch of either the terminal sensory branch of the musculocutaneous or the superficial radial nerve, which may cross over and innervate areas adjacent to or identical with the

usual distribution of the dorsal branch of the ulnar nerve. In all these conditions, a series of diagnostic blocks using a long-acting local anesthetic will help in differentiating the several pain syndromes that may be confused with a continuing neuritis of the dorsal branch of the ulnar nerve.

Radial Nerve

Just as compression neuropathies of the radial nerve occur more frequently than is generally believed, so do the complications of this seldom recognized syndrome. The usual radial nerve palsy associated with fractures of the distal half of the humeral diaphysis is most often a result of the

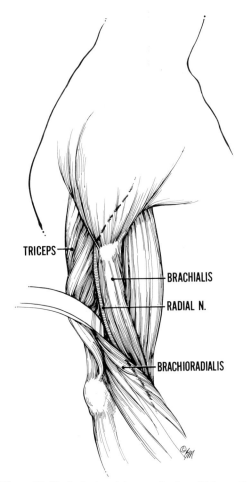

Figure 11–12. A displaced fracture in the middle or distal third of the humerus may commonly be associated with radial nerve paralysis due to entrapment of the radial nerve at the lateral intermuscular septum as the nerve passes from the posterior to the anterior compartment of the brachium on the lateral side of the humerus. (Courtesy of E. Roselius. From Greene, D. P. (ed.): Operative Hand Surgery, New York-London, Churchill Livingstone, 1982.).

fixation of the radial nerve and its consequent compression neuropathy at the lateral intermuscular septum (Fig. 11–12).[55, 106, 131, 139] Because palsy of the radial nerve associated with humeral fracture does not recover normal function in approximately one third of cases, the longstanding complications of this injury and associated radial neuropathy are evident. The complication of prolonged, even irreversible, neuropathy of the radial nerve as a result of compression at the lateral intermuscular septum could well be considered to be a reversible lesion if early decompression were performed, possibly with internal fixation of the humeral fracture.[138]

It should also be remembered that some authors have described a compression neuropathy of the lateral intermuscular septum of the radial nerve in the absence of associated fracture and displacement of the humerus.[111, 117] As the surgeon evaluates a radial tunnel syndrome, if there is a finding of denervation of the extensor carpi radialis longus, brachioradialis, or even occasionally the extensor carpi radialis brevis, it might be prudent to extend exploration of the radial nerve proximal to the radial tunnel, and to decompress the lateral intermuscular septum as the radial nerve pierces it in its course from the posterior to the anterior compartment of the brachium.[107, 151]

Unlike most compression neuropathies in which most patients will note postoperatively an immediate and definite improvement in symptoms, after surgery for the radial tunnel syndrome patients normally note an extended period of similar symptoms without significant improvement following surgical decompression. This delay in resolution of symptoms should not be interpreted as a complication of the surgical decompression, but rather as a

considered norm in the recovery from this syndrome.

The detailed exploration of the radial nerve for radial tunnel syndrome should begin about 2 inches proximal to the radial head to avoid the obvious complication of inadequate release of the radial nerve (Fig. 11–13). Because of its relatively limited exposure, the posterior muscle splitting approach to the radial tunnel is not preferred. Rather, an anterolateral approach to the radial tunnel, which initially isolates the radial nerve between the brachialis and the brachioradialis and then traces the nerve distally, provides the best possible surgical approach to relieve any compressing bands, whether they are located anterior to the radial head or in or about the radial leash of vessels on the deep surface of the extensor carpi radialis brevis or the arcade of Frohse.

At the time of surgery, the aponeurosis of the extensor carpi radialis brevis may be most easily ignored as a possible compressing force on the radial nerve. This occurs because the surgical procedure for exploration of the radial nerve is normally performed with the elbow extended and the forearm in supination. In the supinated position, the compressive band of the aponeurosis of the extensor carpi radialis brevis is loose and folded away from the radial nerve.[43] As a consequence, it does not appear to be a significant factor, unless the forearm is rotated into pronation, often with associated flexion of the wrist, to demonstrate the stout band on the deep surface of the extensor carpi radialis brevis, which often overlies and probably contributes to a compression of the nerve as it enters the proximal rim of the supinator muscle, the so-called arcade of Frohse.

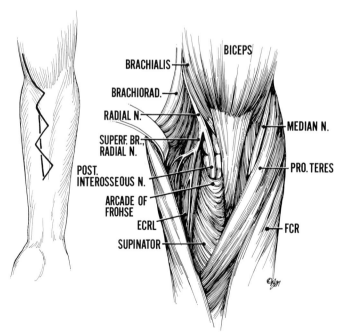

Figure 11–13. Decompression of the radial tunnel is most easily performed from the anterior approach, tracing the radial nerve from between the brachioradialis and brachialis distally through the supinator muscle to ensure complete decompression of the radial nerve and its branches. *FCR,* flexor carpi radialis, *ECRL,* extensor carpi radialis longus. (Courtesy of E. Roselius. From Greene, D. P. (ed.): Operative Hand Surgery, New York-London, Churchill Livingstone, 1982.)

BICEPS

BRACHIALIS

BRACHIORAD.

RADIAL N.

SUPERF. BR.
RADIAL N.

POST.
INTEROSSEOUS N.

ARCADE OF
FROHSE

ECRL

SUPINATOR

MEDIAN N.

PRO. TERES

FCR

A compression neuropathy at the distal border of the supinator muscle, as the deep radial nerve passes from between the two heads of the supinator muscle to the dorsal extensor surface of the forearm, has been described as an area of compression of the radial nerve. Although this site of compression had been predicted, many surgeons have not decompressed this area as part of their usual surgical decompression of the radial tunnel, and continuing symptoms from the radial tunnel syndrome may have produced a few cases resulting from this compression of the deep radial nerve.[43]

Neuritis of the superficial branch of the radial nerve, so-called Wartenberg's syndrome, may also be confused with a persistent radial tunnel syndrome.[197] The superficial portion of the radial nerve is only involved in a radial tunnel syndrome in approximately 50% of cases. When the radial tunnel syndrome includes a compression of the superficial branch of the radial nerve, the dysesthetic or paresthetic symptoms of the superficial branch of the radial nerve are generally relieved within a few days of radial nerve decompression. If the dysesthetic or paresthetic symptoms persist in the distribution of the radial nerve following radial tunnel surgery, it is well to consider a separate compression of the superficial radial nerve, which most commonly occurs as the nerve passes dorsal to the tendon and aponeurosis of the brachioradialis in the distal third of the forearm in its course to the dorsoradial aspect of the hand. This diagnosis can usually be confirmed with a diagnostic local anesthetic block infiltrated subcutaneously along the dorsal edge of the tendon of the brachioradialis in the distal third of the forearm. This site could be defined further if the patient has a positive percussion test over the radial nerve at this same point in the distal third of the forearm.

Wartenberg's syndrome may also be confused with a neuropathy of the musculocutaneous nerve in its distal sensory branch, particularly when the distal sensory branch overlies a portion or even the entire dorsoradial aspect of the hand, usually supplied by the superficial radial nerve. The lateral antebrachial cutaneous nerve, the distal sensory branch of the musculocutaneous, can usually be anesthetized with a diagnostic block of a long-acting local anesthetic by subcutaneous injection just lateral to the biceps tendon and just proximal to the elbow crease, taking care not to infuse the local anesthetic deep between the surfaces of the brachialis and brachioradialis, which would, of course, anesthetize the radial nerve. If a block of the musculocutaneous nerve is successful in relieving paresthetic or dysesthetic pain on the dorsoradial aspect of the wrist, and there is no concomitant palsy of the radial nerve—that is, loss of function of the wrist extensors, finger extensors, or thumb extensors or abductors—it can usually be presumed that there is a variation of the lateral antebrachial cutaneous nerve innervating the dorsal sensory cutaneous area of the hand.

Thus during the postoperative evaluation of a patient who has undergone surgical decompression of an entrapment neuropathy, particularly when the patient's response to the surgical decompression is less than anticipated or desired, both by the patient and the surgeon, the physician must continue to be aware of those conditions that may complicate any entrapment neuropathy. The neuropathy associated with diabetes mellitus, in many cases, not only because of its frequency but also because of its severity, may delay or inhibit the recovery of nerve function following the decompression. The experience with carpal tunnel syndrome is most vivid in this regard. Patients with diabetes, either diagnosed or even undiagnosed, will normally demonstrate a delay in their improvement following relief of the transverse carpal ligament by two to three times the normal 6- to 8-week period in which the usual patient can be expected to regain a large portion of neurologic function. Improvement in patients with severe axonotmesis or even neurotmesis will similarly be delayed, or the patient may be totally unresponsive.

A major peripheral neuropathy will have a similar effect to that of the neuropathy of diabetes mellitus in delaying a favorable response following decompression. My experiences with amyotrophic lateral sclerosis, Charcot-Marie-Tooth, multiple sclerosis, and several other undiagnosed but widespread peripheral neuropathies, have confirmed this.

The "double crush" nerve entrapment syndrome described by Upton and McComas in 1973 is not an uncommon cause of delayed response to decompression of an entrapment neuropathy. Accordingly, a delayed response of a carpal tunnel syndrome might well be looked for at the pronator level. A delayed response to a release of a Wartenberg's syndrome of the radial nerve at the wrist might be found at the radial tunnel, and a delayed response to the decompression of the ulnar tunnel might be found at the cubital tunnel. Particularly in the case of the ulnar nerve, a compression syndrome at the thoracic outlet must be considered as a proximal source of a "double crush," and detailed testing to include somatosensory evoked potentials across the thoracic outlet may be of considerable help in the diagnosis of a "double crush" syndrome along the axis of the ulnar nerve.[62]

References

1. Adson, A. W.: Progressive ulnar paralysis. Minn. Med., 1:455, 1918.
2. Arkin, A. M.: Habitual luxation of the ulnar nerve. J. Mt. Sinai Hosp., 7:208, 1940.
3. Arnold, A. G.: The carpal tunnel syndrome in congestive cardiac failure. Postgrad. Med. J., 53:623, 1977.
4. Ashby, B. S.: Hypertrophy of the palmaris longus. J. Bone Joint Surg., 46B:230, 1964.
5. Backhouse, K. M., and Churchill-Davidson, D.: Anomalous palmaris longus muscle producing carpal tunnel-like compression. Hand, 7:22, 1975.
6. Bakke, J. L., and Wolff, H. G.: Occupational pressure neuritis of the deep palmar branch of the ulnar nerve. Arch. Neurol. Psychiatry, 60:549, 1948.

7. Barnard, L. B., and McCoy, S. M.: The supracondyloid process of the humerus. J. Bone Joint Surg., 28:845, 1946.
8. Baruch, A., and Hass, A.: Anomaly of the median nerve. J. Hand Surg., 2:331, 1977.
9. Beaton, L. E., and Anson, B. J.: The relation of the median nerve to the pronator teres muscle. Anat. Rec., 75:23, 1939,
10. Bendler, E. M., et al.: The bilaterality of carpal tunnel syndrome. Arch. Phys. Med. Rehabil., 58:362, 1977.
11. Blodgett, R. C., Jr., Lipscomb, P. R., and Hill, R. W.: Incidence of hematologic disease in patients with carpal tunnel syndrome. J.A.M.A., 182:814, 1962.
12. Blunden, R.: Neuritis of deep branch of the ulnar nerve. J. Bone Joint Surg., 40B:354, 1958.
13. Blunt, M. J.: The vascular anatomy of the median nerve in the forearm and hand. J. Anat., 93:15, 1959.
14. Bonney, G.: Scalenus medius band. J. Bone Joint Surg., 47B:268, 1965.
15. Brain, W. R., Wright, A. D., and Wilkerson, M.: Spontaneous compression of both median nerves in the carpal tunnel. Six cases treated surgically. Lancet, 1:277, 1947.
16. Brannon, W. E.: Cervical rib syndrome. J. Bone Joint Surg., 45A:977, 1963.
17. Brones, M. F., and Wilgis, E. F.: Anatomical variations of the palmaris longus, causing carpal tunnel syndrome: Case report. Plast. Reconstr. Surg., 62:798, 1978.
18. Broudy, A. S., Leffert, R. D., and Smith, R. J.: Technical problems with ulnar nerve transposition at the elbow: Findings and results of reoperation. J. Hand Surg., 3:85, 1978.
19. Bucher, T. P. J.: Anterior interosseous nerve syndrome. J. Bone Joint Surg., 54B:555, 1972.
20. Buchthal, F., and Rosenfalck, A.: Sensory conduction from digit to palm and from palm to wrist in the carpal tunnel syndrome. J. Neurol. Neurosurg. Psychiatry, 34:243, 1971.
21. Burman, M. A., and Sutro, C. J.: Recurrent luxation of the ulnar nerve by congenital posterior position of the medial epicondyle of the humerus. J. Bone Joint Surg., 21:958, 1939.
22. Butler, B., and Bigley, E.: Aberrant index (first) lumbrical tendinous origin associated with carpal-tunnel syndrome. A case report. J. Bone Joint Surg., 53A:160, 1971.
23. Campbell, J. B., Morantz, R. A., and Post, K. D.: A technique for relief of motor and sensory deficits occurring after anterior ulnar transposition. J. Neurosurg., 40:405, 1974.
24. Cannon, B. W., and Love, J. B.: Tardy median palsy: Median neuritis: Median thenar neuritis amenable to surgery. Surgery, 20:210, 1946.
25. Champion, D.: Gouty tenosynovitis and the carpal tunnel syndrome. Med. J. Aust., 1:1030, 1969.
26. Cherington, M.: Proximal pain in the carpal tunnel syndrome. Arch. Surg., 108:69, 1974.
27. Cherington, M: Ulnar conduction velocity in thoracic outlet syndrome. N. Engl. J. Med., 294:1185, 1978.
28. Childress, H. M.: Recurrent ulnar-nerve dislocation at the elbow. J. Bone Joint Surg., 38A:978, 1956.
29. Childress, H. M.: Recurrent ulnar-nerve dislocation at the elbow. Clin. Orthop., 108:168, 1975.
30. Comtet, J., Quicot, L., and Moyen, B.: Compression of the deep palmar branch of the ulnar nerve by the arch of the adductor pollicis. Hand, 10:176, 1978.
31. Craven, P. R., and Green, D. P.: Cubital tunnel syndrome. Treatment by medial epicondylectomy. J. Bone Joint Surg., 62A:986, 1980.
32. Cseuz, K. A., et al.: Long-term results of operation for carpal tunnel syndrome. Mayo Clin. Proc., 41:232, 1966.
33. Curtis, B. F.: Traumatic ulnar neuritis; transplantation of the nerve. J. Nerv. Ment. Dis., 25:480, 1898.
34. Curtis, R. M. and Eversmann, W. W., Jr.: Internal neurolysis as an adjunct to the treatment of the carpal-tunnel syndrome. J. Bone Joint Surg., 55A:733, 1973.
35. Dale, W. A.: Thoracic outlet compression syndrome. Arch. Surg., 117:1437, 1982.
36. Daube, J. R.: Nerve conduction studies in the thoracic outlet syndrome. Neurology, 25:347, 1975.
37. Denman, E. E.: An unusual branch of the ulnar nerve in the hand. Hand, 9:92, 1977.
38. Doll, D. C., and Weiss, R. B.: Unusual presentations of multiple myeloma. Postgrad. Med., 61:116, 1977.
39. Dupont, C., et al.: Ulnar-tunnel syndrome at the wrist. A

report of four cases of ulnar-nerve compression at the wrist. J. Bone Surg., 47A:757, 1965.
40. Eiken, O., Carstram, N., and Eddeland, A.: Anomalous distal branching of the median nerve. Scand. J. Plast. Reconstr. Surg., 5:149, 1971.
41. Eisen, A.: Early diagnosis of ulnar nerve palsy: An electrophysiological study. Neurology, 24:256, 1974.
42. Engber, W. D., and Cmeiner, J. G.: Palmar cutaneous branch of the ulnar nerve. J. Hand Surg., 5:26, 1980.
43. Eversmann, W. W., Jr., and Green, D. P. (eds.): Operative Hand Surgery, New York, Churchill-Livingstone, 1982, pp. 957–1009.
44. Eversmann, W. W., Jr., and Ritsick, J. A.: Intraoperative changes in motor nerve conduction latency in carpal tunnel syndrome. J. Hand Surg., 3:77, 1978.
45. Farber, J. S., and Bryan, R. S.: The anterior interosseous nerve syndrome. J. Bone Joint Surg., 50A:521, 1968.
46. Fearn, C. B. d'A., and Goodfellow, J. W.: Anterior interosseous nerve palsy. J. Bone Joint Surg., 47B:91, 1965.
47. Felsenthal, G.: Median and ulnar distal motor and sensory latencies in the same normal subject. Arch. Phys. Med. Rehabil., 58:297, 1977.
48. Felsenthal, G.: Comparison of evoked potentials in the same hand in normal subjects and in patients with carpal tunnel syndrome. Am. J. Phys. Med., 57:228, 1978.
49. Felsenthal, G.: Median- and ulnar-evoked muscle and sensory action potentials. Am. J. Phys. Med., 57:167, 1978.
50. Fenning, J. B.: Deep ulnar-nerve paralysis resulting from an anatomical abnormality. A case report. J. Bone Joint Surg., 47A:1381, 1965.
51. Ferner, H.: Ein abnormer verhaluf des nervus medianus vor dem M. pronator teres. Anat. Anz., 84:151, 1937.
52. Fincham, R. W., and Cape, C. A.: Neuropathy in myxedema. A study of sensory nerve conduction in the upper extremities. Arch. Neurol., 19:464, 1968.
53. Folkers, K., et al.: Biochemical evidence for a deficiency of vitamin B_6 in the carpal tunnel syndrome based on a crossover clinical study. Proc. Natl. Acad. Sci. U.S.A., 75:3410, 1978.
54. Froimson, A. I., and Zahrawi, F.: Treatment of compression neuropathy of the ulnar nerve at the elbow by epicondylectomy and neurolysis. J. Hand Surg., 5:391, 1980.
55. Garcia, A., and Maeck, B. H.: Radial nerve injuries in fractures of the shaft of the humerus. Am. J. Surg., 99:625, 1960.
56. Gardner, R. C.: Confirmed case and diagnosis of pseudocarpal-tunnel (sublimis) syndrome. N. Engl. J. Med., 282:858, 1970.
57. Gassmann, N., Segmuller, G., and Stanisic, M.: Carpal tunnel syndrome. Indications, technique and results following epineural and interfascicular neurolysis. Handchirurgie, 9:137, 1977.
58. Gelberman, R. H., Verdeck, W. H., and Brodhead, W. T.: Supraclavicular nerve entrapment syndrome. J. Bone Joint Surg., 57A:199, 1975.
59. Gilliatt, R. W.: Classical neurological syndrome associated with cervical rib and band. Ann. Neurol., 4:124, 1979.
60. Gilliatt, R. W., and Thomas, P. K.: Changes in nerve conduction with ulnar nerve lesions at the elbow. J. Neurol. Neurosurg. Psychiatry, 23:312, 1960.
61. Gilliatt, R. W., et al.: Peripheral nerve conduction in patients with a cervical rib and band. Ann. Neurol., 4:124, 1978.
62. Glover, J. L., et al.: Evoked responses in the diagnosis of "thoracic outlet syndrome." Surgery, 89:86, 1981.
63. Golding, D. N.: Brachial neuralgia and the carpal tunnel syndrome. Br. Med. J., 3:803, 1968.
64. Gori, D. R.: Carpometacarpal dislocation producing compression of the deep branch of the ulnar nerve. J. Bone Joint Surg., 53A:1387, 1971.
65. Gould, J. S., and Wissinger, H. A.: Carpal tunnel syndrome in pregnancy. South. Med. J., 71:144, 1978.
66. Graham, W. P., III: Variations of the motor branch of the median nerve at the wrist. Plast. Reconstr. Surg., 51:90, 1973.
67. Green, E. J., Dilworth, J. H., and Levitin, P. M.: Tophaceous gout. An unusual cause of bilateral carpal tunnel syndrome. J.A.M.A., 237:2747, 1977.
68. Grokoest, A. W., and Demartini, F. E.: Systemic disease and the carpal tunnel syndrome. J.A.M.A., 155:635, 1954.

69. Hartwell, S. W., Jr., and Kurtay, M.: Carpal tunnel compression caused by hematoma associated with anticoagulant therapy. Report of a case. Cleve. Clin., 33:127, 1966.

70. Hayes, C.: Ulnar tunnel syndrome from giant cell tumor of tendon sheath: A case report. J. Hand Surg., 3:187, 1978.

71. Hecht, O., and Lipsher, E.: Median and ulnar nerve entrapment caused by ectopic calcification. J. Hand Surg., 5:30, 1980.

72. Henry, A. K.: Extensile Exposure, 2nd ed., Baltimore, Williams & Wilkins, 1970.

73. Hongell, A., and Mattsson, H. S.: Neurographic studies before, after and during operation for median nerve compression in the carpal tunnel syndrome. Scand. J. Plast. Reconstr. Surg., 5:103, 1971.

74. Howard, F. M.: Ulnar nerve palsy in wrist fractures. J. Bone Joint Surg., 43A:1197, 1961.

75. Howard, F. M., and Shafer, S. J.: Injuries to the clavicle with neurovascular complications. A study of fourteen cases. J. Bone Joint Surg., 47A:1335, 1965.

76. Hunt, J. R.: Tardy or late paralysis of the ulnar nerve. A form of chronic progressive neuritis developing many years after fracture dislocation of the elbow joint. J.A.M.A., 66:11, 1916.

77. Jabaley, M. E.: Personal observations on the role of the lumbrical muscles in carpal tunnel syndrome. J. Hand Surg., 3:82, 1978.

78. James, G. G. H.: Nerve lesions about the elbow. J. Bone Joint Surg., 38B:589, 1956.

79. Jeffery, A. K.: Compression of the deep palmar branch of the ulnar nerve by an anomalous muscle. J. Bone Joint Surg., 53B:718, 1971.

80. Johnson, R. K., and Shrewbury, M. M.: Anatomical course of the thenar branch of the median nerve—usually in a separate tunnel through the transverse carpal ligament. J. Bone Joint Surg., 52A:269, 1970.

81. Jones, R. E., and Gauntt, C.: Medial epicondylectomy for ulnar nerve compression syndrome at the elbow. Clin. Orthop., 139:174, 1979.

82. Kaplan, E. B.: Variation of the ulnar nerve at the wrist. Bull. Hosp. Joint Dis., 24:85, 1963.

83. Kaplan, H., and Clayton, M.: Carpal tunnel syndrome secondary to *Mycobacterium kansasii* infection. J.A.M.A., 208:1186, 1969.

84. Kemble, F.: Electrodiagnosis of the carpal tunnel syndrome. J. Neurol. Neurosurg. Psychiatry, 31:23, 1968.

85. Kessel, L., and Rang, M.: Supracondylar spur of the humerus. J. Bone Joint Surg., 48B:765, 1966.

86. Khunadorn, N., et al.: Carpal tunnel syndrome in hemophilia. N.Y. State J. Med., 77:1314, 1977.

87. Kiloh, L. G., and Nevin, S.: Isolated neuritis of the anterior interosseous nerve. Br. Med. J., 1:850, 1952.

88. King, T., and Morgan, F. P.: The treatment of traumatic ulnar neuritis. Mobilization of the ulnar nerve at the elbow by removal of the medial epicondyle and adjacent bone. Aust. N.Z. J. Surg., 20:35, 1950.

89. Kleinert, H. E., and Hayes, J. R.: The ulnar tunnel syndrome. Plast. Reconstr. Surg., 47:21, 1971.

90. Klofkorn, R. W., and Steigerwald, J. C.: Carpal tunnel syndromes as the initial manifestation of tuberculosis. Am. J. Med., 60:583, 1976.

91. Kopell, H. P., and Thompson, W. A. L.: Pronator syndrome. N. Engl. J. Med., 259:713, 1958.

92. Kremer, M., et al.: Acroparesthesiae in the carpal-tunnel syndrome. Lancet, 2:590, 1953.

93. Kummel, B. M., and Zazanis, G. A.: Shoulder pain as the presenting complaint in carpal tunnel syndrome. Clin. Orthop., 92:227, 1953.

94. Laha, R. K., Lunsford, D., and Dujovny, M.: Lacertus fibrosus compression of the median nerve. Case report. J. Neurosurg., 48:838, 1978.

95. Lain, T. M.: The military brace syndrome: A report of sixteen cases of Erb's palsy occurring in military cadets. J. Bone Joint Surg., 51A:557, 1969.

96. Lake, P. A.: Anterior interosseous nerve syndrome. J. Neurosurg., 41:306, 1974.

97. Lanz, U.: Anatomical variations of the median nerve in the carpal tunnel. J. Hand Surg., 2:44, 1977.

98. Lassa, R., and Shrewbury, M. M.: A variation in the path of the deep motor branch of the ulnar nerve at the wrist. J. Bone Joint Surg., 57A:990, 1975.

99. Layton, K. B.: Acroparesthesia in pregnancy and the carpal tunnel syndrome. Obstet. Gynecol., 65:823, 1958.

100. Leach, R. E., and Odom, J. A.: Systemic causes of the carpal tunnel syndrome. Postgrad. Med., 44:127, 1968.

101. Learmonth, J. R.: Technique for transplanting the ulnar nerve. Surg. Gynecol. Obstet., 75:792, 1942.

102. Lettin, A. W. F.: Carpal tunnel syndrome in childhood. J. Bone Joint Surg., 47B:556, 1965.

103. Levy, M., and Pauker, M.: Carpal tunnel syndrome due to thrombosed persisting median artery. A case report. Hand, 10:65, 1978.

104. Linscheid, R. L., Peterson, L. P. A., and Juergens, J. L.: Carpal tunnel syndrome associated with vasospasm. J. Bone Joint Surg., 49A:1141, 1967.

105. Lipscomb, P. R.: Tenosynovitis of the hand and the wrist: Carpal tunnel syndrome, de Quervain's disease, trigger digit. Clin. Orthop., 13:164, 1959.

106. Lipscomb, P. R., and Burelson, R. J.: Vascular and neural complications in supracondylar fractures in children. J. Bone Joint Surg., 37A:487, 1955.

107. Lister, G. D., Belsole, R. B., and Kleinert, H. E.: The radial tunnel syndrome. J. Hand Surg., 4:52, 1979.

108. Lluch, A. L.: Ulnar nerve entrapment after anterior transposition at elbow. N.Y. State J. Med., 1:75, 1975.

109. Loong, S. C.: The carpal tunnel syndrome: A clinical and electrophysiological study of 250 patients. Proc. Aust. Assoc. Neurol., 14:51, 1977.

110. Loong, S. C., and Seah, S. C.: Comparison of median and ulnar sensory nerve action potentials in the diagnosis of the carpal tunnel syndrome. J. Neurol. Neurosurg. Psychiatry, 34:750, 1971.

111. Lotem, M., et al.: Radial palsy following muscular effort. A nerve compression syndrome possibly related to a fibrous arch of the lateral head of the triceps. J. Bone Joint Surg., 53B:500, 1971.

112. Ludin, H. P., Lutschg, J., and Valsangiacomo, F.: Comparison of orthodromic and antidromic sensory nerve conduction. 1. Normals and patients with carpal tunnel syndrome. E.E.G. E.M.G., 8:173, 1977.

113. Maeda, K., et al.: Anterior interosseous nerve paralysis. Report of 13 cases and review of Japanese literatures. Hand, 9:165, 1977.

114. Mallet, B. L., and Zilkha, K. J.: Compression of the ulnar nerve at the wrist by a ganglion. Lancet, 1:890, 1955.

115. Mangini, U.: Flexor pollicis longus muscle. Its morphology and clinical significance. J. Bone Joint Surg., 42A:467, 1960.

116. Mannerfelt, L., and Hybbinette, C. H.: Important anomaly of the thenar branch of the median nerve. Bull. Hosp. Joint Dis., 33:15, 1972.

117. Manske, P. R.: Compression of the radial nerve by the triceps muscle. Case report. J. Bone Joint Surg., 59A:835, 1977.

118. Marie et Foix, P.: Atrophie isolée de l'éminence thenar d'origine nevritique. Rôle du ligament annulaire anterieur de carpe dans la pathogenie de la lesion. Rev. Neurol., 26:647, 1913.

119. Marinacci, A. A.: Comparative value of measurement of nerve conduction velocity and electromyography in diagnosis of carpal tunnel syndrome. Arch. Phys. Med. Rehabil., 45:548, 1964.

120. Massey, E. W.: Carpal tunnel syndrome in pregnancy. Obstet. Gynecol. Surg., 33:145, 1978.

121. Massey, E. W., O'Brien, J. T., and Georges, L. B.: Carpal tunnel syndrome secondary to carpopedal spasm. Ann. Intern. Med., 88:804, 1978.

122. Maxwell, J. A., Keyes, J. J., and Ketchem, L. D.: Acute carpal tunnel syndrome secondary to thrombosis of a persistent median artery. J. Neurosurg., 38:774, 1973.

123. Mayers, L. B.: Carpal tunnel syndrome secondary to tuberculosis. Arch. Neurol., 10:426, 1964.

124. McDowell, C. L., and Hanceroth, W. D.: Compression of the ulnar nerve in the hand by a ganglion. Report of a case. J. Bone Joint Surg., 59A:980, 1977.

125. McFarland, G. G., and Hoffer, M. M.: Paralysis of the

intrinsic muscles of the hand secondary to lipoma in Guyon's canal. J. Bone Joint Surg., 53A:375, 1971.

126. McGowan, A. J.: The results of transposition of the ulnar nerve for traumatic ulnar neuritis. J. Bone Joint Surg., 32B:293, 1950.

127. McLellan, D. L., and Swash, M.: Longitudinal sliding of the median nerve during movements of the upper limb. J. Neurol. Neurosurg. Psychiatry, 39:566, 1976.

128. Melvin, J. L., Schuckmann, J. A., and Lanese, R. R.: Diagnostic specificity of motor and sensory nerve conduction variables in the carpal tunnel syndrome. Arch. Phys. Med. Rehabil., 54:69, 1973.

129. Michaelis, L. S.: Stenosis of carpal tunnel, compression of median nerve, and flexor tendon sheaths, combines with rheumatoid arthritis elsewhere. Proc. R. Soc. Med., 43:414, 1950.

130. Mittal, R., and Gupta, B.: Median and ulnar nerve palsy: An unusual presentation of the supracondylar process. Report of a case. J. Bone Joint Surg., 60A:557, 1978.

131. Morris, A. H.: Irreducible Monteggia lesion with radial-nerve entrapment. J. Bone Joint Surg., 56A:1744, 1974.

132. Nakano, K. K., Lundergan, C., and Okihiro, M. M.: Anterior interosseous nerve syndromes. Diagnostic methods and alternative treatments. Arch. Neurol., 34:477, 1977.

133. Neblett, C., and Ehni, G.: Medial epicondylectomy for ulnar palsy. J. Neurosurg., 32:55, 1970.

134. O'Brien, M. D., and Upton, A. R. M.: Anterior interosseous nerve syndrome. A case report with neurophysiological investigation. J. Neurol. Neurosurg. Psychiatry, 35:531, 1972.

135. Ochoa, J.: Schwann cell and myelin changes caused by some toxic agents and trauma. Proc. R. Soc. Med., 67:3, 1974.

136. Ogden, J. A.: An unusual branch of the median nerve. J. Bone Joint Surg., 54A:1779, 1972.

137. O'Hara, L. J., and Levin, M.: Carpal tunnel syndrome and gout. Arch. Intern. Med., 120:180, 1967.

138. Omer, G. E.: Injuries to nerves of the extremity. J. Bone Joint Surg., 56A:1615, 1974.

139. Packer, J. W., et al.: The humeral fracture with radial palsy: Is exploration warranted? Clin. Orthop., 88:34, 1972.

140. Papathanassiou, B. T.: A variant of the motor branch of the median nerve in the hand. J. Bone Joint Surg., 50B:156, 1968.

141. Payan, J.: Electrophysiological localization of ulnar nerve lesions. J. Neurol. Neurosurg. Psychiatry, 32:208, 1969.

142. Phalen, G. S.: The carpal-tunnel syndrome: Seventeen years' experience in diagnosis and treatment of six hundred fifty-four hands. J. Bone Joint Surg., 48A:211, 1966.

143. Phillips, R. S.: Carpal tunnel syndrome as a manifestation of the systemic disease. Ann. Rheum. Dis., 26:59, 1967.

144. Poppi, M., et al.: Fractures of the distal radius with ulnar nerve palsy. J. Trauma, 18:278, 1978.

145. Purnell, D. C., Daly, D. D., and Lipscomb, P. R.: Carpal tunnel syndrome associated with myxedema. Arch. Intern. Med., 108:751, 1961.

146. Reimann, A. F., et al.: The palmaris longus muscle and tendon. A study of 1600 extremities. Anat. Rec., 89:495, 1944.

147. Richards, R. L.: Traumatic ulnar neuritis—the results of anterior transposition of the ulnar nerve. Edinburgh Med. J., 52:14, 1945.

148. Riche, P.: Le nerf cubital et les muscles de l'éminence thénar. Bull. Mem. Soc. Anat. Paris, 5:251, 1897.

149. Richier, H. P., and Thoden, U.: Early electroneurographic diagnosis of carpal tunnel syndrome. E.E.G. E.M.G., 8:187, 1977.

150. Richmond, D. A.: Carpal ganglion with ulnar nerve compression. J. Bone Joint Surg., 45B:513, 1963.

151. Roles, N. C., and Maudsley, R. H.: Radial tunnel syndrome. Resistant tennis elbow as a nerve entrapment. J. Bone Joint Surg., 54B:499, 1972.

152. Rolfsen, L.: Snapping triceps tendon with ulnar neuritis. Acta Orthop. Scand., 41:74, 1970.

153. Sabour, M. S., and Fadel, H. E.: The carpal tunnel syndrome—a new complication ascribed to the "Pill." Am. J. Obstet. and Gynecol., 107:1265, 1970.

154. Salgeback, S.: Ulnar tunnel syndrome caused by anomalous muscles. Case report. Scand. J. Plast. Reconstr. Surg., 11:255, 1977.

155. Schiller, F., and Kolb, F. O.: Carpal tunnel syndrome in acromegaly. Neurology, 4:371, 1954.

156. Schjelderap, H.: Aberrant muscle in the hand causing ulnar nerve compression. J. Bone Joint Surg., 46B:361, 1964.

157. Schmidt, H., and Eiken, O.: The anterior interosseous nerve syndrome. Scand. J. Plast. Reconstr. Surg., 5:53, 1971.

158. Schultz, R. J., Endler, P. M., and Huddleston, H. D.: Anomalous median nerve and an anomalous muscle belly of the first lumbrical associated with carpal-tunnel syndrome. J. Bone Joint Surg., 55A:1744, 1973.

159. Seddon, H. J.: Carpal ganglion as a cause of paralysis of the deep branch of the ulnar nerve. J. Bone Joint Surg., 34B:386, 1952.

160. Seyffarth, H.: Primary myoses in the M. pronator teres as cause of lesion of the N. medianus (the pronator syndrome). Acta Psychiatr. Neurol. [Suppl.], 74:251–254, 1951.

161. Sharrard, W. J. W.: Anterior interosseous neuritis. Report of a case. J. Bone Joint Surg., 50B:804, 1968.

162. Shea, J. D., and McClain, E. J.: Ulnar nerve compression syndromes at and below the wrist. J. Bone Joint Surg., 51A:1095, 1969.

163. Sherren, J.: Remarks on chronic neuritis of the ulnar nerve due to deformity in the region of the elbow joint. Edinburgh Med. J., 23:500, 1908.

164. Simpson, J. A.: Electrical signs in the diagnosis of carpal tunnel and related syndromes. J. Neurol. Neurosurg. Psychiatry, 19:275, 1956.

165. Smith, B., and Herbst, B. A.: Anterior interosseous nerve palsy. Arch. Neurol., 30:330, 1974.

166. Smith, J. W.: Factors influencing nerve repair. I. Blood supply to peripheral nerves. Arch. Surg., 93:355, 1966.

167. Smith, J. W.: Factors influencing nerve repair. II. Collateral circulation of the peripheral nerves. Arch. Surg., 93:433, 1966.

168. Spinner, M.: The functional attitude of the hand afflicted with an anterior interosseous nerve paralysis. Bull. Hosp. Joint Dis., 30:21, 1969.

169. Spinner, M.: Cryptogenic infraclavicular brachial plexus neuritis. (Preliminary report.) Bull. Hosp. Joint Dis., 37:98, 1976.

170. Spinner, M.: Injuries to the Major Branches of the Peripheral Nerves of the Forearm, 2nd ed., Philadelphia, W. B. Saunders, 1978.

171. Starreveld, E., and Ashenhurst, E. M.: Bilateral carpal tunnel syndrome in childhood. Neurology, 25:234, 1975.

172. Stellbrink, G.: Compression of the palmar branch of the median nerve by atypical palmaris longus muscle. Handchirurgie, 4:155, 1972.

173. Stern, M., Rosner, L., and Blinderman, E.: Kiloh-Nevin syndrome. Clin. Orthop., 53:95, 1967.

174. Stern, P. J., and Kutz, J. E.: An unusual variant of the anterior interosseous nerve syndrome. J. Hand Surg., 5:32, 1980.

175. Stewart, J. D., and Eisen, A.: Tinel's sign and the carpal tunnel syndrome. Br. Med. J., 2:1125, 1978.

176. Stratton, C. W., Phelps, D. B., and Reller, L. B.: Tuberculoid tenosynovitis and carpal tunnel syndrome caused by *Mycobacterium szulgai*. Am. J. Med., 65:349, 1978.

177. Struthers, J.: On a peculiarity of the humerus and humeral artery. Monthly J. Med. Sci., 8:264, 1848.

178. Struthers, J.: Anatomical and Physiological Observations, Part I, Edinburgh, Sutherland & Knox, 1854.

179. Struthers, J.: On some points in the abnormal anatomy of the arm. Br. Foreign Med.-Chirurg. Rev., 12:523, 1854.

180. Sunderland, S.: Nerves and Nerve Injuries, Baltimore, Williams & Wilkins, 1968.

181. Sunderland, S.: Nerve lesion in the carpal tunnel syndrome. J. Neurol. Neurosurg., Psychiatry, 39:615, 1976.

182. Swanson, A. B., et al.: Ulnar nerve compression due to an anomalous muscle in the canal of Guyon. Clin. Orthop., 83:64, 1972.

183. Taleisnik, J.: The palmar cutaneous branch of the median nerve and the approach to the carpal tunnel. An anatomical study. J. Bone Joint Surg., 55A:1212, 1973.

184. Taylor, A. R.: Ulnar nerve compression at the wrist in rheumatoid arthritis. J. Bone Joint Surg., 56B:142, 1974.

185. Thomas, D. F.: Kiloh-Nevin syndrome. J. Bone Joint Surg., 44B:962, 1962.

186. Thomas, J. E., Lambert, E. H., and Cseuz, K. A.: Electrodiagnostic aspects of the carpal tunnel syndrome. Arch. Neurol., 16:635, 1967.
187. Thomas, P. K.: Motor nerve conduction in the carpal tunnel syndrome. Neurology, 10:1045, 1960.
188. Thomsen, P. B.: Compression neuritis of the ulnar nerve treated with simple decompression. Acta Orthop. Scand., 48:164, 1977.
189. Toshima, Y., and Kimata, Y.: A case of ganglion causing paralysis of intrinsic muscles innervated by the ulnar nerve. J. Bone Joint Surg., 43A:153, 1961.
190. Turner, M. S., and Caird, D. M.: Anomalous muscles and ulnar nerve compression at the wrist. Hand, 9:140, 1977.
191. Uriburu, I. J. F., Morchio, F. J., and Marin, J. C.: Compression syndrome of the deep branch of the ulnar nerve (pisohamate hiatus syndrome). J. Bone Joint Surg., 58A:145, 1976.
192. Vance, R. M., and Gelberman, R. H.: Acute ulnar neuropathy with fractures at the wrist. J. Bone Joint Surg., 60:962, 1978.
193. Vichare, N. A.: Spontaneous paralysis of the anterior interosseous nerve. J. Bone Joint Surg., 50B:806, 1968.
194. Wagman, I. H., and Lesse, H.: Maximum conduction velocities of motor fibers of ulnar nerve in human subject of various ages and sizes. J. Neurophysiol., 15:235, 1952.
195. Wallace, T. J., and Cook, A. W.: Carpal tunnel syndrome in pregnancy. Am. J. Obstet. Gynecol., 73:1333, 1957.
196. Ward, L. E., Bicker, W. H., and Corbin, K. B.: Median neuritis (carpal tunnel syndrome) caused by gouty tophi. J.A.M.A., 167:844, 1958.
197. Wartenberg, R.: Cheiralgia paresthetica (isolierte neuritis des ramus superficialis nervi radialis). Z. Neurol. Psychiatr., 141:145, 1932.
198. Watson-Jones, R.: Leri's pleonosteosis, carpal tunnel compression of the median nerve and Morton's metatarsalgia. J. Bone Joint Surg., 31B:560, 1949.
199. Weins, E., and Lau, S. C. K.: The anterior interosseous nerve syndrome. Can. J. Surg., 21:354, 1978.
200. Wilbourn, A. J.: Case report #7: True neurogenic thoracic outlet syndrome. Am. Assoc. Electromyogr. Electrodiagn. (Rochester, Minn.).
201. Williams, H. T., and Carpenter, N. H.: Surgical treatment of the thoracic outlet compression syndrome. Arch. Surg., 113:850, 1978.
202. Wilson, D. H., and Krout, R.: Surgery of ulnar neuropathy at the elbow: 16 cases treated by decompression without transposition. Technical note. J. Neurosurgery, 38:780, 1973.
203. Wilson, J. N.: Profiles of the carpal canal. J. Bone Joint Surg., 36A:127, 1954.
204. Woltman, H. W., and Learmonth, J. R.: Progressive paralysis of the nervus interosseous dorsalis. Brain, 57:25, 1934.
205. Worster-Drought, C.: Pressure neuritis of the deep palmar branch of the ulnar nerve. Br. Med. J., 1:247, 1929.
206. Wright, I. S.: The neurovascular syndrome produced by hyperabduction of the arms. Am. Heart J., 29:1, 1945.
207. Yamaguchi, D. M., Lipscomb, P. R., and Soule, E. H.: Carpal-tunnel syndrome. Minn. Med., 48:22, 1965.
208. Zoega, H.: Fracture of the lower end of the radius with ulnar nerve palsy. J. Bone Joint Surg., 48B:514, 1966.

12

COMPLICATIONS FOLLOWING SECONDARY OR RECONSTRUCTIVE NERVE REPAIR

Hanno Millesi

GENERAL CONSIDERATIONS

The aim of peripheral nerve repair is to achieve good motor and sensory recovery with useful function. Failure to achieve this may be due to one of the following causes:

1. The involved neurons may not have sufficient power to produce enough axon sprouts and to make them travel over long distances; this may be due to advanced age, general disease, vast retrograde degeneration, and long distance between site of injury and end-organs, as with brachial plexus lesions.

2. Degeneration of end-organs due to a long interval between injury and repair.

3. Obvious errors during surgery (*e.g.*, if a nerve is sutured to a tendon).

4. Poor planning.

5. Selection of improper technique.

6. Postoperative complications; may be subdivided as apparent postoperative complications, which cause clear symptoms and must be treated specifically; and hidden complications, which do not cause characteristic symptoms but result in failure of nerve regeneration.

The diagnosis that something has gone wrong with nerve regeneration is established by clinical examination and neurophysiologic studies. After a sufficient period, based on the distance between site of injury and motor recovery, regeneration is expected to occur. Another symptom of insufficient return of function is a simultaneous action of antagonists, which neutralize each other. Poor or no return of sensibility, along with dysesthesia and paresthesia, indicate a failure of sensory recovery.

It should be noted that dysesthesia and paresthesia represent a complication of peripheral nerve repair, which can be very troublesome for the patient and the physician.

To define complications properly after nerve repair is extremely difficult. It is obvious that lack of nerve regeneration occurring because of advanced age or the coaptation of a nerve stump with a tendon does not represent a complication, but poor planning or the selection of an improper technique can produce real problems. It is difficult to define the turning point beyond which a regeneration neuroma, which always forms after transecting a nerve, becomes a complication. The borderline is nebulous and is actually delineated by the complaints made by the patient.

Complications after peripheral nerve surgery may be in one of the following groups: (1) those occurring during surgery or the final stage of the operation; (2) those of the early postoperative phase; (3) those of the late postoperative phase; (4) those related to pain; (5) other complications; and (6) those related to an eventual donor site.

DELAYED PERIPHERAL NERVE REPAIR

During Surgery or Its Final Stage

In an end-to-end neurorrhaphy, the two stumps have to be approximated and coapted under certain tension. To reduce the tension for the operation and postoperative healing, the adjacent joints are flexed. This flexion has to be maintained. If, at the end of the operation, insufficient care has been taken, a rupture of the suture site may occur.

Early Postoperative Phase

A hematoma represents a serious complication and endangers the result, especially if it is located within the nerve after a tight epineural repair. Such a local hematoma cannot be recognized, so it therefore is extremely important to avoid intraneural bleeding by careful hemostasis using bipolar coagulation. This danger does not exist if the epineurium has been resected and a fascicular or interfascicular repair has been performed. If bleeding of an intraneural vessel occurs, the blood has the possibility of distributing itself over the whole wound.

A wound hematoma is easily diagnosed by the tight tension and swelling in the area of the wound. Occurrence of a wound hematoma is an indication for a revision in the operating roon and for careful evacuation after opening the skin wound, with reclosure.

Rupture of the skin wound may occur as a result of poor preoperative planning, with skin closure under too much tension. It may also be the result of a new injury. If recognized in time, the wound is closed during surgery utilizing a plastic surgical procedure to protect the nerve repair with secondary skin grafting.

Breakdown of the edges of the skin wound occurs if the suturing was done under tension, or if tension were produced by a hematoma or swelling. If the breakdown involves only a small strip of skin, and the skin wound is far from the site of the repair, the result of the nerve repair will not be influenced. If the breakdown of the skin edges occurs in close proximity to the nerve repair, severe consequences can be prevented if excision and wound closure are done using a plastic surgical procedure (local flap rotation with secondary skin grafting). In extreme situations, a distant flap may even be necessary. The decisive point is that the excision of the necrotic part be performed before an infection is established, as long as the necrosis is dry. This means that some time must elapse, but the excision should be performed at the fourth or fifth day after the original surgery. The occurrence of skin necrosis is the result of a technical fault or of poor planning. If the skin in the area of the future nerve repair is scarred and tight, an operation should be performed to provide stable skin coverage.

A severe wound infection is an indication to open the wound immediately to control the infection. The result of a nerve repair will be compromised in most cases, not only because of opening the wound but also because of fibrous tissue formation and constriction of healing. Certainly, severe wound infection as a result of an aseptic leak is extremely rare. A moderate wound infection might develop as the result of formation of a hematoma, rupture of the skin wound, or necrosis of the skin edges. Thus, in case of any of these complications, it is extremely important that the surgeon react immediately to avoid infection.

Late Postoperative Phase

Three to 6 weeks after a neurorrhaphy, with relief of tension by flexion of the adjacent joints, gradual mobilization is started. During this phase the suture site is under tension. By stretching the scar tissue between the cross-sectional areas of the two stumps, they are separated from each other, and the gap fills with additional scar tissue. It is more difficult for the regeneration axon sprouts to penetrate across such a zone of scar tissue. Axons that have already crossed the suture liner could be damaged by stretching of the scar tissue or compressed by consecutive hypertrophy of scar tissue.[9, 10] The scar between the two nerve stumps could be unstable for a long time, and axon damage with axonolysis may be observed several months after the original injury.

A hypertrophy of the epineural and adventitial tissue causes a compression of the suture site, which impedes nerve regeneration. This hypertrophy might be the consequence of tension or of a foreign body reaction against suture material, with formation of granulomas.

Compression of the distal stumps by scar tissue may form an obstacle, preventing further progression of the axon sprouts. The same may occur at the typical sites of an entrapment syndrome. In normal conditions the canal is wide enough and does not cause symptoms. After trauma and nerve repair, there might be a relative narrowing, which stops regeneration at this site.

All these complications do not become apparent. They can be suspected only if regeneration does not occur in proper time, and a Tinel-Hoffmann sign does not proceed (Fig. 12–1). The Tinel-Hoffmann sign is an important finding and can be of great help if interpreted correctly. If the surgeon carries out percussion with the finger at the site of a neuroma at which axon sprouts are present, the patient feels an electric shock-type pain radiating into the area of distribution of the sensory fibers. After nerve repair with the advancement of the axon sprouts into the distal stump, the Tinel-Hoffmann sign moves toward the periphery. During the delayed healing phase, a rather long zone along the distal stump represents a positive Tinel-Hoffmann sign, but there is usually a punctum maximum, corresponding to the bulk of the outgrowing axon sprouts. The Tinel-Hoffmann sign reaches the periphery and gradually disappears when the sensory axon sprouts have reached end-organs. The Tinel-Hoffmann sign (and its movement) is not a parameter of good nerve regeneration because it is positive even if a few axon sprouts move toward the periphery, and it does not relate to the quality of the sensory fibers. On the other hand, if the Tinel-Hoffmann sign does not move, it may be concluded that regeneration has not started or has been

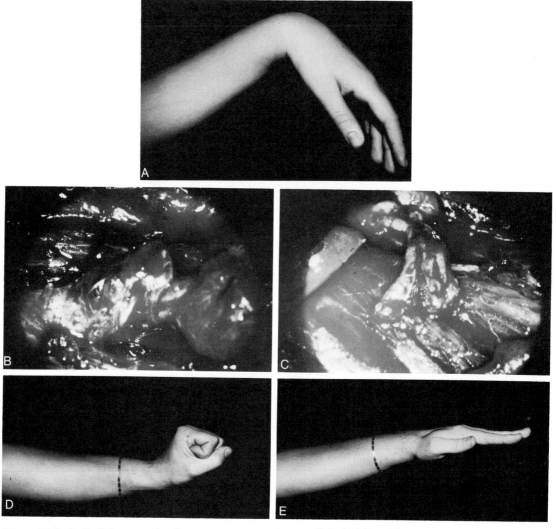

Figure 12–1. *A,* Radial nerve palsy due to an upper arm fracture (left side) in a 15-year-old patient. Continuity was restored by grafting 12-cm long sural nerve segments. The Tinel-Hoffmann sign had advanced to the distal end of the grafts, where it remained. A block at the distal end of the grafts was suspected. *B,* Exploration showed a thickening at the distal end of the grafts; *C,* after resection the cross section of the graft shows good fascicular structure; *D, E,* coaptation of the graft with the distal stump was performed with good return of function.

stopped at a certain level. If the punctum maximum of the Tinel-Hoffmann sign remains constant at the site of the nerve repair, it indicates that most of the axon sprouts could not cross the line of coaptation. A positive Tinel-Hoffmann sign at the level of a crossing scar or at a typical site of an entrapment syndrome indicates that some axon sprouts have had difficulty proceeding at this level. If, after waiting for 3 or 4 months, no advancement occurs, a block should be suspected and re-exploration is indicated.

Complications Related to Pain

It has been explained above that the formation of a neuroma occurs after every transection of a peripheral nerve. In the case of coaptation with a distal stump, the axon sprouts can proceed along the distal stump to reach the end-organ. Along with the advancement of the Tinel-Hoffmann sign, the patient quite often feels pain and discomfort in the area of the original denervation. This can be regarded as an expression of ongoing regeneration; the symptoms disappear when regeneration has finished. Persistent radiating pain and paresthesias indicate that only a minority of axon sprouts have reached the distal stump, and that most have formed a neuroma, which might develop into a painful neuroma and then represent a severe complication. If pain persists, the patient may develop a pain syndrome with lowering of the pain threshold, and finally a centrally fixed pain syndrome results. To avoid this development, an early revision of the suture site is indicated to remove everything that irritates the nerve and blocks the advancement of the axon sprouts. In the early phase of development, the pain syndrome can be cured in this way. After the pain has become centrally fixed, local procedures do not help.

Other Complications

These problems are not directly related to the nerve operation, but can be very severe if they occur and can compromise the result. If an attempt is made to overcome a large defect by vast mobilization and forceful approximation of the nerve stumps, with maximal flexion of the adjacent joints, a prolonged immobilization has to be maintained in a nonphysiologic position. The result can be a pressure sore due to pressure of the plaster cast, Volkmann-like ischemic damage due to a too-tight plaster cast, and joint stiffness.

NERVE GRAFTS

Complications During Surgery or its Final Stage

Modern techniques of nerve grafting attempt to reduce surgical trauma to a minimum. Tension is kept at zero and, consequently, only very few stitches are used to approximate an individual graft to a corresponding fascicle or fascicle group. Thus, the tensile strength at the end of the operation is minimal. With tension at zero, this is sufficient. Animal experiments with rabbits have demonstrated that, 24 hours after such a procedure, the tensile strength reaches values between 17 and 35 g, and after 1 week there is a tensile strength of 100 g for the sciatic nerve. It is therefore extremely important to avoid the application of any force at the end of the operation and during the early postoperative phase. Closing the skin without being aware of the possibility of dislocation of the nerve graft by shearing forces may cause disruption. The same is true for careless cleaning of the skin after skin closure. The immobilization at the end of the operation should be carried out in exactly the position the limb was in during the operation. The utilization of suction drainage should be avoided, because this may also cause dislocation.

Early Postoperative Phase

An interneural hematoma cannot occur after an interfascicular or fascicular nerve grafting procedure because the epineurium has been resected, and eventual bleeding can be distributed within the wound. If a nerve graft has been performed, there is the possibility of intraneural hematoma formation and, in addition, the danger of vascular occlusion with resultant necrosis of the graft. In addition to these special complications, all the other complications that have been listed for neurorrhaphy may also occur.

In my experience with interfascicular nerve grafts, I have had to reintervene several times because of the formation of a large hematoma caused by breakdown of skin edges and, in one case, caused by disruption of the skin wound when the patient fell 10 days after surgery. All these cases were immediately explored. It is interesting to note that in none of these cases were the nerve grafts displaced or disrupted. After evaluation of the hematoma and after providing a proper skin cover, the course was uneventful.

Late Postoperative Phase

Nerve grafts may become necrotic and slough; however, this theoretic possibility has not been observed in clinical practice. If a nerve graft does not survive, it undergoes a rather slow microbiotic process, leading to fibrosis. In one case of complete failure of a grafting procedure in a young patient, the revision revealed total fibrosis of the whole graft, which was resected and replaced by new grafts and led to final useful recovery (see Fig. 12–1). The situation was recognized because of the persisting positive Tinel-Hoffmann sign at the proximal end of the graft.

After free grafting of cutaneous nerve grafts of the size of the sural nerve in a proper recipient site, the grafts survive well, including their Schwann cells. At re-exploration after several months, the grafts do not show fibrosis and can be easily recognized individually. If, as in the experiments of Bratton and colleagues, the central zone of the graft loses its normal structure, which can be recognized only as "ghostlike," the survival was not optimal, and this can be regarded as a complication.[4, 6] However, in these experiments, there was still some return of function.

Nerve grafts may become adherent to muscle and this means chronic irritation and eventual outgrowth of axons into a denervated muscle, resulting in failure. I have seen this with the ulnar nerve in its distal course, in which the nerve is close to the flexor carpi ulnaris muscle. Contact of nerve grafts with a muscle without covering by fascia should be avoided. Grafts of the median nerve at the wrist tend to become adherent to tendons, and this was the reason for some of my failures. Adhesions can be avoided by performing the nerve repair in a second stage, after the tendons have been restored, and by creating a tunnel for the nerve grafts without contact with flexor tendons.

The typical complication for nerve grafting procedures is the fibrosis to the distal site of coaptation. The possibility of a block at the distal end of a graft during the time the axon sprouts need to proceed along the graft was discussed very early in the literature.[5, 7, 11, 12] The axon sprouts cannot proceed easily into the distal stump. The Tinel-Hoffmann sign, which has moved along the graft, stops at the distal site of coaptation. If this occurs a re-exploration is indicated, with resection of this distal suture site. Before the introduction of microsurgery, such a block at the distal site occurred constantly if the graft was longer than 3 or 4 cm. Thus, the regular resection of the distal suture site in cases of longer nerve grafts was recommended.[3] After the development of microsurgical techniques, a block at the distal end of the graft occurred only in a minority of cases.[8] In the vast majority the distal site of coaptation was crossed easily, even in long grafts. In my first series of 50 cases, a block at the distal site of coaptation, making reoperation necessary, was observed in seven cases (14%). With increasing experience and technical developments, this rate dropped to an insignificant value. Bosse has drawn attention to the problem of the distal suture site and recommends planning the nerve graft in two stages, performing only the proximal coaptation at the first operation and leaving the distal end of the graft open.[1, 2] The distal connection is then carried out at the second operation. According to my experience, a block at the distal end of the suture site occurs extremely rarely. If it does occur it may be recognized easily by the behavior of the Tinel-Hoffmann sign. Performing the proximal and distal coaptations in one stage has the enormous advantage that most care can be devoted to identifying corresponding parts of the two stumps and connecting them by individual nerve grafts.

As with the neurorrhaphy, the graft or the distal stump can be compressed by a crossing scar. A graft across the ulnar nerve sulcus at the distal end of the humerus may be exposed to the same irritation as the ulnar nerve itself. Regeneration may also be prevented by compression of the distal stump at the typical sites of entrapment syndromes.

Complications Related to Pain

The problems already discussed for neurorrhaphy are also relevant to nerve grafting procedures. In contrast to neurorrhaphies, the occurrence of painful neuromas after nerve grafting is extremely rare. This is why I have used the restoration of continuity as the treatment of painful neuroma after peripheral nerve lesions. In five cases with painful neuroma of the median and ulnar nerve in the forearm due to war injuries, with loss of continuity and recurrent failure of other techniques, the pain syndrome could be controlled in four of them. In a series of eleven cases of painful neuromas of branches of the superficial radial nerve at the wrist and in the dorsum of the hand, the pain syndrome was controlled in all but one by restoration of continuity by nerve graft.

Other Complications

The incidence of other complications is extremely low, because immobilization is not maintained in an extreme position and lasts only for 8 to 10 days.

Complications Related to the Donor Site

The excision of a cutaneous nerve as the nerve graft causes the formation of a regeneration neuroma at the site of transection. There will be a positive Tinel sign at this level. In addition, the patient will realize a relative loss of sensibility for the sural nerve in the distribution of this nerve—for example, for the lateral ankle and along the lateral margin of the foot. The loss of sensibility is usually incomplete because the sural nerve has no autonomous zone. By the time axon sprouts grow in from the neighboring areas, there will be some discomfort and dysesthesia. This is a normal development and cannot be regarded as a complication. After some time sensibility will improve, but it will never reach normal values. The patient must be informed before the operation about these events.

At the site of resection a painful neuroma may develop, and this must be regarded as a serious complication. Some cases have been described in the literature.[13] It is necessary to do everything to avoid this. As a rule, the sural nerve is excised in its whole length with transection below the popliteal fossa, even if only a short segment is desired. In this case, the level of transection is rather high underneath the fascia and is well protected by muscles, without direct contact with muscular tissue. With this precaution, I have not yet seen one case with a painful neuroma in my whole series of nerve grafts performed since 1964.

NEUROLYSIS

Complications During Surgery and its Final Stage

During internal neurolysis, the surgeon is constantly exposed to the temptation to do too much. Internal neurolysis proceeds in stages, which aims to decompress the nerve fascicles from constricting fibrous tissue. The operation starts with an epifascicular epineurotomy. If this does not lead to decompression, the epifascicular epineurium is excised (epifascicular epineurectomy) and, if this is not sufficient, some fibrotic interfascicular epineural tissue is removed. New fibrous tissue will form. The basis for the operation is the hope that the newly formed fibrous tissue will not exert a constricting effect. This can only be achieved by minimizing the surgical trauma: just enough should be done to achieve decompression, sparing the nonfibrotic parts between the fascicles with the vessels. After internal-neurolysis, the involved nerves should be placed in good soft tissue, away from any zone of irritation. This is achieved with the ulnar nerve by transposing it to the volar side of the elbow joint or into a subcutaneous bed, or along the median nerve underneath the flexor muscles.

A complication may develop by dislocation of the nerve from the desired position during skin closure and immobilization.

Early Postoperative Phase

Hematoma, skin rupture, breakdown of skin, and infections are devastating complications with neurolysis.

Last Postoperative Phase

Chronic irritations by adhesions to muscle or tendon impede regeneration after neurolysis and cause paresthesias and dysesthesias. By the translocation of the nerve after neurolysis, a new site of irritation or constriction may have been created. This refers especially to the ulnar nerve, which can be irritated by Struthers' ligament or by the medial intermuscular septum, or at the level of its entry into the subfascial compartment at the forearm in cases of subcutaneous translocation.

Complications

Nerve lesions in continuity occur frequently at the site of an irritative nerve lesion, characterized by a superficial pain with light touch and a deep continuing pain that worsens with change of weather and cold and decreases only when the patient is externally distracted. In contrast to causalgic pain, this type of pain is not influenced by humidity or emotional stimuli. Such an irritative nerve may, in rare cases, develop after an internal neurolysis. One reason may be the formation of small neuromas within the nerve in which interconnecting branches had been transected. A re-exploration is indicated to make sure that all irritative factors are excluded. Small neuromas are excised, and the small branch that goes into the neuroma is coagulated by bipolar coagulation. If this revision is not successful, cervical chordotomy is considered.

DELAYED BRACHIAL PLEXUS REPAIR

The surgical treatment of brachial plexus lesions consists of two phases. In phase 1, within 6 months after the accident, attempts are made to neurotize denervated nerve territories. This is done early if spontaneous recovery is unlikely to occur. According to the amount of damage nerve tissue has suffered, neurolysis and restoration of continuity by nerve grafts are performed. Neurorrhaphy is rarely possible. All complications listed previously may also occur in brachial plexus surgery.

Complications of the Final Stage of Operation

One major complication during exposure of the brachial plexus is the bleeding from the subclavian artery. A lesion to the artery during dissection is likely to occur in patients who had rupture of the artery at the time of the original trauma with surgical reconstruction or ligature. In such cases the anatomic situation is completely changed, and it is difficult to get a clear idea of the individual structures. The best way to avoid arterial bleeding is to locate the artery and the individual parts of the brachial plexus in the periphery beyond the area of injury on normal tissue and to dissect along the artery into the area of injury. In the few cases in which this complication was seen, there was no problem in closing the hole in the artery by arterial sutures. The same might happen to a vein graft that bridges an arterial defect to the subclavian vein.

In the depth of the supra- and infraclavicular dissection, there is danger of damaging one of the vessels that is in close relation to the lower roots, the arteria cerebralis, the arteria cervicalis ascendens, and the arteria thoracica suprema. During the isolation of the inferior cord and roots C8 and T1, there is theoretically the possibility of a lesion of the pleura.

If an intercostal nerve transfer is performed, each individual costal nerve has to be isolated underneath the rib. If the periosteum is carefully detached and the rib lifted, there is enough space to isolate the nerve without coming into close contact with the pleura. However, there is the possibility of an injury to the pleura. If this happens, the best way to deal with this complication is to resect the segment of the corresponding rib and to close the hole in the pleura by sutures. If there is a major defect, though, suturing has a poor chance of success and may increase the opening. In this case, the best method is to utilize a dermis graft and to suture it onto the defect in a watertight manner. Drainage of the pleural cavity is mandatory.

As in nerve grafting in general, dislocation of the graft may occur during osteosynthesis if an osteotomy of the clavicle has been performed. The clavicular origin of the major pectoralis muscle and the origin of the minor pectoralis muscle at the processus coracoideus is sometimes detached and may have to be reinserted. This maneuver may result in dislocation of the grafts if not performed carefully.

After the operation is finished, immobilization is maintained using a plaster cast that includes the head, the chest, and the whole arm. Necessarily, the head and body have to be lifted to apply the plaster to the dorsal side of the head and body, and special attention must be exercised during this phase to maintain the relative position of the head and chest.

The operation for brachial plexus surgery takes many hours. The head is turned to the site of the injury, and this means it is in an extreme position. Under certain conditions, after a cranial cerebral trauma, the cerebral situation could deteriorate after surgery. I have seen this in one case in which central neurologic symptoms occurred and subsided very slowly. Each case with cranial cerebral as well as brachial plexus lesions should therefore be studied before operation to evaluate an eventual risk in this regard.

Early Postoperative Phase

A small hematoma may occur if postoperative drainage was inadequate due to the fact that a huge wound cavity has been created. This occurs especially in cases that have had a rupture of the subclavian artery at the original injury, with or without reconstruction. The occurrence of a small hematoma does not influence the result. In this case, the hematoma is evacuated after 10 days by percutaneous puncture. An extensive hematoma is an indication for re-exploration.

In cases of root avulsion and formation of a meningocele, there is danger that a fistula may form. If the meningocele is recognized during operation, it is resected at its base and the communication with the subarachnoidal space is carefully closed in a watertight manner. In spite of careful management, a fistula may occur at the third or fourth postoperative day. In all cases that I have seen there was only a limited amount of secretion, and it subsided spontaneously after a few days. The only therapeutic measures taken were observation of the electrolyte and fluid balances and protection against infection by antibiotics. In rare cases, a re-exploration with closure of the fistula might be necessary. Infection is fortunately a very rare complication. In a series of 104 cases, infection occurred only twice. In one case it occurred after formation of a hematoma that had not been evacuated, and in another case it was in the form of an osteomyelitis of the clavicle after osteotomy.

During the late postoperative phase, the possible complications are similar to the ones that occur after nerve grafting.

Complications Related to Pain

A certain percentage of brachial plexus cases develop a pain syndrome that is already established when the patient undergoes brachial plexus surgery. If the cause of the pain syndrome was compression of parts of the brachial plexus, pain relief might be achieved by surgery. This does not manifest itself immediately. Sometimes after the operation the patient complains of more severe pain. Usually the area of maximal pain moves slowly toward the periphery, and the pain disappears gradually. If pain continues to be a problem, neurosurgical procedures such as cervical chordotomy should be considered.

Patients with a brachial lesion with preserved continuity, who have had no pain problem before the operation, may develop pain, dysesthesia, and paresthesia in the periphery as a result of the operation. This is regarded as a positive sign and usually the symptoms disappear with return of function.

Because the patient has to be immobilized for 8 to 10 days and the arm is anesthetized, there is the possibility of a pressure sore caused by the plaster, and care must be taken to avoid this. The same is true for the back, where the skin over the spina scapulae and acromion is exposed to external pressure.

Complications in relation to the donor site of nerve grafts are the same as those outlined above.

References

1. Bosse, J. P.: Personal communication at the Fifth International Symposium on Microsurgery, Guaruja, May 15–18, 1979.
2. Bosse, J. P.: Discussion remark. *In* Gorio, A., Millesi, H., and Mingrino, S. (eds.): Posttraumatic Peripheral Nerve Regeneration (Experimental Basis and Clinical Implications), New York, Raven Press, 1981, p. 374.
3. Bsteh, F. X., and Millesi, H.: Zur Kenntnis der zweizeitigen Nerveninterplantation bei ausgedehnten peripheren Nervendefekten. Klin. Med. (Mosk.), 12:571, 1960.
4. Bratton, B. R., et al.: Experimental interfascicular nerve grafting. J. Neurosurg., 51:323, 1979.
5. Davis, L., and Cleveland, D. A.: Experimental studies in nerve transplants. Ann. Surg., 99:271, 1934.
6. Kline, D. G., Hudson, A. R., and Bratton, B. R.: Use of grafts to repair serious gaps. *In* Gorio, A., Millesi, H., and Mingrino, S. (eds.): Posttraumatic Peripheral Nerve Regeneration (Experimental Basis and Clinical Implications), New York, Raven Press, 1981, pp. 339–342.
7. Lewis, D.: Some peripheral nerve problems. Boston Med. Surg. J., 188:975, 1923.
8. Millesi, H.: Zum Problem der Überbrückung von Defekten peripherer Nerven. Wien. Med. Wochenschr., 118:182, 1968.
9. Millesi, H.: Healing of nerves. Clin. Plast Surg., 4:459, 1977.
10. Millesi, H., Berger, A., and Meissl, G.: Experimentelle Untersuchungen Zur Heilung durchtrennter peripherer Nerven. Chir. Plastica, 1:174, 1972.
11. Stookey, B.: The futility of bridging nerve defects by means of nerve flaps. Surg. Gynecol. Obstet., 29:287, 1919.
12. Therkelsen, J., and Pool, J. L.: Stored nerve grafts for two-stage sciatic nerve repair in dogs. J. Neuropathol. Exp. Neurol., 16:383, 1957.
13. Wilgis, E. F. S.: Discussion remark. *In* Millesi, H. (ed.): Indication, Technique, and Results of Nerve Grafting, Sonderheft, Handchirurgie, 1977.

13

COMPLICATIONS AND PITFALLS IN MODERN UPPER LIMB TETRAPLEGIA SURGERY

Erik Moberg

Many methods have been tried to restore some of the upper limb function lost in tetraplegia. Up until a decade ago, an almost general resistance against such trials prevailed, and the changing attitude is certainly not completely accepted. However, there is a rapidly growing number of research studies in the field (see references), most of them with very positive results.[6, 7, 8, 10, 11, 12, 13, 14, 17]

The new way of thinking in reconstructive upper limb tetraplegia surgery, based mainly on the presence or absence of tactile gnosis, is different from earlier approaches which were based almost entirely on motor considerations. Therefore, complications reported or known from surgery performed more than 15 years ago and all the pitfalls from methods now abandoned will not be discussed.

Many early trials were done in the belief that the experiences from reconstructive hand surgery in polio could be applied in tetraplegia. Such thinking disregards modern concepts of kinesthesia.[13] Table 13–1, which summarizes the loss in different conditions, makes this point of view self-explanatory.

The first factor to determine is whether afferents are available in regard to grip. Disregarding this is one of the more common causes of failure in this type of surgery.

I will not review all the different surgical methods used in the last decade, but a few words and illustrations are necessary as a background. The surgery works with restoration of active elbow extension and a hand grip.[1, 3, 5, 8, 10, 17] For the elbow extension, three techniques are proposed: (1) the transfer of the posterior part of the deltoid to the triceps tendon with the help of free toe tendon grafts (Fig. 13–1); (2) the same transfer, but with the bridging performed by a reflected strip of the triceps tendon;[2] or (3) the use of the transferred biceps directly to the triceps tendon.[2, 10, 17]

The construction of an active hand grip (it is much more a case of construction rather than of reconstruction) is dependent on the extent of the loss, on what is left and available for use. If the elbow extensor procedure can be standardized, the hand grip procedure can be almost as variable as

Table 13–1. LOSS OF UPPER LIMB FUNCTION IN TETRAPLEGIA COMPARED WITH THAT IN POLIO

	Normal	Polio	Tetraplegia
Reliable ligaments	45	45	3 ?
Muscles for motion or transfer	37	4–8	1–2–3
Tactile gnosis	Normal	Normal	Greatly reduced
Proprioception	Normal	Normal	or absent

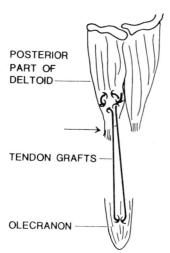

Figure 13–1. Lost elbow extension can be restored by a transfer of the posterior part of the deltoid, which is then elongated with tendon grafts. (Reproduced with permission from Moberg, E.: The Upper Limb in Tetraplegia. Stuttgart, Thieme, 1978.)

POSTERIOR PART OF DELTOID

TENDON GRAFTS

OLECRANON

the number of patients. Therefore, a few examples will illustrate the following discussion.

To discuss all the variations and procedures to be used, as well as to compare results, it has been necessary to construct a new classification. The old one, built on cervical levels, is too crude. Each arm must be classified separately, and the available sensory function and number of useful muscles must be determined.

The simplest method is shown in Figure 13–2.[10] If not only vision is available to lead the gripping function but also in at least one of the hands the thumb has some tactile gnosis (two-point discrimi-

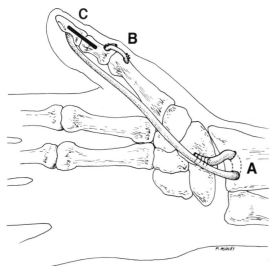

Figure 13–2. A thumb key grip can be constructed with wrist extension as motor through a tenodesis (A) of the flexor pollicis longus tendon to the radius followed by stabilization of distal thumb joint with a 2 mm steel pin (C) and of the metacarpophalangeal joint with a mobile tenodesis (B).

nation at least 10 mm) and wrist extension power is moderate (at least grade 3), a simple key grip can be given to *both* hands. For one of them, vision will control the grip; for the other, cutaneous sensibility. Vision can only control one hand. If more is available, it will be a question of active pronation, finger flexion, finger extension or, in a few cases, even some intrinsic stabilization and perhaps opposition. Generally, the last-mentioned function should not be aimed for, because it is less useful and requires a group of motors.[12, 13]

My discussion is based on personal experience in more than 130 hand grip and over 60 elbow extensor constructions. Together with corrections and procedures performed in more than one stage, this represents 300 to 400 operations. To this should be added a vast number of cases reported by colleagues and collaborators.

Today, fortunately, true surgical complications (e.g., wound infections, decubital ulcers from plaster, tendon ruptures, fever from other sources, shoulder-hand-finger syndrome, thrombosis, and embolism or heart failure) are quite rare. All this is very reassuring when one has to perform surgery on the already greatly incapacitated patient. However, these problems do exist, and will be discussed below.

The real causes of disappointments and pitfalls in this type of surgery involve unsatisfactory evaluation, false indications, the different procedures on hand and arm not performed in optimal order, and inadequate or even destructive follow-up treatment. As mentioned above, a new way of thinking is necessary, and this includes the examination. Everyone who performs this surgery must gain experience and this, of course, requires enough patients to work with.

GENERAL COMPLICATIONS

Such impaired body systems as those seen in cases of paraplegia and tetraplegia will no doubt result in complications in combination with those from anesthesia and surgery. In one of the two patients I have had in whom a functional loss had occurred, a good key grip was obtained through hand surgery. Under general anesthesia later, when an elbow extensor procedure on the same arm was performed, further compression of the spinal cord occurred, no doubt due to an unstable cervical spine, and this caused the level of injury to be lowered about half a segment. This experience has made me prefer a brachial plexus block whenever possible. In another case, a similar loss occurred, but it was 3 years after surgery and happened spontaneously. I felt that this also was due to further compression, but a number of reports have clarified the occurrence of posttraumatic cystic degeneration of the cord.[15] (My other case of functional loss was a failure to achieve elbow extension, and the surgery weakened the deltoid. Significant other improvement was achieved in both arms.)

Fever not originating from the field of surgery has occurred several times, probably from the lungs or the urinary tract. Lung ventilation is, of course, below normal. In one case I felt that it was a question of atelectasis, but it was reported as a slight pulmonary embolism. The symptoms disappeared rapidly. I have heard reports of serious delirium tremens complications, but I have not seen them myself.

As with any other surgical procedure, the period after surgery requires extra observation, foresight, and care to avoid the risks always involved with the rest of the body. The treatment during this period, therefore, should take place in a special paraplegic ward and not in a general one.

TRUE SURGICAL COMPLICATIONS

Wound Infection. All my operations have healed by primary intention except for two early cases of elbow extensor construction, in which hematomas in the deltoid region had to be evacuated, leading to slightly draining secondary healing. This did not influence the final results. Meticulous hemostasis and suction drainage prevented this complication.

Migration of K-wires, used to stabilize the distal thumb joint, has led in a number of early cases to small infections at the thumb tip if the wires were not removed in time. This migration problem will be discussed later in this section.

The very low overall infection risk in this type of surgery is encouraging, because obviously the bacterial skin flora in tetraplegic patients may present a greater risk in regard to infection than in most other surgery because of the difficulty with personal hygiene. One report, however, mentioned difficulties with skin healing, said to be caused by poor vascularity.[2]

Pressure Lesions. Because so much of the skin area is involved in the treatment, there is a great reduction in protective cutaneous sensibility. It must be remembered that correct answers to pinprick and cotton wool tests do not mean that the quality of sensibility is high enough to ensure adequate reaction to plaster pressure. Obviously, therefore, the use of plaster of Paris or of pressure during splinting can involve great risks for cutaneous necrosis without signaling pain reactions. Michaelis recommended that plaster should be removed daily for inspection.[9] I have not found this to be necessary, and I keep the plaster splint in place for elbow extensor procedures up to 6 weeks without change. For the hand operations, the same is done for up to 3 to 4 weeks. A longer period is almost never indicated. However, I insist that the surgeon must apply the plaster personally, and observe it until it hardens; only he knows through his own examination the quality and limits of the patient's sensibility regions. All plasters must be judiciously padded—not too much, not too little, all according to the regions.

Only three times have I had personal experience with such pressure sores. In one case it had nothing to do with the plaster. A rubber band traction splint, used preoperatively to reduce an old finger contracture, produced a small skin necrosis on the middle finger that healed without functional loss. In another case, an elbow splint caused a necrotic area of 3 × 3 cm, which also healed without functional loss. In the third case, a heavy man with an elbow splint, who was at home several weeks after surgery, found swelling and blisters over the fourth and fifth fingers on awakening one morning. During the night, the weight of the arm and the plaster, which ended above the wrist, had caused pressure lesions and necrosis. The fourth finger healed without loss. In the fifth the necrosis went into the proximal interphalangeal joint, causing joint infection. It was found best to amputate the immobile and insensitive finger. The risk in this case could have been foreseen, and the patient should have been warned before going home. Such mishaps will discourage patients, and this man has not yet returned for the planned further surgery, which no doubt could have been helpful to him. However, he got a most useful elbow extensor. Again, it must be stressed that this surgery requires foresight far beyond that for most other routine work.

Pin Migration. In a few early cases Kirschner wires used to stabilize the distal thumb joint had a tendency to migrate out at the tip of the digit (see Fig. 13–2C). This occurred after a delay of a few months up to several years. When it was noticed that this was going to happen and the pin caused some discomfort, it was easy to remove through a small incision. If desired for stability, a new pin could be inserted. By no means can an advanced flexion deformity (a Froment's sign thumb) be accepted, because this will give insufficient grip. If the pin ends are left very blunt and the distal end is under the periosteum, the migration problem should not occur. Other surgeons have avoided this migration by the use of a threaded pin.[1, 16] I still use the K-wire, because the joint ligaments slowly shorten and, after a year or two, if the pin is taken out, the distal thumb joint has only about 20° of passive mobility left. Patients feel that such thumbs are best for gripping action, better than with the totally stiff distal joint, and much better than the ones with more flexion. Another reason is that the bigger threaded pins more easily produce a bony fusion of the joint, which should make the procedure less reversible. In only one case have I seen the 2-mm K-wire cause bony healing in the form of a narrow bony "tube," visible on x-ray around the wire.

A semantic difference will often cause a surgical complication here. In the United States the European 2 mm K-wires are named Steinmann's pins. This difference can lead to the use of 1.5 or even 1 mm wires, which are too weak and will break.

THE SHOULDER-HAND-FINGER SYNDROME

This syndrome, a frightening complication in all major hand surgery, could be a frequent occurrence in this type of surgery. The normal pumping function of the moving tissues, which acts through the valves of the veins and the lymphatic vessels and causes the return of fluids from the hand, is greatly reduced because of the paralysis. The shoulder, as well as the arm and hand, are affected. The formation of edema, organizing into diffuse scar tissue with stiffening of joints, should be common. However, it is easier to solve this problem than might be expected.

In the elbow, a compression dressing that includes the whole hand is used for the first 5 to 7 days after surgery to prevent edema. If edema occurs, it is more difficult to resolve than when found in other hand surgery. The hand tissues at the time of surgery and after the first few months are more fibrous than normal, which prevents new swelling, and also there are a few degrees less mobility in the finger joints, but this is less important than in the normal hand. The conclusion is that the precautions taken have been sufficient to rule out the danger of the shoulder-hand-finger syndrome in tetraplegia surgery. I do not know of a single case in which this factor has caused a final result below expectations. Some authors claim that the sympathetic nervous system is the scapegoat of this complication, but this is debatable.

SLACKENING OF PERFORMED TENODESIS

Such slackening occurs easily, and care is necessary to prevent it. One of the great difficulties is to get surgeons to understand how long tendon construction needs to "ripen." As soon as they are solid, they are usually stable. For tenodesis, the dorsal one over the thumb metacarpophalangeal joint, the perfect technique has not been found. One wants a passive joint flexion of about 20 to 30°. My first trials were to fix the dorsal tendon to the metacarpal with one or two sutures through holes in the bone, pressing the raw tendon against bone to produce adhesions. When this often turned out to be insufficient, I used four sutures. This also failed and, at reoperation, it was found that the central surface of the tendon was solidly fixed to the bone. However, in the middle of the tendon, a new gliding pathway had developed. Thus, a technique was tried similar to that used for fixation of the flexor pollicis longus tenodesis (see Fig. 13–2A). Two holes were made through the cortex of the metacarpal head, the extensor pollicis tendon was cut proximally and made to form a sling through the holes and back to itself, and then distally sutured. Even if this sling is reinforced by a small tendon graft, failures can occur. In a few cases a bony fusion may be made, but in many cases the patient does not like two stiff joints in the thumb. The technical problems must be solved in such a way that a stiff joint is avoided. On the other hand, too much slack means quite a reduction in grip power. With a new and as yet unpublished method, these difficulties can be avoided. The flexor pollicis

longus tendon is taken out of its normal pathway. The thumb metacarophalangeal joint is taken out at this level, moved under nerves and vessels to the pisiform region and further through the canal of Guyon, under the flexor tendons in the volar compartment of the wrist to radius. Here it is anchored in the same way as in the original method. This new method will be published in a report from the Philadelphia meeting, March 1984, "Another Decade in Tendon Surgery."

Other slackening of tenodesis is rare, and easier to prevent or handle. In five or six cases, the flexor pollicis longus tenodesis to the radius had slackened, usually caused by too vigorous and too early propulsion of the wheelchair. In such cases, it was quite easy to shorten the tendon distally in the thumb by another operation using local anesthesia. The protracted tendon was anchored with a pull-out wire suture fixed around the nail. Immobilization followed for 4 weeks. Heavy pull on the tenodesis construction is now postponed to at least 2 months after surgery.

The use of the very thin extensor pollicis brevis tendon was tested in some early cases—for example, for an extensor tenodesis. The results were unsatisfactory, and the tendon in question seemed too thin for most purposes. The only exception seems to be in its use for thumb abduction-extension motored by the brachioradialis muscle. Because this function needs long training, the tendon is probably not subjected to much strain early but will get ample time for fixation.

The most serious slackening problem occurs in the deltoid transfers, in which the ripening process takes several months. If the elbow flexion starts too early, much extension power is lost and will never be regained. In a very frank study about complications in this surgery, Bryan wrote that "The hardest lesson to learn has been the need to mobilize the elbow slowly. Moberg advised 10° per week."[1] Even this can occasionally be too much. It remains to be seen if a new technique, devised by Castro and Pitá, will be helpful in shortening the time in question.[2]

The number of late adjustments has not turned out to be a great problem. With added experience, especially in follow-up treatment, which can never become routine, these problems can be considerably reduced.

EVALUATION AND INDICATIONS OF PROBLEMS

If the real surgical complications are few and can generally be treated, and the necessity of surgical rehabilitation of the hand in tetraplegia is evident, the difficulties with an adequate approach and correct thinking must be resolved. There seem to be two main errors: (1) to try to imitate normal hand function that, due to the enormous loss, is an impossible task (see Table 13–1); (2) to try to perform too much in one session.

Table 13–1 shows that the loss, except for that in a very few cases (different in different countries, but about the same in Scandinavia and the United States) includes the sensibility qualities, factors of paramount but hitherto unrecognized importance.[10, 12, 13] In spite of all that the patient and surgeon could wish, the little left is only enough for one or two simple functions. For example, opposition of the thumb should not be a goal, because this function requires a number of active muscles working together, and also because this grip is far less useful than the key grip. The latter requires only one active muscle, and this is often all one can obtain. It has turned out that the fusion of the wrist to get more muscles for transfer is a serious mistake. Active extension of the wrist is the base on which gripping function should be built. Also, the flexor carpi radialis works better where it is, and should not be transferred. Arthrodesed joints should be limited to the very few needed. Often the grip can be given only to one hand owing to lack of afferent impulses. If tactile gnosis is absent, the patient has to rely only on vision, which, as a rule, can supply only one hand efficiently.

This is not the place for a thorough discussion of the ways to evaluate cases for surgery, and the different indications. It should only be stressed that experience is required, and some errors are still impossible to avoid. The patient is teaching the surgeon new facts almost every day. With growing experience, the surgeon will find that, in the earlier cases, in spite of good results, still a bit more could have been gained by a more precise indication. It is a fascinating surgery, opening up new views for other hand surgery.

Naturally, patients like to reduce the time for the total surgical rehabilitation as much as possible, and also like to get more dexterous than is realistically possible at each session. The power to train and to make useful what is done is much below the standard in other hand surgery. It must be remembered that it is less often the question of relearning old functions; rather, and more importantly, it is a problem of finding totally new applications for the remaining sensory and motor functions. The training must usually be limited to one single function each time, and the patient's total energy must be concentrated on this. Nothing should divert him, which means that other surgery and other treatment (e.g., hip or bladder) must either be finished before or postponed until the upper limb procedures have been completed. Trying to "help" the patient by performing two different procedures at the same time usually produces no or poor results. Still worse, it easily results in a total loss of conditions for repair and correction. The possibilities that existed before are often definitely lost. Very frank reports of such experiences have been given by Bryan.[1] I have not tried to perform the elbow extensor procedure bilaterally in the same session, because this makes the patient totally helpless for several months and the training most difficult.

My own method is quite to the contrary: to start with slow advancement. For example, I require that the elbow flexion after a deltoid transfer be almost completely regained before the hand procedure is started. I have found that the hand procedure can be performed with good result when elbow flexion has reached the 90° position.

It is very disappointing to perform the wrong type of operation, or to operate on a patient not suitable for surgery at all. All details of the necessary examination must be performed personally by the surgeon.[12, 17] I have never seen a case in which vital information about sensibility, motor function, and psychology could be obtained from the available hospital records. Nonoperative rehabilitation never requires this, and most examinations were generally left to others. The new way of thinking has changed this; the responsibility is that of the surgeon, who also has a need for the new classification to be able to compare results.

References

1. Bryan, R. S.: The Moberg deltoid-triceps replacement and key-pinch operations in quadriplegia. Preliminary experiences. Hand, 9:3, 1977.
2. Castro-Sierra, A., and Lopez-Pitá, A.: A new surgical technique to correct triceps paralysis. Hand, 15:42, 1983.
3. DeBenedetti, M.: Restoration of elbow extension power in the tetraplegic patient using the Moberg technique. J. Hand Surg., 4:1, 1979.
4. Freehafer, A. A.: Flexion and supination deformities of the elbow in tetraplegics. Paraplegia, 15:221, 1977.
5. Hentz, V. R., and Keoshian, L. A.: Changing perspectives in surgical hand rehabilitation in quadriplegic patients. Plast. Reconstr. Surg., 60:4, 1979.
6. House, J. H., Gwathmey, F. W., and Lundsgaard, D. K.: Restoration of strong grasp and lateral pinch in tetraplegia due to spinal cord injury. J. Hand Surg., 1:152, 1976.
7. Lamb, D.W.: Current situation in the management of the upper limb in tetraplegia. Rehab. Med., 1:135, 1979.
8. McDowell, C. L., Moberg, E., and Smith, A. G.: International conference on surgical rehabilitation of the upper limb in tetraplegia. J. Hand Surg., 4:4, 1979.
9. Michaelis, L. S.: Orthopaedic Surgery of the Limbs in Paraplegia, Berlin, Springer, 1964.
10. Moberg, E.: Surgical treatment for absent single-hand grip and elbow extension in quadriplegia. J. Bone Joint Surg., 57A:196, 1975.
11. Moberg, E.: Editorial. Hand, 9:205, 1977.
12. Moberg, E.: The Upper Limb in Tetraplegia: A New Approach to Surgical Rehabilitation. Stuttgart, Thieme, 1978.
13. Moberg, E. The role of cutaneous afferents for position sense and kinaesthesia. Brain, 106:1, 1983.
14. Report from the committee on spinal cord injuries, International Federation of Societies for Surgery of the Hand. Paraplegia, 19:386, 1981.
15. Session on posttraumatic cystic degeneration of the cord. Paraplegia, 19:67, 1981.
16. Smith, A. G.: Early complications of key grip hand surgery for quadriplegia. Paraplegia 19:123, 1981.
17. Zancolli, E.: Functional restoration of upper limbs in traumatic quadriplegia. In Zancolli, E. (ed.): Structural and Dynamic Basis of Hand Surgery, 2nd ed., Philadelphia, J. B. Lippincott, 1979.

14

COMPLICATIONS IN FRACTURES OF THE PHALANGES AND METACARPALS

Richard S. Idler,
Douglas Schreiber,
and James W. Strickland

The most common complications related to fractures of the phalanges and metacarpals are malunion, nonunion, infection, and arthrofibrosis. Other frequently seen problems include tendon adherence at the fracture site, traumatic skin loss, difficulties with wound healing, sensory loss, reflex sympathetic dystrophy, and persistent pain. Depending on the nature of the injury, it is not uncommon for multiple complications to exist simultaneously; however, for simplicity's sake, an attempt will be made to examine each type of complication separately and to stress the characteristic features of each.

The surgeon caring for phalangeal and metacarpal fractures must be aware of factors that can lead to complications, and must make every effort to control those factors that will lead to the best possible result for the patient. The patient's age, the presence of chronic systemic disease, social pressures, and economic factors may prevent the patient from cooperating fully in his own care. The surgeon must compensate by careful attention to planning and technique, and must watch for and recognize complications as they occur. Timely and appropriate therapy should be planned, keeping the patient's well-being foremost in mind.

MALUNION

Management of fractures of the phalanges and metacarpals demands adherence to the same basic principles of fracture treatment required by other long bones. Due to the smaller size of these structures and the necessity of maintaining digital joint mobility, great attention must be paid to accurate reduction and to the judicious management of soft tissues adjacent to the fracture. If the injury has not been correctly diagnosed because of inadequate clinical and roentgenographic evaluation, or if the fracture has been inadequately reduced, improperly immobilized, or neglectfully followed, it may heal in an angulated or rotated position (Fig. 14–1). Open reduction and internal fixation of these fractures will not necessarily ensure success. Malunion may result from inaccurate reduction or inadequate techniques of fixation. Insufficient stabilization and improper immobilization or attempts at early motion may result in loss of reduction and in eventual malunion (Fig. 14–2).

Malunion is uncommon in closed nonarticular fractures of the distal phalanx. Open fractures with interruption of the overlying pulp and nail bed are more likely to be unstable and develop a malunion. In the presence of a unilateral skin wound, late angulation of the distal bony fragment may occur as a consequence of scar contracture. In fingertip injuries with underlying terminal phalangeal fractures, K-wire internal fixation may be required to provide adequate stability for soft tissue reconstruction. Malunion of the distal phalanx can produce a permanent nail bed deformity. Despite the objectionable cosmetic consequence of angular or rota-

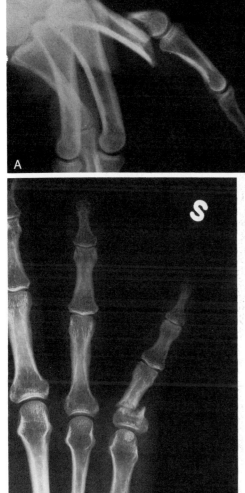
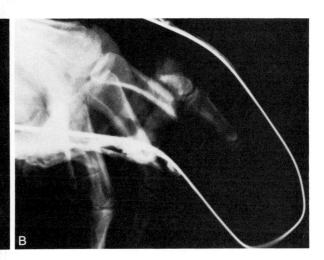

Figure 14–1. A, B, Inadequate reduction and immobilization of a displaced fracture of the neck of the proximal phalanx. This unstable fracture was poorly reduced and inadequately immobilized in an anterior posterior aluminum foam splint-cast combination. Failure to maintain reduction and to follow the patient adequately resulted in a malunion. *C,* Malunion with an angulatory deformity of a fracture of a base of the proximal phalanx of the small finger. Considerable long-term disability resulted from the abducted position of this digit.

tional malunion of the distal phalanx, function is usually unimpaired and late intervention is seldom warranted.

Fractures involving the proximal and middle phalanges often result in angular and rotational malalignment. The deformity following fracture of the middle phalanx is dependent on the fracture level. If it is distal to the insertion of the flexor digitorum superficialis, the angulation will be volar. If it is proximal to this insertion, the angulation will usually be dorsal. Fractures of the proximal phalanx tend to angulate volarly, although this may be modified by the vector of the injuring force (Fig. 14–3).

When phalangeal fractures unite with a uniplanar anterior posterior deformity, apparent limitations of flexion or extension may be noted at the adjacent joint. As little as 25° of volar angulation of the proximal phalanx may prevent the fingertip from reaching the palm and limit proximal interphalangeal joint extension by relative lengthening of the extensor tendon.[1] Volar angulation of the middle phalanx may result in the combination mallet finger and swan-neck deformity described by Bowers.[2] In both instances, bony realignment and the restoration of muscle tendon balance in the digit may be achieved by an opening wedge osteotomy. This should be augmented with bone grafting and internal fixation.

Impacted transverse phalangeal fractures often present as biplanar angular deformities with volar angulation and rotation. If this is not corrected, the digit may deviate out of its normal plane of flexion and extension, with resultant digital overlap. Roentgenograms often do not demonstrate this deformity adequately, and a thorough clinical examination is more valuable. With the fingers in extension, one

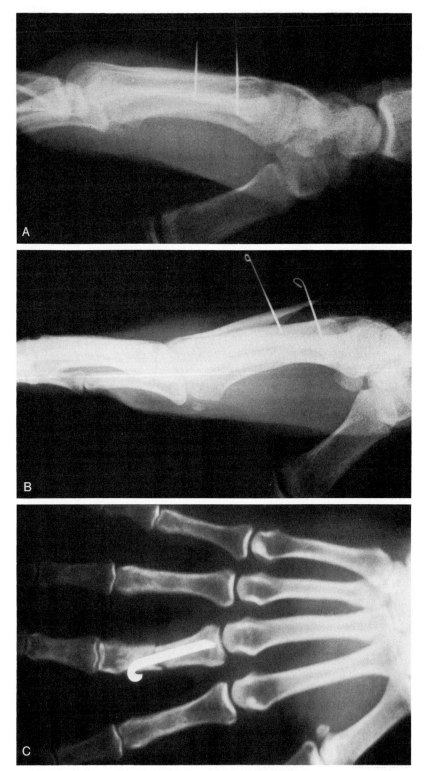

Figure 14–2. A, B, Inadequate open reduction and internal fixation. This oblique fracture of the proximal metacarpal was inadequately fixed with two vertically placed parallel Kirschner wires, which led to secondary displacement. More secure fixation techniques would have obviated the need for additional procedures in this case. *C,* Angulatory deformity of the proximal phalanx following improper use of a small Rush pin for internal fixation.

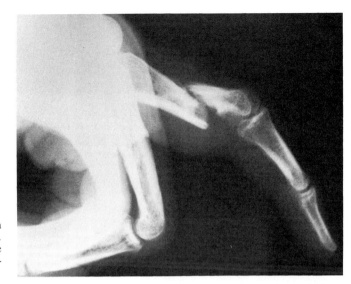

Figure 14–3. Typical volar angulation of a short oblique fracture of the proximal phalanx. If not adequately reduced, imbalance of the flexor and extensor forces may result in impaired digital function.

may observe the nail beds to check alignment. If the fingernails all appear to lie on the same level plane, rotational malalignment is probably not present. Minor rotational deformities may not become apparent until the finger is checked in flexion.[3] The fingers should be examined as a group and flexed together into a fist. Evidence of digital overlap suggests the presence of rotational malalignment (Fig. 14–4).

The prevention of malunion in phalangeal fractures requires an accurate initial reduction followed by secure immobilization and frequent, careful clinical and roentgenographic follow-up. Once rotational malunion is established, an osteotomy is necessary to correct it (Fig. 14–5). This osteotomy need not be done at the site of fracture, but may be better performed at the level of the proximal metaphysis at which union is more certain. When injury produces comminution or loss of bone in the proximal or middle phalanges, angulation in multi-

ple planes, including rotational malalignment, may result. Under these circumstances, closed treatment is often inadequate in achieving and maintaining alignment. An open reduction with internal fixation is necessitated. Power tools and proper bone-holding instruments facilitate the procedure. Fracture fragments may be stabilized with Kirschner wires, interosseous wires, small fragment bone screws, plates, or a combination of these.

If there is a sufficient amount of bone loss, length should be maintained by an interpositional bent Kirschner wire or by the use of an external fixation device. Grafting of the defect may be carried out as early as 7 to 10 days after injury, as described by Freeland and colleagues, or delayed until wound healing is complete and tissue equilibrium has been achieved.[4] In severe injuries, late bone grafting after complete healing of the soft tissues may be the wiser course of action.

If corrective osteotomy is required, special atten-

Figure 14–4. Rotational malalignment of the fifth finger following improper reduction of a proximal phalangeal fracture. In full digital flexion, the overlapping of the fifth finger is dramatically demonstrated.

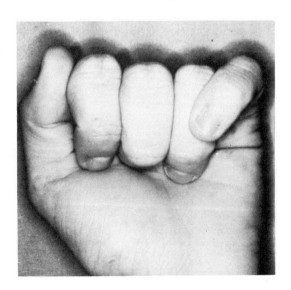

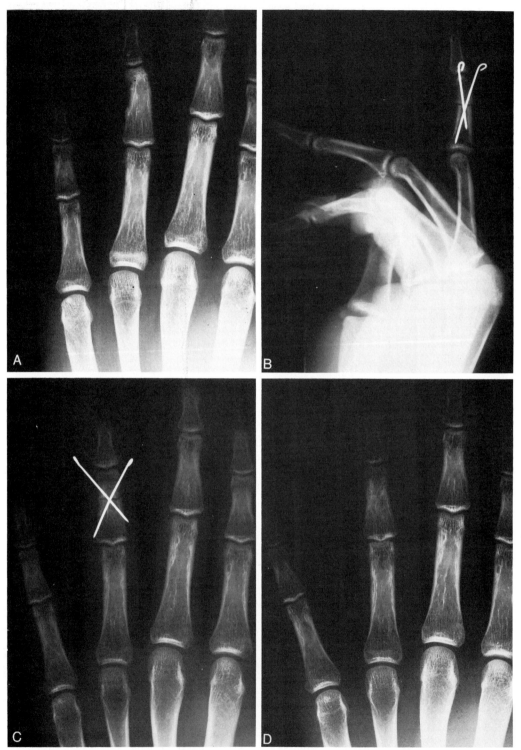

Figure 14–5. Correction of malunion by osteotomy. *A,* Angulatory and rotatory malunion of an oblique fracture through the distal third of the middle phalanx; *B, C,* corrective osteotomy with stabilization by Kirschner wires; *D,* appearance of healed phalanx following osteotomy.

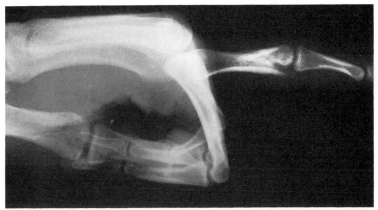

Figure 14–6. Bony joint block following malunion of oblique proximal phalangeal fracture. This distal oblique fracture of the proximal phalanx healed with a projecting palmar spike from the proximal fragment, which mechanically prevented proximal interphalangeal joint flexion. Ostectomy of the protruding spike or occasionally osteotomy is necessary to restore joint motion.

tion must be paid to the adjacent soft tissues because of the diminished vascularity that may have resulted from the original injury. Cancellous bone grafting is recommended as an adjunct to healing of the osteotomy.[5] Bone graft taken from the distal radius or proximal ulna is often adequate for small defects.

If a larger amount of graft is needed, the ilium provides an excellent donor site.

Malunion of oblique phalangeal and metacarpal fractures may produce an osseous bone spike protruding volarly or dorsally, which impales the adjacent tendons or forms a mechanical block to

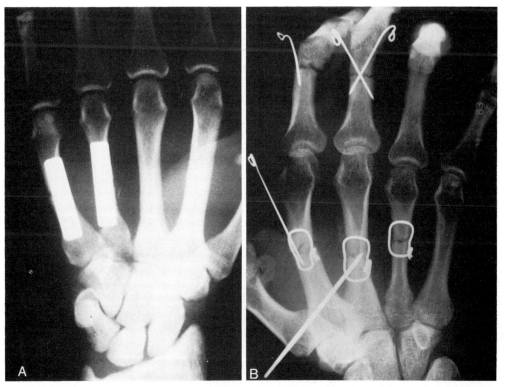

Figure 14–7. Internal fixation of multiple metacarpal fractures. *A,* Fixation of fractures of the fourth and fifth metacarpals by means of skeletal plates; *B,* the use of circumferential interosseous wires supplemented by Kirschner wires for fractures of the second, third, and fourth metacarpals. Although often managed conservatively, widely displaced or unstable metacarpal fractures may require open reduction and fixation to restore alignment and rotation.

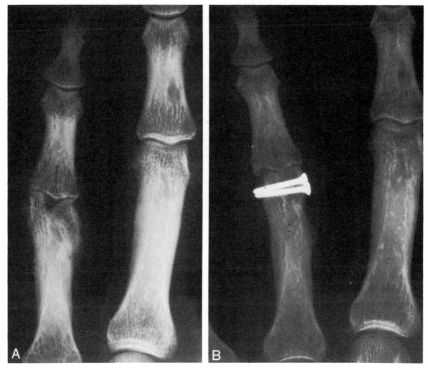

Figure 14–8. Articular incongruity with malunion of proximal phalangeal condylar fragment managed by osteotomy. *A,* A depressed and rotated condylar fragment of the proximal phalanx with early malunion at 6 weeks; *B,* correction by osteotomy and screw fixation.

complete joint motion (Fig. 14–6). Late attritional tendon ruptures can result from this deformity. If no other rotational or angulatory deformity exists, a simple ostectomy of this spike should restore satisfactory joint motion or tendon gliding.[6]

The possibility of complications associated with metacarpal shaft fractures should not be underestimated. These fractures tend to angulate dorsally because of the pull of the intrinsic muscles and, if healing occurs in this position, the involved metacarpal heads will become prominent in the palm. As a result of the mobility of the fifth carpometacarpal joint, angulation up to 20° can be accepted in this metacarpal without loss of the normal transverse metacarpal arch.[7] If the third or fourth metacarpals heal with dorsal angulation, the transverse metacarpal arch will be reversed and impair function of the hand.

Rotational malalignment is a common finding in oblique or badly displaced metacarpal fractures of the thumb, index, or little fingers. Fractures involving the central metacarpals are frequently stabilized by the soft tissue attachments to the adjacent border metacarpals; however, this will not be the case in the presence of multiple metacarpal fractures. In these injuries, open reduction and internal fixation may prevent the need for later derotational osteotomy (Fig. 14–7). An effort should be made to minimize soft tissue and periosteal dissection to avoid potential joint arthrofibrosis and tendon adherence. Secure fixation achieved with the use of

interfragmental screws or small plates may permit an early motion program that will minimize the complications of soft tissue healing.

Fractures of the metacarpal necks are often dorsally angulated with displacement of the metacarpal head into the palm, but rarely to a significant degree. They can usually be reduced adequately using closed technique. Special attention must be paid to fractures involving the second, third, and fourth metacarpal necks to avoid loss of the normal transverse metacarpal arch. Correctional osteotomy is seldom required, especially in fractures of the fifth metacarpal neck, in which 40° of angulation is felt to be acceptable.[7] Osteotomy at the level of the metacarpal neck is hard to immobilize without transfixing the adjacent metacarpophalangeal joint, which may lead to disabling joint stiffness.

Anatomic reduction is required in intra-articular fractures of the phalanges and metacarpals. Malunion across an articular surface will almost invariably lead to a painful stiff joint, which will compromise performance of the entire digit (Fig. 14–8).

In distal interphalangeal (DIP) joint fractures closed manipulation often yields satisfactory results, but open reduction is required for certain injuries. Displaced fractures of the condyles of the middle phalanx should be perfectly reduced and stabilized with small Kirschner wires or interfragmental screws. Attempts to accomplish K-wire fixation percutaneously are usually unsuccessful. The dorsal lip avulsion fracture seen in mallet finger injuries must

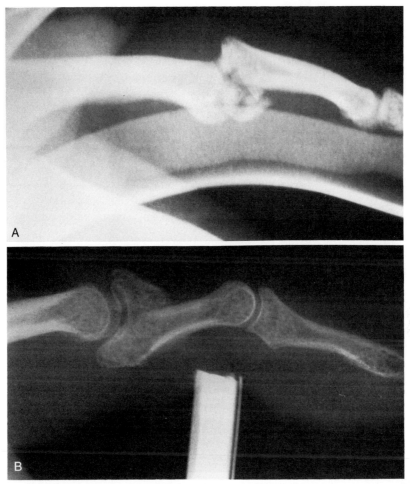

Figure 14–9. Malposition and malunion of articular fractures and fracture dislocations at the proximal interphalangeal joint. *A,* Chronic dorsal displacement of the base of the middle phalanx following a comminuted articular fracture of the palmar phalangeal base. This complication with almost inevitable joint destruction frequently results from inadequate reduction, inadequate immobilization, or inadequate follow-up x-rays following these difficult injuries. *B,* Comminuted intra-articular fracture at the base of the middle phalanx, which has healed with substantial displacement, angulation, and shortening. Whether managed by open or closed techniques, these fractures require accurate reduction and frequent monitoring to return satisfactory joint function.

be approached surgically if it is large enough to allow volar subluxation of the distal phalanx, or if it remains displaced after closed reduction with the DIP joint held in extension. Volar lip fractures seen with avulsion of the flexor digitorum profundus in football jersey injuries likewise require surgical treatment, with reinsertion of the tendon unit. Various procedures have been used for correction of the established mallet finger or neglected profundus tendon avulsion, often with less than satisfactory results. Arthrodesis is the most predictable salvage procedure.

Intra-articular fractures of the proximal interphalangeal and metacarpophalangeal joints may heal in less than anatomic alignment in spite of open reduction and internal fixation. This is especially true when the fractures are comminuted. Perhaps the most frustrating of all injuries is the fracture dislocation of the proximal interphalangeal joint, for which there is a multitude of treatment protocols.

Even in the best of hands, the results following this injury are frequently disappointing (Fig. 14–9). If an intra-articular fracture results in a painful and stiff joint, fusion or arthroplasty is indicated depending on the requirements and wishes of the patient. Attempts at intra-articular correctional osteotomies have not led to predictably satisfactory results in our hands if the process of post-traumatic arthritis has commenced.

Bennett's fractures should be opened, anatomically reduced, and internally stabilized if they cannot be restored by closed manipulation and percutaneous Kirschner wire fixation. If this fracture is treated with less than perfect reduction, painful arthritis will develop, requiring later surgical arthrodesis or interpositional arthroplasty (Fig. 14–10).

Intra-articular fracture of the base of the fifth metacarpal, also known as the baby Bennett's fracture, is an unstable injury with displacement produced by deforming external forces. Like the Ben-

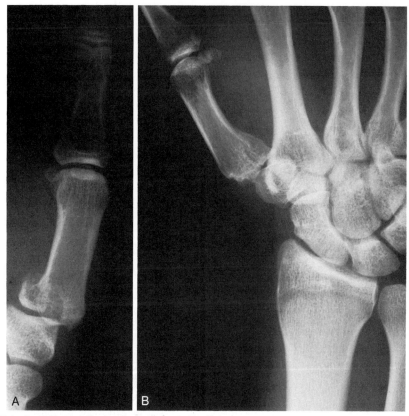

Figure 14–10. Malunion following Bennett's fracture. *A,* Typical appearance of unreduced Bennett's fracture, with lateral and proximal displacement of the major fragment; *B,* articular incongruity of the first metacarpal base following failure to achieve anatomic reduction.

nett's fracture, this injury requires an anatomic reduction and internal fixation using either closed or open technique. The late result of improper treatment is painful arthritis, requiring arthrodesis or interpositional arthroplasty of the carpometacarpal joint (Fig. 14–11).[8]

NONUNION

Nonunion in the phalangeal or metacarpal fracture may result from inadequate reduction, improper immobilization, interposition of soft tissue, loss of bone, or infection. Nonunion in fractures of the distal phalanges following crush injuries occurs not infrequently, but the fragments are usually small and are well supported by the overlying fingernail, if present. This form of nonunion rarely requires treatment, and pain may reflect the adjacent soft tissue damage rather than unhealed bone. Nonunions occasionally occur at the base of the distal phalanx and may be symptomatic at this level, where the fingernail is a less effective external splint. These fractures will usually heal with immobilization by Kirschner wires inserted percutaneously across the un-united fracture. If nonunion persists, bone grafting is required.[9]

As with other long bones, nonunion of phalangeal fractures occurs more frequently at the diaphyseal

level. Treatment of these nonunions requires rigid internal fixation and cancellous bone grafting. In our experience, cancellous graft obtained from the distal radius has usually been adequate. In cases of loss of bone with shortening or loss of bone secondary to chronic infection, the area of nonunion should be excised and replaced with a properly formed dowel graft. In such cases, an iliac crest bone graft is a better source.

Nonunion of the metacarpals occurs most frequently with involvement of the central rays. Here, relatively simple transverse or short oblique fractures may be held in distraction because of the ligamentous connections between adjacent bones. Also, soft tissue interposition can easily occur. If a painless fibrous nonunion results, no treatment is indicated. A painful nonunion should be treated with bone grafting and rigid internal fixation. Ray resection is an appropriate treatment in persistent painful nonunion of the index or little finger metacarpals, with marked stiffness and contractures involving the remainder of the digit.

INFECTION

In view of the multiple lacerations and minor injuries that occur to the hand in everyday use, its ability to withstand infection is remarkable. How-

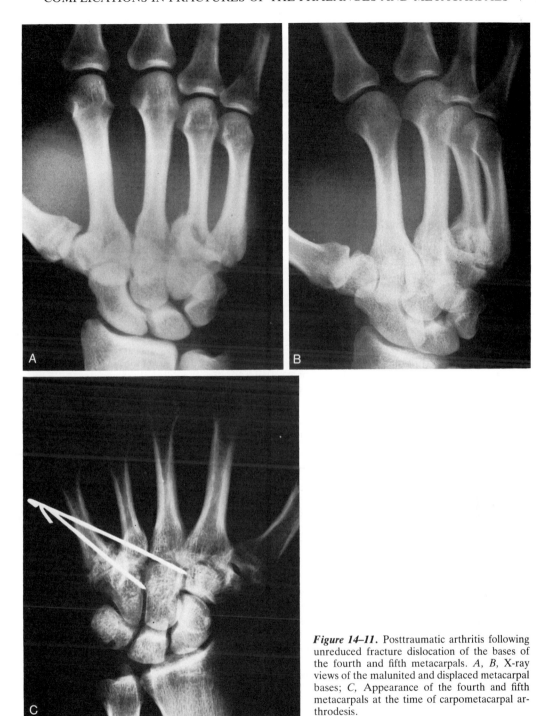

Figure 14–11. Posttraumatic arthritis following unreduced fracture dislocation of the bases of the fourth and fifth metacarpals. *A, B,* X-ray views of the malunited and displaced metacarpal bases; *C,* Appearance of the fourth and fifth metacarpals at the time of carpometacarpal arthrodesis.

ever, when associated with significant contamination and soft tissue injury, compound fractures are at high risk of developing infection. This is especially true when a compound injury occurs in the presence of a human bite, burn, or overlooked foreign body.

The avoidance of infection is predicated on adequate stabilization of the fracture, complete surgical débridement of devitalized tissue, removal of all foreign material, and delayed closure of wounds contaminated by human and animal oral secretions. In straightforward compound fractures without extensive soft tissue injury, the initial débridement and fixation of the fracture may be safely performed on an outpatient basis, and the patient may be released on a short course of broad-spectrum prophylactic antibiotics. In severe compound fractures, it may be necessary to admit the patient to the hospital for treatment with intravenous antibiotics until soft tissue coverage has been obtained and the danger of infection has been reduced.

The treatment of osteomyelitis in metacarpals and phalangeals is similar to that employed in the treatment of chronic infection involving any bone. If a nonunion is present it is desirable to obtain stabilization, putting the adjacent soft tissues at rest and allowing the body's own defense mechanisms to concentrate on the bone infection. An infected nonunion will neither heal nor become uninfected while gross motion is present. A sequestrum or involucrum should be surgically removed unless it provides stability to the infected phalanx or metacarpal. A draining sinus should be appropriately excised along with the underlying necrotic bone and covered with good local tissues, if possible.

Even if infection in a compound fracture does not lead to osteomyelitis, it may evolve into a purulent tenosynovitis if the wound communicates with a tendon sheath. Purulent tenosynovitis is truly a surgical emergency, and requires immediate incision and drainage of the tendon sheath. Failure to institute early decompression of the sheath leads to tendon necrosis.

ARTHROFIBROSIS

Joint stiffness to some degree is an almost constant complication of fractures of the phalanges and metacarpals. The fundamental factors producing stiffness and loss of joint motion in the hand are edema, fibrosis, and immbolization (Fig. 14–12).

Stiffness in the hand following fracture can be minimized by properly reducing and immobilizing the fracture, preventing hematoma and infection, applying a mildy compressive dressing, and elevating the injured extremity. When open reduction is performed, meticulous hemostasis should be obtained to minimize postoperative bleeding. Prophylactic antibiotics should be administered to minimize the risk of infection. The hand should be immobilized in a secure mildly compressive dressing, which places the joints of the hand in a position that minimizes the impact of arthrofibrosis. We favor a position of wrist dorsiflexion of 20 to 30°, metacarpophalangeal joint flexion of 45 to 60°, and interphalangeal joint flexion of 0 to 10°.

We have found that problems with stiffness and contracture significantly increase if immobilization is prolonged beyond 4 weeks.[10] The advantage of secure internal fixation using interfragmental screws and plates is that early motion can be initiated as soon as pain lessens, thus minimizing the complications of soft tissue healing such as arthrofibrosis and tendon adherence.

An attempt should always be made to regain motion using conservative measures before approaching the stiff hand surgically. The key to nonsurgical mobilization is active and passive range-of-motion exercises under the supervision of a compassionate and well-trained therapist. Force must always be applied slowly and continuously during passive exercise, and must not increase the swelling

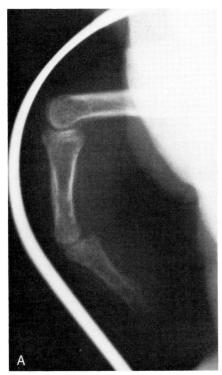
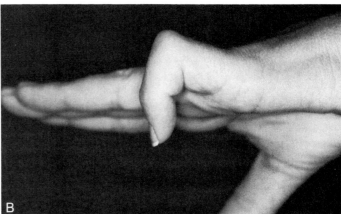

Figure 14–12. Arthrofibrosis of the proximal interphalangeal joint following improper immobilization of a proximal phalangeal fracture. *A,* X-ray appearance of the "90°-90°" method of immobilization of the digit following fracture of the base of the proximal phalanx (not visualized); *B,* a fixed 80° flexion contracture of the proximal interphalangeal joint is shown 3 months after treatment shown in *A.*

or pain of the joints. Early active exercises are paramount for mobilization of the digit, and the use of functional electrical stimulation and biofeedback are beneficial. Local nerve blocks and stellate ganglion blocks are also very helpful, and will often allow the patient to overcome an early plateau in therapy. Passive taping programs and dynamic splinting will allow the patient to continue to make progress once secure bone stability has been achieved.

Continued efforts may be necessary to control swelling while the patient is undergoing therapy. Individually fashioned compressive finger and hand stockinettes can be utilized to supplement elevation of the extremity. In some instances, systemic or locally administered steroid preparations are helpful in controlling swelling.

When a plateau in therapy is reached and the amount of motion in the involved digit or digits is unacceptable, the stiff joint should be approached surgically. Before operating, it is important to try to determine by clinical and roentgenographic examination which structures are the contracting factors. Potential limiting factors include the skin across the joint; adherence of the extensor, intrinsic, or flexor tendons, contracture of collateral ligaments or volar plate, and bony exostoses.

When the proximal interphalangeal joint becomes contracted in a position of extension, the pathology is usually located dorsally. Dorsal scar contracture, skin adherence, adherence of the extensor mechanism to the underlying fracture, or dorsal capsular contracture may limit flexion of the joint. A dorsal surgical approach is utilized, and a systematic examination with release of tightened or adherent structures is performed. As might be expected, the more anatomic structures involved, and the more extensive the surgical release, the greater the likelihood that motion gained in surgery will be lost over time.

Contracture of the proximal interphalangeal joint in flexion may occur as the result of volar scar contracture, volar plate or collateral ligament contracture, flexor tendon adherence, and flexor myostatic contracture. Other possibilities include adherence of the spiral oblique retinacular ligament to the collateral ligament and bony obstruction or exostosis. A volar approach through a Bruner-type incision is utilized under these circumstances, with the same methodical systematic exploration and release of tight or adherent structures. Whenever possible, operations for relief of joint contracture should be done under local anesthesia to allow the patient to mobilize the joint actively following release. If the procedure is performed under a general anesthetic, the flexor system can be approached at the level of the palm or wrist to apply manual traction.

Contracture of the metacarpophalangeal joint usually occurs in a position of extension that is favored by distention of the joint or by adjacent soft tissue swelling. In the position of extension, the collateral ligaments are relaxed. Because of the cam action present with flexion at the metacarpophalangeal joint, contracture of the collateral ligaments in this relaxed position prevents full flexion. One should remember that, although normal metacarpophalangeal joints passively flex to 90°, most functions of the hand do not require flexion of the index and middle fingers beyond 75° or of the ring and little fingers beyonds 80°. Thus, it is not necessary to achieve 90° of active motion of metacarpophalangeal joints to have a useful hand. If 75° of active motion is achieved, surgical intevention is unwarranted.

Extensor tenolysis and dorsal capsulotomy of the metacarpophalangeal joint demand a careful technique. Injudicious resection of the radial collateral ligament of this joint leads to postoperative ulnar drift. Care must be taken to maintain the integrity of the extensor mechanism while performing tenolysis or capsulectomy; otherwise, decentralization of the extensor mechanism over the metacarpophalangeal joint will result. As in capsulectomy of the proximal interphalangeal joint, a well-supervised program of active and passive range of motion with passive and dynamic splinting must be followed to ensure a good result postoperatively.

Joint contractures may also be due to irreparable damage within the joint itself. This can often be determined by preoperative roentgenographic examination. In these instances, releasing the collateral ligaments and other tight or adherent structures will be unlikely to improve motion over time, and will not alter the preoperative pain. Here, salvage may be attempted either through an arthrodesis or arthroplasty. The choice of which procedure to use depends not only on the condition of the soft tissue about the joint but also on the desires and needs of the patient.

One of the most difficult problems to manage is the first web contracture, with the thumb fixed in adduction secondary to contacture of the intrinsic musculature, joint capsule, subcutaneous tissues, and overlying skin. When these structures are released, a gap is created that must be supplemented with adequate skin coverage and padding. This can usually be obtained with a local rotation flap and split-thickness skin graft to the resultant defect. Occasionally, a groin pedicle flap or cross-arm flap is required. In addition, it is wise to fix the thumb metacarpal in a position of opposition with a threaded K-wire or external fixator to prevent recurrence of the deformity.

TENDON ADHERENCE

It is not uncommon for tendons to be lacerated or transected in association with fractures. This combination results in a high likelihood of tendon adherence, with limitation in digital motion (Fig. 14–13). Whenever possible, tendon repair is performed at the time of fracture reduction and stabilization. An attempt is also made to restore any disruption of the pulley system. The patient should

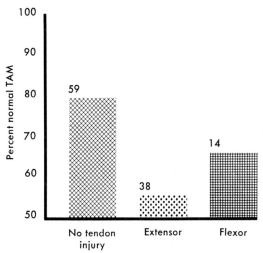

Figure 14–13. Significant influence of tendon injuries on nonarticular fractures of the proximal phalanx. Extensor tendon injuries were more prejudicial than flexor tendon injuries in this series. Proximal phalangeal fractures without tendon injury returned approximately 80% of the normal digital total active range of motion *(TAM)*, while fractures in association with flexor tendon injuries returned 67% and those with concomitant extensor tendon damage returned only 55%. (From Strickland, J. W., et al.: Factors influencing digital performance after phalangeal fracture. *In* Strickland, J. W., and Steichen, J. B. [eds.]: Difficult Problems in Hand Surgery, St. Louis, C. V. Mosby, 1982.)

always be forewarned of the possible necessity for secondary tenolysis under these circumstances.

Even when tendons are not lacerated, adherence at the fracture site may occur. This may involve either the flexor tendons, extensor tendons, or both, depending on the level and severity of the injury (Fig. 14–14).[10] This is particularly true in the presence of malalignment or displacement, which results in an osseous spike that impales the tendon. Alternatively, if adherence does not occur, attritional rupture may. Even with nondisplaced fractures and occasionally in the absence of fracture, a "turret" exostosis may occur and interfere with excursion of the overlying tendon.

Flexor tendon adherence is most likely to occur in fractures through the proximal and middle phalanges with volar angulation. The volar periosteum of the phalanges forms the floor of the fibro-osseous flexor sheath. With angulation, the tendon may become impaled on an osseous spike or caught in the abundant callus of secondary bone healing. An anatomic reduction of the fracture will minimize this complication. Limiting immobilization to less than 4 weeks will decrease the severity of the tendon adhesions.

Adherence of the extensor mechanism occurs frequently with concomitant extensor lacerations and underlying fractures. The integrity of the extensor mechanism should be restored at the time of primary fracture treatment and, whenever possible,

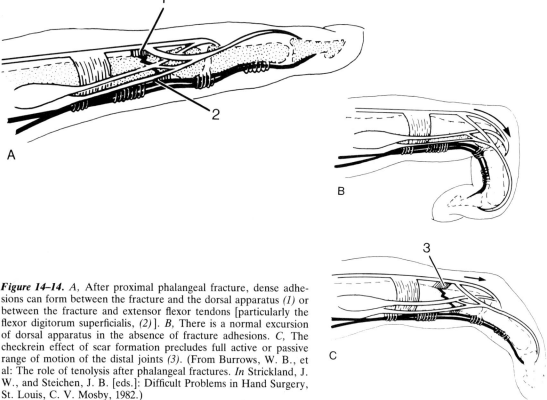

Figure 14–14. A, After proximal phalangeal fracture, dense adhesions can form between the fracture and the dorsal apparatus *(1)* or between the fracture and extensor flexor tendons [particularly the flexor digitorum superficialis, *(2)*]. *B,* There is a normal excursion of dorsal apparatus in the absence of fracture adhesions. *C,* The checkrein effect of scar formation precludes full active or passive range of motion of the distal joints *(3).* (From Burrows, W. B., et al: The role of tenolysis after phalangeal fractures. *In* Strickland, J. W., and Steichen, J. B. [eds.]: Difficult Problems in Hand Surgery, St. Louis, C. V. Mosby, 1982.)

C·C· PATEL

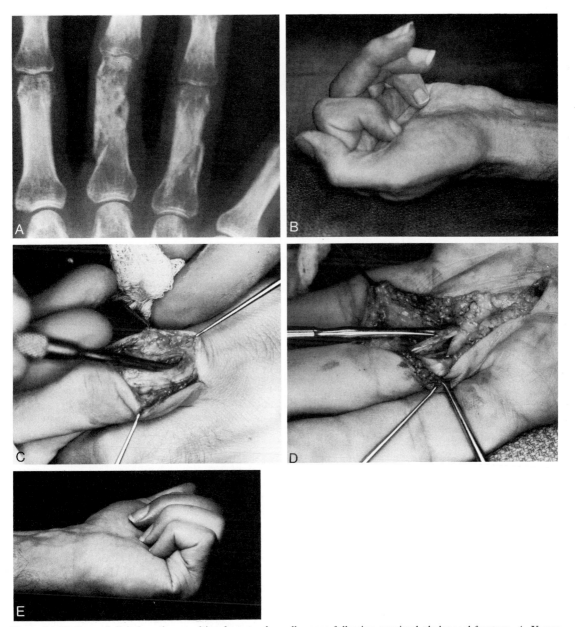

Figure 14–15. Loss of digital motion resulting from tendon adherence following proximal phalangeal fracture. *A*, X-rays of acceptably reduced and well-healed fractures through the midportion of the proximal phalanges of the long and ring fingers; *B*, extension contractures and decreased total active flexion in the middle and ring fingers several months after healing; *C*, tenolysis of the dorsal apparatus by individual mobilization of the central tendon and lateral bands; *D*, tenolysis of the flexor digitorum superficialis from adhesions to bone as well as intertendinous adhesions between the superficialis and profundus tendons; *E*, markedly improved range of motion in the involved digits following tenolysis. (From Burrows, W. B., et al: The role of tenolysis after phalangeal fractures. *In* Strickland, J. W., and Steichen, J. B. [eds.]: Difficult Problems in Hand Surgery, St. Louis, C. V. Mosby, 1982.)

the periosteum should be closed to provide an interposing tissue layer between the extensor mechanism and fracture. Motion is initiated at 4 weeks once adequate extensor tendon healing has occurred, but even with early motion the need for tenolysis is frequent.

A stable reduction with early motion offers the best insurance against loss of tendon excursion.

Open reduction can potentially increase the risk of tendon adherence unless early motion is instituted. A delay in open reduction of greater than 2 weeks following fracture can be expected to increase the risk of tendon adherence greatly. If open reduction is to be followed by early motion, fixation must be adequate or loss of reduction may result, with even greater problems of tendon adherence.

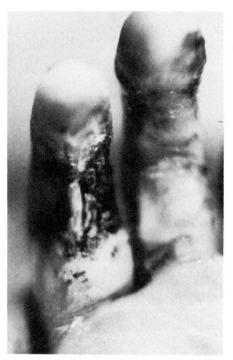

Figure 14–16. Severe skin necrosis with exposed flexor tendon following improper immobilization of a phalangeal fracture by compressing the digit too tightly against a rigid palmar splint.

If tendon-bone adhesions do occur and result in a significant limitation of digital joint motion, tenolysis may be required, particularly when an appropriate period of conservative mobilization has not proved to be successful. The procedure is best carried out under local anesthesia so that the patient can actively demonstrate the complete release of all restraining adhesions (Fig. 14–15). Joint releases may also be required at the time of tenolysis to ensure maximum restoration of joint function.

SKIN NECROSIS

Loss of skin in phalangeal and metacarpal fractures may occur as part of the initial injury. Skin necrosis as a complication of treatment may occur from overly vigorous attempts to attain immediate primary closure of contused soft tissues. It is better to leave the wound open while the injured extremity is elevated and immobilized in a compressive dressing for 24 to 36 hours. Delayed primary closure may then be possible, without risk of further skin necrosis. Complications of necrosis can occur with improper early application of tight constrictive dressings or casts to an injured hand (Fig. 14–16). A classic example is dorsal skin loss over the metacarpophalangeal and proximal interphalangeal joints resulting from the use of a box-type or 90-90 plaster cast for immobilization of a boxer's fracture. We have been impressed with the safety and advantages of using plaster splints within compressive dressings instead of full circular plaster casts. Compression can be adjusted as needed, and it is possible to take down the dressing easily and examine the injured part without loss of reduction. Although no technique will totally safeguard against complications of pressure necrosis, close observation of the patient and of the injured part is the only way to minimize them. Any complaints of discomfort within a dressing should be closely examined, particularly if the patient complains of a burning-type pain. This is commonly associated with either pressure necrosis or the early onset of a reflex sympathetic dystrophy.

Skin traction may lead to significant complications (Fig. 14–17). The use of improper technique and lack of patient cooperation in follow-up led to an unfortunate complication of circumferential skin necrosis around the distal aspect of the digit. Skin traction cannot be used to reduce a fracture, but only to maintain a reduction. Traction must never be supplied in such a manner that the distal fingertip

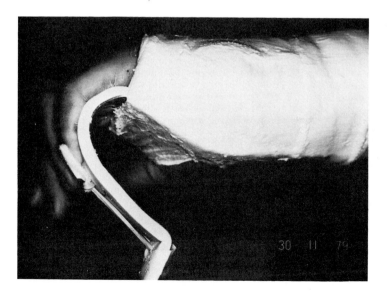

Figure 14–17. Complications following skin traction in an effort to reduce an unstable fracture of the base of the middle phalanx. This photograph illustrates the potential skin problems that may result from excessive pressure against the palmar surface of the digit when traction forces are used to pull the finger against an unyielding splint. This particular patient went on to a superficial slough of distal phalangeal skin.

cannot be examined. Finally, one must have a cooperative patient who understands the possible complications of this form of treatment, and will accept responsibility along with the physician in their avoidance. Complications inherent with skin traction can now be avoided by using skeletal traction made possible with commercially available external minifixators.

SENSORY LOSS

Sensory loss usually occurs in association with open displaced fractures of the phalanges. It may also be noted in closed fractures associated with a crush component. Early diagnosis requires a complete neurologic examination of the injured extremity prior to instituting therapy. Sensory loss associated with closed fractures should be treated expectantly. When sensory loss is present in an open fracture, the fracture should be stabilized and the injured nerve explored. If its continuity has been disrupted, repair should be performed at the same time.

Sensory return following nerve injuries depends on the nature of the injury, the patient's age, and the anatomic location of the injury. Anesthesia over the radial aspect of the little finger does not constitute the same amount of disability as does anesthesia over the ulnar aspect of the thumb or radial side of the index finger. Return of two-point discrimination less than 10 mm should be considered a good result, and should contraindicate exploration or revision of a previous neurorrhaphy. Failure of sensory return within the expected time limit may be an indication for surgical intervention. Sensory loss with two-point discrimination greater than 10 mm that is troublesome to the patient may require neurolysis, excision of neuroma with primary repair, or nerve grafting. The prospect for return of useful function in the anesthetized digit that has sustained a fracture and associated tendon injury is poor. In such instances, early or delayed amputation may be the best treatment.

PAIN

Pain is to be expected after fractures of the phalanges and metacarpals. It is only when this pain persists for an unusually prolonged length of time that it becomes a complication.

Cold intolerance is often present after phalangeal and metacarpal fractures. This varies in intensity from annoying to incapacitating. In general, it should be treated symptomatically with avoidance of cold and expectant support for the patient. In all but the rare patient, it resolves completely by 2 years. If disabling symptoms persist, digital sympathectomy may provide prolonged or permanent relief. In the occasional patient, amputation may be necessary.

Painful neuromas may also form after phalangeal fractures with associated nerve injuries. Expectant support and desensitization programs will be sufficient in most cases. In some cases, transcutaneous nerve stimulation is of benefit. When the pain persists, surgical intervention may be necessary. Exploration of the nerve may demonstrate only scar entrapment, which requires an external neurolysis with or without transposition of the nerve to a less prominent area or more satisfactory bed. A neuromatous incontinuity may require internal neurolysis, or excision of the neuroma with nerve grafting. Disabling hyperesthesias are sometimes only responsive to proximal transection of the nerve and placement of the proximal end into a protected soft tissue bed.

The problem of arthralgia has been mentioned previously. Painful joints may be treated with fusion, arthroplasty, or amputation, depending on the status of the adjacent soft tissues and on the desires and needs of the patient.

REFLEX SYMPATHETIC DYSTROPHY

Reflex sympathetic dystrophy tends to occur in the patient with a low pain threshold and a dependent personality. It often does not develop immediately but surfaces gradually to dominate the clinical picture. Early signs of impending problems are failure of the patient to mobilize uninvolved digits as instructed, and the appearance of symptoms of vasospasm. Osteoporosis becomes visible on x-ray at 5 to 8 weeks. The pain does not conform to any peripheral nerve distribution but instead is generalized and often ill defined.

There are two principles in the treatment of reflex sympathetic dystrophy: relief of pain and active use of the involved extremity. Relief of pain must be obtained before use of the extremity can begin. The long-term use of narcotics must be avoided in these chronic problems. In our expeirence, transcutaneous nerve stimulation has been helpful when instituted early. The stimulus amplitude should be controlled by the patient, because overly intense stimuli can produce additional pain. Stellate ganglion blocks, preferably performed in a series of three to five blocks followed by intensive therapy while the block is in effect, have also been beneficial in our experience. Other centers have reported beneficial results with reserpine and guanethidine Bier blocks.

These patients may have emotional and psychiatric problems that must not be overlooked. The attending physician and treating therapist must invest additional time with these patients and be emotionally supportive. Appropriately administered psychotropic drugs and antidepressants may be indicated. Passive modalities to improve circulation, decrease edema, and prepare the patient for active participation in the treatment program should be started early. Attention should also be paid to general body condition, and the patient should be kept ambulatory and as active as possible. The most important phase of active exercise, assisted by dynamic splints and desensitization, requires that the patient begin to assume increasing responsibility.

References

1. Coonrad, R. W., and Pohlman, M. H.: Impacted fractures in the proximal portion of the proximal phalanx of the finger. J. Bone Joint Surg., 51A:1291, 1969.
2. Bowers, W. H.: Mallet deformity of fingers after phalangeal fracture: Case report of treatment by the Fowler procedure. J. Bone Joint Surg., 59A:525, 1977.
3. Kaplan, E. B.: Treatment of fractures of metacarpals and proximal phalanx by skeletal traction. Bull. Hosp. Joint Dis., 5:99, 1944.
4. Freeland, A. E., Jabaley, M. E., and Chaves, A. M.: Delayed primary bone grafting in the hand and wrist after traumatic bone loss. J. Hand Surg., 7:423, 1982.
5. Abbott, L. C., et al.: The evaluation of cortical and cancellous bone grafting material. J. Bone Surg., 29:381, 1947.
6. Clinkscales, G. S., Jr.: Complications in the management of fractures in hand injuries. South. Med. J., 63:704, 1970.
7. Hunter, J. M., and Cowen, N. J.: Fifth metacarpal fractures in a compensation clinic population: A report on one hundred and thirty-three cases. J. Bone Joint Surg., 52A:1159, 1970.
8. El-Bacha, A.: The carpometacarpal joints (excluding the trapeziometacarpal). In Tubiana, R. (ed.): The Hand, Vol. 1, Philadelphia, W. B. Saunders, 1981, pp. 162–167.
9. Itoh, Y., Uchinishi, K., and Oka, Y.: Treatment of pseudoarthrosis of the distal phalanx with the palmar midline approach. J. Hand Surg., 8:80, 1983.
10. Strickland, J. W., et al.: Factors influencing digital performance after phalangeal fracture. In Strickland, J. W., and Steichen, J. B. (eds.): Difficult Problems in Hand Surgery, St. Louis, C. V. Mosby, 1982, pp. 126–139.

15

COMPLICATIONS OF DIGITAL LIGAMENT INJURY

William H. Bowers

"The skeleton deprived of its ligaments dislocates, its form and the power of its muscles negated."[1] The stabilizing function of the interphalangeal ligament structure is thus implied by noting the consequences of its disruption—deformity and loss of power. It is worth noting that interphalangeal ligaments do not *provide* motion, they *allow* motion. They provide a stable link that allows the efficient transmission of muscular force across the joint. The capsular structure is differentiated into collateral ligaments, volar capsular ligament (volar plate), and their subsets so that motion in a given plane is highly, partially, or minimally restricted. These capsular ligaments are "tuned" constantly by normal joint motion. This tuning maintains their optimum length and suppleness.

Injury and its consequent healing response interfere greatly with this sophisticated restrictive-permissive function. Depending on the specifics of the structure injured, the type of injury, and the healing event, motion may be allowed in previously restricted planes (instability) or limited in previously unrestricted planes (contracture). Asymmetry of capsular tension as a result of inadequate healing or too much scarring may cause uneven joint surface tracking and uneven joint compressive forces. (Figure 15–1 illustrates the natural history of capsular injury.) This may eventuate successively in loss of full power, a chronically swollen and painful joint, and arthrosis. In this sense, joint laxity, contracture, deformity, arthrosis, pain, and loss of strength, job, hobby, or happiness may be complications of digital ligament injury. Treatment in any form is invariably an additional insult to tissue, and has its own particular consequences. These may include infection, broken pins or wires, injury to uninjured structures, dystrophic pain syndromes, stiffness of adjacent joints, or diagnostic inadequacies leading to the wrong treatment entirely.

The above discussion presents a classic learning sequence (anatomy, natural history of injury, and intervention) that must now be described in detail if we are to think about how these injuries are to be managed.

FUNCTIONAL ANATOMY

Osseous Structure

Both joints' proximal articular surfaces are bicondylar. The condyles have a prominent and important volar lateral flare, most pronounced at the proximal interphalangeal joint (Fig. 15–2). On the lateral surface of this condyle a shallow crater marks the extensive origin of the cordlike proper collateral ligament. Coextensive with this is the origin of the accessory collateral or "suspensory" ligament of the volar plate. Articular cartilage covers a volar-tilted 180° surface. The proximal interphalangeal joint's *distal* articular face presents a prominent intercondylar ridge separating two shallow articular depressions (Fig. 15–3). From the lateral side the general shape is concave to contract an arc of approximately 80° on the convex proximal articular surface. The confluence of the intercondylar ridge and the dorsal margin of the articular concavities produces a distinctly elevated dorsal tubercle, at which the central slip of the extensor tendon inserts. Less distinct, at the distal interphalangeal joint, the dorsal margin of the distal articular face is referred to as the dorsal ridge and provides a broad but thin attachment surface for the extensor tendon. At both joints the distal articular face has a broad cartilage-covered volar facet, which is often incorrectly assumed to be the attachment surface for the volar plate. The meniscal leaf of the volar plate articulates with this

145

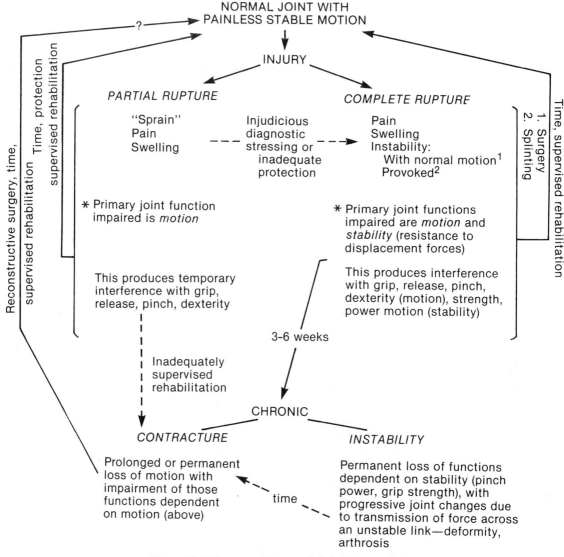

NORMAL JOINT WITH
PAINLESS STABLE MOTION

?

INJURY

PARTIAL RUPTURE

"Sprain"
Pain
Swelling

Injudicious
diagnostic
stressing or
inadequate
protection

COMPLETE RUPTURE

Pain
Swelling
Instability:
  With normal motion[1]
  Provoked[2]

* Primary joint function
impaired is *motion*

* Primary joint functions
impaired are *motion* and
stability (resistance to
displacement forces)

This produces temporary
interference with grip,
release, pinch, dexterity

This produces interference
with grip, release, pinch,
dexterity (motion), strength,
power motion (stability)

3-6 weeks

Inadequately
supervised
rehabilitation

CHRONIC

CONTRACTURE

INSTABILITY

Prolonged or permanent
loss of motion with
impairment of those
functions dependent
on motion (above)

time

Permanent loss of functions
dependent on stability (pinch
power, grip strength), with
progressive joint changes due
to transmission of force across
an unstable link—deformity,
arthrosis

Reconstructive surgery, time,
supervised rehabilitation

Time, protection
supervised rehabilitation

1. Surgery
2. Splinting

Time, supervised rehabilitation

Figure 15–1. The natural history of digital ligament injury.

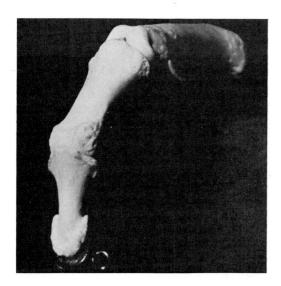

Figure 15–2. The prominent volar lateral flare is seen clearly
in this end-on view of the proximal interphalangeal joint.

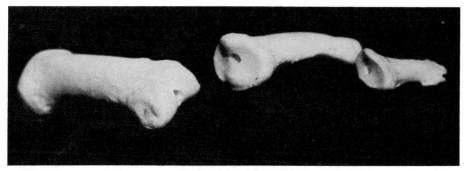

Figure 15–3. The disarticulated digit shows the proximal phalanx condylar depression where the collateral ligament originates. The various articular facets of the distal face of the PIP joint are clearly seen. The phalangeal perspective dramatizes the size difference between the two joints.

facet. The central plate's attachment is well onto the volar metaphysis of the distalward phalanx. Just lateral to this area are volarlateral tubercles. Beginning here and going around the volarlateral corner, the volar plate and proper collateral ligament attach successively in a dense fashion. This corner is designated as the "critical corner" for its importance in both volar and lateral joint stability, both of which can be lost by a force concentration at this point (Fig. 15–4).[2]

Capsular Structure

The joint capsular structure is intricate and highly differentiated to provide stability throughout its single arc of motion. Dynamic assistance is offered dorsally and volarly by the enveloping tendon structure. The extensor digitorum communis inserts on the dorsal ridge at the distal interphalangeal joint from collateral ligament to collateral ligament, and is confluent with the capsule in its entirety. The extensor central slip attachment at the proximal interphalangeal joint is confined to the dorsal tu-

bercle. The capsule is confluent with the tendon centrally, and thins dorsolaterally to underlie the extensor lateral bands.

The proper collateral ligaments are short, cord-like, and strong, originating in the proximal phalanx lateral condylar depression and inserting a millimeter or two distally on the lateral volar tubercles of the distalward phalanx, where they are confluent with the distal lateral margins of the volar plate ("critical corner"; see Fig. 15–4).

The proximal interphalangeal joint volar plate proximally resembles a swallowtail, with each tail (proximal rein, check ligament) coming firmly from bone just inside the walls of the second annular pulley (A2) at its distal margin (Fig. 15–5). This proximal volar plate attachment is coextensive with the proximal attachment of the first cruciate pulley, which straddles the sharp distal margin of the A2 pulley.[2, 3] Each limb of the cruciate pulley proceeds distally and volarly around the flexors; the two cross in the midvolar line to insert on the contralateral side of the volar plate at its thick central portion. This arrangement provides, in essence, a bilateral twin-tailed proximal origin of the volar plate—one

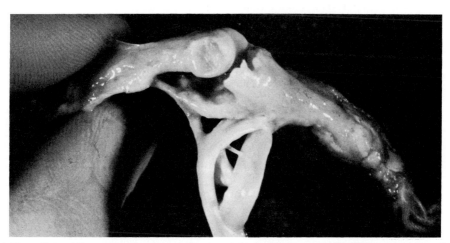

Figure 15–4. The collateral ligament-volar plate confluence at the "critical corner" In addition, the twin-tailed nature of the volar plate can be seen. The accessory collateral "suspensory" ligament of the volar plate has been removed.

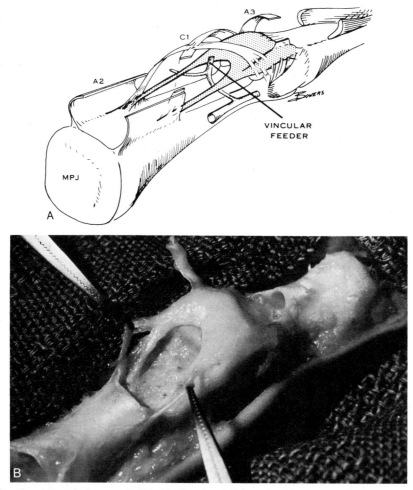

Figure 15–5. Drawing *(A)* and photograph *(B)* showing the oblique volar view of the proximal interphalangeal joint volar plate, collateral ligament, and sheath relationships. Note especially the relationship of the C1 pulley to the volar plate.

tail directly into bone, the other crossing over the flexor sheath, whose tension may be influenced by the volume of the contents of the flexor sheath.[4] The limbs of the proximal attachment (swallowtail) bridge the retrocondylar recess.

Through the resulting hiatus the transverse arterial feeders proceed medially under the floor of the flexor sheath, join, and form the major vincular vessel, which then passes volarly through the arch of the swallowtails to the flexor tendons. Distally, the volar plate is attached strongly only at its lateral margin on the volar lateral surface of the critical corner. The central 80% is meniscoid, and the meniscal leaf faces the articular facet at the base of

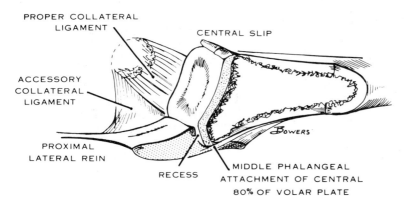

Figure 15–6. Intra-articular view of hemisection of volar plate showing the relationship of the accessory collateral ligament to the proper collateral ligament and volar plate. In addition to the meniscal recess separating the volar plate and volar articular facet, the insertion of the central volar plate on the metaphysis of the middle phalanx is clearly seen.

the distalward phalanx. The attachment of this central portion is by a thin extension onto the roughened area of the volar metaphysis under the flexor digitorum superficialis insertion. The meniscal recess or space adjacent to the articular facet and facing the meniscal portion of the central plate is shown in Figure 15–6. The subcondylar portion of the volar plate averages 1.5 mm thick, and increases the moment arm of the flexors up to 35% over that offered by the condylar radius alone.[2] Its absence by excision or retraction would affect the joint posture, not only by loss of a static restraint but by decreasing the flexion turning moment of the tendons.

Differences in Proximal and Distal Interphalangeal Joints

The major osseous difference at the proximal and distal joints is size. The contact surface area of a typical proximal interphalangeal joint is 100 mm², compared to 40 mm², at the distal interphalangeal joint. The distal interphalangeal joint volar plate differs from that at the proximal joint in several respects. Its proximal portion resembles the swallowtail configuration at the proximal interphalangeal joint but, when these tails are followed serially, it appears that the flexor digitorum superficialis absorbs the swallowtail-like anchors of the distal interphalangeal joint volar plate without their insertion into bone.[3] The meniscal recess is much more distinct at the distal interphalangeal joint. The flexor digitorum superficialis has no attachment to the proximal interphalangeal joint volar plate, whereas at the distal interphalangeal joint the flexor digitorum profundus blends intimately with the plate, fanning over its surface from one lateral insertion to the other.

The other major difference between the two joints is the relationship of the oblique retinacular ligament of Landsmeer. This ligament's proximal attachment is intimately related to the proximal origin of the volar plate just at the distal margin of the A2 pulley. It passes volar to the proximal interphalangeal joint axis of motion and joins the lateral bands to end dorsal to the distal interphalangeal joint axis of motion. Its consistent presence and significance are debated but, as described, it should act as a ligament coordinating interphalangeal flexion and extension—tightening as the proximal interphalangeal joint is extended and extending the distal interphalangeal joint as its tension increases. The volar capsular structures resemble one another in providing attachment for the third and fifth annular pulleys and in providing a subsheath approach for vincular feeder vessels (Fig. 15–7). Both volar plates are suspended from the phalangeal condyles by the accessory collateral ligaments. These collateral, or suspensory, ligaments are quite distinct from the proper collateral ligaments, although their condylar origin is coextensive.

Collateral Ligament-Condylar Relationships

A final anatomic comment deals with the lateral volar flares of the condyles at the interphalangeal joints. At the *metacarpo*phalangeal joint, the collateral ligament's origin is eccentric with regard to the curvature of the articular surface. Thus, it tightens as rotation occurs around the increased radius of the volar curve. Lateral stability is present in flexion, but sufficient laxity for rotational and lateral movements is available in extension. The lateral volar flares or bulges of the phalangeal condyles at the interphalangeal joints serve the same purpose (see Fig. 15–2). In full extension, the joint is stabilized by the combined *accessory* collateral ligament-volar plate confluence that cups the lateral condylar flare tightly, providing a taut volar half of

Figure 15–7. The entire two-joint volar plate-collateral ligament-tendon sheath relationship.

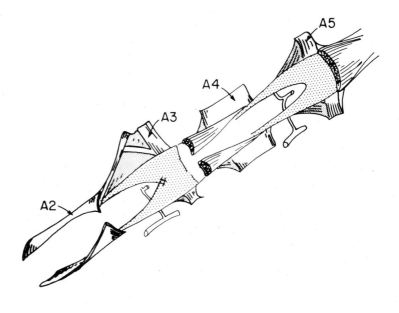

the capsule much as the posterior capsule of the knee provides lateral stability at the joint in full extension. As flexion begins, lateral instability is immediately noted. The position of most instability (i.e., most capsular laxity) is from 30 to 60° of flexion. This is an arc when neither the accessory collateral ligament-volar plate complex nor the collateral ligaments are taut. It is not surprising that this arc of motion is the *last* to be lost as a traumatic joint becomes stiff. The joint again becomes stable to lateral stress at about 80°, at which point the collateral ligaments are tightened by the *lateral* flares of the phalangeal condyles.

MANAGEMENT OF CAPSULAR INJURY

The natural history of capsular injury has been shown in Figure 15–1. Table 15–1 presents complications of injuries to specific structures in the proximal and distal interphalangeal (PIP; DIP) joints. The second column refers to the usually named components of the interphalangeal joint capsules. Each structure's presumed function is listed in the third column, and the fourth and fifth columns list *functional* complications if the structure either heals with laxity (instability) or with excessive scarring (contracture).

Table 15–1. COMPLICATIONS OF SPECIFIC STRUCTURAL INJURIES

Joint(s) Involved	Structure	Function	Impairment	
			Chronic Contracture	*Chronic Instability*
Proximal Interphalangeal Joint	Radial (ulnar) collateral ligament	Resists lateral displacement in pinch and grip functions; provides stable linkage for force transmission across joint	Extension contracture (limited flexion)	Lateral instability in pinch, grip; asymmetric tracking (deformity with muscle-generated forces, leading to arthrosis)
	Volar plate	Provides static resistance to hyperextension; increases moment arm of flexors; stabilizes joint to lateral stress in full extension	Flexion contracture (limited extension); occurs rarely as a result of *primary* volar plate injury—secondary contracture is more common	Hyperextension habitus of joint (swan-neck); locking in hyperextension; recurrent dorsal dislocation; extension contracture
	Accessory collateral ligament	Works with volar plate to stabilize joint to lateral stress in full extension	Flexion contracture (limited extension)	?
	Oblique retinacular ligament of Landsmeer	?	Flexion contracture (limited extension)	?
Distal Interphalangeal Joint	Oblique retinacular ligament of Landsmeer	Extends DIP joint by static link as PIP joint	Extension contracture (loss of flexion)	?
	Radial (ulnar) collateral ligament	Resists lateral displacement in pinch and grip functions; provides stable linkage for force transmission across joint	Extension contracture	Lateral instability in pinch, grip; asymmetric tracking (deformity) with muscle generated forces leading to arthrosis
	Volar plate	Static resistance to hypertension; increases moment arm of flexors; stabilizes joint to lateral stress in full extension	Flexion contracture	Rare hyperextension or dorsal subluxation because strong protection is offered by flexor digitorum profundus
Both	Dorsal capsule	Blends intimately with central slip (PIP joint) and extensor digitorum communis (DIP joint)	Extension contracture	Usually associated with tendon rupture at PIP joint (central slip) and DIP joint (mallet finger)

Acute Capsular Injury

The rationale for management of digital ligament injury is theoretically simple. In practice, however, inattention to details, short cuts, treatment modifications, and judgment error produce unsatisfactory results all too frequently. Some principles that I have found helpful follow:

As in all physician-managed injuries, an explanation—in advance—of the recovery process is in order. Persistent joint swelling and slow recovery of the extremes of motion are predictable consequences of this injury. It is well to suggest a period of 4 to 6 months as a reasonable time that must elapse before patient or physician judge an end result, even when all goes well.

Sprains

Ligament injuries without loss of stability are to be diagnosed as quickly as possible. The goal of treatment is a quick return to function by protection for comfort and supervised motion as soon as possible thereafter. Unnecessary immobilization may produce the complication of prolonged contracture. The joint *will* have reduced motion for a variable period of time, and will thus be subject to reinjury. Failure to protect the partial rupture adequately may allow a subsequent trivial injury to complete the rupture, which may then go undiagnosed. At the very least, reinjury adds significantly to the total insult and will prolong the recovery. Buddy taping to an adjacent finger is admirably suited to this task.

Ligament Disruption

Diagnosis. *Ensure by sufficient diagnostic effort that the correct diagnosis is known.* The overriding consideration is stability, and its loss must be ascertained early. Clues are everywhere: the history of displacement, the fleck of bone where ligament or volar plate attach, comparative stress testing of joint structures with or without digital block anesthesia, the asymmetry of articular relationships on injury and, particularly, postreduction roentgenograms, stress roentgenograms, and arthrography. One must pursue the diagnosis until certainty exists about which structures are disrupted.

Attaining Normal Stability. When stability is lost the *treatment plan must provide the potential for reestablishment of normal stability.* This may take the form of splinting so that the injured structures are firmly in contact, or surgical exploration, if necessary, to achieve the same result.

I use two tests to help decide on the need for adding the insult of surgery to the insult of injury. The first is that of articular congruity. Inability to achieve a gross reduction of joint displacement is a primary indication for open reduction. If a closed reduction is thought to be obtained, however, the post-reduction roentgenogram must be examined in true anteroposterior and true lateral projections for perfect congruity. The lack of this essential element is an indication that something more must be done (perhaps surgery) before splinting is begun. The second test is that of unprovoked instability. The injured digit, if not examined and reduced immediately after injury, will often require digital block anesthesia for this test. After reduction the patient is asked to carry the digit through a full range of motion. If the digit tracks asymmetrically, deforms, or the reduction is lost, severe capsular disruption or structural interposition exists, and surgical exploration is indicated. A further clue that the potential for reestablishment of normal stability is lacking is the presence of widely displaced articular marginal fragments on the post-reduction roentgenograms. This is a relative indication for surgery, and judgment must be exercised.

Protection and Mobilization. Once the diagnosis of instability has been made and the potential for its reestablishment is assured, the *capsular ligament must be protected long enough to allow it to resume its stabilizing function.* However, the *joint must be mobilized early enough to avoid prolonged or permanent loss of motion* due to immobilization, scarring, or both. Here, opinion varies considerably. Some advise 2, 3, or even 5 weeks of immobilization followed by protected motion. Most agree that unprotected motion can be safely begun at 6 weeks. The choice can be simplified by considering the reliability of protected motion. In complete PIP volar plate disruption, stability can usually be ensured by well-applied and supervised extension block splinting for 2 to 3 weeks, and buddy taping for the remainder of the 6-week period. At the DIP, buddy taping is not applicable, and splinting should be more complete and for a longer period of time. In complete collateral ligament injuries there is usually dorsal or volar capsular injury as well. If motion is begun earlier than 3 weeks, frequent reassessment of articular congruity must be made to ensure that articular surface incongruity does *not* develop.

The use of buddy taping early in collateral ligament injuries has a theoretical problem in that joints of adjacent digits lie at different levels. The injured digit, forced to track in tandem with its neighbor, may undergo undesirable rotational forces that could influence the ultimate stability of these ligaments with their associated hemicapsular disruption. An alternative is the "controlled passive motion" technique of Duran and Houser, modified to become "controlled active motion" for digital hemicapsular disruptions.[5]

I favor immobilization of complete collateral ligament ruptures, surgically repaired or not, by immobilization for 3 weeks. The digit is then splinted statically for an additional 3 weeks during which time, under supervision, active motion of the isolated joint is begun. A reliable patient can perform this at home. At 6 weeks unprotected motion is allowed.

General Comments

The various combinations of multiple capsular structure disruption are limited to the varieties of dislocations—dorsal, lateral, or volar (in order of frequency). The indications for surgery do not change from those noted above, nor do the principles of intelligent postinjury management. Of note in the rather rare volar dislocation at the PIP joint is the often associated central slip rupture. This must be recognized, if present. Treatment may either be by splinting or surgery. The complication of boutonnière eventuates if the injury goes unrecognized.

A further comment regards PIP and DIP joint collateral ligament injuries. These structures are small, short, thick, and strong, with highly specialized attachments to both phalanges. When ruptured by avulsion fracture, the ligament can often be restored adequately because the ligament structure itself is intact. If ruptured within the substance of the ligament, a small, short, thick, highly specialized structure becomes two or more swollen sources of scar. The swelling and softening that go with the inflammatory response, and the contracture that accompanies scar maturation, render it impossible to repair the collateral ligaments *at these two joints* such that the resultant structure will be predictably normal in length, strength, or function. I thus recommend that, when necessary either to reduce a joint displacement openly or to remove an interposed ligament, surgical trauma be minimized. Collateral ligament repair should be limited to approximation of the fragments. This should be done with as few small sutures as are consistent with maintaining position until the immobilizing techniques are in place. The injury is then managed as the instability demands. This approach is consistent with all known mechanisms of healing, and avoids the additional surgical insult of certain modalities, such as drill holes, nonabsorbable sutures, and wires.

Chronic Capsular Derangements

Chronic Capsular Contracture

The management of contracture in the stable congruous joint is nonoperative early in the postinjury period (less than 8 months). I favor the use of serial casting and active motion with alternating static splints in the extremes of motion. When the joint is no longer inflamed, the technique of joint mobilization is to be preferred to dynamic splinting.[6] Wedging forces in these small joints are mentioned only to be condemned. The former technique avoids the undesirable joint compression forces and splint management problems of the latter, but requires a skilled hand therapist. Contractures that do not respond to this program are usually old (greater than 8 months) or have undiagnosed components of incongruity or capsular instability. These are best managed by joint reconstruction, replacement, or both.

When a stable joint fails to respond to nonoperative measures and the obligatory wait for the joint structures to return to a stable metabolic state has elapsed (6 to 8 months after injury), operative release of the contracture can be considered. Excellent approaches to this technique have been published, typified by the methodical approach of Curtis.[7] One must remember that all satisfactory techniques call for the recreation of capsular instability, again requiring careful postoperative supervision. Extensive contractures require collateral ligament release or excision, and flexion contractures generally require accessory collateral ligament excision and volar plate release at the proximal attachments. In both cases, flexor and extensor tenodesis must be considered as part of the contracture until proven otherwise.

Chronic Joint Capsular Instability

The management of late instability is usually operative. There is little evidence that closed management can successfully restore stability or congruity unless one is willing to accept the inevitability of loss of motion. This may be an acceptable compromise in the DIP joint, thumb metacarpophalangeal joint, and, under certain circumstances, in the index PIP joint.

The operative management of chronic volar plate instability is generally successful.[8] This is not surprising when one considers that the static stabilizing function of this structure is operative only in full extension and is augmented by the dynamic forces of both flexor tendons. The collateral ligaments are not reinforced by other structures. They must move freely over the condyles while offering symmetric stability to the deforming forces of motion throughout the arc. In addition, the proper collateral ligaments must provide static resistance to deforming forces generated in grip and pinch.

There are several methods for the restoration of the chronically lax collateral ligament.[9-12] To achieve stability at no expense to motion, the eccentric origin and insertion of the collateral ligament must be reproduced. The tension of the repair must be such that, at the end point of collagen maturation, the new ligament is long enough to allow its excursion over the lateral volar flare of the phalangeal condyle in flexion yet tight enough to provide midrange (30 to 60°) stability. Here, perhaps, one can consider tradeoffs. In the ulnar side digits, collateral ligament repair must allow full motion or power grip will be diminished. The tension thus should be set with the joint in 90° of flexion. In the radial side digits, stability is the prime requirement, and tension should be adjusted in the range in which the joint is normally most unstable (the 30 to 60° range).

Final Comment

If you arrive at this point and realize that you have not been told how to manage—in a stepwise fashion—any specific injury to a complication-free end result, my aim will have been partially accomplished. The task will be completed if you now read with the intent to think about principles, not methods. It is indeed rare that a significant digital ligament injury does not, during its management, perplex the thinking surgeon and therapist. More work must be done before a cookbook can be written.

References

 1. Eaton, R. G.: Joint Injuries of the Hand, Springfield, IL, Charles C Thomas, 1971.
 2. Bowers, W. H., et al.: The proximal interphalangeal joint volar plate. I. An anatomical and biomechanical study. J. Hand Surg., 5:79, 1980.
 3. Landsmeer, J. M. F.: Atlas of Anatomy of the Hand, Edinburgh, Churchill-Livingstone, 1976, pp. 189–199, 239–249.
 4. Landsmeer, J. M. F.: The proximal interphalangeal joint. Hand, 7:30, 1975.
 5. Duran, R. J., and Houser, R. G.: Controlled passive motion following flexor tendon repair in zones 2 and 3. In A.A.O.S. Symposium on Tendon Surgery in the Hand, St. Louis, C. V. Mosby, 1975, pp. 105–114.
 6. Maitland, G. D.: Peripheral Manipulation, 2nd ed., Boston, Butterworth, 1977, pp. 187–197.
 7. Curtis, R. M.: Capsulectomy of the interphalangeal joints of the fingers. J. Bone Joint Surg., 36A:1219, 1954.
 8. Bowers, W. H.: The proximal interphalangeal joint volar plate. II. A clinical study of hyperextension injury. J. Hand Surg., 6:77, 1981.
 9. Lane, C. S.: Reconstruction of the unstable proximal interphalangeal joint: The double superficialis tenodesis. J. Hand Surg., 3:368, 1978.
10. Palmer, A. K., and Linschied, R.: Chronic recurrent dislocation of the proximal interphalangeal joint of the finger. J. Hand Surg., 3:95, 1978.
11. McCue, F. C., et al.: Athletic injuries of the proximal interphalangeal joint requiring surgical treatment. J. Bone Joint Surg., 52A:937, 1970.
12. Redlar, I., and Williams, J. T.: Rupture of a collateral ligament of the proximal interphalangeal joint of the fingers. J. Bone Joint Surg., 49A:322, 1967.

16

COMPLICATIONS OF FRACTURES, DISLOCATIONS, AND LIGAMENTOUS INJURIES OF THE WRIST

Julio Taleisnik

FRACTURES OF THE DISTAL RADIUS AND ULNA

"Learn to see in another's calamity the ills which you should avoid." Syrus Publilius, 42 B.C. Maxim 120.

In spite of the benign reputation of fractures of the distal radius, the injury itself or its treatment may result in significant residual disability. In a study of 2132 Colles' fractures by the physicians of the Workmen's Compensation Board of the New York State Department of Labor, only 62, or 2.9%, were considered to have no permanent loss of function.[10] In most series the complication rate varies between 20 and 25%[68] to 31%.[39, 68, 71] Compli-

cations may be due to the injury itself or may be the result of its treatment, and can occur early or late in the course of treatment. Early complications take place within the initial few weeks following injury, when consolidation is not firm enough to preclude reduction by manipulation or by surgical means.[54] Late complications are those present after the fracture has healed.

Depending on the structure(s) involved, complications may be osseous, articular, neurologic, tendinous or vascular (Table 16–1). The significant factors in obtaining a satisfactory end result are numerous; three are most important: accurate reduction, adequate immobilization, and early and persistent active use of all parts not involved by the

Table 16–1. COMPLICATIONS OF FRACTURES OF DISTAL RADIUS AND ULNA

Structure	Early	Late
Bones	Inadequate reduction Inadequate immobilization Associated injuries (carpus, forearm, elbow)	Malunion Nonunion
Joints	Carpal ligamentous injury Radioulnar Radiocarpal	Carpal instability (RC, MC) Radioulnar RC arthrosis Fingers
Nerves	Contusion Entrapment } Immediate or Compression } early secondary	Carpal tunnel syndrome Guyon canal syndrome
Tendons	Entrapment	Rupture
Vascular	RSD early Intrinsic contracture, early	RSD late Intrinsic contracture late

injury or constrained by immobilization.[10] Significant also are the control of edema and relief of pain to allow the patient comfortable use of the extremity. An accurate evaluation of the nature and extent of the initial injury are also important, because although undisplaced extra-articular fractures are expected to do well, they may result in unexpected, at times significant, disability. Conversely, a poor anatomic result may coexist with very satisfactory function, a characteristic almost unique to these

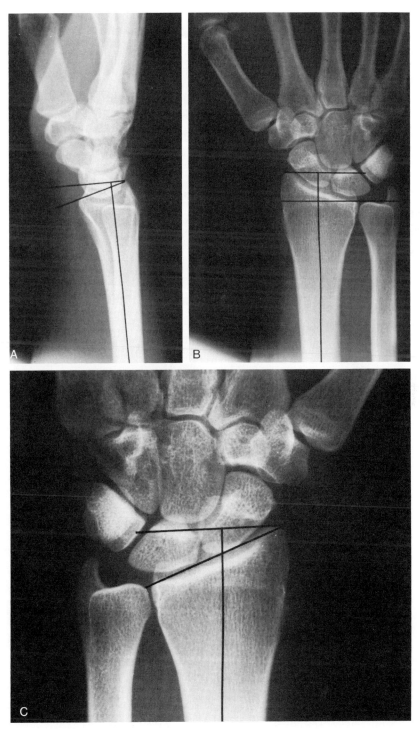

Figure 16–1. Measurements of normal volar tilt *(A),* radial length *(B),* and inclination *(C).*

Table 16–2. CLASSIFICATION OF COLLES' FRACTURES (FRYKMAN)*

| | Distal Ulnar Fracture | |
	Absent	Present
Extra-articular	I	II
Intra-articular (RC)	III	IV
Intra-articular (RU)	V	VI
Intra-articular (RC + RU)	VII	VII

*Modified from Dobyns, J. H., and Linscheid, R. L.: Fractures and dislocations of the wrist. *In* Rockwood, C. A., Jr., and Green, D. P. (eds.): Fractures, Philadelphia, J. B. Lippincott, 1975.

fractures, and attributed by Gartland and Werley to "the innate ability of the wrist joint to overcome and compensate for residual bony deformity."[30, 68, 71, 124, 177] Although a perfect anatomic result cannot be taken as a guarantee of good function, there is agreement that, in accordance with sound orthopedic principles, a better anatomic restoration will most likely result in a more satisfactory function.[3, 10, 68, 76, 172]

Frykman's classification (Table 16–2) has prognostic value in that those fractures in the higher groups are more likely to develop complications. In a review of 565 fractures seen at the Mayo Clinic there were 177 complications, of which 69 developed in Frykman's groups VII and VIII.[39] This was also Frykman's experience: intraarticular fractures, particularly if including the distal radioulnar joint, or if penetrating the radiocarpal joint with simultaneous fractures of the distal ulna, had less favorable prognosis.

The following discussion of complications of fractures of the distal radius and ulna will be limited to those problems arising directly as a consequence of the fracture or its management, excluding complications common to the treatment of other orthopedic conditions (*e.g.,* postoperative infections, infections in open injuries, soft tissue loss accompanying open fractures). No attempt will be made to separate complications secondary to Colles'-type fractures from those following Barton's or Smith's varieties. In my opinion, complications following different types of fractures of the distal radius are similar and subject to management that is dictated by the complication, rather than by the original fracture.

Radiographic Evaluation: The Normal Wrist

Three anatomic radiographic parameters are important in evaluating radioulnocarpal relationships: volar tilt, radial inclination or angulation, and radial length (Fig. 16–1).[58, 71] *Volar tilt* is determined in lateral radiographs, and is measured as the angle between a line perpendicular to the long axis of the radius and a line tangential to the plane of the distal articular surface of the radius. The tilt is 0° when this articular surface is perpendicular to the long

axis of the shaft of the radius. The normal volar tilt is given a + sign and averages +11° in most series, although it may be as low as −7° and as high as +28°.[49, 58, 71, 76, 108, 169, 172] *Radial inclination* is represented by the angle between a line perpendicular to the long axis of the radius and a line tangential to the distal articular surface of the radius in posteroanterior roentgenograms. It averages 22°, but may be as low as 12° or as high as 30°.[49, 71, 76, 108, 169, 172] *Radial length* is the distance in millimeters between two lines parallel to each other, traced at the tip of the radial styloid and along the head (not the styloid) of the ulna; it averages 9 mm.[169]

Osteoarticular Complications

For most patients, closed reduction of fractures of the distal radius followed by immobilization in plaster are sufficient. Usually, these fractures reduce easily and can be maintained in some volar flexion and ulnar deviation, with the forearm pronated. If excessive force is required in pronounced volar flexion, other positions may be tried. Frequently, reduction in supination and ulnar deviation is successful.[169, 170] Smith's fractures are probably best treated by reduction and by immobilization in supination.[207] When maintenance of reduction requires non-physiologic volar flexion, ulnar deviation, or both, finger function is potentially compromised,

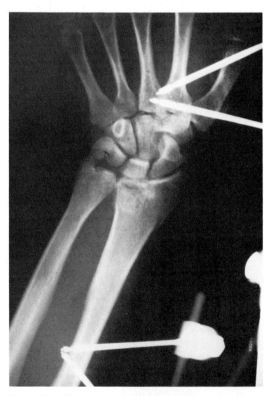

Figure 16–2. Comminuted fracture of distal radius treated with external fixation. (Courtesy of Dr. B. A. Ewald.)

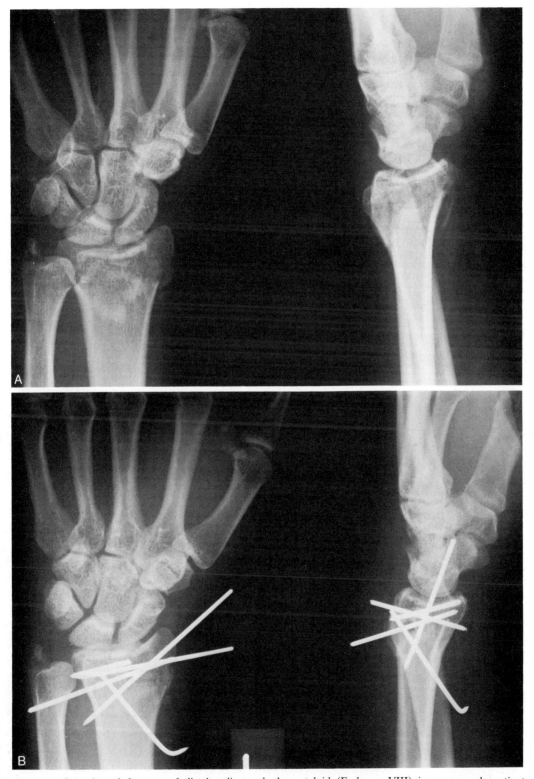

Figure 16–3. Comminuted fracture of distal radius and ulnar styloid (Frykman VIII) in young male patient. *A,* Preoperative radiographs; *B,* Treatment by open reduction and internal fixation with multiple Kirschner wires.

and the danger of entrapment of the median nerve in the carpal tunnel increases. For this reason, and exclusively in the elderly, one may infrequently elect to forego anatomic restoration for the sake of maintenance of hand and shoulder function. In most cases, however, if the initial manipulation is not satisfactory, or extreme positions are needed to maintain reduction, and in comminuted intra-articular and very unstable fractures, as well as in the presence of extensive soft tissue injury, external or internal fixation must be considered (Figs. 16–2 and 16–3). The stability of a fracture of the distal radius is always suspect when there is comminution of the volar cortex. This is usually the buttress on which a successful manipulation can be performed.

Opinions are divided as to which of the normal radiographic parameters is most important to correct for a satisfactory restoration of function. Some authors believe that the volar tilt is most important.[3, 55, 58, 71, 118] Others favor restoration of radial inclination and length, or of all three parameters.[10, 28, 30, 64, 79, 83, 93, 124, 216] Fernandez observed that deformities became symptomatic when there was angulation of 25 or 30° in *either plane,* or with a loss of radial length greater than 6 mm, particularly in the younger, more active patients.[64]

In Dowling and Sawyer's experience, no one anatomic characteristic was obviously associated with good or poor function; there was no correlation except in the extremely good or extremely bad

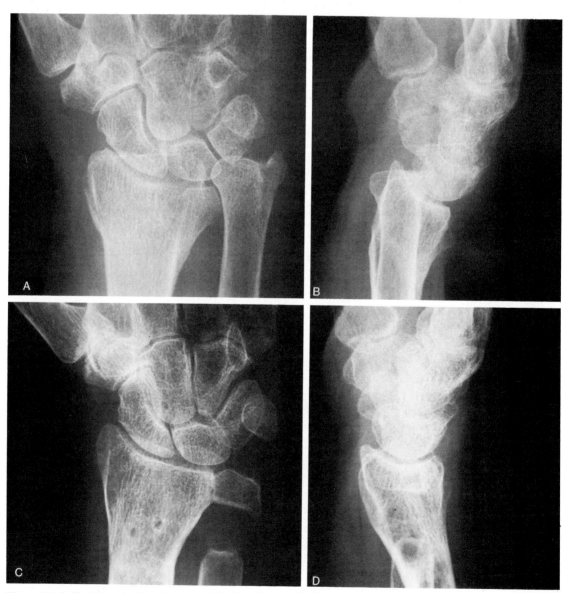

Figure 16–4. Healed malunited fracture of distal radius. *A,* Radioulnar dislocation, with loss of radial height and inclination; *B,* reversed palmar tilt, dorsal radiocarpal instability; *C,* postoperative PA radiograph after osteotomy of distal radius, bone grafting, and Lauenstein procedure of distal ulna; *D,* postoperative lateral view shows residual negative palmar tilt, but radiocarpal stability has been restored.

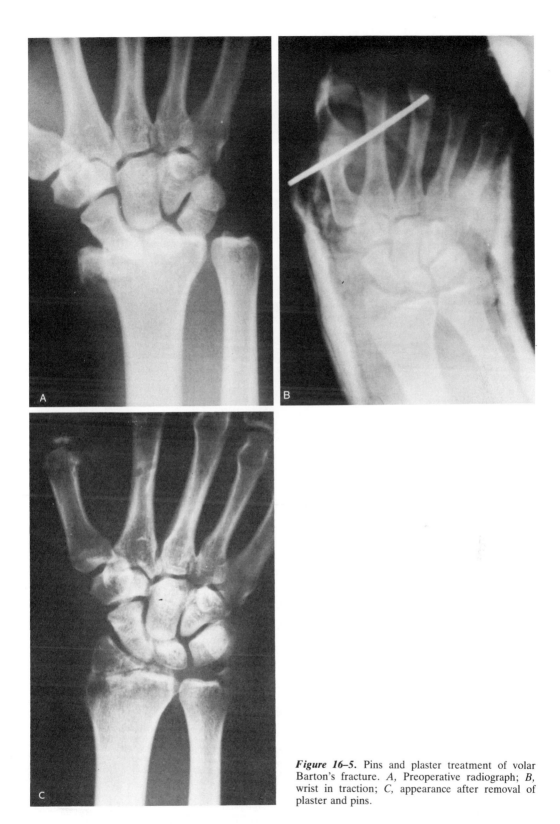

Figure 16–5. Pins and plaster treatment of volar Barton's fracture. *A,* Preoperative radiograph; *B,* wrist in traction; *C,* appearance after removal of plaster and pins.

results although, in general, in the excellent recovery, either the volar tilt had been better restored, or, if any single anatomic element was poorly corrected, the other two tended to be average or above average.[58] Therefore, it is apparent that anatomic

restoration must be attempted, particularly in the young and vigorous patients, because residual loss of volar tilt may interfere with carpal function, changes in radial inclination and length could result in radioulnar derangement, and a combination of all three could contribute to disturb the function of the musculotendinous units crossing the wrist (Fig. 16–4).

When internal or external fixation is needed, the selection of the procedure will vary with the nature of the fracture and according to the operator's experience; external fixators (Roger Anderson, Hoffman, Ace-Colles (see Fig. 16–2), pins and plaster, percutaneous pinning, screws and plates, and Rush rods, may be used (Figs. 16–5 to 16–8).[5, 15, 33, 38, 40, 49, 58, 67, 79, 83, 84, 88, 103, 118, 121, 123, 148, 159, 160, 172, 178, 185, 191] Internal or external fixation may cause additional complications, however. Some are similar to complications arising from the operative intervention of any fractures (*e.g.*, infections); some are specific to the wrist, particularly damage or irritation to the cutaneous branches of the radial nerve.[113] After the fracture has consolidated with persistent, unsightly, and disabling angulation, it may be corrected by an open wedge osteotomy with a pyramidal bone graft obtained from the distal ulna or iliac crest (see Fig. 16–4).[26, 64]

Associated osteoarticular injuries other than involvement of the radiocarpal and radioulnar joints are relatively infrequent. Usually the examiner's attention is drawn to the obvious deformity of the

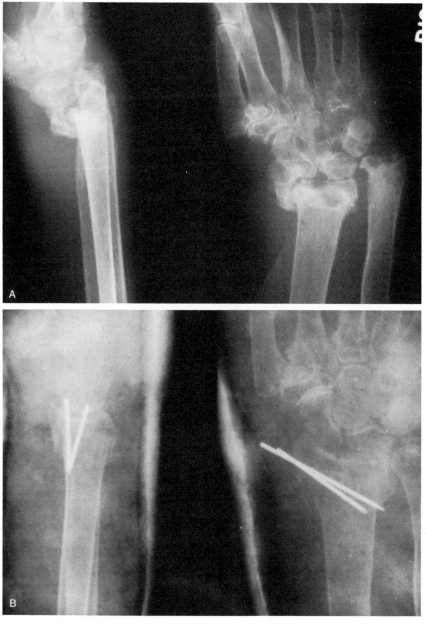

Figure 16–6. Comminuted volar Barton-type fracture. *A*, Preoperative radiographs; *B*, appearance after reduction and blind pinning.

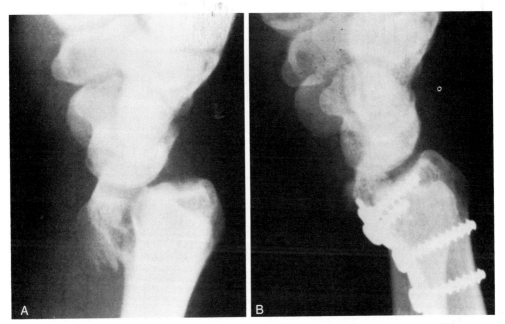

Figure 16–7. Volar Barton's fracture *(A)* treated by operative reduction and plating *(B)*.

wrist. Therefore, less obvious lesions to the elbow, carpus, or hand may be overlooked (Fig. 16–9). It is sound orthopedic practice to examine the joints proximal and distal to the wrist, radiographically if necessary, for fractures, subluxations or dislocations of the elbow, particularly the head or neck of the radius, or of the carpus, especially the scaphoid.

Fractures involving the radiocarpal joint, with disruption of the joint anatomy, should be aggressively treated. Restoration of the articular surfaces is mandatory, particularly in the young individuals. This is best accomplished by direct visualization of the joint and internal fixation with pins, screws, or plates, according to the type of fracture and the operator's experience (see Figs. 16–3 and 16–7). When arthrosis develops as a late complication and is strictly limited to the radiocarpal space, it may be treated using partial arthroplasties, limited arthrodesis, or a combination of both. A fusion incorporating the distal radius, the scaphoid, and the lunate is useful to eliminate painful function, while at the same time preserving the midcarpal joints that have remained uninvolved for a residual and limited but useful and stable range of motion (Fig. 16–10). As for all limited arthrodesis, outside configuration and dimensions of the portion of the wrist to be fused should be preserved to avoid mechanical interference with the neighboring uninvolved carpal joints that are left free to move.[220, 221]

Most associated skeletal injuries disturb the radioulnar relationship.[55] This may be due to an obvious fracture (of the ulnar styloid, head, or neck of the ulna or, less frequently, the ulnar shaft) or to a more subtle injury to the radioulnar support, allowing dorsal (or, less often, palmar) subluxation or dislocation of the head of the ulna.

After the fracture of the radius has been reduced, it is imperative to spend a few minutes assessing the radioulnar relationship. This is usually best done by direct palpation of the radioulnar area; radiographs may help, although in the subtle instabilities these may appear entirely normal. This is the type of injury that is extremely easy to miss and is bound to sublux completely or dislocate dorsally during a period of immobilization in a cast that is usually applied in pronation (Fig. 16–11). If there is any question as to the stability of the radioulnar support, the ulna should be reduced against the distal radius, and a transverse Kirschner wire used for fixation. Early or late posttraumatic involvement of the distal radioulnar joint is a frequent cause of pain, particularly during forearm rotation.

In spite of the early disability and the radiographic changes involving the distal radioulnar joint, many of these patients, particularly the elderly, will progress to a satisfactory level of function if treated conservatively (Fig. 16–12). Initially, intermittent splinting, a gradual exercise program, local injections of steroid preparations, and systemic medications, as needed, are helpful. Except for gross disruptions and for the very active younger patients, it is usually advantageous to postpone surgical treatment for posttraumatic osteoarthritis of the distal radioulnar joint for at least 6 months, preferably longer. When symptoms persist, or when they are creating a continuous disability, several surgical procedures are available for their treatment: excision of the distal ulna, distal ulnar implants, radioulnar fusion with ulnar osteotomy (the Lauenstein procedure), and osteotomy of the ulna with (Milch) or without (Baldwin) restoration of ulnar continuity (Figs. 16–13 and 16–14).[4, 7, 13, 14, 18, 45–48, 53, 77, 87, 131–133, 197, 208]

Text continued on page 166

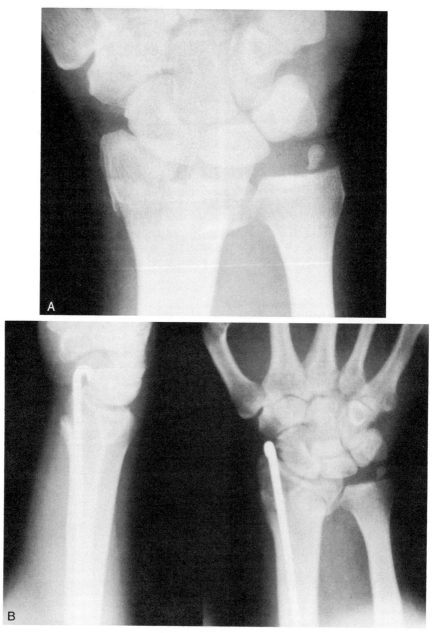

Figure 16–8. *A,* Frykman type VIII fracture of distal radius; *B,* treatment by reduction and manipulation in traction, and fixation with a single Rush rod.

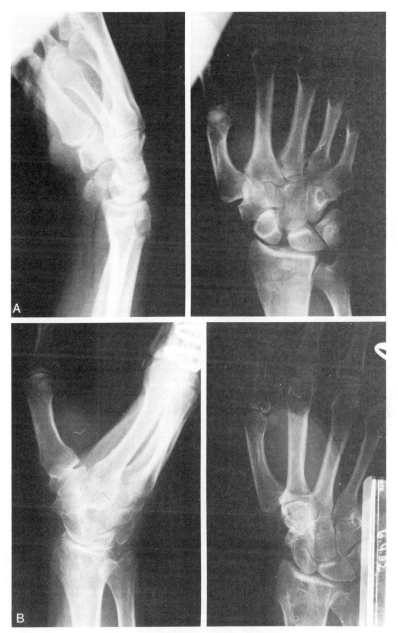

Figure 16–9. *A,* Fracture of distal radius—there is a rotatory subluxation of the scaphoid, missed initially; *B,* persistent subluxation of the scaphoid later treated by fusion between scaphoid, trapezium and trapezoid.

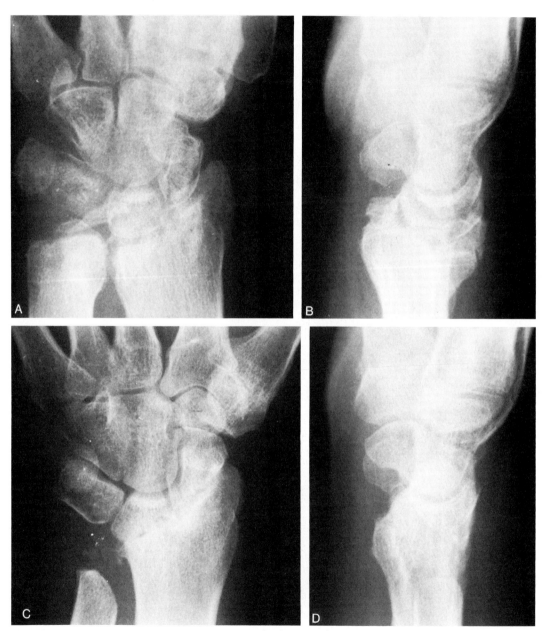

Figure 16–10. A, B, Neglected, unreduced, comminuted intra-articular fracture of distal radius; C, D, after radioscapho-lunate fusion and excision of distal ulna.

Figure 16–11. Dorsal subluxation of distal ulna, noticed after essentially undisplaced fracture of distal radius had healed.

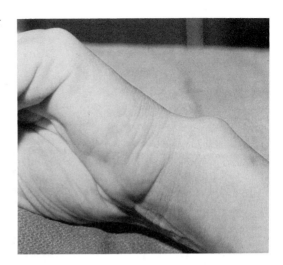

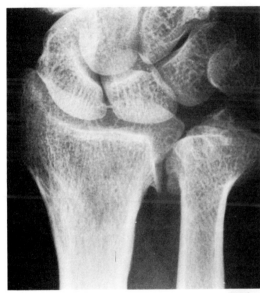

Figure 16–12. Osteoarthritis of distal radioulnar joint.

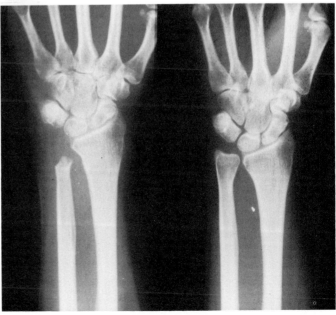

Figure 16–13. Excision of distal ulna for painful distal radioulnar joint (Darrach procedure).

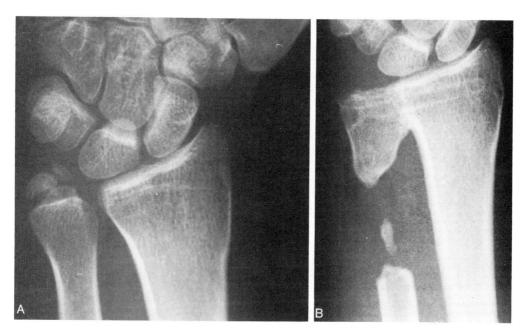

Figure 16–14. Preoperative *(A)* and postoperative *(B)* radiographs of painful distal radioulnar joint treated by radioulnar fusion and by osteotomy of distal ulna (Lauenstein procedure).

Late osteoarthritis involving the distal radioulnar joint is more frequent than radiocarpal osteoarthritis.[39]

Carpal instability as a late complication must be kept in mind. In 1972, Linscheid and colleagues described loss of carpal alignment of proximal or distal carpal rows following malunion of fractures of the distal radius.[114] Dorsal or volar radiocarpal subluxations or secondary instability at the midcarpal level may occur.[114, 200] These forms of instability are best treated by corrective osteotomy of the distal radius (Fig. 16–15). Ligamentous disruption causing rotatory subluxation of the scaphoid may occur (see Fig. 16–9).[39] It is important to distinguish true isolated rotatory subluxation of the scaphoid accompanying fracture of the distal radius from scapholunate dissociations that may be part of a larger injury complex, in which the fracture of the radius enters the radiocarpal joint space between the scaphoid and lunate fossae of the distal radius, allowing the fragment bearing the scaphoid facet to migrate away from that related to the lunate (Fig. 16–16). This may represent a reduced or incomplete form of transstyloid perilunate fracture-dislocation.

Nonunions of fractures of the distal radius are exceedingly rare, even in the presence of comminution. Severe osteoporosis, in addition to comminution, may need to be present for nonunions to develop. This rare complication requires treatment by bone grafting and internal fixation. Because of the disruption of the distal radioulnar joint alignment that uniformly accompanies nonunion, treatment of the distal radioulnar joint by a Lauenstein or Darrach procedure may be done at the same time, allowing for better opposition of radial fragments and for the use of the bone excised from the ulna as a graft (Fig. 16–17).

Neurological Complications

Fractures of the distal radius are a leading cause of acute carpal tunnel syndromes.[1, 11, 119, 129, 186] In 1933, Abbot and Saunders proposed a classification of median nerve injuries accompanying fractures of the distal radius into four groups: (1) *primary injuries,* which are immediately apparent at the time of the fracture; (2) *secondary injuries,* which follow partial or unstable reductions and malunions; (3) *delayed injuries,* which are present months or at times years after the fracture has healed; and (4) *injuries accompanying forced manipulative reduction and immobilization in pronounced flexion and ulnar deviation.*[1] If the onset of symptoms is immediate, a direct injury, by contusion or entrapment, should be suspected. Cooney and collaborators cautioned against the use of excessive force for the manipulation of these fractures.[39] In their series the inci-

Figure 16–15. Dorsal carpal instability (DISI) secondary to malunited fracture of distal radius. *A,* Zigzag alignment; *B,* Postoperative appearance following dorsal open wedge osteotomy of distal radius, bone grafting, and internal fixation.

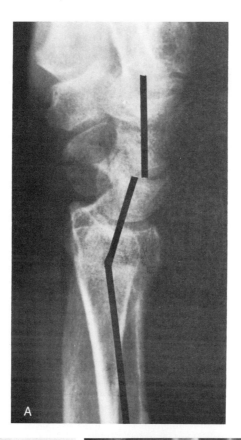

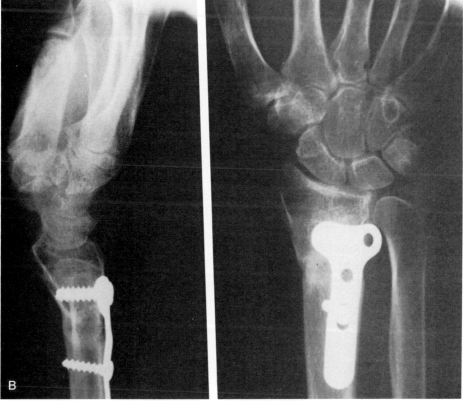

Figure 16–15. See legend on opposite page.

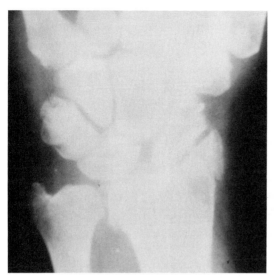

Figure 16–16. Distal radial fracture with depressed scaphoid facet and scapholunate dissociation, which may represent a reduced or incomplete transstyloid perilunate fracture-dislocation.

dence of median neuropathies was lower when appropriate relaxation was obtained with brachial or general anesthesia, suggesting that the force used for reduction under local anesthesia alone may have been a contributing factor to the nerve injury.

A persistent immediate loss of nerve function is extremely rare. Actually, most symptoms of nerve involvement will diminish after the fracture has been reduced.[68] Rather than the presence of symptoms,

it is their progress after reduction and their degree that is important. Most compression neuropathies appear more gradually and somewhat later, and are secondary to edema, hemorrhage, bony fragments, or bony deformity within the carpal canal exerting unacceptable pressures on the nerve and on its blood supply. A wick catheter has been used, inserted within the carpal tunnel, to quantitate these pressures and to aid in distinguishing median neuropathies due to nerve contusion from those due to compression.[11] The distinction is largely academic, however, because in most emergency situations the decision to proceed with a surgical exploration of the nerve is a matter of clinical judgment. In many instances, when swelling is present, immobilization with a sugar tong or a thumbhole splint is preferable, at least until the initial edema has subsided.

There is a direct relationship between median nerve compression at the carpal tunnel and the attitude of the wrist within the cast, in particular the so-called Cotton-Loder position.[1, 119] When the symptoms of nerve compression are mild, a release of constricting bandages, or a modification of the position of immobilization with control of edema and at times the injection of a steroid preparation into the carpal tunnel, may suffice.[119] An operative intervention should be considered when symptoms, particularly burning pain, are severe and persist, or worsen, even after cast modification and release of circular constrictions. The rapid onset of motor deficit is a clear-cut indication of nerve distress and should prompt immediate release of the nerve. Maintenance of reduction should not be a deterrent to surgery. If loss of alignment occurs, the fracture

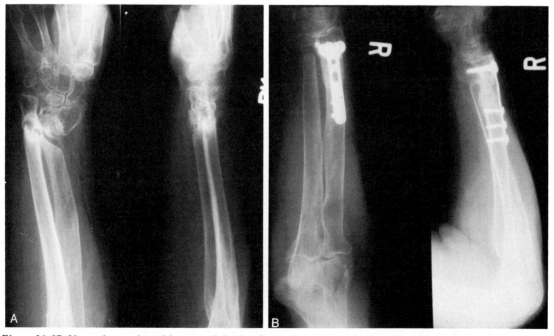

Figure 16–17. Unusual nonunion of fracture of distal radius and ulna *(A)* treated by bone graft and internal fixation of the radius and by a Lauenstein procedure for the distal ulna *(B)*.

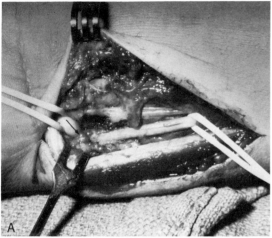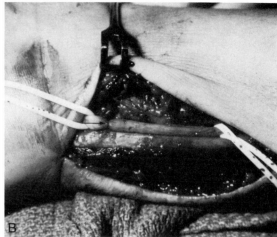

Figure 16–18. Ulnar nerve compression accompanying fracture of distal radius and ulna in a 14-year-old patient. *A,* Fibrous band across ulnar nerve *(arrow); (B),* crease remains in nerve after its release *(arrow).*

should be stabilized by some means of internal fixation at the time of exploration of the nerve; in the long run this will facilitate the management of the fracture while the nerve is allowed to recover.

The ulnar nerve is involved much less frequently in fractures of the distal radius alone.[17, 173, 228] It should be anticipated in some young patients with fractures of the distal ulna with severe angulation or displacement, particularly if accompanied by puckering of the skin at the site of deformity (Fig. 16–18). Simultaneous lesions to median and ulnar nerves are extremely rare.[52, 175, 214] The radial nerve is exceptionally involved by the fracture itself but may be injured in the course of treatment.[113]

Compression neuropathies of later onset are treated by surgical release of the carpal tunnel or the canal of Guyon. If a fracture has healed with residual angulation, this may need correction by a suitable osteotomy for the lasting relief of a nerve compression syndrome.[17]

Complications Involving Tendons

Tendon entrapments involve most usually the extensor pollicis longus, and are rare.[95, 141, 174] Inability to reduce a fracture of the distal radius should suggest soft tissue or tendon interposition.[174] Other tendon problems are usually of late onset. Rupture of the extensor pollicis longus is by far the most frequent complication involving a tendon (Fig. 16–19).[24, 34, 128, 179, 212, 224] Although in many cases, the ruptures can be localized to an area of bone roughness or to a bony spur, this complication has been known to occur after undisplaced fractures. Engkvist and Lundborg observed that rupture of the extensor pollicis longus is usually a late complication, seen approximately 8 weeks following the original injury; they suggested that this tear is secondary to increased pressure within an intact tendon sheath, restricting blood flow to the area of the extensor pollicis longus that winds around Lis-

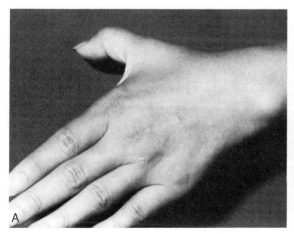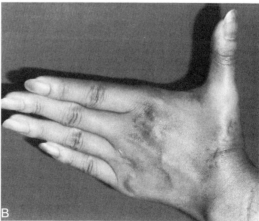

Figure 16–19. A, Loss of EPL after Colles' fracture; *B,* functional result following transfer of EIP to EPL.

ter's tubercule, a portion of the tendon that is normally poorly vascularized.[61]

Other less frequent complications involving tendons include de Quervain's tenosynovitis, trigger finger, and rupture of flexor tendons.[21, 30, 39, 98, 128] Attrition and rupture of the extensor digitorum quinti and other extensor tendons are also possible, particularly when the distal ulna remains prominent or following Darrach procedures.[55, 146] Because of the nature of this tendon injury, direct end-to-end repair is usually not possible. In cases treated early, the interposition of a tendon graft is the procedure of choice. When this cannot be done, activation by remote or side-to-side transfer may be used (see Fig. 16–19). Salvage procedures, such as tenodeses and fusions, are available in selected cases, particularly when the tendon injury results in the loss of function of a single digital joint.

Reflex Sympathetic Dystrophy

This all-inclusive term is used to encompass diverse clinical disorders, with various names such as major and minor causalgia, Sudeck's atrophy, shoulder-hand syndrome, and posttraumatic edema, having as common features the presence of excessive pain and vasomotor and trophic changes following injuries to the limb.[16, 105, 150, 193, 194] Reflex sympathetic dystrophy is a most unpredictable and devastating complication of fractures of the distal radius.[110] The diagnosis must be suspected in patients complaining of pain that is more severe than expected for the nature of the injury, and that is accompanied by excessive swelling, stiffness, discoloration, and evidence of sympathetic disturbance (vaso- and pseudomotor changes; Fig. 16–20).[16]

Actually, all these symptoms and signs are part of the normal response to injury. When this response is disproportionately intense it becomes pathologic.[55] The patient's unwillingness or inability to use the hand soon after the injury should alert the treating physician to the impending catastrophe. An aggressive approach to these early manifestations offers the best assurance of success, even if hospitalization and continuous supervision and treatment are required, until useful function is regained.[68, 105] It is the initial management that is most important in preventing this complication, which should be corrected as soon as suspected and before it produces irrevocable changes.

The patient's emotional and psychological make-up is an important factor—if not in the appearance, at least in the prolongation and aggravation of the reflex sympathetic dystrophy.[150, 193, 194] The experienced practitioner may at times recognize these personality patterns and institute an early program involving active patient participation, designed to forestall the development of the syndrome. Actually, this is a problem that is encountered with enough frequency in upper extremity injuries to justify an aggressive preventive approach for *all* these patients.[55]

Untreated, the initial swelling, stiffness, and discoloration progress to contractures that cannot be reversed, passively or actively, without excruciating exacerbation of pain (Fig. 16–21). The pain itself becomes constant, burning in quality, and frequently aggravated by external physical (temperature) changes or emotional factors.[150] There is radiation of pain to joints proximal to the wrist, including the shoulder (the shoulder-hand or shoulder-hand-finger syndrome[136–138, 193, 194]). Radiographs show a striking osteoporosis, largely limited to the

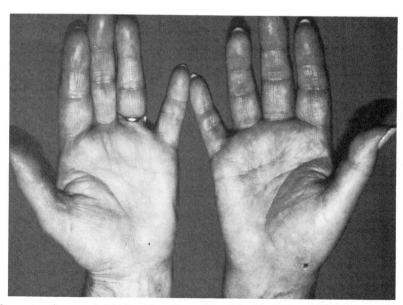

Figure 16–20. Vasomotor changes of right hand in patient with minimally displaced fracture of radius shortly after cast was removed.

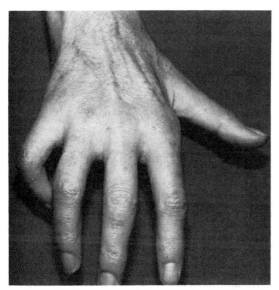

Figure 16–21. Fixed contracture in late reflex sympathetic dystrophy.

small bones of the wrist and hand, particularly the carpus and metaphyseal areas of the long bones (Fig. 16–22).

This initial stage may last 3 to 6 months, and is followed by an intermediate period of increasing contractures, with some diminution of pain and swelling, unless and until passive manipulation of the joints involved is attempted.[16, 68, 193, 194] The skin and nails show dystrophic changes, the hands are cold, and a palmar fasciitis may be seen (Fig. 16–23). In the late stages, there are residual fixed contractures and a permanent, irretrievable loss of function although fortunately the level of discomfort and pain has by that time decreased to tolerable or disappeared altogether.

It must be emphasized again that the best treatment is early and aggressive treatment. Once recognized as an impending reflex sympathetic dystrophy, the patient and family should be made aware of the problem and its potential catastrophic consequences.

The limb is *actively* elevated and held elevated by the ambulatory patient. The use of slings should be discouraged.[68, 107, 136–138] While the patient is at bed rest, it is also best to recruit his active participation, demanding that the arm be kept elevated without the use of constraining hanging devices. The patient should be continuously aware of the need for this active contribution to the care of his problem. All joints that are free should be exercised. It is important to stress those motions most likely to be restricted: shoulder abduction and internal rotation, flexion of the proximal joints of the fingers, and extension of the middle joints. This, in effect, places the hand in a position opposite to the claw stance that these patients tend to assume for comfort and relief of pain (see Fig. 16–21).

Of course, fingers and thumb must be actively

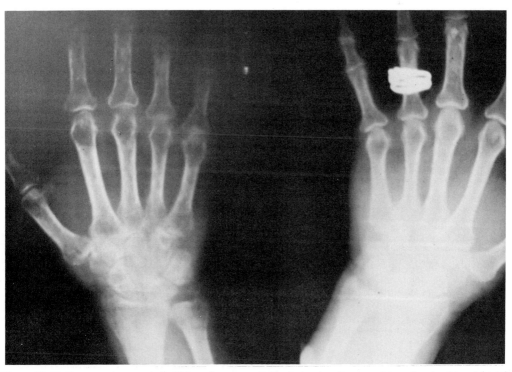

Figure 16–22. Severe osteoporosis (left) in reflex sympathetic dystrophy. Compared to uninvolved hand (right).

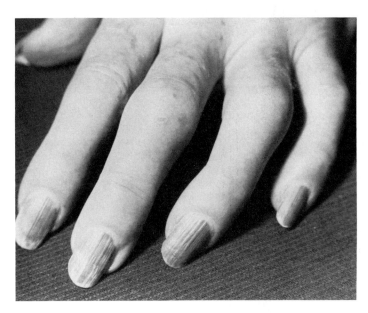

Figure 16–23. Dystrophic nail changes in reflex sympathetic dystrophy.

taken through their full ranges of motion as soon as possible. To assist the patient in carrying out this program, one or more of several measures designed to relieve pain may be used, depending on the stage of the disease and the level of symptoms: sympathetic and somatic nerve blocks, antidepressants, sympatholytic medications, transcutaneous nerve stimulation, regional intravenous or intra-arterial reserpine or intravenous guanethidine (available in Europe but not available for this particular use in the United States).[44, 85, 110, 150, 157, 163] Sympathectomy must be reserved for those patients who achieve significant but temporary relief of their symptoms after sympathetic blocks.[105, 150] High dosages of steroids used during a brief period of 7 to 10 days may assist in triggering a helpful response during the initial stage of reflex sympathetic dystrophy, or whenever pain and swelling interfere with a rehabilitation program.[193, 194] Both dynamic and passive splinting should be used to assist the patient to regain motion, to counteract the tendency toward contractures, and to decrease those contractures that are already present.

Watson[219] has suggested a "loading technique" designed to involve the patient actively in the rehabilitation of the extremity. Patients are asked to scrub a 1-yard area of a kitchen-type floor with a wooden scrub brush for 10 minutes, three times daily. They are instructed to apply their body weight on the shoulder and arm. In addition, these patients must carry, within their homes, a small suitcase or bag loaded with books, or other weights, to the maximum tolerable for the involved hand. It is also extremely important to emphasize to patient and family that this is a longstanding problem that requires, most of all, cooperation, patience and work from the patient himself.

Vascular Complications

Direct vascular impairment is extremely rare in closed fractures of the distal radius and ulna. It is usually associated with the soft tissue injuries that accompany open fractures. Volkmann's contracture is also infrequent in fractures of the wrist. Vascular changes in these patients are most often limited to the intrinsic compartments of the hand and are the result of edema, prolonged immobilization, or muscle ischemia.[180, 181]

Posttraumatic ischemic intrinsic contracture of the hand was first described by Finochietto in a young patient following a crushing injury of the hand with metacarpal fractures.[65] Finochietto pointed out that his patient's ability to flex his fingers varied with the position of the metacarpophalangeal (MP) joints, and described what has since been recognized as the test for intrinsic-plus or intrinsic tightness conditions.[22, 180, 181, 227] In the presence of an intrinsic muscle contracture, greater flexion of the proximal interphalangeal (PIP) joint is possible only when the MP joints are allowed to flex; conversely, if the MP joints are held in extension, flexion of the PIP joints is severely limited or altogether impossible. This condition should be suspected early in the presence of edema, when flexion of the digits is decreased. It may be misdiagnosed as a cellulitis.[184] Initially in the progression of this syndrome, the hand assumes an "intrinsic-minus" position; as fibrosis and contractures of the interossei take place, the fingers adopt the reverse, "intrinsic-plus" attitude.[184] The diagnosis is usually suspected on clinical grounds alone, and is based on the limitation of finger motion described and on the excessive and rapidly indurating edema.

Just as for reflex sympathetic dystrophies, this

condition is best treated when treated early and aggressively. Edema must be controlled, circular or constricting dressings and casts removed or modified, and the patient instructed about a well-supervised exercise program. While control of edema takes place, active and gentle range of motion is encouraged. As soon as swelling decreases enough to allow more strenous exercises, patients are encouraged to flex the fingers fully and to actively assume intrinsic-plus and minus (claw) positions. At this stage, assumption of an intrinsic-minus attitude is an effective "intrinsic stretch" exercise.

If measures to control edema and resume motion fail to control the problem, the interosseous compartments should be surgically released.[180, 181, 184] This is usually performed through longitudinal dorsal incisions in the intermetacarpal spaces. Decompression of median or ulnar nerves at the wrist is not needed, because in most cases there are no sensory changes accompanying the ischemic intrinsic contractures.[184] However, should there be any suggestion of median or ulnar nerve dysfunction, a release of the carpal tunnel and of the canal of Guyon could be performed at the time of the compartmental release. Late contractures are treated by proximal (at the musculotendinous intrinsic junction), distal (at the level of the extensor hood), or combined intrinsic releases.[22, 86, 115, 180, 181, 227]

INJURIES TO THE CARPUS

To those about to diagnose sprained wrist—don't.*

Sprain of the wrist is a diagnosis which is less and less tenable.†

Although these admonitions regarding the diagnosis of wrist sprain were directed to the frequently missed fractures of the scaphoid, they are just as relevant to the entire spectrum of carpal injuries. The diagnosis of sprain must be strictly reserved to the painful wrist only after a thorough evaluation, including clinical examination and all radiographic techniques, and even surgical exploration, have failed to demonstrate a specific clear-cut injury. Many of the complications seen may be avoided if the nature and extent of the original trauma are promptly recognized, and if the correct treatment is instituted at the proper time. The tendency of carpal injuries to progress to complications is a reflection of the highly sophisticated anatomic arrangement of the wrist, which permits a stable range of motion, equaled only by the shoulder and hip joints, in a streamlined articulation without the protection of large bulky muscular support. Many complications seen in the carpus are common to those occurring in other areas (*e.g.*, infections, reflex sympathetic dystrophy, intrinsic contrac-

tures). This section will discuss only those problems specific to the carpus. These complications are secondary to carpal fractures, to carpal dislocations and fracture dislocations, and to carpal instabilities and their treatment.

Carpal Fractures

The Scaphoid

Most complications of carpal injuries are related to the scaphoid because of three anatomic and functional characteristics of this bone: its position as a link or bridge across the midcarpal joint, its pattern of blood supply, and its shape and relationships. The loss of carpal support following scaphoid fractures or dissociations creates the potential for scaphoid nonunions and for some patterns of carpal instabilities. Compromise of the intraosseous blood supply may lead to avascular changes. Finally, the scaphoid surfaces are predominantly articular, with large areas of contact with the radius, lunate, capitate, trapezium, and trapezoid. This allows the development of mono- or multiarticular periscaphoid osteoarthritis following fractures, healed or ununited, or scaphoid dislocations and subluxation.

Nonunions of Scaphoid Fractures. In many cases these occur because of the patient's or physician's neglect. Most recent fractures of the scaphoid show surprisingly little limitation of motion and minimal loss of grip strength.[96, 154] It is therefore not surprising that many patients, particularly the young athletes, delay seeking medical attention, believing their injury to be "just a sprain." This, and the physician's failure to recognize the true nature of the lesion, or to treat it adequately, are main contributors to the development of nonunion (Fig. 16–24). Although the diagnosis of fracture of the scaphoid can be suspected on clinical grounds, it can only be conclusively demonstrated by radiographic means. In 1905, 10 years after Roentgen's discovery of x-rays, Codman and Chase recommended radiography of the wrists in *ulnar deviation*, "for this extends the scaphoid bone, that is, it lifts the distal end so that it comes nearer the plane of the proximal end."[37] Ulnar deviation and some dorsiflexion designed to bring the normally volar flexed scaphoid to a plane parallel to the x-ray plate are now routinely recommended (Fig. 16–25).[20, 89, 126, 142, 155, 165, 187, 190]

Most important, however, is to realize that, in some instances, a fracture of the scaphoid may not be radiographically visible until 2 or more weeks have elapsed since the original trauma. Therefore, when an injury to the scaphoid is strongly suspected but is not demonstrable in routine initial roentgenographic studies, it is prudent to immobilize the wrist in a splint and to repeat radiographs in 2 to 3 weeks, at a time when resorption between fracture fragments may widen the fracture line enough to allow its detection.[8, 19, 23, 36, 92, 97, 126, 135, 167, 182, 183, 187, 210, 222]

---

*Punch; quoted by Todd, Br. J. Surg., 9:7, 1921.
†Spees and Skillern, Int. Clin. (Phila.), 27:263, 1917.

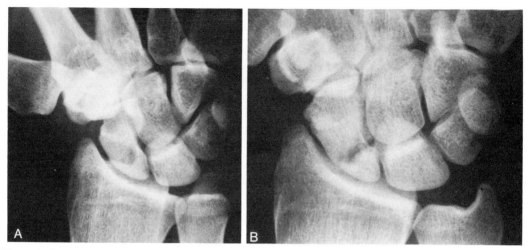

Figure 16–24. *A,* Linear fracture of scaphoid, unrecognized in these initial radiographs; *B,* appearance 1 year later.

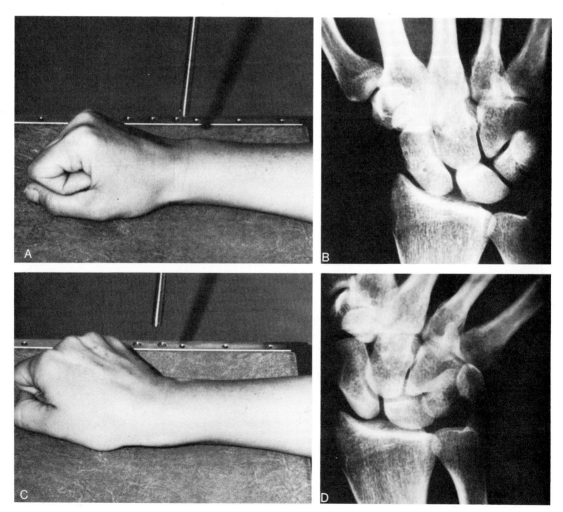

Figure 16–25. PA scaphoid views. *A,* Hand position; *B,* radiographic appearance; *C,* same in ulnar deviation; *D,* radiographic appearance.

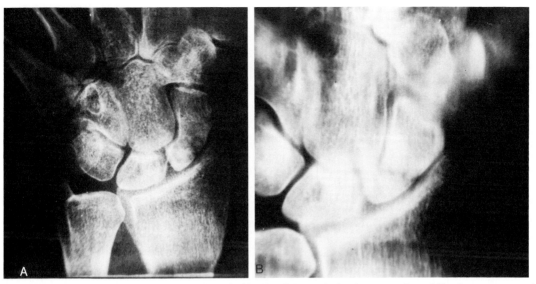

Figure 16–26. *A,* Fracture of proximal third of scaphoid, after 7½ months in plaster cast immobilization, appears to be healed through its medial 60%. *B,* laminogram taken on the same date as *A* shows persistent nonunion.

Terry and Ramin have called attention to a small radiolucent area next to the scaphoid, normally present in the routine posteroanterior projection, the scaphoid fat stripe.[206] Preservation of this space after injury is a strong indication against a fracture of the scaphoid. Conversely, in a retrospective review, Cetti and Christensen found an abnormal fat stripe in 73 of 78 fractures of the scaphoid.[32]

In difficult cases, laminographs, trispiral tomography, and isotope scanning may be used (Fig. 16–26).[41] A normal scan excludes a fracture. Increased focal activity supports the presence of an injury, even if the fracture is not visible in routine radiographs at the time.[70, 102] Bone scans may also provide information on the vascularity of the fracture fragments.[111] Bipartite scaphoids, if they indeed exist, are extremely rare, and may be considered in the differential diagnosis only when there is a foolproof negative history for injury—when the two scaphoid fragments are of near normal density, with clear-cut edges, rounded corners, a smooth jointlike space, particularly if this appearance is present bilaterally, and without osteoarthritic changes—in a patient who is asymptomatic or becomes rapidly asymptomatic.[19, 54, 151] Loss of scaphoid support renders the carpus unstable.[66, 74, 109] The lunate becomes dorsiflexed; the radius, lunate, and scaphoid are no longer colinear, but are aligned in "Z formation"— a collapse pattern variously called "crumpling," "concertina," or DISI (dorsal intercalary segment instability) deformity (Fig. 16–27).[66, 74, 114]

When present, this type of instability should raise suspicion as to the true nature of the original injury, because this may well represent a reduced transscaphoid perilunate fracture dislocation. An attempt may be made to correct this dorsiflexion instability by nonsurgical means when it is seen accompanying

the acute fresh fracture of the scaphoid. Restoration of alignment can be tried by positioning of the wrist (in ulnar deviation or radial deviation with some degree of dorsiflexion), although this is difficult and fails in most instances. Even if successfully per-

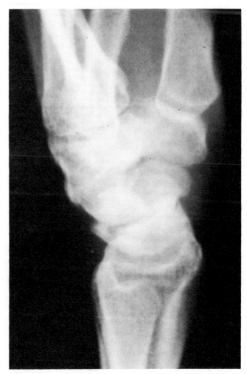

Figure 16–27. Dorsal intercalary segment instability (DISI) accompanying a fracture of the scaphoid.

formed, correction by manipulation is unreliable because the restoration of carpal stability without internal fixation is intrinsically precarious. A DISI alignment must, therefore, be corrected more securely, either by percutaneous pinning of the lunate to the radius in neutral flexion or, preferably, by simultaneous open reduction and internal fixation of the scaphoid fracture and of the displaced lunate.[55]

A scaphoid fracture is considered a nonunion when it has been present for at least 6 months, and when the opposing fracture surfaces show some sclerotic changes.[55] Many patients with ununited scaphoids that are stable and are without carpal collapse may not require any treatment, for they are and may remain essentially symptom-free.[19, 51, 116, 126, 127, 171] There is no evidence to suggest that the incidence of posttraumatic osteoarthritis is increased in these patients.

The choice of treatment for the symptomatic nonunions depends on multiple factors: the location of the fracture within the scaphoid, the presence of avascular changes, the degree of comminution and collapse, the extent and severity of degenerative changes of the periscaphoid surfaces, the patient's age, and the physician's own experience. Although prolonged immobilization alone may reverse the nonunion, this is not recommended because of the potential economic hardship caused to these patients (usually young adults), and because there are alternative methods, both surgical and nonsurgical, which promise a more reliable solution to the problem in an abbreviated time.[15, 162, 195]

For nonunions with good alignment and without osteoarthritis occupying the middle third, but preferably the proximal third or proximal pole of the scaphoid, pulsing electromagnetic field stimulation (PEMF) may be used to great advantage.[69] In the always troublesome fractures of the proximal third, when the proximal fragment is 30% of the scaphoid or less, the use of PEMF for an average of 4.3 months was shown to result in healing in 67% of patients with long-standing nonunions. (Fig. 16–28).[69] Persistent nonunion in proximal third fractures, when the fragment is at least a full third of the scaphoid, may be managed by a Russe-type bone graft (Fig. 16–29).[166, 167] For these injuries it is helpful to add to the bone graft an internal fixation with K-wires or staples placed from the distal scaphoid across the fracture and the proximal fragment

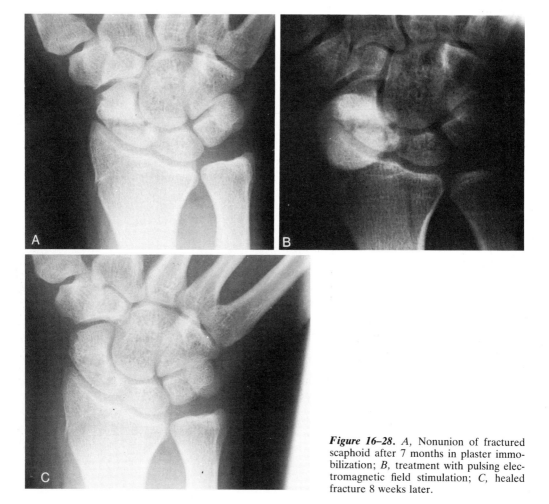

Figure 16–28. A, Nonunion of fractured scaphoid after 7 months in plaster immobilization; B, treatment with pulsing electromagnetic field stimulation; C, healed fracture 8 weeks later.

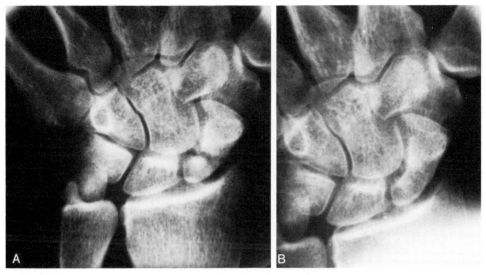

Figure 16–29. *A,* Nonunion of fracture of proximal third of scaphoid; *B,* 5 months after a volar bone graft procedure (Russe), the fracture is healed.

and into the lunate. If the fracture fails to unite after surgery, or for proximal fragments that are too small to accept a bone graft, and in the absence of carpal instability, the fragment may be excised and replaced by a Silastic spacer.[201]

Undisplaced nonunions of the middle third of the scaphoid without carpal instability or osteoarthritic changes may also be treated with PEMF or with a Russe-type bone graft. Whenever the scaphoid is exposed through a volar incision, attention should be given to the repair of volar ligaments that may need to be divided during the surgical approach. If left unrepaired, a potential for immediate or delayed instability is introduced.[55, 201] When there is comminution or volar flexion of the distal scaphoid fragment with a DISI alignment of the carpus, the fracture is best treated by the insertion through a volar approach of a wedge-shaped bone graft, designed to restore length to the "crumpled" scaphoid.[66] Cystic and avascular changes are not contraindications to bone graft procedures.[143]

The Herbert screw is a promising recent addition to the surgical armamentarium for the treatment of these fractures.[90] Avascular necrosis of the proximal fragment, or of a fragment that is too small for a stable fixation, and the presence of osteoarthritic changes, are contraindications for the use of screw osteosynthesis.

Avascular Necrosis. The diagnosis of avascular necrosis is strictly roentgenographic and should be made with caution. The increased density of the proximal fragment may be more apparent than real, produced by rotation to a position of greater thickness.[74] For a valid diagnosis of avascular necrosis, this should be visualized in all projections. The more proximal the fracture, the greater the risk of avascularity of the proximal fragment, a fact well explained by studies of the intraosseous blood sup-

ply to the scaphoid.[72, 202] Although avascular necrosis may delay union in fresh fractures, it is not necessarily an indication of impending nonunion. Its presence should not change the approach to the treatment of these fractures. Fractures do heal in spite of avascular proximal fragments, but protected immobilization should be continued beyond fracture healing, until the avascular bone has been largely replaced. Collapse of the proximal fragment is unusual.[55] The use of PEMF stimulation may be helpful for these patients. When nonunion and avascular necrosis coexist, a Russe bone graft is indicated; if required, satisfactory stabilization may be obtained with two or more Kirschner wires.

Osteoarthritis (or Posttraumatic Degenerative Changes). This may involve any of the large artic-

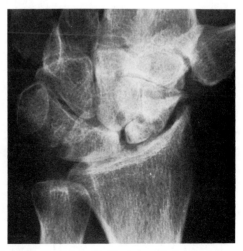

Figure 16–30. Osteoarthritic changes first noticed between scaphoid and tip of radial styloid.

ular surfaces of the scaphoid. Scaphotrapeziotrapezoid (STT) osteoarthritis may occur following distal articular fractures.[41, 55] When painful and unresponsive to nonsurgical management (*e.g.*, steroid injections, intermittent splinting), degenerative changes of the STT joint are best treated by an arthrodesis limited to this articulation.[221] Most frequently, degenerative changes are confined to the styloid-scaphoid space (Fig. 16–30). In these patients it is useful to localize the precise area that is the source of their pain by injections of small amounts of a local anesthetic into the involved articulation. In these cases, a limited radial styloidectomy performed subperiosteally through the anatomic snuffbox may be of help.[213] Some authors consider styloidectomy to be an essential part of the treatment of nonunions, although this procedure does not seem to improve on the results of bone

grafting alone, except in those cases with localized styloidscaphoid osteoarthritis.[187] Furthermore, if performed carelessly, or if excessive, radial styloidectomies may be a factor in the development of subsequent carpal instability and, most importantly, may preclude the later use of a scaphoid implant.[55, 201]

When periscaphoid osteoarthritis is more extensive, involving not only the styloid-scaphoid joint, but also the scaphotrapezium, scaphocapitate spaces, or both, a scaphoid implant may be used, or else the wrist may be arthrodesed from the radius to the distal carpal row or to the second and third metacarpal bases. In 1970, Swanson presented his initial experience using a silicone rubber implant for replacement of the scaphoid.[196] This replacement arthroplasty is indicated for those patients with or without nonunion, but with extensive painful os-

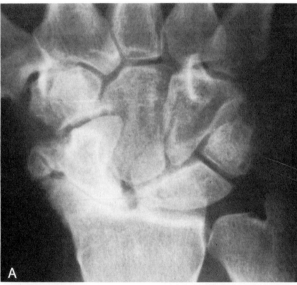
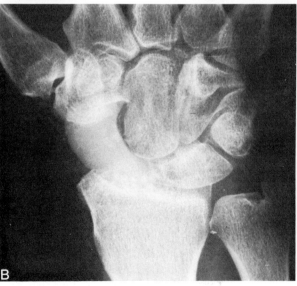
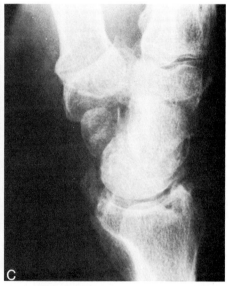

Figure 16–31. A, Severe radioscaphoid degenerative osteoarthritis; *B, C,* Postoperative radiographs after excision of the scaphoid and insertion of a silicone rubber implant. This wrist has remained symptom-free in spite of residual dorsiflexion alignment of the carpus in the lateral view.

teoarthritis strictly limited to the periscaphoid joints. When carpal alignment is satisfactory, scaphoid replacement arthroplasty alone is a very useful procedure (Fig. 16–31). In a long-term evaluation of 607 cases of lunate and scaphoid arthroplasties, Herndon and associates found subluxation of the implant to be their main complication. This is most likely to occur when carpal collapse coexists with the scaphoid problem. Therefore, when instability is present, provisions should be made during surgery for a load-bearing column to transmit forces across the wrist directly to the radius. This can be accomplished by a lunocapitate fusion done simultaneously with the insertion of the scaphoid implant.[220] Partial arthrodeses including the scaphoid are also helpful for osteoarthritis limited to one or two joint spaces; depending on the area involved, these fusions may span the radioscaphoid or radioscapholunate spaces, or may be limited to the articulation between scaphoid and capitate, scaphoid, lunate and capitate, or scaphoid and trapezium.[78, 220, 221]

The Lunate

Kienböck's Disease. This is the major complication of fractures of the lunate. Other complications are secondary to the surgical treatment of the established lunatomalacia.

Fractures of the lunate are rarely recognized acutely. This is due to the position of the lunate in the center of the carpus and the characteristics of the fracture itself, frequently along a frontal plane obscured by the superimposition of other carpal bones. Left to their own evolution, these fractures progress into full-blown Kienböck's disease with distressing frequency.[55] Just as with the scaphoid, in many instances the original injury seems benign and the initial trauma rather minimal. Patients are young

and active, and tend to dismiss this as a simple wrist sprain. Even if medical advice is sought immediately, the diagnosis may not be made until the most traditional changes of Kienböck's disease have finally developed (flattening of the lunate, fragmentation, and sclerosis; Fig. 16–32). Furthermore, even if the patient *is* examined early and the correct diagnosis is established, treatment by immobilization alone will, in most instances, be entirely ineffective in stopping the progression of lunate fragmentation and collapse.

In spite of this, early diagnosis and treatment still offer the best chance for a satisfactory final result. The diagnosis should be suspected in young adults who present with pain, stiffness, and some swelling and tenderness over the lunate, at times following trivial dorsiflexion injuries. In contrast with scaphoid fractures, these patients exhibit greater limitation of motion and a striking weakness of grip.[201] Routine early radiographs may be entirely negative, except for the presence of an ulna-minus variant of wrist configuration.

Hultén, in 1928, published a study of distal radioulnar relationships in normal and Kienböck's wrists.[94] In 51% of the normal individuals, the distal articular surfaces of the radius and ulnar head were found to be at the same level, the so-called zero variant. The ulna-minus variant (ulnar head proximal to the radius) was seen in only 23%. Conversely, patients with Kienböck's disease showed predominantly an ulna-minus variant. The presence of this set of circumstances (young adult, dorsiflexion injury, severe loss of grip strength, tenderness over the lunate, and an ulna-minus radiographic variant) should alert the physician to the possibility of Kienböck's disease. The wrist must be immobilized and repeat radiographs obtained within 2 to 3 weeks. If still inconclusive, and if symptoms persist,

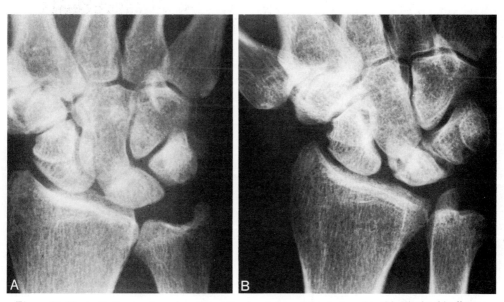

Figure 16–32. A, B, Progressive sclerosis and fragmentation of lunate in wrist with Kienböck's disease.

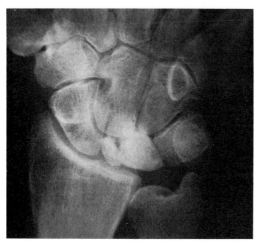

Figure 16–33. Kienböck's disease. The loss of carpal height through foreshortening of the scaphoid and distal migration of the triquetrum on the hamate is apparent.

additional studies are justified, including tomograms, CAT scans and bone scans.[55, 73]

Ståhl was a proponent of prolonged immobilization for the treatment of this condition; this may be successful particularly in the very young patients, but only after many months in a cast.[188] Even under ideal conditions, however, the relentless "nutcracker" effect between capitate and radius will continue to subject the lunate to compression, even within the cast.[55, 201] This suggests that a technique that could unload the lunate and neutralize the nutcracker effect may succeed by allowing the injured lunate to heal without undue pressures. This could be accomplished either by distraction with a radiometacarpal fixator, or by preventing carpal collapse, which could be obtained by holding the scaphoid in a longitudinal dorsiflexed stance by blind pinning to the trapezium and trapezoid. The lunate unloading, if combined with PEMF to stimulate vascular supply, may still offer the best hope of restoration of lunate architecture.

Complications of Treatment. The search for a reliably successful treatment for Kienböck's disease continues. Simple excision of the lunate has been abandoned because of the significant resultant disability.[31, 57, 75, 122, 164] At present, there are three main methods for the treatment of Kienböck's disease with lunate collapse: the joint leveling procedures (ulnar lengthening and radial shortening), the implant resection arthroplasty using a silicone rubber implant, and the use of limited arthrodesis.[9, 35, 78, 156, 176, 196]

In addition to the complications common to other surgical procedures (*e.g.*, infection, nonunion), there are some problems entirely peculiar to the nature of the disease and its treatment. Collapse of the weakened lunate by pressure between capitate and radius is made possible by the shortening of the carpal height allowed by volar flexion of the scaphoid on the radial side, and by the distal migration

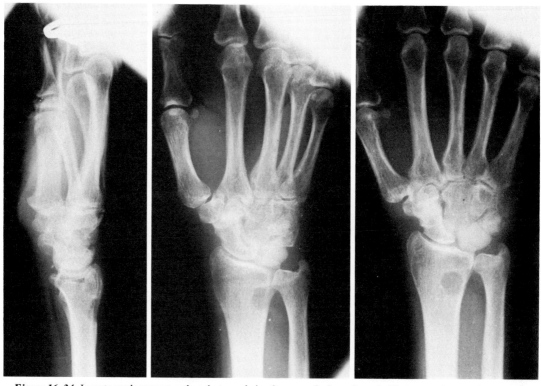

Figure 16–34. Lunate replacement arthroplasty and simultaneous fusion of scaphoid to trapezium and trapezoid.

of the triquetrum on the hamate medially (Fig. 16–33). If the lunate is replaced by a silicone rubber implant, although some compression of the implant may occur without displacement, the natural result of loading will be a shift of the implant into a collapsed stance and its eventual dislocation. Careful reconstruction of the volar capsule or preservation of the volar cortex of the lunate as a palmar buttress may be effective to avoid the dislocation, but do not prevent the development of a carpal instability pattern, particularly if a severe loss of carpal height existed preoperatively.[12]

Chuinard and Zeman proposed to fuse the capitate to the hamate to prevent proximal migration of the capitate.[35] This, in most instances, will be ineffective, because volar flexion of the scaphoid, and distal migration of the triquetrum on the hamate, will continue to allow carpal collapse in spite of the capitate-hamate fusion. A reasonable alternative is to fuse the scaphoid in a longitudinal alignment either to the trapezium and trapezoid, or to the capitate, providing a load-bearing column that bypasses the weakened lunate or its replacement (Fig. 16–34).[219]

The Triquetrum and Pisiform

Complications of fractures of the triquetrum and pisiform are exceedingly rare. Nonunion may oc-cur.[60] Avascular necrosis has not been reported. If the fracture involves the triquetrum-pisiform articular facet, late painful osteoarthritis may develop. The diagnosis should be suspected in patients who complain of pain that is well localized to the pisiform area. There is tenderness at the pisotriquetral level, best elicited by palpation from the ulnar side of the carpus. Painful crepitus by passive side-to-side motion of the pisiform on the triquetrum while the wrist is passively held in volar flexion is pathognomonic.[153] Contraction of the flexor carpi ulnaris against resistance, particularly if the wrist is in dorsiflexion, aggravates the pain, Occasionally, symptoms suggestive of irritation of the ulnar nerve or artery may be present. Radiographs obtained with the hand in slight dorsiflexion and in 30 to 45° of supination, and carpal tunnel views, will demonstrate arthritic changes at the pisotriquetral joint level. Excision of the pisiform is the treatment of choice for this problem.

The Capitate

Isolated fractures of the capitate are rare. This bone is more susceptible to fractures through the neck, usually found in association with other carpal fractures, or fracture dislocations of the carpus.[54] Most frequent is the scaphocapitate fracture syndrome, which consists of a fracture of the neck of

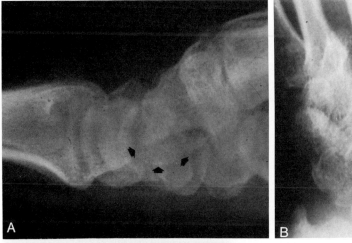
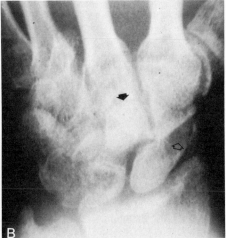
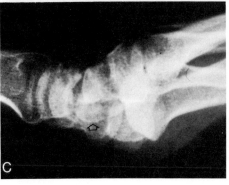

Figure 16–35. Scaphocapitate fracture syndrome. *A,* Head of capitate rotated 90° *(arrows)* lies palmar to body of capitate; *B,* arrows point to head of capitate and scaphoid fracture; *C,* 2-year follow-up. Ununited malrotated capitate head *(arrow)* remains unchanged. The patient is free of symptoms.

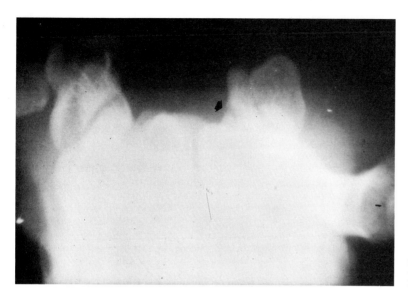

Figure 16–36. Fracture at base of hamate hook (*arrow*; carpal tunnel projection).

the capitate with rotation of the head, associated with a fracture of the waist of the scaphoid (Fig. 16–35).[2, 62, 63, 130, 192, 215] The main complication for this injury is lack of recognition; attention is usually drawn to the more obvious fracture of the scaphoid, while the injury to the capitate remains undetected. Although this may not necessarily lead to disability, accurate reduction and internal fixation is the treatment of choice.[201, 215] Avascular necrosis is extremely unusual and may be treated by intercarpal fusion across the lunocapitate joint, or by excision of the necrotic head and its replacement with an "anchovy"-type arthroplasty.[101, 104, 117, 145, 158] The very rare nonunions of capitate fractures may be treated, if symptomatic, by bone grafting, if the articular surface of the head is satisfactory. If not, a fusion spanning the midcarpal joint and the nonunion may be done.[55]

The Hamate

There are two main varieties of fractures of the hamate, those within the body and those involving the hamular process (hook).[131] Complications arising from these fractures are reduced to two: osteoarthritis involving the hamate-metacarpal joints, following intra-articular fractures of the body, and nonunions of fractures of the hook of the hamate. Osteoarthritis is very infrequent and, when present, rarely symptomatic enough to warrant surgical treatment. Nonunion of fractures of the hamulus are a source of disability, and create a potential for additional complications—ulnar neuropathy and tears of the flexors to the little finger. Fractures of the hook may be easily missed. This injury should be suspected, particularly in golfers, but also in tennis, baseball, and squash players who complain of a deep ill-defined pain referred to the ulnar half of the wrist.[29, 147, 189, 211] There is tenderness to palpation of the hook, but also along the dorsum of the hamate, a feature that may be a source of

confusion.[189] The tip of the hook is found distal and radial to the pisiform, along a line traced from the pisiform to the head of the third metacarpal.[82] Because the canal of Guyon is closely related to the hamulus, fractures at this level may be accompanied by ulnar nerve involvement.[6, 173] Ruptures of flexor tendons may occur by attrition against the rough irregularity of the fracture site.[43]

The diagnosis is radiographic, but requires special projections (Fig. 16–36). A carpal tunnel view and an oblique radiograph with the hand in 45° of supination and the wrist in some radial deviation and dorsiflexion are useful.[6, 147] For both projections, several views in slightly different degrees of rotation may be required before the fracture is identified. Tomograms are helpful when the diagnosis is strongly suspected by the history of the injury and the clinical findings, and when all radiographs have remained inconclusive.[144] With few exceptions, the recommended treatment has been excision of the ununited fragment, even in fractures through the very base of the hook.[25, 29, 59, 135, 147, 189, 211, 225]

Carpal Dislocations and Fracture-Dislocations

In this group are included those severe injuries that result in complete dislocation of one or more carpal bones, with or without simultaneous fractures of the carpus, radius, or ulna. Excluded are the more subtle patterns of carpal subluxation, the so-called carpal instabilities. Carpal dislocations and fracture-dislocations may be classified into three main groups:

1. Frequent dislocations and fracture-dislocations. Included in this group are the dorsal perilunate dislocations, volar dislocations of the lunate, and dorsal transscaphoid perilunate fracture-dislocations (Figs. 16–37, 16–38, and 16–39).

2. Infrequent dislocations and fracture-disloca-

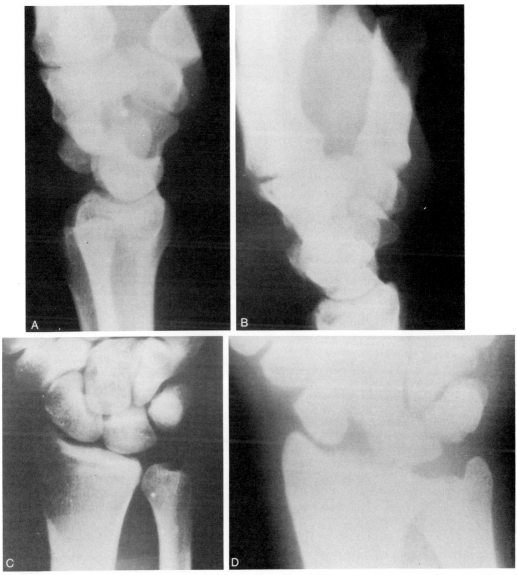

Figure 16–37. *A,* Dorsal perilunate dislocation; *B,* postreduction (lateral view); *C,* postreduction (PA view); *D,* Late (2 weeks) appearance of scapholunate dissociation.

tions. These include the exceptional volar perilunate dislocations, the dorsal dislocation of the lunate, and the dislocation of isolated carpal bones (*e.g.,* scaphoid, scaphoid and lunate, triquetrum; Fig. 16–40).

3. Variants.[80] These represent those dislocations and fracture dislocations with extension of the injury to include the radius (transradial styloid perilunate fracture-dislocations) or the triquetrum (transscaphoid, transtriquetral perilunate fracture-dislocations), or a fracture of the capitate (transscaphoid, transcapitate, dorsal perilunate fracture-dislocations leading to scaphocapitate fracture syndromes; Figs. 16–41 and 16–42).

Although the nomenclature appears confusing at first, it is entirely descriptive in that it follows the path of injury as it progresses around and across those carpal (and radial) structures that are involved. Injuries that closely hug the lunate follow the "lesser arc" and comprise the lunate dislocations and the perilunate dislocations (Fig. 16–43). In the "greater arc injuries," there are one or more fractures of perilunate bones accompanying the dislocation—for example, transscaphoid perilunate, transscaphoid transcapitate perilunate, and transscaphoid transtriquetral perilunate fracture-dislocations (see Fig. 16–43).[99] These injuries represent a continuum of progressive bony and ligamentous damage.[125] The final outcome depends on the position of the hand at impact, the point of application

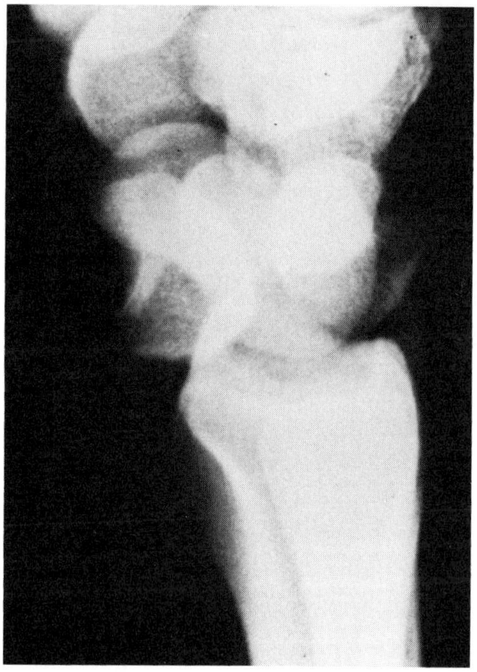

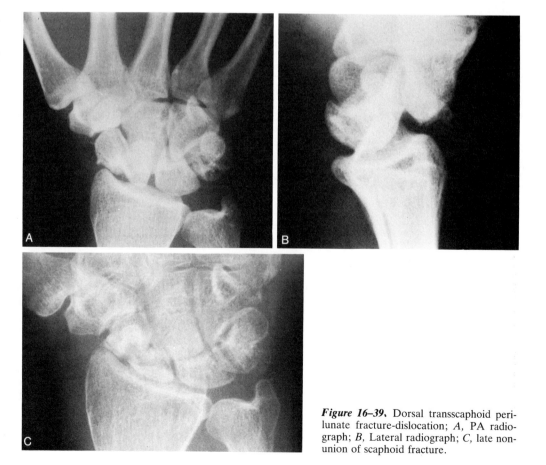

Figure 16–38. Palmar dislocation of the lunate (the "spilled teacup" sign).

of the load to the hand, and the magnitude and duration of the force, particularly in relation to the relative strength of the carpal bones and ligaments.[125, 199]

The following discussion will be largely limited to the complications arising from the more frequent dislocations and fracture-dislocations and their frequent variants.

Dorsal Perilunate Dislocation

The lunate remains under the protective dome of the radius while the remaining carpus dislocates dorsally (see Fig. 16–37). The first possible complication, lack of recognition, is fortunately extremely infrequent, and is altogether avoided by careful roentgenographic evaluation. The true nature of the injury is easier to discern in the lateral projection; the distal concave fossae of the lunate is seen to be empty, because the head of the capitate is dislocated and lies dorsal to the lunate. The scaphoid is volar-flexed, with its proximal pole dorsal to the dorsal rim of the radius. This is part of the second complication, a rotatory subluxation of the scaphoid, which is a frequent sequela of reduced perilunate dislocations.[26, 27, 120, 209, 217, 222] It may lead to a perma-

Figure 16–39. Dorsal transscaphoid perilunate fracture-dislocation; *A,* PA radiograph; *B,* Lateral radiograph; *C,* late nonunion of scaphoid fracture.

Figure 16–40. Simultaneous dislocation of scaphoid and lunate. (From Taleisnik, J., Malerich, M., and Prietto, M.: Palmar carpal instability secondary to dislocation of scaphoid and lunate: Report of case and review of the literature. J. Hand Surg., 7:606, 1982.)

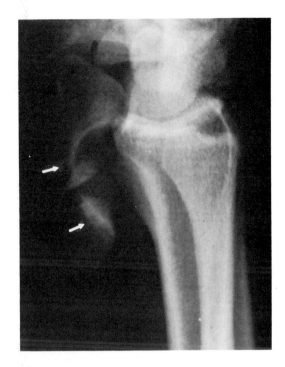

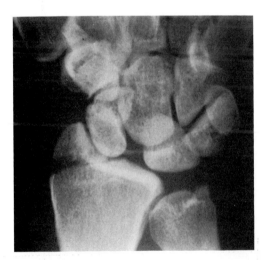

Figure 16–41. Transradial styloid, perilunate fracture-dislocation.

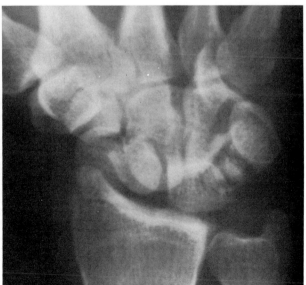

Figure 16–42. Transscaphoid, perilunate, transtriquetral fracture-dislocation.

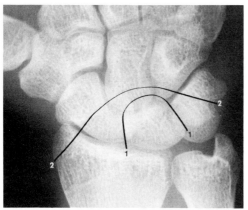

Figure 16–43. Lesser (1) and greater (2) arcs of potential perilunate injuries.

nently unstable carpus unless corrected early. This complication arises because of the severe ligamentous damage that occurs between the scaphoid and lunate during perilunate dislocations. Unless the scaphoid is securely stabilized to the lunate after reduction, it will tend to sublux again into volar flexion and away from the lunate (see Fig. 16–37D). Therefore, after the gross perilunate displacement has been reduced, usually by manipulation alone, and preferably under satisfactory anesthesia and relaxation, the alignment of the scaphoid must be critically assessed. It may appear to be satisfactory initially, only to sublux very rapidly, even within the cast used for postreduction immobilization.

Only rarely does the reduced scaphoid remain in satisfactory alignment. In most cases, if the initial reduction is acceptable, it must be secured by percutaneous or open pin fixation.[81] If manipulative reduction is not possible, however, or if it is unacceptable, an open reduction should be done, preferably through simultaneous volar and dorsal approaches.[56, 80, 198] This allows satisfactory visualization of reduction, and affords the opportunity to repair the invariably large rent that is present on the volar capsule.[80, 198]

If scaphoid subluxation recurs after removal of initial pin fixation, or if the residual secondary rotatory subluxation of the scaphoid is not diagnosed or treated until more than 3 weeks after the initial injury, the surgical reduction of the rotated scaphoid must be complemented by a ligament reconstruction, or by a limited arthrodesis between the reduced scaphoid, trapezium, and trapezoid.[106, 152, 221]

Osteoarthritis is a late complication, and is usually limited to the styloid-scaphoid space unless extensive cartilaginous damage occurred initially, in which case degenerative changes may be more widespread to include the lunocapitate and radiolunate joints predominantly. Treatment for this particular problem is included in the discussion of complications of fractures of the radius and scaphoid.

Median neuropathy, acute or delayed, is also a

potential complication of perilunate dislocation. Its management is identical to that recommended for median nerve entrapments following fractures of the distal radius. Exploration of the nerve during the first few days following an injury affords the unequaled opportunity to evaluate the extent of the volar capsular damage and to repair it.[55]

Transscaphoid Perilunate Fracture-Dislocation

This lesion is similar to the perilunate dislocation, except that the injury occurs through the scaphoid rather than at the scapholunate junction (see Fig. 16–39). The complications are similar to those seen in perilunate dislocations (*i.e.*, lack of recognition, median nerve compression, and late osteoarthritis); however, instead of a rotatory subluxation of the scaphoid, there is a very unstable fracture of the scaphoid. Rarely, manipulative reduction results in an anatomic alignment. Because of the inherent, ever-present instability, however, progress must be assessed at weekly intervals for several weeks.[27]

Most frequently, though, stability must be regained by internal fixation of the fracture of the scaphoid with Kirschner wires or a screw, depending on the surgeon's preference and experience. Failure to fix the scaphoid fracture results in a distressingly high number of nonunions (see Fig. 16–39C).[97, 140] If the scaphoid is stabilized early, a bone graft may be unnecessary *unless* the fracture is comminuted. When a bone graft is not contemplated, the fracture may be exposed and fixed using a lateral approach through the anatomic snuffbox. When a bone graft is needed, the fracture is best exposed through an anterior (Russe's) approach.[167] An uncommon mistake is to attempt stabilization by bone grafting alone (Fig. 16–44). This will inexorably fail. After the injury has been stabilized, later complications

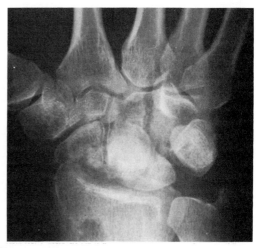

Figure 16–44. Transscaphoid perilunate fracture-dislocation, treated initially by reduction and bone grafting through a palmar approach (Russe). This resulted in prompt recurrence of the dislocation. The radiograph shows carpal alignment 4 weeks after the injury.

are similar to those discussed for fractures of the scaphoid.

Volar Dislocation of the Lunate

This results from the same mechanism of injury that produces a dorsal perilunate dislocation, except that the damage is more extensive, allowing the lunate to dislocate in a palmar direction while the head of the capitate relocates in line with the radius.[26, 27, 55, 59, 80, 81, 120, 204, 217, 218] Again, lateral radiographs are diagnostic and show the distal concave surface of the lunate empty of capitate, facing forward—the "spilled teacup" sign (see Fig. 16–38).[81] The complications that may arise are similar to those seen after perilunate dislocations; carpal instabilities, however, and median neuropathies are more likely to occur, and are more severe when present. Avascular necrosis of the lunate after dislocation is exceedingly rare because the lunate retains an important source of blood supply through the intact palmar radiolunate ligament.[27, 55, 120, 140, 168] This must be kept in mind if an operative reduction is required through a palmar approach: extreme care must be exercised during the exposure and reduction of the lunate to avoid damage to this all-important ligament.

Whether the reduction is accomplished through closed manipulation or surgically, radiocarpal alignment must be protected by internal fixation with Kirschner wires until stability has been restored. In some instances this may not be enough and, on removal of fixation, a slow drift of the scaphoid may be seen in subsequent radiographs. In such cases the scaphoid must again be surgically reduced

and firmly stabilized by ligament reconstruction or preferably by scaphotrapezium-trapezoid arthrodesis.[106, 152, 221]

Variants

The two most frequent variants involve the addition to the common fracture-dislocation of a trans-radial styloid fracture or a fracture through the triquetrum (see Figs. 16–41 and 16–42). All these injuries are extremely unstable, and demand accurate reduction and internal fixation. The complications arising are similar to those already discussed for other forms of dislocations and fracture-dislocations of the carpus—namely, instability, malunion, median neuropathies, and late osteoarthritis.

Posttraumatic Carpal Instabilities

Posttraumatic carpal instabilities are carpal injuries in which loss of normal alignment of the carpal bones develops early or late.[114] Carpal instabilities may be static or dynamic.[200] Static instabilities show a loss of carpal alignment in routine films; this radiographic and clinical deformity cannot be actively corrected by the patient (Fig. 16–45). Conversely, in dynamic instabilities, patients are able either to assume a position of radiocarpal collapse or to return the wrist to normal alignment at will. Routine radiographs are normal, unless obtained after the patient has subluxed the carpus; only then can the loss of alignment be appreciated, either in a dorsal (dynamic DISI) or volar (dynamic VISI) direction (Fig. 16–46). In most cases, dynamic insta-

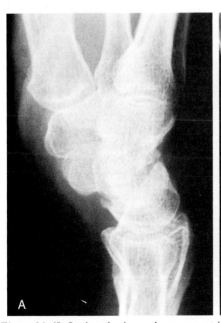
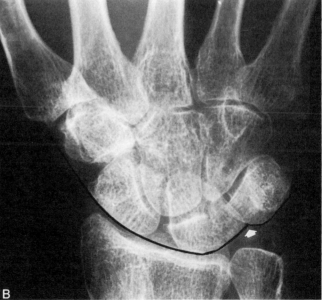

Figure 16–45. Static volar intercalary segment instability (VISI) deformity. *A,* Lateral radiograph: scaphoid and lunate are both palmar-flexed; *B,* PA view shows broken carpal condyle profile ("Shenton's line of the wrist") at LT space *(arrow).* The scaphoid is volar-flexed and the triquetrum is "low" (distal) on the hamate.

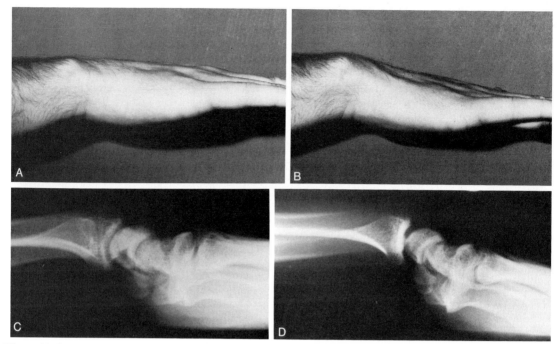

Figure 16–46. Dynamic VISI deformity. *A,* Appearance of the hand in neutral alignment; *B,* the patient can actively depress the carpus—this is accompanied by a painful, loud "snap"; *C,* radiocarpal alignment in neutral; *D,* dynamic VISI deformity.

bilities are secondary to a loss of ligamentous midcarpal support. The continuous synchronous gliding of proximal and distal carpal rows has changed in these patients to an abrupt subluxation as the hand is brought into potentially unstable positions, usu-

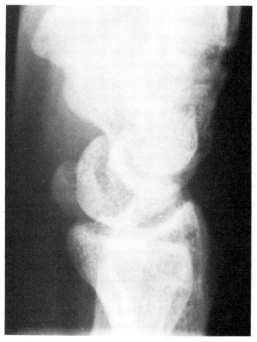

Figure 16–47. Static DISI deformity.

ally in ulnar deviation with the forearm in pronation (see Fig. 16–46).[112, 200] The subluxation is accompanied by an audible "snap" that can be readily palpated at the triquetrohamate joint level.

Linscheid and associates described two major instability patterns, both determined in lateral radiographs by the alignment of the lunate, the intercalary segment in the radiolunocapitate link. When the lunate assumes a position of dorsiflexion, either because of trauma or disease (rheumatoid arthritis), the instability is called DISI for dorsal intercalary segment instability (Fig. 16–47). In VISI deformities, the lunate is volar-flexed (volar intercalary segment instability; see Fig. 16–45*A*).

Rotatory subluxation of the scaphoid or scapholunate dissociation is the most frequent type of static dorsiflexion instability (Fig. 16–48). Normally the lunate tends to dorsiflex, a tendency that is counterbalanced by the volar flexion action of the scaphoid.[100] A ligamentous tear between scaphoid and lunate frees the lunate to its natural dorsiflexion tendency. In this injury, the dissociated scaphoid loses the palmar tethering provided to its proximal pole by the deep palmar radioscapholunate ligament.[198] The proximal pole subluxes dorsally and the net effect is one of scaphoid volar flexion, with its longitudinal axis now perpendicular to that of the radius.

In regard to static volar flexion instabilities, the current belief, although still speculative, is that these instabilities are due to a dissociation between lunate and triquetrum, a mechanism that effectively delivers the lunate to the now unopposed volar

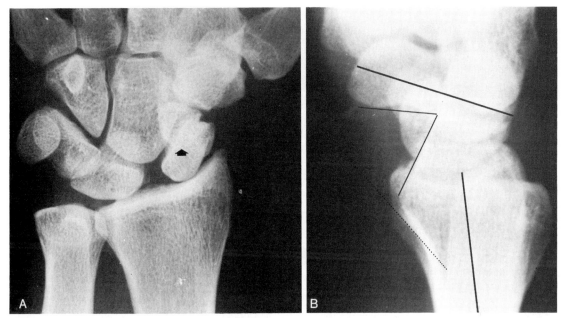

Figure 16–48. Rotatory subluxation of the scaphoid. *A,* AP radiograph—note the "cortical ring sign" *(arrow),* foreshortened scaphoid, and widened scapholunate space; *B,* lateral radiograph showing longitudinal axis of scahpoid "perpendicular" to that of radius, dorsiflexion of lunate, and "V"-shaped angle made by palmar outlines of scaphoid and radial styloid. The long axis of the scaphoid and a line tangential to the palmar flare of the radius *(dashed line)* intersect at an acute angle.

flexion influence of the scaphoid (see Fig. 16–45).[161, 203] A third instability pattern is typified by a dorsal carpal subluxation of the carpus, and a fourth is seen in posteroanterior (PA) radiographs as an ulnar shift or translocation of the carpus (Fig. 16–49).[226]

The main complication arising from the treatment of posttraumatic carpal instabilities is the lack of recognition of the existence of an instability pattern, and of the actual location of the source of the instability. In the first case, the injury is dismissed as "just a sprain." In the second, the injury is recognized but treatment may be erroneously applied to an area not responsible for the collapse deformity. A second set of complications is secondary to the actual treatment of the injury. The third group of complications includes those that are common to all the other wrist injuries, such as median nerve compressions, late osteoarthritis, persistent instabilities, and reflex sympathetic dystrophy. These have already been discussed.

Lack of Recognition of an Instability Pattern

Dorsiflexion Instability (Scapholunate Dissociation). This is the most frequent form of carpal instability. The diagnosis may be suspected on clinical grounds alone, in patients with a voluntary recurrent carpal snap, usually reproduced in palmar flexion, when the proximal pole of the perpendicular scaphoid is forced dorsally past the dorsal rim of the radius. In some patients an unstable scaphoid can be manipulated by the examiner into a subluxed position while, at the same time, the patient's symptoms are reproduced. The diagnosis is, however, entirely based on radiographic findings (see Fig. 16–48).

Anteroposterior Views. These are obtained with the hand in supination.[209] They show widening of the scapholunate space when compared to the opposite uninjured wrist, foreshortening of the scaphoid, and a cortical "ring" produced by the distal pole of the volar-flexed scaphoid seen end-on.[42]

Lateral Views. These show the following: the longitudinal axis of the scaphoid is perpendicular to the long axis of the radius; the volar outline of the scaphoid and the volar margin of the radial styloid meet to form a "V" rather than a "C" pattern; the longitudinal axis of the scaphoid and a line tangential to the volar flare of the radius intersect at a sharp angle rather than being almost parallel to each other; and the lunate is dorsiflexed.[50, 66, 74, 114, 199]

Tangential Posteroanterior Radiographs (Moneim). These are designed to avoid the overlap of scaphoid and lunate that is present in routine PA projections.[139] When the ulnar border of the hand is elevated 20° off the table, the x-ray beam aligns with the scapholunate joint, allowing any abnormal widening to become more apparent.

Palmar Flexion Instabilities (Lunotriquetral Dissociations). These are more frequently seen in rheumatoid patients.[55, 56, 114, 161, 203] There are a number of radiographic findings (see Fig. 16–45).

PA Views. These show the following: the convex proximal outline of the carpal condyle is no longer smooth, but is interrupted by a step-off between

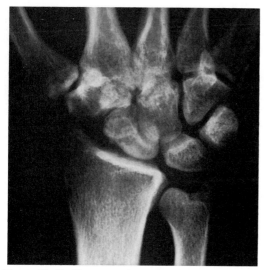

Figure 16–49. Ulnar carpal translocation. The lunate is opposite the ulnar head.

lunate and triquetrum, with the triquetrum now appearing closer to the ulnar head; lunate and scaphoid are volar-flexed (the scaphoid is foreshortened), and the triquetrum is dorsiflexed in a "low" or distal position in relation to the hamate.[161, 223]

Lateral Views. These show the following: the lunate is tilted in volar flexion; the scaphoid is perpendicular to the long axis of the radius, just as in rotatory subluxation of the scaphoid, except that here there is no scapholunate dissociation because both scaphoid and lunate are volar-flexed together. When the ligamentous injury is suspected on clinical grounds but cannot be demonstrated in routine radiographs, arthrograms should be obtained.

Midcarpal Instabilities. These are always dynamic (see Fig. 16–46). They should be suspected in pa-

tients who can actively collapse their wrists into DISI or VISI by ulnar or radial deviation with the forearm and hand in pronation.[112] Cineradiographs, or lateral radiographs obtained with the wrist in ulnar or radial deviation both before and after the "snap" is elicited, should confirm the diagnosis.

Treatment should be directed to the source of the instability pattern. When these patients' injuries are seen as complications, their injuries are no longer fresh and demand reconstructive stabilizing procedures. Rotatory subluxation of the scaphoid may be treated by ligament reconstruction or by a limited fusion, usually performed between the reduced scaphoid and the trapezium and trapezoid (Fig. 16–9).[106, 152, 221] Similarly, midcarpal instabilities may be treated by ligament reconstruction or by a limited arthrodesis between triquetrum and hamate; this will effectively render the midcarpal joint stable (Fig. 16–50).[112] There is very little experience in the treatment of the VISI deformities, probably because these forms of carpal instability produce relatively minor disability. A strip of flexor carpi ulnaris left attached distally has been threaded across the lunate from palmar to dorsal, and anchored on the dorsal rim of the radius to tenodese the volar-flexing lunate in a neutral alignment (Fig. 16–51).[200] The same result may be obtained by a capsulodesis between the dorsal rim of the radius and the dorsal pole of the reduced and realigned lunate, effectively tethering this dorsal pole proximally and preventing lunate volar flexion. A limited arthrodesis between the reduced lunate and the triquetrum or capitate, or more reliably between lunate, triquetrum, capitate, and hamate, may also be used.

Complications of Treatment of Carpal Instabilities

Ligament Reconstruction. These procedures usually involve the drilling of bones to pass tendon

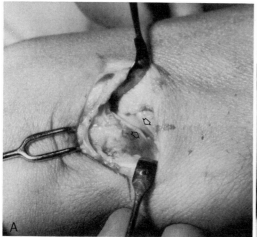
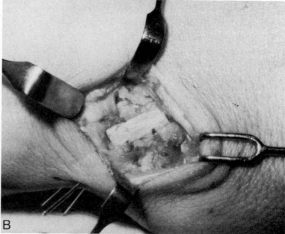

Figure 16–50. Operative views of triquetrohamate fusions. *A,* Triquetrohamate joint *(arrows)*; *B,* partial triquetrohamate arthrodesis: cancellous bone fills the cavity; a cortical graft is slotted across the joint; three Kirschner wires were used for fixation.

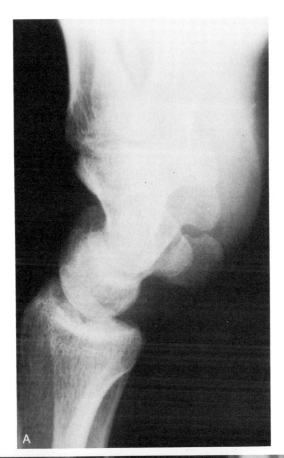

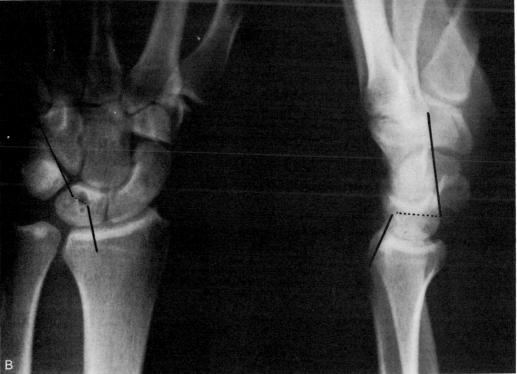

Figure 16–51. *A,* VISI deformity, *B,* postoperative radiographs. Lines show the diagrammatic course of a strip of flexor carpi ulnaris used to tenodese the lunate in a neutral alignment.

grafts to tether or tenodese the subluxing carpal units. There are two main drawbacks: (1) the low coefficient of elasticity of tendon grafts in comparison with that of the ligaments they are attempting to replace; and (2) the difficulty present in gauging the exact tension for the reconstructed ligament. Therefore, if the new ligament (tendon graft) is inserted as tight as is required for correction of the underlying carpal displacement, the postoperative range of motion will be very limited. As the patient exercises to regain a functional range, however, one of three outcomes may be seen: (1) a rupture of the reconstructed ligament, and consequently a recurrence of deformity; (2) a fracture through the wall of the tunnel that was drilled for the tendon graft; or (3) a progressive narrowing of the joint space spanned by the newly reconstructed ligament and the eventual development of osteoarthritic changes.

Limited Arthrodesis. Complications here may be those that are seen in other fusions (*e.g.*, nonunion, infection, malunion) or may be very specific to the carpus itself. These usually result from insufficient correction or from interference of the fused unit with the function of neighboring carpal joints, and lead to late osteoarthritic changes of those articulations that were left surrounding the arthrodesed unit.

References

1. Abbott, L. C., and Saunders, J. B. de C. M.: Injuries of the median nerve in fractures of the lower end of the radius. Surg. Gyn. Obstet., 57:517, 1933.
2. Adler, J. B., and Shaftan, G. W.: Fractures of the capitate. J. Bone Joint Surg., 44A:1537, 1962.
3. Ahstrom, J. P., Jr.: Treatment of Colles' fractures by posterior splint immobilization. Orthop. Rev., 11:147, 1982.
4. Albert, S. M., Wohl, M. A., and Rechtman, A. M.: Treatment of the disrupted radio-ulnar joint. J. Bone Joint Surg., 45A:1373, 1963.
5. Anderson, R., and O'Neil, G.: Comminuted fractures of the distal end of the radius. Surg. Gynecol. Obstet., 78:434, 1944.
6. Andress, M. R., and Peckar, V. G.: Fractures of the hook of the hamate. Br. J. Radiol., 43:141, 1970.
7. Apfelbach, G., Weinstein, L., and Moshein, J.: Ulnar resection for malunited Colles' and Smith's fractures. Bull. Northwest. Univ. Med. School, 27:1, 1953.
8. Archambault, J. L.: Resined fiberglass cast for carpal navicular fractures. Physician Sports Med., 8:83, 1980.
9. Axelson, R.: Behandling av Lunatomalaci, Aktiebolag, Göteborg, Elanders Boktrycker, 1971.
10. Bacorn, R. W., and Kurtzke, J. F.: Colles' fracture. A study of two thousand cases from the New York State Workman's Compensation Board. J. Bone Joint Surg., 35A:643, 1953.
11. Bauman, T. D., et al.: The acute carpal tunnel syndrome. Clin. Orthop., 156:151, 1981.
12. Beckenbaugh, R. D., et al.: Kienböck's disease: The natural history of Kienböck's disease and consideration of lunate fractures. Clin. Orthop., 149:98, 1980.
13. Berg, E.: Indications for and results with the Swanson distal ulnar prosthesis. South Med. J., 69:858, 1976.
14. Blaimont, P., et al.: La résection de l'extrémité distale du cubitus dans les séquelles des fractures de l'avant-bras et du poignet. Acta Orthop. Belg., 29:641, 1963.
15. Böhler, L.: Técnica del Tratamiento de las Fracturas, 3rd ed., Vol. 1. (Translated from the German, 7th ed., by Schneider, G., and Jimeno-Vidal, F.) Barcelona, Editorial Labor S. A., 1954.
16. Bonica, J. J.: Causalgia and other reflex sympathetic dystrophies. Postgrad. Med., 53:143, 1973.
17. Bourrel, P., and Ferro, R. M.: Nerve complications in closed fractures of the lower end of the radius. Ann. Chir. Main, 1:119, 1982.
18. Boyd, H. B., and Stone, M. M.: Resection of the distal end of the ulna. J. Bone Joint Surg., 26:313, 1944.
19. Boyes, J. H.: Bunnell's Surgery of the Hand, 5th ed., Philadelphia, J. B. Lippincott, 1970.
20. Bridgman, C. F.: Radiography of the carpal navicular bone. Med. Radiogr. Photogr., 25:104, 1949.
21. Broder, H.: Rupture of flexor tendons associated with a malunited Colles' fracture. J. Bone Joint Surg., 36A:404, 1954.
22. Bunnell, S.: Ischaemic contracture, local, in the hand. J. Bone Joint Surg., 35A:88, 1953.
23. Burnett, J. H.: Fracture of the (navicular) carpal scaphoid. N. Engl. J. Med., 211:56, 1934.
24. Calberg, G., et al.: Rupture du tendon long extenseur du pouce après fracture du poignet. Acta Orthop. Belg., 27:493, 1961.
25. Cameron, H. U., Hastings, D. E., and Fournasier, V. L.: Fracture of the hook of the hamate: A case report. J. Bone Joint Surg., 57A:276, 1975.
26. Campbell, R. D., Jr., Lance, E. M., and Yeoh, C. B.: Lunate and perilunar dislocation. J. Bone Joint Surg., 46B:55, 1964.
27. Campbell, R. D., Jr., et al.: Indications for open reduction of lunate and perilunate dislocation of the carpal bones. J. Bone Joint Surg., 47A:915, 1965.
28. Campbell, W. C.: Malunited Colles' fractures. J.A.M.A., 109:1105, 1937.
29. Carter, P. R., Eaton, R. G., and Littler, J. W.: Ununited fracture of the hook of the hamate. J. Bone Joint Surg., 59A:583, 1977.
30. Cassebaum, W. H.: Colles' fracture: A study of end results. J.A.M.A., 143:963, 1950.
31. Cave, E. F.: Kienböck's disease of the lunate. J. Bone Joint Surg., 21:858, 1939.
32. Cetti, R., and Christensen, S.-E.: The diagnostic value of displacement of the fat stripe in fracture of the scaphoid bone. Hand, 4:75, 1982.
33. Chapman, D. R., et al.: Complications of distal radial fractures: Pins and plaster treatment. J. Hand Surg., 5:509, 1982.
34. Christophe, K.: Rupture of the extensor pollicis longus following Colles' fracture. J. Bone Joint Surg., 35A:1003, 1953.
35. Chuinard, R. G., and Zeman, S. C.: Kienböck's disease: An analysis and rationale for treatment by capitate-hamate fusion. Orthop. Trans., 4:18, 1980.
36. Cleveland, M.: Fracture of the carpal scaphoid. Surg. Gynecol. Obstet., 84:769, 1947.
37. Codman, E. A., and Chase, H. M.: The diagnosis and treatment of fracture of the carpal scaphoid and dislocation of the semilunar bone. With a report of thirty cases. Ann. Surg., 41:321, 1905.
38. Cole, J. M., and Obletz, B. E.: Comminuted fractures of the distal end of the radius treated by skeletal transfixion in plaster cast. An end result study of 33 cases. J. Bone Joint Surg., 48A:931, 1966.
39. Cooney, W. P., Dobyns, J. H., and Linscheid, R. L.: Complications of Colles' fractures. J. Bone Joint Surg., 62A:613, 1980.
40. Cooney, W. P., Linscheid, R. L., and Dobyns, J. H.: External pin fixation for unstable Colles' fractures. J. Bone Joint Surg., 61A:840, 1979.
41. Cooney, W. P., Ripperger, R. R., and Linscheid, R. L.: Distal pole scaphoid fractures. Orthop. Trans., 4:18, 1980.
42. Crittenden, J. J., Jones, D. M., and Santarelli, A. G.: Bilateral rotational dislocation of the carpal navicular. Radiology, 94:629, 1970.
43. Crosby, E. B., and Linscheid, R. L.: Rupture of the flexor profundus tendon of the ring finger secondary to ancient fracture of the hook of the hamate. J. Bone Joint Surg., 56A:1076, 1974.
44. Dabezies, E. J., Gould, J., and Murphy, J.: Intravenous

reserpine for treatment of reflex sympathetic dystrophy: A preliminary report. Presented at the American Society for Surgery of the Hand, 35th Annual Meeting, Atlanta, 1980.

45. Darrach, W.: Anterior dislocation of the head of the ulna. Ann. Surg., 56:802, 1912.

46. Darrach, W.: Partial excision of lower shaft of ulna for deformity following Colles' fracture. Ann. Surg., 57:764, 1913.

47. Darrach, W.: Fractures of the lower extremity of the radius. Diagnosis and treatment. J.A.M.A., 89:1683, 1927.

48. Darrach, W., and Dwight, K.: Derangements of the inferior radio-ulnar articulation. Med. Rec. 87:708, 1915.

49. DePalma, A. F.: Comminuted fractures of the distal end of the radius treated by ulnar pinning. J. Bone Joint Surg., 34A:651, 1952.

50. Destot, E.: Injuries of the Wrist: A Radiological Study. (Translated by Atkinson, F. R. B.) London, Ernest Benn, 1925.

51. Dickinson, J. C., and Shannon, J. G.: Fractures of the carpal scaphoid in the Canadian Army. Surg. Gynecol. Obstet., 79:225, 1944.

52. Dickson, F. D.: Peripheral nerve injuries associated with fractures of the long bones. South Med. J., 19:37, 1926.

53. Dingman, P. V. C.: Resection of the distal end of the ulna (Darrach operation). J. Bone Joint Surg., 34A:893, 1952.

54. Dobyns, J. H., and Linscheid, R. L.: Fractures and dislocations of the wrist. In Rockwood, C. A., Jr., and Green, D. P. (eds.): Fractures, Philadelphia, J. B. Lippincott, 1975, p. 345.

55. Dobyns, J. H., and Linscheid, R. L.: Complications of treatment of fractures and dislocations of the wrist. In Epps, C. H., Jr. (ed.): Complications in Orthopaedic Surgery, Vol. 2, Philadelphia, J. B. Lippincott, 1978.

56. Dobyns, J. H., et al.: Traumatic instability of the wrist. In American Academy of Orthopaedic Surgeons: Instructional Course Lectures, Vol. 24, St. Louis, C. V. Mosby, 1975.

57. Dornan, A.: The results of treatment of Kienböck's disease. J. Bone Joint Surg., 31B:518, 1949.

58. Dowling, J. J., and Sawyer, B., Jr.: Comminuted Colles' fractures. Evaluation of a method of treatment. J. Bone Joint Surg., 43A:657, 1961.

59. Dunn, A. W.: Fractures and dislocations of the carpus. Surg. Clin. North Am., 52:1513, 1972.

60. Durbin, F. C.: Nonunion of the triquetrum. J. Bone Joint Surg., 32B:388, 1950.

61. Engkvist, O., and Lundborg, G.: Rupture of the extensor pollicis longus tendon after fracture of the lower end of the radius. A clinical and microangiographic study. Hand, 11:76, 1979.

62. Fenton, R. L.: The naviculo-capitate fracture syndrome. J. Bone Joint Surg., 38A:681, 1956.

63. Fenton, R. L., and Rosen, H.: Fracture of the capitate bone: Report of two cases. Bull. Hosp. Joint Dis., 11:134, 1950.

64. Fernandez, D. L.: Correction of post-traumatic wrist deformity in adults by osteotomy, bone-grafting and internal fixation. J. Bone Joint Surg., 64A:1164, 1982.

65. Finochietto, R.: Retracción de Volkmann de los músculos intrínsecos de las manos. Bol. Trab. Soc. Cir. Buenos Aires, 4:31, 1920.

66. Fisk, G.: Carpal instability and the fractured scaphoid. Ann. R. Coll. Surg., 46:63, 1970.

67. Forgon, M., and Mammel, E.: The external fixateur in the management of unstable Colles' fracture. Int. Orthop., 5:9, 1981.

68. Frykman, G.: Fractures of the distal radius including sequelae—shoulder-hand-finger syndrome, disturbance in the distal radio-ulnar joint and impairment of nerve function. A clinical and experimental study. Acta Orthop. Scand. (Suppl.), 108, 1967.

69. Frykman, G. K., et al.: Pulsing electromagnetic field treatment of nonunions of the scaphoid. A preliminary report. Orthop. Trans., 6:160, 1982.

70. Ganel, A., et al.: Bone scanning in the assessment of fractures of the scaphoid. J. Hand Surg., 4:541, 1979.

71. Gartland, J. J., and Werley, C. W.: Evaluation of healed Colles' fractures. J. Bone Joint Surg., 33A:895, 1951.

72. Gelberman, R. H., and Menon, J.: The vascularity of the scaphoid bone. J. Hand Surg., 5:508, 1980.

73. Gentaz, R., et al.: La maladie de Kienböck approche tomographique: Analyse de 5 cas. Nouv. Presse Med., 1:1207, 1972.

74. Gilford, W. W., Bolton, R. H., and Lambrinudi, C.: The mechanism of the wrist joint, with special reference to fractures of the scaphoid. Guy's Hosp. Rep., 92:52, 1943.

75. Gillespie, H. S.: Excision of the lunate bone in Kienböck's disease. J. Bone Joint Surg., 43B:245, 1961.

76. Golden, G. N.: Treatment and prognosis of Colles' fracture. Lancet, 1:511, 1963.

77. Gonçalves, D.: Correction of disorders of the distal radioulnar joint by artificial pseudoarthrosis of the ulna. J. Bone Joint Surg., 56B:462, 1974.

78. Graner, O., et al.: Arthrodesis of the carpal bones in the treatment of Kienböck's disease, painful ununited fractures of the navicular and lunate bones with avascular necrosis, and old fracture-dislocations of carpal bones. J. Bone Joint Surg., 48A:767, 1966.

79. Green, D. P.: Pins and plaster treatment of comminuted fractures of the distal end of the radius. J. Bone Joint Surg., 57A:304, 1975.

80. Green D. P.: Carpal dislocations. In Green, D. P. (ed.): Operative Hand Surgery, Vol. 1, New York, Churchill Livingstone, 1982.

81. Green, D. P., and O'Brien, E. T.: Classification and management of carpal dislocation. Clin. Orthop., 149:55, 1980.

82. Greene, M. H., and Hadied, A. M.: Bipartite hamulus with ulnar tunnel syndrome. Case report and literature review. J. Hand Surg., 6:605, 1981.

83. Griffin, T. W., Jr., and Huster, R. H.: Rush rod fixation of Colles' fracture in the elderly. J. Bone Joint Surg., 57A:1030, 1975.

84. Hammond, G.: Comminuted Colles' fracture. Am. J. Surg., 78:617, 1949.

85. Hannington-Kiff, J. G.: Relief of Sudeck's atrophy by regional intravenous guanethidine. Lancet, 1:1132, 1977.

86. Harris, C., Jr., and Riordan, D. C.: Intrinsic contracture in the hand and its surgical treatment. J. Bone Joint Surg., 36A:10, 1954.

87. Hartz, C. R., and Beckenbaugh, R. D.: Long-term results of resection of the distal ulna for post-traumatic conditions. J. Trauma, 19:219, 1979.

88. Heim, U., and Pfeiffer, K. M.: Small Fragment Set Manual: Technique Recommended by the ASIF Group, New York, Springer-Verlag, 1974.

89. Henry, M. G.: Fractures of the carpal scaphoid bone in industry and in the military service. Arch. Surg., 48:278, 1944.

90. Herbert, T. J.: Management of the fractured scaphoid bone using a new surgical technique. Orthop. Trans., 6:464, 1982.

91. Herndon, J. N., et al.: A long-term evaluation of 607 cases of lunate and scaphoid arthroplasty. Presented at the 32nd Annual Meeting of the American Society for Surgery of the Hand, Las Vegas, 1977.

92. Hill, N. A.: Fractures and dislocations of the carpus. Orthop. Clin. North Am., 1:275, 1970.

93. Hobart, M. H., and Kraft, G. L.: Malunited Colles' fracture. Am. J. Surg., 53:55, 1941.

94. Hultén, O.: Über anatomische Varationen der Handgelenkknochen. Acta Radiol. Scand., 9:155, 1928.

95. Hunt, D. D.: Dislocation of the extensor pollicis longus tendon in Smith's fracture of the radius. A case report. J. Bone Joint Surg., 51A:991, 1969.

96. Jaekle, R. F., and Clark, A. G.: Acute fractures of the carpal scaphoid. Surg. Gynecol. Obstet., 68:820, 1939.

97. Jahna, H.: Behandlung und Behandlungsergebnisse von 734 Frischen einfachen Brüchen des Kahnbeinkörpers der hand. Wien. Med. Wochensch., 51/52:1023, 1954.

98. Jahna, H.: Erfahrungen und nachuntersuchungser gebnisse von 47 de Quervainschen verrenkungsbrüchen. Arch. Orthop. Unfallchir., 57:51, 1965.

99. Johnson, R. P.: The acutely injured wrist and its residuals. Clin. Orthop., 149:33, 1980.

100. Johnston, H. M.: Varying positions of the carpal bones in the different movements of the wrist. Part I. Extension, ulnar and radial flexion. J. Anat., 41:109, 1907.

101. Jonsson, G.: Aseptic bone necrosis of the os capitatum. Acta Radiol., 23:562, 1942.

102. Jørgensen, T. M., et al.: Scanning and radiology of the carpal scaphoid bone. Acta Orthop. Scand., 50:663, 1979.
103. Kapandji, A.: L'ostéosynthèse par double embrochage intra-focal. Traitement fonctionnel des fractures non articulaires de l'extrémité inférieure du radius. Ann. Chir., 30:903, 1976.
104. Kimmel, R. B., and O'Brien, E. T.: Surgical treatment of avascular necrosis of the proximal pole of the capitate. Case report. J. Hand Surg., 7:284, 1982.
105. Kleinert, H. E., Wayne, L., and Kutz, J. E.: Post-traumatic sympathetic dystrophy. Orthop, Clin. North Am., 4:917, 1973.
106. Kleinman, W. B., Steichen, J. B., and Strickland, J. W.: Management of chronic rotary subluxation of the scaphoid by scaphotrapezio-trapezoid arthrodesis. J. Hand Surg., 7:25, 1982.
107. Knapp, M. E.: Treatment of some complications of Colles' fracture. J.A.M.A., 148:825, 1952.
108. Kristiansen, A., and Gjersøe, E.: Colles' fracture. Operative treatment, indications and results. Acta Orthop. Scand., 39:33, 1968.
109. Landsmeer, J. M.: Studies in the anatomy of articulation. I. The equilibrium of the "intercalated" bone. Acta Morphol. Nederl. Scand., 3:287, 1961.
110. Lankford, L. L.: Reflex sympathetic dystrophy. In Green, D. P. (ed.): Operative Hand Surgery, Vol. 1. New York, Churchill Livingstone, 1982.
111. Lichtman, D. M., and Alexander, C. E.: Decision making in scaphoid nonunion. Orthop. Rev., 11:55, 1982.
112. Lichtman, D. M., et al.: Ulnar midcarpal instability. Clinical and laboratory analysis. J. Hand Surg., 6:515, 1981.
113. Linscheid, R. L.: Injuries to radial nerve at wrist. Arch. Surg., 91:942, 1965.
114. Linscheid, R. L., et al.: Traumatic instability of the wrist: Diagnosis, classification and pathomechanics. J. Bone Joint Surg., 54A:1612, 1972.
115. Littler, J. W.: The physiologic and dynamic function of the hand. Surg. Clin. North Am., 40:259, 1960.
116. London, P. S.: The broken scaphoid bone. The case against pessimism. J. Bone Joint Surg., 43B:237, 1961.
117. Lowry, W. E., and Cord, S. A.: Traumatic avascular necrosis of the capitate bone. Case report. J. Hand Surg., 6:245, 1981.
118. Lucas, G. L., and Sachtjen, K. M.: An analysis of hand function in patients with Colles' fracture treated by Rush rod fixation. Clin. Orthop., 155:172, 1981.
119. Lynch, A. C., and Lipscomb, P. R.: The carpal tunnel syndrome and Colles' fractures. J.A.M.A., 185:363, 1963.
120. MacAusland, W. R.: Perilunar dislocation of the carpal bones and dislocation of the lunate bone. Surg. Gynecol. Obstet., 79:256, 1944.
121. MacFarlane, J. A., and Thomas, R. H.: Fixed skeletal traction in the treatment of certain fractures at the wrist. Can. Med. Assoc. J., 36:10, 1937.
122. Marek, F. M.: Avascular necrosis of the carpal lunate. Clin. Orthop., 10:96, 1957.
123. Marsh, H. O., and Teal, S. W.: Treatment of comminuted fractures of the distal radius with self-contained skeletal traction. Am. J. Surg., 124:715, 1972.
124. Mason, M. L.: Colles' fracture. A survey of end-results. Br. J. Surg., 40:340, 1953.
125. Mayfield, J. K.: Mechanism of carpal injuries. Clin. Orthop., 149:451, 1980.
126. Mazet, R., and Hohl, M.: Conservative treatment of old fractures of the carpal scaphoid. J. Trauma, 1:115, 1961.
127. Mazet, R., and Hohl, M.: Fractures of the carpal navicular: Analysis of 91 cases and review of the literature. J. Bone Joint Surg., 45A:82, 1963.
128. McMaster, P. E.: Late ruptures of extensor and flexor pollicis longus tendons following Colles' fracture. J. Bone Joint Surg., 14:93, 1932.
129. Meadoff, N.: Median nerve injuries in fractures in the region of the wrist. Calif. Med., 70:252, 1949.
130. Meyers, M. H., Wills, R., and Harvey, J. P.: Naviculo-capitate fracture syndrome: Review of the literature and case report. J. Bone Joint Surg., 53A:1383, 1971.
131. Milch, H.: Fracture of the hamate bone. J. Bone Joint Surg., 16:459, 1934.
132. Milch, H.: Cuff resection of the ulna for malunited Colles' fracture. J. Bone Joint Surg., 23:311, 1941.
133. Milch, H.: So-called dislocation of the lower end of the ulna. Ann. Surg., 16:282, 1942.
134. Milch, H.: Treatment of disabilities following fractures of the lower end of the radius. Clin. Orthop., 29:157, 1963.
135. Milford, L.: The hand. In Edmonson, A. S., and Crenshaw, A. H. (eds.): Campbell's Operative Orthopaedics, 6th ed., Vol. 1, St. Louis, C. V. Mosby, 1980.
136. Moberg, E.: The shoulder-hand-finger syndrome as a whole. Acta Chir. Scand., 109:284, 1955.
137. Moberg, E.: The shoulder-hand-finger syndrome. Surg. Clin. North Am., 40:367, 1960.
138. Moberg, E.: Shoulder-hand-finger syndrome, reflex dystrophy. Causalgia. Acta Chir. Scand., 125:523, 1963.
139. Moneim, M. S.: The tangential posteroanterior radiograph to demonstrate scapholunate dissociation. J. Bone Joint Surg., 63A:1324, 1981.
140. Morawa, L. G., Ross, P. M., and Schock, C. C.: Fractures and dislocations involving the navicular-lunate axis. Clin. Orthop., 118:48, 1976.
141. Morrissy, R. T., and Nalebuff, E. A.: Distal radial fracture with tendon entrapment. A case report. Clin. Orthop., 124:205, 1977.
142. Mouchet, A.: Fractures isolées due scaphoïde carpien. Presse Med., 6:122, 1934.
143. Mulder, J. D.: Pseudoarthrosis of the scaphoid bone (abstract). J. Bone Joint Surg., 45B:621, 1963.
144. Murray, W. T., et al.: Fracture of the hook of the hamate. Am. J. Roentgenol., 133:899, 1979.
145. Newman, J. H., and Watt, J.: Avascular necrosis of the capitate and dorsiflexion instability. Hand, 12:176, 1980.
146. Newmeyer, W. L., and Green, D. P.: Rupture of digital extensor tendons following distal ulnar resection. J. Bone Joint Surg., 64:178, 1982.
147. Nisenfield, F. G., and Neviaser, R. J.: Fracture of the hook of the hamate. A diagnosis easily missed. J. Trauma, 14:612, 1974.
148. Nonnenmacher, J., Wagnon, J., and Kempf, I.: Notra conception actuelle du traitemente des fractures du poignet par compression-extension de l'adulte. Acta Orthop. Belg., 47:870, 1981.
149. Nonnenmacher, J., et al.: Traitement des fractures du poignet per brochage dynamique. Acta Orthop. Belg., 47:877, 1981.
150. Omer, G. E., and Thomas, S. R.: The management of chronic pain syndromes in the upper extremity. Clin. Orthop. 104:37, 1974.
151. O'Rahilly, R.: A survey of carpal and tarsal anomalies. J. Bone Joint Surg., 35A:626, 1953.
152. Palmer, A. K., Dobyns, J. H., and Linscheid, R. L.: Management of post-traumatic instability of the wrist secondary to ligament rupture. J. Hand Surg., 3:507, 1978.
153. Palmieri, T. J.: Pisiform area pain treatment by pisiform excision. J. Hand Surg., 7:477, 1982.
154. Pennsylvania Orthopedic Society, Scientific Research Committee: Evaluation of treatment for non-union of the carpal navicular. J. Bone Joint Surg., 44A:169, 1962.
155. Perschl, L.: Zur röntgenologischen Diagnostik der frischen Kahnbeinbrüche der Hand. Roentgenpraxis, 10:11, 1938.
156. Persson, M.: Causal treatment of lunatomalacia. Further experiences of operative ulna lengthening. Acta Chir. Scand., 100:531, 1950.
157. Porter, J. M., et al.: Effect of intra-arterial injection of reserpine on vascular wall catecholamine content. Surg. Forum, 22:183, 1972.
158. Rand, J. A., Linscheid, R. L., and Dobyns, J. H.: Capitate fractures: A long-term follow-up. Clin. Orthop., 165:209, 1982.
159. Rasquin, C., et al.: Traitement des fractures du poignet par fixateur externe. Indications et premiers résultats. Acta Orthop. Belg., 45:678, 1979.
160. Rauis, A., et al.: Bipolar fixation of fractures of the distal end of the radius. Int. Orthop., 3:89, 1976.
161. Reagan, D. S., Linscheid, R. L., and Dobyns, J. H.: The lunotriquetral sprain. Presented at the 36th Annual Meeting of the American Society for Surgery of the Hand, Las Vegas, 1981.

162. Rehbein, F.: Zur konservativen Behandlund der veralteten Kahnbeinbrüches und der Kahnbeinpseudarthrose der Hand. Arch. Klin. Chir., 260:356, 1948.
163. Rijnders, W., and Gerritse, R.: The use of regional intravascular sympathetic (R.I.S.) block with guanethidine (Ismelin) as an adjunct to the treatment of post-traumatic disturbances of function of the hand. Presented at the 37th Annual Meeting of the American Society for Surgery of the Hand. New Orleans, 1982.
164. Roth, F. B.: Aseptic necrosis of the lunate bone: A case report with a study of the pathological changes. J Bone Joint Surg., 25:683, 1943.
165. Rothberg, A. S.: Fractures of the carpal navicular. Importance of special roentgenography. J. Bone Joint Surg., 21:1020, 1939.
166. Russe, O.: Behandlungsengebnisse der spongiosaauffüllung bei Kahnbeinpseudarthrosen. Z. Orthop., 81:466, 1951.
167. Russe, O.: Fracture of the carpal navicular. Diagnosis, nonoperative treatment and operative treatment. J. Bone Joint Surg., 42A:759, 1960.
168. Russell, T. B.: Intracarpal dislocations and fracture dislocations. A review of fifty-nine cases. J. Bone Joint Surg., 31B:524, 1949.
169. Sarmiento, A.: The brachioradialis as a deforming force in Colles' fractures. Functional bracing in supination. J. Bone Joint Surg., 57A:311, 1965.
170. Sarmiento, A., et al.: Colles' fractures. Functional bracing in supination. J. Bone Joint Surg., 57A:311, 1975.
171. Sashin, D.: Treatment of fractures of the carpal scaphoid. A report of sixty-four cases. Arch. Surg., 52:445, 1946.
172. Scheck, M.: Long-term follow-up of treatment of comminuted fractures of the distal end of the radius by transfixion with Kirschner wires and cast. J. Bone Joint Surg., 44A:337, 1962.
173. Shea, J. D., and McClain, E. J.: Ulnar nerve compression syndrome at and below the wrist. J. Bone Joint Surg., 51:1095, 1969.
174. Shively, J. L., and Lesnick, D. S.: Distal radius fracture with tendon entrapment. Orthopaedics, 5:1330, 1982.
175. Siegel, R. S., and Weiden, I.: Combined median and ulnar nerve lesions complicating fractures of the distal radius and ulna. Two case reports. J. Trauma, 8:1114, 1968.
176. Simmons, E. H., and Dommissee, G.: An investigation into the pathogenesis and treatment of Kienböck's disease. Presented at the 35th Annual Meeting of the American Society for Surgery of the Hand, Atlanta, 1980.
177. Smaill, G. B.: Long-term follow-up of Colles' fracture. J. Bone Joint Surg., 47B:80, 1965.
178. Smith, B. L.: Treatment of comminuted distal radius fractures using pins and plaster. Contemp. Orthop., 3:629, 1981.
179. Smith, F. M.: Late rupture of extensor pollicis longus tendon following Colles' fracture. J. Bone Joint Surg., 28:49, 1946.
180. Smith, R. J.: Intrinsic muscles of the fingers. Function, dysfunction and surgical reconstruction. In American Academy of Orthopaedic Surgeons: Instructional Course Lectures, Vol. 24, St. Louis, C. V. Mosby, 1975.
181. Smith, R. J.: Intrinsic contracture. In Green, D. P. (ed.): Operative Hand Surgery, Vol. 1, New York, Churchill Livingstone, 1982.
182. Soto-Hall, R., and Haldeman, K. O.: The conservative and operative treatment of fractures of the carpal scaphoid (navicular). J. Bone Joint Surg., 23:841, 1941.
183. Speed, K.: Fractures and dislocations of the carpus. Calif. Med., 72:93, 1950.
184. Spinner, M., et al.: Impending ischemic contracture of the hand. Early diagnosis and management. Plast. Reconstr. Surg., 50:341, 1972.
185. Sponsel, K.: Colles' fracture. Minn. Med., 47:175, 1964.
186. Sponsel, K. H., and Palm, E. T.: Carpal tunnel syndrome following Colles' fracture. Surg. Gynecol. Obstet., 121:1252, 1965.
187. Sprague, B., and Justis, E. J.: Nonunion of the carpal navicular: Modes of treatment. Arch. Surg., 108:692, 1974.
188. Ståhl, F.: On lunatomalacia (Kienböck's disease): Clinical and roentgenological study, especially on its pathogenesis and late results of immobilization treatment. Acta Chir. Scand. (Suppl.), 126:1, 1947.

189. Stark, H. H., et al.: Fracture of the hook of the hamate in athletes. J. Bone Joint Surg., 59A:575, 1977.
190. Stecher, W. R.: Roentgenography of the carpal navicular bone. Am. J. Roentgenol., 37:704, 1937.
191. Stein, A. H., and Katz, S. F.: Stabilization of communited fractures of the distal inch of the radius: Percutaneous pinning. Clin. Orthop., 108:174, 1975.
192. Stein, F., and Siegel, M. W.: Naviculocapitate fracture syndrome. A case report: New thoughts of the mechanism of injury. J. Bone Joint Surg., 51A:391, 1969.
193. Steinbrocker, O.: The shoulder-hand syndrome. Am. J. Med., 3:402, 1947.
194. Steinbrocker, O., and Argyros, T. G.: The shoulder-hand syndrome: Present status as a diagnostic and therapeutic entity. Med. Clin. North Am., 46:1533, 1958.
195. Stewart, M. J.: Fractures of the carpal navicular (scaphoid): A report of 436 cases. J. Bone Joint Surg., 36A:998, 1954.
196. Swanson, A. B.: Silicone rubber implants for the replacement of the carpal scaphoid and lunate bones. Orthop. Clin. North Am., 1:299, 1970.
197. Swanson, A. B.: Implant arthroplasty for disabilities of the distal radioulnar joint. Use of a silicone rubber capping implant following resection of the ulnar head. Orthop. Clin. North Am., 4:373, 1973.
198. Taleisnik, J.: The ligaments of the wrist. J. Hand Surg., 1:110, 1976.
199. Taleisnik, J.: Wrist, anatomy, function, and injury. In American Academy of Orthopaedic Surgeons: Instructional Course Lectures, Vol. 27, St. Louis, C. V. Mosby, 1978.
200. Taleisnik, J.: Post-traumatic carpal instability. Clin. Orthop., 149:73, 1980.
201. Taleisnik, J.: Fractures of the carpal bones. In Green, D. P. (ed.): Operative Hand Surgery, Vol. 1, New York, Churchill Livingstone, 1982.
202. Taleisnik, J., and Kelly, P. J.: The extraosseous and intraosseous blood supply of the scaphoid bone. J. Bone Joint Surg., 48A:1125, 1966.
203. Taleisnik, J., Malerich, M., and Prietto, M.: Palmar carpal instability secondary to dislocation of scaphoid and lunate: Report of case and review of the literature. J. Hand Surg., 7:606, 1982.
204. Tanz, S. S.: Rotation effect in lunar and perilunar dislocation. Clin. Orthop., 57:147, 1968.
205. Tanzer, L., and Horne, J. G.: Dorsal radiocarpal fracture dislocation. J. Trauma, 20:999, 1980.
206. Terry, D. W., and Ramin, J. E.: The navicular fat strip: A useful roentgen feature for evaluating wrist trauma. Am. J. Roentgenol., 124:25, 1975.
207. Thomas, F. B.: Reduction of Smith's fracture. J. Bone Joint Surg., 39B:463, 1957.
208. Thomas, T. H., and Mathewson, M. H.: Habitual anterior subluxation of the head of the ulna treated by Baldwin's operation. A case report. Hand, 14:67, 1982.
209. Thompson, T. C., Campbell, R. D., Jr., and Arnold, W. D.: Primary and secondary dislocation of the scaphoid bone. J. Bone Joint Surg., 46B:73, 1964.
210. Thorndike, A., Jr., and Garrey, W. E.: Fractures of the carpal scaphoid. N. Engl. J. Med., 222:827, 1940.
211. Torisu, T.: Fracture of the hook of the hamate by a golf swing. Clin. Orthop., 83:91, 1972.
212. Trevor, D.: Rupture of the extensor pollicis longus tendon after Colles' fracture. J. Bone Joint Surg., 32B:370, 1950.
213. Trojan, E.: Grafting of ununited fractures of the scaphoid. Proc. R. Soc. Med., 67:1078, 1974.
214. Turner, J.: Über nervenschädigungen beim typischen radiusbruch. Arch. Klin. Chir., 128:422, 1924.
215. Vance, R. M., Gelberman, R. H., and Evans, E. F.: Scaphocapitate fractures: Patterns of dislocation, mechanism of injury, and preliminary results of treatment. J. Bone Joint Surg., 62A:271, 1980.
216. Van der Linden, W., and Ericson, R.: Colles' fracture. How should its displacement be measured and how should it be immobilized? J. Bone Joint Surg., 63A:1285, 1931.
217. Wagner, C. J.: Perilunar dislocations. J. Bone Joint Surg., 38A:1198, 1956.
218. Wagner, C. J.: Fracture-dislocations of the wrist. Clin. Orthop., 15:181, 1959.

219. Watson, H. K.: Personal communication, 1980.
220. Watson, H. K., Goodman, M. L., and Johnson, T. R.: Limited arthrodesis. Part II: Intracarpal and radiocarpal combinations. J. Hand Surg., 6:223, 1981.
221. Watson, H. K., and Hempton, R. F.: Limited wrist arthrodesis. I. The triscaphoid joint. J. Hand Surg., 5:320, 1980.
222. Watson-Jones, R.: Fractures and Joint Injuries, 4th ed., Vol. 2, Baltimore, Williams & Wilkins, 1960.
223. Weber, E. R.: Biomechanical implications of scaphoid waist fractures. Clin. Orthop., 149:83, 1980.
224. Weinberg, E. D.: Late spontaneous rupture of the extensor pollicis longus tendon following Colles' fracture. J.A.M.A., 142:979, 1950.
225. Wissinger, H. A.: Resection of the hook of the hamate. Plast. Reconstr. Surg., 56:501, 1975.
226. Youm, Y., et al.: Kinematics of the wrist. I. An experimental study of radioulnar deviation and flexion-extension. J. Bone Joint Surg., 60A:423, 1978.
227. Zancolli, E. A.: Structural and Dynamic Bases of Hand Surgery, 2nd ed., Philadephia, J. B. Lippincott, 1979.
228. Zoëga, H.: Fractures of the lower end of the radius with ulnar nerve palsy. J. Bone Joint Surg., 48B:514, 1966.

17

COMPLICATIONS FOLLOWING AMPUTATIONS OF PARTS OF THE HAND

Paul W. Brown

The surgeon has three goals in dealing with wounded hands: the preservation or restoration of function, comfort or the absence of pain, and as normal an appearance as possible. These objectives are brought into particularly sharp focus when the wound includes amputation of digits or anticipation of amputation. It is seldom possible to achieve all three: Almost always one can be achieved—occasionally two, but very rarely all three. Priorities for each must be assigned; these will depend on many variables, each of which must be given a relative value. These include the nature of the wound, which digits are involved, dominant or nondominant hand, and the nature of the patient and his particular requirements. The patient's requirements will vary with age, sex, vocation, avocation, personality, ethnic and culture factors, and the patient's own assessment of such intangibles as beauty and disability. Economic factors may necessarily influence surgical decisions. Least tangible, most abstract, and most important is the patient's motivation to return the hand to useful function.

Some patients will be quite practical about the matter, and will pragmatically elect function over appearance if a choice must be made. Others will be adamant in demanding that all digits be preserved, even though they will be without function and may handicap the remainder of the hand. To them appearance and body image—often based on ethnic values—are more important than function. The choice is difficult: the patient must be a party to it but may be poorly equipped for this while in a state of emotional shock and fresh from the scene of the accident. Pressure from relatives and vain hopes for surgical miracles may influence both the patient and the surgeon. Unless the indications for amputation, or acceptance of amputations already

incurred, are very clear and mutually agreed on, it is better to try to preserve or to reattach parts and to make definitive decisions later, when perspectives are clear and emotionalism has subsided.

Complications of amputations of the hand may be caused by attempting to save too much or too little, by improperly selecting an appropriate level of amputation, or by problems concerning the amputation stump itself.

SAVING TOO MUCH

Severed digits may be reattached provided several criteria are met. The patient must agree to it, having first understood what is entailed in the surgery and its possible risks and complications. The amputations must have been incurred no more than 12 hours previously, and the severed parts must have been kept clean and iced. The state of the digits of the hand must be compatible with reattachment; severe crush and mangling injuries detract from the chance of successful revascularization and useful function. There must be a trained microsurgical team immediately available, as well as adequate operating and nursing facilities. Compromise on any of these points will lead to complications: digits that do not survive; danger of infection to the rest of the hand; digits that will not function, entailing a protracted hospital stay and added expense; and, above all, a delay in early return of the injured hand to useful function.

Most hands, except for those of some professionals such as musicians, can perform all functions well lacking a finger or two. A common complication of digital reattachment is a viable but poorly functioning finger that impedes manual function. The deci-

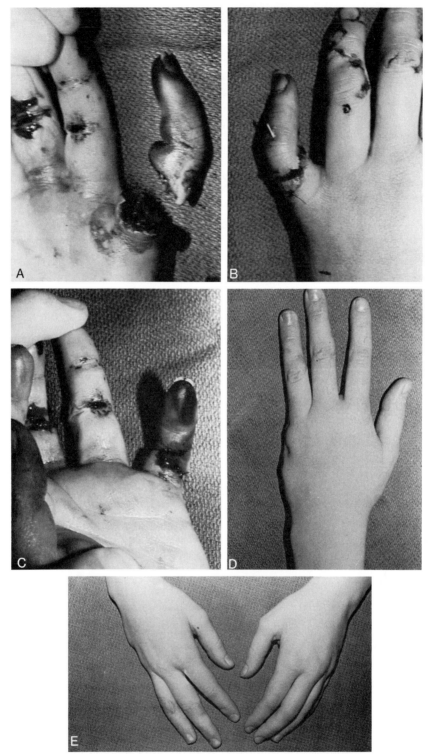

Figure 17–1. *A,* This young woman amputated her small finger in an automobile accident, and despite advice to the contrary, she strongly argued for reattachment; *B,* reattachment was accomplished, and the finger maintained good circulation for 3 days, but circulation became deficient on the third day despite attempts to re-establish blood flow; *C,* by the sixth day it was obvious the finger was non-viable; *D,* resection of the distal two thirds of the fifth metacarpal was done; *E,* the patient reported that "no one notices that I'm missing my left small finger." She has modified her typing and piano playing successfully, and there is no significant functional loss.

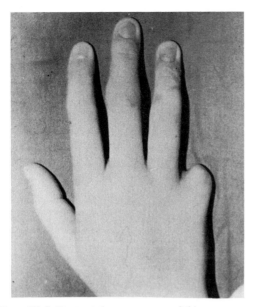

Figure 17–2. Contrast the appearance of this young woman's hand with that shown in Figure 17–1. The missing finger is obvious. Resection of the fifth metacarpal gives a better appearance than retention of a stump, which serves no useful purpose except for those whose hands require maximum strength and leverage in gripping tools such as heavy wrenches and shovels.

sion to reattach parts should be preceded by a realistic appraisal of the alternative—a projection of what the functional and cosmetic result would be if the amputation were accepted and the hand returned to early use.

Successful reattachment of single digits, thumbs excepted, usually represent a triumph of technique over judgment. Rarely do reattached fingers function well enough to be smoothly incorporated into hand coordination, and rarely do they serve the hand as well as it would function without the impaired finger.

There is considerable question as to how short a finger can be and still be useful. If appearance is paramount, one can accept salvage of a distal segment with poor sensibility, motion, or comfort. If function is given precedence, then it is better to have a shorter finger with good sensibility. A common complication is the fingertip or distal segment that is badly damaged but still viable, which becomes a clumsy detriment to the hand.

A finger with at least half of the middle phalanx and useful proximal interphalangeal joint flexion is a useful digit if the stump is comfortable and has good sensibility. Index and little finger stumps shorter than that represent functional complications; most such hands are better served by resection of the entire digit and of two thirds of the metacarpal (Fig. 17–1). Many patients find short index and

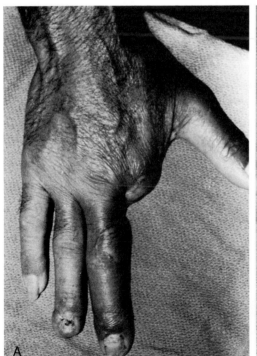

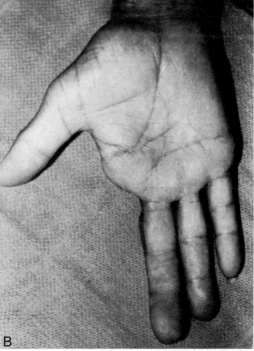

Figure 17–3. *A, B,* Hand of a male laborer whose right index finger had been destroyed in a crush injury and amputated through the metacarpophalangeal joint. He found the second metacarpal head something of a nuisance, because "I'm always bumping it on something." The hand would look better and be more dextrous if the distal two thirds of the second metacarpal were resected, but strength of grasp would be somewhat diminished. For this patient's occupation, which entails lifting heavy castings, ray resection would probably be a mistake.

small finger stumps a nuisance. They should be considered as minor complications, easily remedied.

Retention of proximal segments of any of the fingers is generally not advisable, except in those who require great strength of grasp in their work (Fig. 17–2). Disarticulation of the index or little finger through the metacarpophalangeal joint results in a knob (the metacarpal head), which is unattractive and is constantly being bruised (Fig. 17–3). Metacarpophalangeal disarticulation of the middle or ring fingers causes a hole in the hand, a minor problem to which most patients accommodate well (Figs. 17–4 and 17–5). The gap decreases as the adjacent fingers gradually lean toward each other.

Thumbs have a higher priority for salvage than other digits but the same basic principle applies: better a short comfortable stump with good sensibility than a longer unhappy one. There is a common misconception that thumb length must be preserved at all costs; this philosophy leads to complications of poorly functioning thumb stumps. Patients with such stumps, which are shortened and covered with good skin, will quickly return the hand to good function, and consistently report that they can use the shortened thumb much better than they could the longer but unsatisfactory thumb (Fig. 17–6).

PAINFUL AMPUTATION STUMPS

Patients who are well motivated to use their hands quickly accommodate to a comfortable amputation stump. Within a month or so of the amputation, the shortened digit is assimilated into normal hand function and coordination. Not so for the painful stump—as long as it remains painful it will never be useful. The patient will divorce the digit from all patterns of hand usage, and will develop defensive patterns of motor activity to protect the stump from the painful stimuli of touch and pressure. This not only will prolong rehabilitation of the damaged hand but will prevent the patient from ever using the hand well until the discomfort is relieved. Worse,

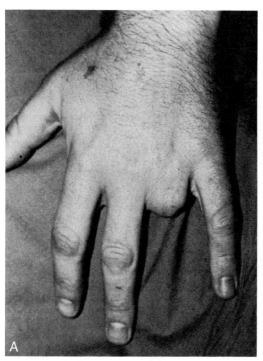
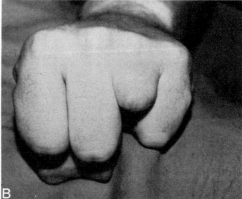
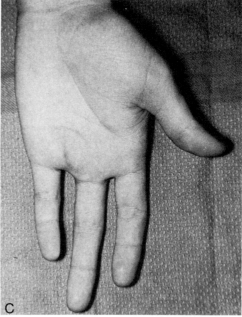

Figure 17–4. *A, B,* Hand of a male office worker who suffered a ring avulsion with amputation through the proximal phalanx of the ring finger—he felt that "the hole in my hand" was noticeable and a nuisance in that small objects such as coins "fell out"; *C,* resection of the stump of the head and neck of the fourth metacarpal allowed the two adjacent fingers to close the gap partially with better appearance and function.

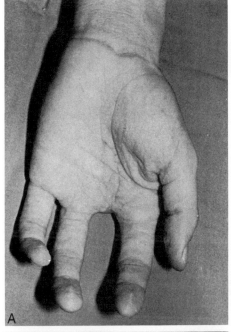
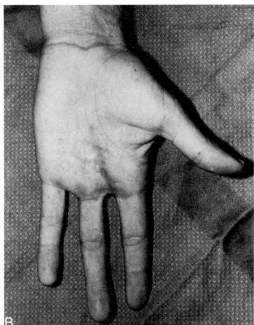
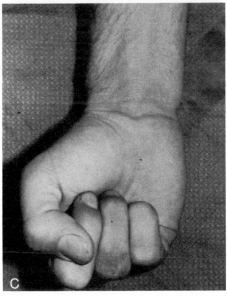

Figure 17-5. *A*, Hand of an electrician whose left middle finger had been disarticulated at the metacarpophalangeal joint following a gunshot wound of the finger—he was dissatisfied with the appearance, and complained of small objects falling out of his hand. *B, C,* The third metacarpal was removed through its base, and the second ray and index finger transposed. This patient reported that the missing finger was "noticed by no one," and that nuts and bolts no longer trickled out of his hand. He also found the narrow hand allowed him to work in tight spaces more easily.

it may lead to a fixed pain pattern—causalgia—and even to reflex sympathetic dystrophy.

The cause of the pain may be a neuroma that has formed at the severed end of the digital nerve, and that is generally adherent to the cicatrix at the end of the stump. Such neuromas tend to be larger and more bulbous than those that form at the end of digital nerves 1 or 2 cm proximal to the stump. Avoidance of this complication is simple enough. At the time of amputation the digital nerve should be transected at least 1 cm proximal to the amputation level, and even more proximal if it is anticipated that there will be much scarring in the stump.

The painful amputation neuroma is easy to diag-

nose. Usually the patient can point to a very discrete area of maximum sensitivity to percussion in the end of the stump. The eraser end of a lead pencil is useful as a percussion tool to localize the neuroma. Occasionally two painful neuromas will be found, one for each digital nerve.

Some amputation stumps will not have a specific point of tenderness but will be diffusely painful over the entire end of the stump, or even throughout the entire distal segment of a shortened digit. Such stumps are generally covered with rather poor quality skin, which is often thin and adherent to the underlying bone. Such a complication is generally the result of trying to preserve too much length at

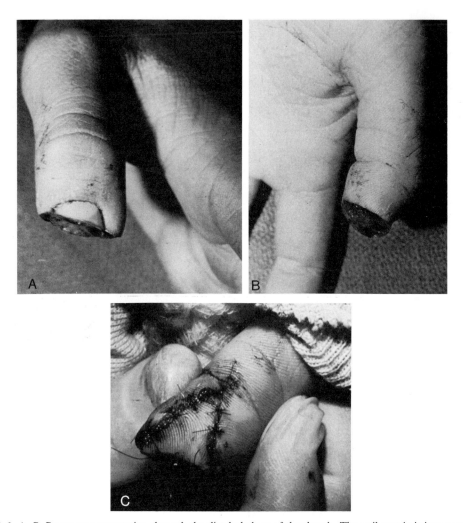

Figure 17–6. A, B, Power saw amputation through the distal phalanx of the thumb. The nail matrix is intact and the nail will regrow, but loss of the phalangeal tuft and the tactile pad deprives the growing nail of support—the nerve will curve volarward over the end of the stump. C, Distal advancement of a (V-Y) flap will gain some length and somewhat improve the situation. Such a local advancement flap should retain good sensibility; without good sensation the thumb stump could be functionally improved by shortening, covering the stump with normally sensible skin and sacrificing the nail.

the expense of coverage of the stump with good quality skin. A contributor to this type of painful stump is the split-thickness skin graft for the fingertip amputation, in which a portion of the distal phalanx is exposed and the graft has become adherent to the bone (Fig. 17–7). The problem may be improved by replacement of the poor quality skin with a full-thickness skin transfer. Shortening the finger for this complication would give a comfortable stump, but only at the expense of the fingernail.

More difficult pain problems arise from neuromas of the common digital nerves in hands in which amputation has extended into the metacarpals. A painful neuroma in the palm will cripple the entire hand, and the patient will tend to become very protective of the hand. Such a condition is more likely to progress to causalgia than the finger stump neuroma. The earlier the neuroma is localized and resected, the less chance there is of such a serious complication developing. Once the sequence of painful stimuli, defensive patterns, and reflex dystrophic changes have developed, removing the stimulus—that is, the painful neuroma—may no longer be adequate to break what has become a vicious circle. The mechanism for the development of this pattern is not well understood but personality factors seem to play a part, because the condition appears more frequently in patients with passive-aggressive traits, in insecure patients who hold themselves in poor esteem, and in patients who are poorly motivated to return to work. The well-motivated and well-adjusted patient may develop a painful neuroma in the palm, but seems to respond better to resection of the neuroma and will seldom develop the fixed pain patterns seen in causalgia.

DYSVASCULAR DIGITS

A fairly common complication of amputated digits that have been reattached is their intolerance to cold due to impaired vascularity or to a combination of impaired vascularity and sensibility. The reattached finger may be classified as a "success" because it has good motion and at least fair sensibility and appearance but may, nevertheless, remain a source of discomfort and annoyance to the patient during cold weather or when working in water. Even though blood supply is adequate to sustain viability, there is enough impairment in perfusion and sometimes in sympathetic response that the finger develops a condition similar to Raynaud's phenomenon. Whether the finger should be retained or amputated depends on the severity of symptoms, the functional impairment of the hand, and the patient's own assessment of the situation.

Digital stumps that have had severe vascular compromise, even though viable and functional, may develop the same problem. Such a stump is rarely a satisfactory one, and the complication is best dealt with by ray resection in the case of index or little fingers or by metacarpophalangeal disartic-

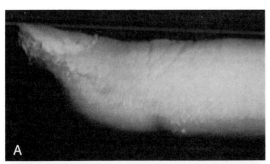
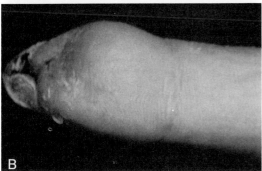

Figure 17–7. *A, B,* Oblique skiving injury of digit, with loss of most of tactile pad with bone and nail intact. This fingertip amputation was covered with split thickness skin, the worst of the possible choices. A more satisfactory stump would have resulted if the wound had been allowed to close by itself, by a local advancement flap, or by a cross finger flap.

ulation for middle or ring fingers. The dysvascular thumb stump is a more difficult problem; unless the symptoms are very severe, the stump is best accepted as it is. Experimental work on stripping sympathetic fibers from digital arteries offers some promise for decreasing the severity of cold sensitivity problems.

FINGERNAIL COMPLICATIONS

Transverse amputations through the fingertip, fingernail, and a portion of the bony phalangeal tuft create an amputation complication for which there is really no satisfactory answer. The stump will heal spontaneously or will heal with a skin graft, but the loss of length of the tactile pad leaves no base for the distal half of the nail, which continues to grow from the uninjured matrix and will curve volarward to form a hook or talon that interferes with function, is difficult to trim, catches on clothing, and is unsightly. The stump is made more functional by removing the nail and its matrix, but a cosmetic defect is created that may be unacceptable to the patient. Attempts to add to the length of the stump are seldom successful.

Amputations that cut through the nail base require the removal of the remainder of the nail and all of the matrix. The matrix must be entirely removed, dissecting down to the underlying bone. Often small pieces of matrix are retained that allow the regrowth of nail remnants. To remove these requires dissection to the bone and thorough curettage. Some recommend cauterization with phenol, but this is not too effective because it may delay healing of the wound.

ADAPTATION

Accommodation to loss of part of the hand is governed by many factors, some of which may be influenced by the surgeon and some of which may not. Acceptance of physical impairment depends to a large degree on the patient's personality. Some are devastated by finger loss and are quite literally crippled by it, while others accept it with aplomb and aggressively return their hand to useful function. Dependent types may equate impairment with disability, using it as an escape from unpleasant work or life situations. Payment of disability benefits often delays rehabilitation and return to work; the self-employed consistently return to work earlier than those whose income is assured as long as they are "disabled." Compensation boards, unions representing their members' "rights," and attorneys tend to exaggerate impairment, delay return to work, and impede adaptation by the patient. On the other hand, employers who are interested only in maximum production immediately on return to work are reluctant to allow an amputee to return until convinced that there is no significant disability or that there will not be an increased liability risk.

Employers who allow an injured worker to return to light work while still accommodating to the loss can markedly facilitate acceptance of the amputation by the worker, and thereby aid in rehabilitation.

Thus, the key to successful rehabilitation of a hand with missing digits is the patient's desire to use it, the motivation to return the hand to useful function. Motivation is a complex distillation of many personality traits; patients of strong character reject the concept of disability, whereas those of weaker makeup may welcome disability if they can use it as an escape from the unpleasant, a protection from a hostile environment, or an opportunity for reward. A common and sometimes avoidable complication of amputations of fingers is the patient who sees himself as crippled. There are many, however, who, with some guidance and stimulation from their physician, can be led, cajoled, or pushed into accepting their impaired hands as only inconvenient and not as a disability.

It is the responsibility of the surgeon to do everything possible to help the patient rehabilitate the hand. If involvement with the process ends with wound healing, the surgeon is merely a surgical technician but, if there is continued involvement with the patient's recovery until nothing more can be done, the surgeon is truly a physician. The surgeon will be disappointed with the outcome in some patients, and these will have unavoidable complications—but there will also be gratification from others who do return their hands to productivity as the result of both the surgeon's skills and interest in the end result; and these patients may well have had potential complications that never occurred.

Bibliography

Bertelsen, A., and Capener, N.: Fingers, compensation, and King Canute. J. Bone Joint Surg., 42B:390, 1960.

Brown, P. W.: The Role of motivation in patient recovery. Conn. Med., 42:555, 1978.

Brown, P. W.: Less than ten: A report from surgeons with missing fingers. J. Hand Surg., 71:31, 1982.

Brown, P. W.: The rational selection of alternatives in upper extremity amputation. Orthop. Clin. North Am., 12:843, 1981.

Chase, R. A.: The severely injured upper limb. To amputate or reconstruct: That is the question. Arch. Surg., 100:382, 1970.

Conolly, W. B., and Goulston, E.: Problems of digital amputation: A clinical review of 260 patients and 301 amputations. Aust. N. Z. J. Surg., 43:118, 1973.

Gruneberg, R., and Spence, A. J.: Finger amputations and the ability to work. Hand, 6:236, 1974.

Harvey, F. J., and Harvey, P.: A critical review of the results of primary finger and thumb amputations. Hand, 6:157, 1974.

Kleinert, H. E., Jablon, J., and Tsai, T. M.: An overview of replantation and results of 347 replants in 245 patients. J. Trauma, 20:390, 1980.

London, P. S.: Simplicity of approach to treatment of the injured hand. J. Bone Joint Surg., 43B:454, 1961.

Ratliff, A. H. C.: Amputation of the distal part of the thumb. Hand, 4:190, 1972.

Scott, F. A., and Howar, J. W.: Recovery of function following replantation and revascularization of amputated hand parts. Presented at the Annual Meeting of the American Association for the Surgery of Trauma, Phoenix, Arizona, February 19, 1980.

White, W. L.: Why I hate the index finger. Orthop. Rev., 9:23, 1980.

Wild, G. B.: Amputation hastens return to work. Occup. Health (Lond.), 24:97, 1972.

18

COMPLICATIONS FOLLOWING REPLANTATION AND REVASCULARIZATION

Frank A. Scott

Since the advent of microvascular surgery, guidelines for replantation and revascularization of amputated or severely injured extremities have been fairly well established. Advances in microsurgical techniques and instrumentation have led to relatively predictable survival rates. Several centers have reported survival rates between 85 and 95%.[1-5]

Recovery of hand function has been studied, and expectations following replantation are known.[4-8] Various objective criteria to evaluate hand function, such as active and passive range of motion, sensibility, and strength, demonstrate certain problems associated with the successful replantation or revascularization of these injured parts. Whether some of these problems should be considered to be complications, by strict definition, or to be fairly predictable end results, is an issue that is difficult to define. This chapter will discuss these complications and those measures that can be taken to minimize and improve loss of function.

In addition, several important questions should be considered. What constitutes a "good" result following replantation surgery? What should be considered a "complication"? What should be considered a "failure"? Each case must be considered on its own merit. A "good" result in one patient may not be considered acceptable in another individual, depending on motivation, occupation, and other social factors. Each patient's expectations are different.

The social costs of replantation must also be considered. These include wages lost, medical expenses, rehabilitation costs, insurance payments and premiums, and many other factors difficult to quantitate. Is the replantation effort going to improve overall hand function? The emphasis of replantation must be directed at recovery of function, as well as

survival. A sensate gripping hand, in most cases, is better than an upper extremity prosthesis. No replantation is without "complication." Most replantations, despite "complications," are functionally better than the equivalent amputation if the selection criteria and indications have been considered preoperatively.

Complications following replantation and revascularization may be divided into early complications, those that occur during the immediate postoperative period (within 2 weeks), and late complications, which include those criteria used to evaluate recovery of function.

EARLY COMPLICATIONS

Acute complications frequently manifest as failure of survival of revascularized tissue. Survival rates should be at least 80%, and most series reflect 80 to 90% survival rates.[1-5] Factors that affect survival rates include stringent patient selection, meticulous microsurgical techniques, including the more liberal use of vein grafts, and careful postoperative monitoring.[4, 5, 9, 10]

Arterial Insufficiency

A healthy replanted digit demonstrates a rapid capillary refill, pink color, and warmth. Skin temperature readings may be slightly increased compared to those of an adjacent uninjured digit, secondary to inflammation associated with the injury and ischemia. Acute arterial insufficiency is characterized by pale color, absent or diminished capillary refill, loss of tissue turgor, and a sudden drop in skin temperature. Skin temperature monitoring should be performed postoperatively, and readings should remain above 30° C. It has been shown that digits with temperatures below 30° C are not likely to survive.[11] Perfusion fluorometry is also being used to assess circulation, and can predict both arterial insufficiency and venous congestion before dermal changes become evident.[12] The fluorometer allows for an objective measurement of tissue fluorescence, requires a smaller dose of fluorescein, can monitor tissue elimination of dye (*e.g.,* as in venous congestion), and allows for repeated testing at close intervals.

Arterial insufficiency may be due to thrombosis at the anastomosis or vasospasm. The first 10 postoperative days are most critical. Over 80% of vascular occlusions occur within the first 2 days, although sporadic cases of vascular occlusion have been reported at day 12 and day 14.[13–15]

When signs of acute arterial insufficiency occur, the dressing should be checked for constriction, which may be secondary to hardened bloody drainage or secondary to an improperly applied dressing. The extremity should be lowered to below the heart level, and systemic status should be checked to rule out a peripheral vascular shutdown. This may be secondary to blood loss or to inadequate fluid intake. Vasospasm may be responsible for decreased peripheral perfusion secondary to cool room temperature, anxiety, nicotine, or caffeine. The latter two agents are restricted postoperatively, and the patient is hospitalized on strict bed rest in a warm room and kept relaxed. If vasospasm is suspected or the dressing needs to be changed in the first few days, a stellate ganglion block or peripheral nerve block should be performed to minimize sympathetic stimulation. I have monitored a skin temperature drop of 2° C associated only with a dressing change. Dressings should not be changed during the first 5 days, unless absolutely necessary. Indwelling catheters for continuous regional nerve block nerve anesthesia with concomitant sympathetic effect have been recommended.[16] These are used occasionally to minimize arterial spasm proximal to the anastomosis in an attempt to increase flow across the anastomosis.

If acute arterial insufficiency develops, the conservative measures discussed should be used. If these fail, the patient should be considered for return to the operating room, where all anastomoses should be explored. Re-exploration must be done as soon as possible after recognition of arterial inflow disturbance. This underlies the importance of skin temperature monitoring or fluorometry to detect early circulatory problems. Salvage after re-exploration has been reported to be from 34 to 50%.[15, 17] The longer the interval from replantation (*i.e.,* after 72 hours), the less likely re-exploration will benefit tissue survival. Similarly, if deterioration has been gradual, the salvage rate is less rewarding. At re-exploration, the thrombosed anastomosis should be excised, the vessel ends should be resected until normal intima and vessel wall are seen,

and reversed interposition vein grafts should be inserted. Another option is to harvest a vascular pedicle from an adjacent uninjured digit.

Another form of arterial insufficiency is manifested by the "no reflow" phenomenon. Despite a patent arterial anastomosis (intraoperatively or later), the distal capillary bed fails to open. The digit may revascularize initially, but progressive arterial insufficiency develops. This occurs most commonly in association with prolonged ischemia or crush injury. It is felt to be due to cellular swelling, intravascular coagulation, and increased interstitial fluid.

Postoperative anticoagulation protocols vary considerably, and it is impossible to verify the efficacy of various regimens with respect to survival rates. Many replantation centers utilize full heparinization, low-molecular-weight dextran, dipyridamole, or aspirin. In a sharp amputation, I feel that aspirin 10 gr twice daily is adequate. In crushing or avulsion injuries, full heparinization may be utilized. During the replantation procedure an intravenous heparin bolus, 3000 to 5000 units, is usually given at the completion of the first arterial anastomosis.

All the postoperative regimens discussed are essential to minimize the frequency of arterial insufficiency, but it must be emphasized that the primary factor responsible for a patent anastomosis is a technically perfect repair. Normal vessel ends must be accurately and atraumatically coapted, without tension. Tension at the anastomosis will frequently lead to thrombosis. Reversed vein graft interposition is indicated in any situation in which the vessel repair may be under tension. Vein grafts should not be inserted too long, because kinking may occur and thrombus develop.

Venous Insufficiency

Venous insufficiency manifests initially with very brisk capillary refill, a bright pink color that soon develops a bluish purple hue, and a more subtle but progressive drop in temperature. Leung has described a clinical sign to detect early venous congestion, called the "throbbing sign."[18] The replanted digit is lightly squeezed between the examiner's thumb and index finger. As the pressure is released and a pink color returns to the replanted digit, a throb can be palpated, secondary to adequate arterial inflow in the presence of poor venous outflow. Similar conservative measures should be instituted immediately on recognition of venous obstruction. Dressings should be noted for constriction or hardened blood, and alternate sutures may need to be removed and the extremity elevated. Indications for re-exploration are also similar to those for arterial occlusion. In the presence of progressive signs of venous insufficiency, all vascular anastomoses should be explored. Results following late exploration after several hours of venous congestion are not good.

The frequency of venous thrombosis versus arterial thrombosis has been variably reported. Morrison and O'Brien documented that arterial thrombosis was the cause of failure in 60% and venous thrombosis in 20% of cases.[13] Several other centers reported a higher frequency of venous thrombosis as a cause of replantation failure.[3, 19]

Infection

Infection following digital replantation is infrequent. In our series of 100 patients, no acute infections were noted, despite grossly contaminated injuries.[5] This is most likely because of thorough débridement, frequent irrigation, often for multiple hours during surgery, and loose closure of wounds. Prophylactic pre-, intra-, and postoperative antibiotics are also administered.

In major limb replantation, however, infection is a primary cause of failure. Myonecrosis with secondary infection may develop. Ischemia time is critical to minimize myonecrosis and its metabolic effects. Restoration of arterial input is of prime importance, even if a temporary shunt needs to be established while skeletal fixation is accomplished.[12] It also allows for assessment of distal muscle perfusion, which may lead to further débridement of questionable muscle tissue. Fasciotomies must always be performed in major limb replantation to prevent compartment syndrome and minimize myonecrosis. The most important factor in prevention of infection is thorough débridement of all nonviable tissue.

Bleeding

Postoperative hemorrhage has not been a major complication in my experience. Routine heparinization is not used with my patients, which is most likely responsible for excess postoperative bleeding. Aspirin 10 gr twice daily is the only form of anticoagulation routinely administered. Occasionally, in crushed or avulsed tissue that has been revascularized, in which the risk of thrombosis is greater, I will heparinize the patient. The dressing must be able to accommodate bleeding without causing constriction. Loose wound closure will also allow for drainage of blood. Ligation of significant bleeders prior to skin closure should also be performed.

Edema

A mild amount of edema is expected following replantation, secondary to local tissue injury, suboptimal venous drainage, and ischemic changes. Edema is most marked in 48 to 72 hours, and the replanted part must be watched carefully during this period. Causes of external pressure, such as tight dressings and sutures, should be corrected. Uncontrolled edema will lead to venous congestion. The optimum posture for the extremity following replantation is elevation on several pillows, with the forearm supinated and the elbow extended.

Gangrene

Any of the previously discussed complications can ultimately progress to failure of replantation or revascularization, and to gangrene of all or part of the digit or extremity. In digital replantation, dry gangrene usually develops. The nonviable tissue does not require revision immediately, and it is prudent to delay amputation until other conditions, including other replanted digits, have stabilized.

In major limb replantation, circulatory failure and infection often lead to wet gangrene, and immediate amputation is indicated to avoid systemic complications.

LATE COMPLICATIONS

Chen has stated that "survival without restoration of function is not success."[20] Return of function is the ultimate goal of any replantation effort. Many of the late complications to be discussed are reflected in loss of function. It again should be emphasized that some of these "complications" are actual goals, which represent realistic expectations of the replantation effort.

Loss of Motion

The greatest challenge in replantation surgery is the restoration of joint motion and tendon gliding.[3–5, 7] It is impossible to isolate the various factors responsible for loss of motion, but these include joint problems (e.g., capsular contracture and intra-articular injury), flexor and extensor adhesions or disruption, intrinsic adhesions, and contracture.

Several series have analyzed return of motion following replantation.[3, 5, 21] We studied total active motion (TAM), and noted that the average finger TAM was 120°, which would be considered poor motion.[5] Eighty-four percent of fingers were rated poor with respect to motion. TAM was correlated with the level of injury, type of wound, and age. Age of the patient did not significantly alter the results but, in general, younger patients developed better motion. Avulsion amputations did produce the poorest range of motion, because flexor and extensor tendons were often avulsed from the forearm. The most significant factor responsible for recovery of motion was the level of amputation (Fig. 18–1). Injuries at the metacarpophalangeal joint, proximal phalanx, and proximal interphalangeal joint produced the poorest finger TAM in both replantation and revascularization patients. Thumb injuries at the same level also produced poor TAM. In the revascularization group, the relationship of fracture and flexor tendon injury to resultant TAM demonstrated that TAM with fracture was 167° and

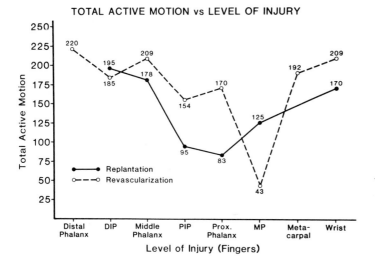

Figure 18–1. Graph demonstrates total range of motion postoperatively with respect to level of injury. (From Scott, F. A., Howar, J. W., and Boswick, J. A.: Recovery of function following replantation and revascularization of amputated hand parts. J. Trauma, 21:207, 1981.)

TAM without fracture was 202°. TAM with the flexor tendon intact was 196°, compared to 160° with flexor tendon laceration.[5] In general, revascularization patients develop better motion (see Fig. 18–1) because some of these digits had intact flexor or extensor tendons or no fracture. Chen and colleagues considered that range of motion exceeding 60% of normal was a criterion for an excellent result.[6] In general, active range of motion approximates 50% of normal.

There are several reasons for this reduced motion. The most common level for amputation or injury in our series was the proximal phalanx of the finger or thumb.[5] This level also produced the poorest range of motion. An injury at this level results in a zone II flexor tendon injury, a proximal phalanx fracture, and injury to the intrinsic hood and extensor tendon. Injury to one of these structures alone is known to produce potential problems with respect to recovery of motion. Poor results in 50% of flexor tendon injuries with concomitant arterial repair were reported in one series.[22] With concomitant fracture and extensor tendon laceration, these problems are compounded. It is more difficult to start early flexor-controlled mobilization with or without dynamic traction because of the increased risk of fracture site motion, extensor disruption, and flexor rupture. Tamai emphasized that the criteria used for flexor tendon repair cannot be strictly applied to replanted digits "because digit replantation is not only an injury to the flexor tendon, but includes all tissues of the finger that have been repaired at the same time and at the same level."[21] In many of these injuries, the segmental blood supply to the flexor tenorrhaphy may have been compromised, leading to tendon disruption, or to elongation of the repair. Every effort must be made at surgery to perform a meticulous and strong tendon repair to minimize the possibility of postoperative rupture and scarring. Postoperative motion must be started earlier than classic protocols suggest. Gentle active and passive exercises are often started as soon as

pain and swelling permit. Postoperative therapy includes an individualized and carefully supervised protective exercise program and early dynamic splinting. Later, static splinting and passive stretching are added.

Active interphalangeal joint extension is difficult to develop with injuries at this zone II level. Adhesions of the extensor hood and intrinsics to the proximal phalanx fracture are responsible for this loss of proximal interphalangeal (PIP) joint extension. It is important to splint these joints prophylactically while they are extended. This is usually accomplished with a dorsal night static extension splint. During the day, a dynamic extension splint with a metacarpophalangeal (MP) block is used to protect extensor repairs and to promote active flexion. Revascularized digits appear to be more reactive to color changes and swelling with initiation of traction therapy, and close monitoring is needed. Rigid bone fixation is important to allow for early motion. If Kirschner wires are used, they should not violate adjacent joints or interfere with the extensor mechanism.

For amputations distal to the PIP joint, active range of motion was better. In our series and others, middle phalanx injuries produced a satisfactory range of motion.[5, 23] If the central extensor tendon insertion is preserved and the flexor sublimis insertion is intact, almost full PIP and MP motion can be expected. Distal joint extension is usually limited; however, good function results.[23] The injury of a 35-year-old man who sustained a power saw amputation of his left index, long, and ring fingers through the middle phalanx is shown in Figure 18–2A. Good flexion is seen postoperatively (Fig. 18–2B) with full PIP extension and distal joint extensor lag (Fig. 18–2C).

Transmetacarpal, wrist, and distal forearm amputations also recover better motion than proximal phalanx level injuries (see Fig. 18–1). Tendon gliding problems do not generally develop to the same extent, and a functional range of motion results.

Similar problems with recovery of motion are noted with thumb amputations.[5] However, if carpometacarpal joint motion is intact and the rotatory function of the thumb preserved, MP and IP joint stiffness are not as important as in the fingers. Restoration of length and sensibility of the thumb are of paramount importance and recovery of motion, although ideal, is not essential for thumb function. One study on thumb replantation emphasized that stiffness of the thumb does not significantly alter pinch or grasp function in the presence of normal carpometacarpal motion.[24] However, Schlenker and associates noted that patients felt that limitation of motion accounts for decreased usefulness more so than loss of sensibility, and 12

of 64 patients underwent 16 secondary procedures to improve thumb function.[25] They concluded that MP and IP arthrodesis should be avoided.

Flexor Tendon Adhesions

Restoration of tendon gliding is most difficult following replantation and revascularization. The reasons for this have been discussed. As in isolated zone II flexor repairs, tendon adhesions within the digital sheath limit tendon excursion. Adhesions in the proximal palm, carpal tunnel, and distal forearm are less of a problem and respond more favorably to active and passive therapy.

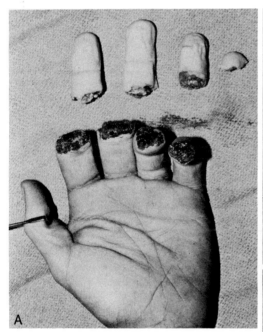

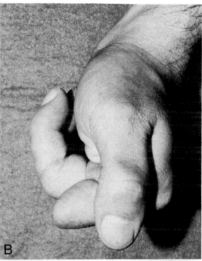

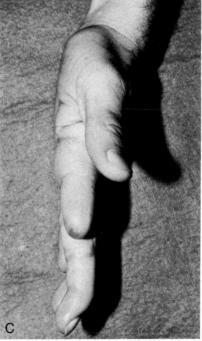

Figure 18–2. *A,* Power saw amputation of index, long, and ring fingers through middle phalanges, left hand, in a 35-year-old barber; *B,* excellent PIP joint flexion is evident postreplantation; *C,* full PIP extension recovered with active DIP extensor lag noted.

One of the most common secondary procedures after successful replantation is flexor tenolysis. This is usually combined with digital joint capsulectomy, and is generally not performed until 6 months after injury. Before consideration of surgery, the patient should demonstrate a failure to improve motion with aggressive splinting and exercise, but should also demonstrate enough cooperation and rehabilitation potential to maintain postoperatively whatever motion is realized at surgery.

On occasion, flexor tenolysis may be combined with extensor tenolysis, but generally one should concentrate on one surface at a time. Dependent on the particular problem, extensor or flexor tenolysis may be performed initially. In our series and others, tenolysis was the most frequently performed secondary procedure.[5, 12]

Two-staged flexor tendon reconstruction is sometimes required at the time of tenolysis. Often, the dense scarring around the repair site compromises the healing of the tenorrhaphy and, after excision of the scar, the repair site may appear weak, attenuated, and likely to rupture or, on occasion, does rupture during tenolysis. One must be prepared to insert a Silastic rod and reconstruct pulleys, if necessary.

Primary insertion of Silastic rods has been used during the initial replantation or revascularization procedure if the damaged condition of the flexor tendon(s) is severe, or when the damage to surrounding tissue is expected to interfere with tendon healing and gliding, or in avulsion injuries in which a flexor tendon is avulsed from the musculotendinous junction of the forearm.[5, 17, 26] This eliminates the necessity of a first-stage procedure later, and also maintains the intact pulley system and prevents flexor sheath collapse. There have been no infections in our series.[5]

Flexor Tendon Rupture

Rupture of a repaired flexor tendon after replantation appears to be more common than following an isolated flexor tendon injury and repair. This may be due to earlier mobilization, poorer blood supply at the repair site, and the complexity of a multiple structure injury. Every attempt should be made to perform an accurate and strong repair.

As discussed, rupture may also occur following tenolysis. In both circumstances, two-stage tendon reconstruction may be indicated. Again, first-stage Silastic rod insertion may be accompanied by joint capsulotomy. In our study, these staged procedures resulted in an increase of 56° of TAM for replanted and 72° for revascularized fingers.[5] Figure 18–3 illustrates the result following flexor reconstruction in a 31-year-old architect. The injury and the immediate result, with marked IP joint stiffness of the index finger and significant limitation of long finger motion, are shown (Fig. 18–3A and B). The replanted index finger required a two-stage flexor reconstruction followed by tenolysis of the flexor

graft. The revascularized long finger required flexor tenolysis and later an extensor tenolysis and PIP contracture release. A functional range of motion resulted (Fig. 18–3C and D). This particular patient required three postreplantation surgical procedures and multiple dynamic and static splints to achieve this result. Such a case demonstrates the difficulties and long-term rehabilitation effort that is often needed to obtain maximum motion and tendon gliding.

Extensor Adhesions

Adhesions at the level of extrinsic extensor repair occur for the same reasons that flexor adhesions develop. Similar problems are noted with loss of active extension compared to passive joint extension. Although loss of active MP joint extension may be evident after replantation, in most cases it can be recovered without the need for tenolysis. Restoration of PIP extension, in my opinion, is the greatest challenge of replantation rehabilitation. This problem will be discussed further with regard to intrinsic adhesions. Although extensor adhesions do limit PIP extension, primary extensors of the PIP joint are the intrinsic muscles.

Extrinsic extensor tenolysis is occasionally indicated with satisfactory return of MP joint extension. Whether this procedure should be performed prior to flexor tenolysis depends on individual priorities, including the severity of flexor adhesions and of joint contracture. Rupture of extrinsic tendon repair is not common following replantation or revascularization.

Intrinsic Adhesions

Because proximal phalanx amputations are the most common level of injury, intrinsic adhesions are a frequent complication. PIP joint extension is difficult to restore with amputation at this level. The intrinsic mechanism together with the extrinsic extensor tendon form a hood over the proximal phalanx fracture. Dense adhesions develop between these structures, which virtually eliminate any excursion of the intrinsic hood. Progressive PIP joint flexion contracture may develop, and attenuation of the central slip may occur.

Tenolysis of the extensor and intrinsic mechanisms at the proximal phalanx level does not produce as reliable long-term recovery of extension as does extrinsic extensor tenolysis. Initial posttenolysis active PIP extension is good, but it is difficult to maintain this extension with time. Night static extension splints should be used to maintain passive PIP extension. Dynamic PIP extension splints with MP extension block can be used during the day, but this does not develop active extensor power and should only be a supplement to an aggressive active PIP extension exercise program.

With middle phalanx amputations, as discussed earlier, PIP extension is preserved but loss of active

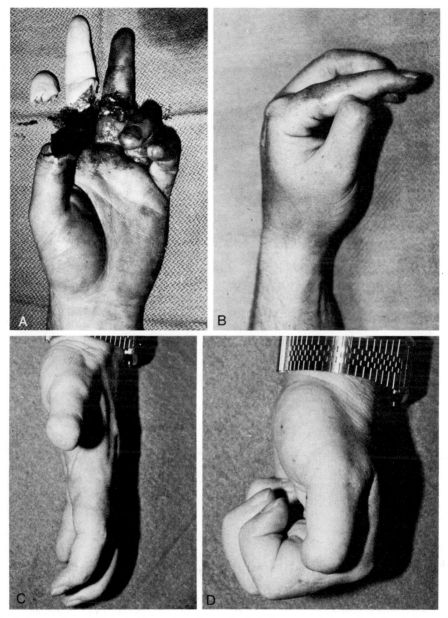

Figure 18–3. A, Amputation of left index finger through proximal phalanx, amputation of left thumb tip, and incomplete amputation of left long finger through proximal phalanx; *B,* immediate result following replantation of left index finger and revascularization of left long finger; *C, D,* motion resulting after flexor reconstruction and extensor tenolysis.

DIP motion is usually evident. May and co-workers documented an average range of 9° at the distal joint.[23] Attempts at tenolysis of the extensor and intrinsic mechanism over the middle phalanx have not substantially improved distal joint extension.

Intrinsic Contracture

Major limb amputations and those injuries proximal to the midpalm not uncommonly develop intrinsic tightness. This is most likely a result of muscle ischemia, but can also be caused by direct injury or crush. Intrinsic tightness manifests as contracture of the thumb web space, MP joint contracture, and loss of active IP joint flexion. Often these contractures require release.[27]

Joint Contracture and Ankylosis

Joint contracture and ankylosis result from direct injury (dislocation or fracture), tendon adhesions, muscle paralysis, and inadequate splinting. Certain intra-articular injuries develop degenerative changes requiring later arthrodesis or implant arthroplasty. Arthrodesis is often performed at the time of replantation, when primary severe joint destruction is present. On occasion, primary Silastic implant arthroplasty is done under these conditions. Primary PIP implant arthroplasty has yielded only fair results.[5, 12] Primary MP implant arthroplasty results in better motion.

Secondary implant arthroplasty provides satisfactory results for MP joint reconstruction, and less rewarding motion at the PIP joint.

Capsulectomy for joint contracture without severe articular destruction is frequently performed, often in conjunction with tendon reconstruction. Volar plate and collateral ligament release are utilized through a palmar approach for flexion deformities of the PIP joint.[28] MP extension contractures are released through standard dorsal approaches. Postoperative splinting (dynamic and static) is used to maintain optimum joint position and motion.

Arthrodesis is commonly indicated for IP joint disease or contracture. There appears to be no increase in the frequency of delayed union or nonunion as compared to that in patients undergoing similar procedures for conditions not related to replantation.

Loss of Sensibility

Recovery of sensibility following replantation has been generally satisfactory, especially with digital replantation. Morrison and colleagues reported that 90% of their patients developed a two-point discrimination between 4 and 15 mm.[17] Urbaniak noted protective sensation in 90%, at least 15 mm in 66%, and 10 mm or less in 50% of patient.[29] In our series, 40% of replanted digits developed less than 6 mm of two-point discrimination, 8% developed 6 to 10 mm, and 18% developed 11 to 15 mm.[5] Thirty-four percent of replanted digits developed only protective sensibility. Results for revascularized digits were better, with 70% developing less than 6 mm two-point discrimination. Several authors have stated that nerve recovery following replantation is comparable to nerve recovery following an isolated nerve repair.[5, 14, 29] Gelberman and associates demonstrated that sensory return was correlated with the restoration of digital vascularity.[30] With a pulse pressure of 85% or greater, two-point discrimination was usually less than 6 mm. Other factors related to recovery of sensibility include age, level, and type of injury.[30] Every attempt should be made to repair nerves at the time of replantation. The results of primary neurorrhaphy in replantation are better than the results of secondary repair.[3] An accurate epineural or group fascicular repair can be performed in most cases. Those nerves requiring grafting should be repaired later electively. It is my impression that restoration of sensibility following nerve grafts in replanted digits is not as good as primary repair.[5]

Paralysis of Muscles

Major limb replantations (at or proximal to the wrist) may result in intrinsic paralysis, including thenar and hypothenar muscles. Tendon transfers may be necessary to improve function.

Neuroma

Neuromata may result from repair or lack of repair of severed nerve(s). Standard techniques and indications for treatment should be considered. Kleinert and Tsai, and Morrison and co-workers, have reported patients with severe pain and paresthesias, which required amputation of the digit to relieve these symptoms.[2, 17]

Cold Intolerance

Cold intolerance is an almost universal symptom following replantation.[3, 5, 7, 8, 30, 31] In our series, 100% of replantation patients reported cold symptoms, and in revascularization patients, 49% reported significant cold symptoms.[5] Urbaniak stated that this problem usually resolves in 2 years.[29] Some patients, especially those living in colder climates, report a lesser degree of symptoms indefinitely.

Nonunion and Malunion

The incidence of nonunion and malunion does not seem to be high. In our series, 7 of 100 patients developed nonunion at the amputation site.[5] There were 7 nonunions in 149 hand units (nonunion rate of 5%). Four of these seven patients underwent bone grafting for nonunion. This was usually for stabilization of deformity rather than for pain. Morrison and associates also reported one nonunion and ten malunions in 100 patients, none of which required treatment.[17] Urbaniak reported a nonunion rate of less than 5%.[29] Phelps and Lilla reported delayed bone healing in replantation.[31] Tamai also reported delayed bone healing, with an average of 2.3 months in clean amputations and 2.8 months in crush amputations.[21] Five of seven digits with nonunion required bone grafting. Delayed bone healing is less of a problem when compression fixation is used.[2]

Not all malunions or nonuions require treatment. If a nonunion is painful or unstable, it may require internal fixation and bone grafting. In some of our patients, a painless nonunion was a source of motion, and no treatment was required. Each case of malunion must be considered individually, because rotational malalignment and angulation may not be significant if adjacent digits are missing or are also malaligned. Derotation osteotomy, on occasion, is indicated. Open reduction, internal fixation, and bone grafting should be considered before tendon and joint reconstruction, which may require early postoperative motion.

Loss of Strength

It is anticipated that reduction of grip and pinch will result from these mutilating injuries. In our series, the average return of grip strength in replantation patients was 53% as compared to the uninjured hand, and in revascularization patients it was 65%.[5] Pinch strength was recorded at 50% of the uninjured hand in replantation patients and 59% in revascularization. These measurements, of course, reflect the influence of a number of factors, such as tendon and joint function, digit(s) amputated, and patient motivation. They do, however, reflect hand impairment in general.

SINGLE-DIGIT REPLANTATION AND REVASCULARIZATION

There has been much discussion regarding whether single digit amputations should be replanted. Many series have recommended that in most circumstances single-digit amputations or severe single digital injuries not be replanted or revascularized.[5, 9, 13] Thumb amputations are excluded from this single-digit amputation category. In the presence of three normal uninjured fingers, a replanted or revascularized finger does not usually recover satisfactory function, and often this digit will interfere with overall hand function and result in more impairment than if the digital amputation had been closed primarily. This is especially true with index finger amputations.

The patient in Figure 18–4 is a 52-year-old carpenter who incompletely amputated his left nondominant index finger in a saw, resulting in a comminuted proximal phalanx fracture, both flexor tendon lacerations, and disruption of both neurovascular bundles. Revascularization was successful but a stiff, insensitive, and cold-intolerant digit resulted. There is a great tendency for patients to bypass an injured index finger. Similar problems may develop with any other digit, although they appear to be more exaggerated with index and little finger amputations at the proximal phalanx level.

All factors need to be considered in the decision not to replant a single finger. Amputations distal to the PIP joint recover much better function, and consideration should be given to a replantation of a single-digit amputation at this level.[5, 23] Cosmesis and patient desires also need to be considered. One must adopt an individualized approach to the single-digit amputation, and the general philosophy not to proceed with replantation must remain flexible.

Ability to Return to Work

Certainly a general indication of how functional a replantation becomes is the patient's return to work data. Type of employment and length of time off work are important. We studied these factors in our patients, who did not include children, nonworking teenagers, housewives, or retired persons.[5] Eighty-eight percent of replantation patients returned to work within an average of 4.4 months. Two thirds, however, returned to a different job, and one third returned to the same job. Some patients required formal job re-education. In the revascularization group, 97% of patients studied returned to work, with 73% returning to the same job and 27% assuming a new job. Average time off work was 3.9 months. One of the most important factors in avoiding the "disability disease" that frequently affects workers is an early return-to-work policy. These figures reflect an aggressive attempt to return patients to work in some capacity and to motivate these individuals to be productive while, in many instances, involved in postoperative rehabilitation programs. It is important that early return to work be considered as an important aspect of the total rehabilitation effort.

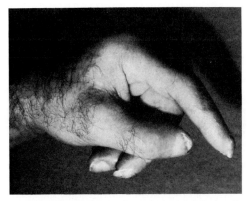

Figure 18–4. Incomplete amputation of left index finger in a 52-year-old carpenter, with resultant stiffness, cold intolerance, and loss of sensibility.

References

1. Berger, A., et al.: Replantation or amputation: A basic discussion after three years of replantation work. Int. J. Microsurg., 1:18, 1979.
2. Kleinert, H. E., and Tsai, T. M.: Microvascular repair in replantation. Clin. Orthop., 133:205, 1978.
3. Weiland, A. J., Villarreal-Rios, A., and Kleinert, H. E.: Replantation of digits and hands: Analysis of surgical techniques and functional results in 71 patients with 86 replantations. J. Hand Surg., 2:1, 1977.
4. Yoshizu, T., Katsumi, M., and Tajima, T.: Replantation of untidily amputated finger, hand, and arm: Experience of 99 replantations in 66 cases. J. Trauma, 18:194, 1978.
5. Scott, F. A., Howar, J. W., and Boswick JA: Recovery of function following replantation and revascularization of amputated hand parts. J. Trauma, 21:204, 1981.
6. Chen, C., Qian, Y., and Yu, Z.: Extremity replantation. World J. Surg., 2:513, 1978.
7. Kleinert, H. E., Jablan, M., and Tsai, T. M.: An overview of replantation and results of 347 replants in 245 patients. J. Trauma, 20:390, 1980.
8. Manktelow, R. T., and McKee, N. H.: Digital replantation: A functional assessment. Can. J. Surg., 22:47, 1979.
9. Kleinert, H. E., et al.: Digit replantation—selection, technique, and results. Orthop. Clin. North Am., 8:309, 1977.
10. Gould, J. S., Gould, S. H., and Caudill-Babkes, E. L.:

Interpositional microvascular vein grafting. Hand, 11:332, 1979.

11. Stirrat, C. R., et al.: Temperature monitoring in digital replantation. J. Hand Surg., 3:342, 1978.

12. Wilson, C. S., et al.: Replantation of the upper extremity. Clin. Plast. Surg., 10:85, 1983.

13. Morrison, W. A., O'Brien, B. M., and MacLeod, A. M.: Evaluation of digital replantation. A review of 100 cases. Orthop. Clin. North Am., 8:295, 1977.

14. O'Brien, B. M.: Microvascular reconstructive surgery. Edinburgh, New York, Churchill Livingstone, 1977, p. 171.

15. Scott, F. A., and Boswick, J. A.: Replantation and revascularization of amputated hand parts. *In* Boswick, J. A. (ed.): Current Concepts in Hand Surgery, Chap. 24., Philadelphia, Lea & Febiger, 1983, p. 192.

16. Phelps, D. B., Rutherford, R. B., and Boswick, J. A.: Control of vasospasm following trauma and microvascular surgery. J. Hand Surg., 4:109, 1979.

17. Morrison, W. A., O'Brien, B. M., and MacLeod, A. M.: Digital replantation and revascularization: A long-term review of one hundred cases. Hand, 10:125, 1978.

18. Leung, P. C.: The "throbbing sign"–an indication of early venous congestion in replantation surgery. J. Hand Surg., 4:409, 1979.

19. Leung, P. C.: An analysis of complications in digital replantations. Hand, 12:25, 1980.

20. American Replantation Mission to China: Replantation surgery in China. Plast. Reconstr. Surg., 52:476, 1973.

21. Tamai, S.: Digit replantation. Clin. Plast. Surg., 5:195, 1978.

22. Lester, G. D., et al.: Primary flexor tendon repair followed by immediate controlled immobilization. J. Hand Surg., 2:441, 1977.

23. May, J. W., Tosh, B. A., and Gardner, M.: Digital replantation distal to the proximal interphalangeal joint. J. Hand Surg., 7:161, 1982.

24. Chow, J. A., Bilos, Z. J., Chunprapaph, B.: Thirty thumb replantations: Indications and results. Plast. Reconstr. Surg., 64:626, 1979.

25. Schlenker, J. D., Kleinert, H. E., and Tsai, T. M.: Methods and results of replantation following traumatic amputation of the thumb in sixty-four patients. J. Hand Surg., 5:63, 1980.

26. Lendvay, P. G.: Replacement of the amputated digit. Br. J. Plast. Surg., 26:398, 1973.

27. Morrison, W. A., O'Brien, B. M., and MacLeod, A. M.: Major limb replantation. Orthop. Clin. North Am., 8:343, 1977.

28. Scott, F. A., and Boswick, J. A.: Palmar arthroplasty for the treatment of the stiff swan-neck deformity. J Hand Surg 8:267–272, 1983.

29. Urbaniak, J. R.: Replantation of amputated parts: Technique, results and indications. *In* American Academy of Orthopaedic Surgeons: Symposium on Microsurgery–Practical Use in Orthopaedics, St. Louis, C. V. Mosby, 1979, pp. 64–82.

30. Gelberman, R. H., et al.: Digital sensibility following replantation. J. Hand Surg., 3:313, 1978.

31. Phelps, D. B., Lilla, J. A., and Boswick, J. A.: Common problems in clinical replantation and revascularization in the upper extremity. Clin. Orthop., 133:11, 1978.

19

COMPLICATIONS FOLLOWING CRUSH INJURIES

Alan E. Seyfer
Monroe I. Levine

Crushing and compression injuries of the hand and upper extremity are quite common in today's mechanized society. Although often unobtrusive initially, the injury can result in serious regional and systemic complications, which endanger the life of the patient and the function of the extremity. The purpose of this chapter is to present a practical approach to the management of crushing trauma, with emphasis on minimizing the local and systemic sequelae of this devastating injury.

Figure 19–1. The severe crush injury combines disruption of soft tissues with skeletal instability. Such extensive destruction requires aggressive rehabilitation if function is to be salvaged.

THE CRUSH WOUND

Mechanism of Injury

The crushing force may consist of many interacting components. However, direct compression of tissues and shearing forces directed across bones, arteries and other tissue interfaces seem to be the most devastating. Muscle, tendon, and nerve fibers may be avulsed, arteries and capillaries torn, and

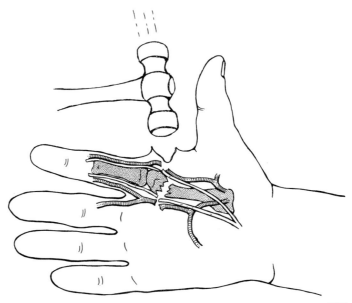

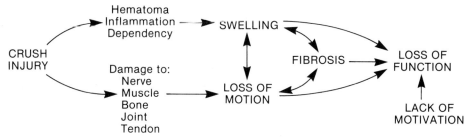

Figure 19–2. Schematic of the interrelated sequence of events that can complicate the crush injury. All the factors listed here are important, but one of the most critical is the motivation of the patient. A lack of motivation can frustrate the best rehabilitative efforts. Note the close correlation of factors leading to loss of function.

bones shattered. Frequently, the skin envelope is opened, adding a potent stimulus to the inflammatory reaction and increasing the risk of sepsis (Fig. 19–1). In a severe crush, this destructive sequence may involve both compressive and shearing elements, whether due to the classic wringer-type injury, impact of a heavy object, or other well-known mechanisms.

Local Consequences

The local tissue response to crushing is one of severe inflammation, followed by repair and regeneration. Shortly after injury, the inflammatory cycle is initiated and the vascular endothelium becomes extremely permeable. Soft tissues are inundated by a protein-rich transudate that fills the interstitium. Injured cells undergo a period of cloudy swelling, during which there is an accumulation of subcellular metabolites.[16] On a larger scale, blood vessels are opened, with direct bleeding into the tissues, which further increases the volume of the injured structures. This hematoma is, in fact, a devitalized tissue and, aside from prolonging inflammation, increases the prospect of infection.[4] Such bleeding and edema, especially when associated with direct tissue injury in the vicinity of joints and tendons, immobilizes the gliding structures and predisposes to organization and fibrosis. The end result is permanent loss of motion, unless the repair phase is favorably modified by aggressive wound care and rehabilita-

tion. This includes débridement, irrigation, stabilization of skeletal elements, elevation, and early motion.

An exaggerated scenario would be a severe open crush wound of the hand that is improperly débrided, with malpositioning of bony elements, placed in a poor functional position, without elevation, and allowed to remain inactive. Although this is the "worst case" scenario, any one element, improperly treated, can lead to the same devastating result.

In this setting, the inadequate débridement can lead to a rampant destructive infection, and the swelling secondary to these insults is accentuated by allowing the hand to hang in the dependent position. The poorly reduced fractures are followed by shortening, disruption of articular balance, and musculotendinous inefficiency. Lack of motion robs both injured and uninjured structures of movement, and further prolongs the swelling. Again, the overall result can be permanent loss of function and a debilitated hand or upper extremity.

Another critically important consideration is the motivation of the patient, which often outweighs other factors (Fig. 19–2). A well-motivated patient can profit from rehabilitative efforts and be reintegrated into the mainstream of society despite anatomic shortcomings.[5]

Emphasis should be primarily on the functional return of the patient to society, restitution of function to the injured part and, to a lesser extent, anatomic perfection. These efforts should be pur-

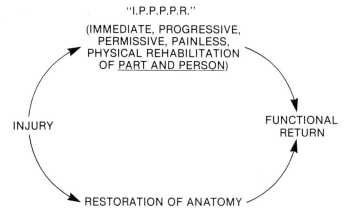

Figure 19–3. Emphasis is always on prevention of complications and on the *recovery of function*, both of the injured hand as well as of the whole patient. Anatomic perfection, although a useful goal, is not always possible.

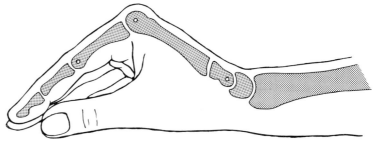

Figure 19–4. The "protected" position, which minimizes adverse contractures and keeps the hand in the "ready" position and from which daily therapy can be started most easily. In this illustration, the thumb should actually be slightly further away from the fingertips.

sued concurrently from the very start, rather than sequentially, as is often the case (Fig. 19–3).

These complications represent only a few of the many problems that can occur in a crush injury. In approaching the crush wound, therefore, it is extremely important to minimize such difficulties early in the course of treatment if any useful function is to be restored.

General Principles of Management

The goals of treatment are to preserve life and limb and to restore function. Accordingly, it is vital to rule out serious injuries to other systems that threaten the life of the patient. After this is accomplished, attention may be turned to the injured extremity.

Stiffening of the small joints of the hand is by far the most common and serious local complication. Also, prolonged immobilization is the single most preventable cause of this stiffness. Thus, the guiding principle in the management of the crush wound is maintenance of motion and preservation of the function of uninjured parts of the hand. Immobilization is done only as absolutely necessary, and for as short an interval as required by safe principles of

wound care.[3] Preferably, only the injured area is immobilized, allowing active range of motion to all other structures. If the hand must be immobilized, it should be maintained in the "protective" position, with metacarpophalangeal joints at 90° flexion, interphalangeal joints in extension, and the thumb in palmar abduction (Fig. 19–4). This position will best minimize adverse contracture of periarticular structures, and will enhance the prospect for full recovery of motion.[23]

In general, open wounds are débrided in the operating room and left open for delayed closure. At the initial débridement unstable fractures are internally fixed, and crucial decisions are made for the potential reconstruction of the soft tissues (see below).

It is helpful to divide crush injuries into *components,* and to discuss each injured system and its management in turn. It must be emphasized that varying degrees of trauma exist in each individual and in each organ system. Thus, in a specific patient, a *mixed injury* is the rule. Within this context, we have arbitrarily divided each injury into mild, moderate, and severe (Table 19–1). Each component will be discussed in these terms, along with the natural history of the injury and its potential complications. Following this outline, methods of min-

Table 19–1. CLASSIFICATION OF CRUSH INJURIES TO THE HAND

Injured Organ or System	Mild	Moderate	Severe
Skin	Contusion; partial thickness injury	Laceration; avulsed areas about 1 cm diameter	Large portions of full-thickness skin missing
Blood vessels	Capillary disruption	Arteriolar disruption; major vessels intact	Major arterial injury; impending loss of portion of hand
Nerves	Stretch injury; axonal flow disrupted; neurapraxia-axonotmesis; first to second-degree injury	Nerve fibers disrupted; groups in order; third-degree injury	Nerve fibers and groups disrupted; neurotmesis; trunk severed; fourth- to fifth-degree injury
Muscle	Contusion	Muscular fascicles disrupted	Muscular groups disrupted or severed; large areas of necrosis
Tendon	Tendon exposed; paratenon intact	Paratenon loss; tendon damaged but in continuity	Loss of tendon substance
Joints	Stable	Unstable; subluxation, tendency to dislocate	Significant loss of articular surface
Bone (fractures)	Stable	Unstable without loss of bone	Loss of bone

imizing these local complications will be presented. The systemic complications of the crushing injury will then be discussed.

COMPLICATIONS RELATED TO SKIN INJURY

Coverage of deeper structures with well-vascularized serviceable skin is one of the first priorities. Because open wounds prolong inflammation, predispose to scarring, and can result in desiccation of vital tissues, this closure is accomplished as soon as it is safely possible. However, it is not imperative to do this on the day of injury, because coverage may be most safely done in a delayed manner.

Natural History

Mild Injury

In the mild crushing injury, the skin is usually intact or has areas of contusion, which represent dermal hematomas. Areas of abrasion, representing partial thickness injury, are also seen. This type of wound usually heals without functional loss within 10 to 14 days, as long as infection does not supervene in the abraded areas.

Moderate Injury

The skin is intact with severe contusion or, in the older or immunosuppressed individual, the upper layers may be sheared off at the dermal level. Lacerations may be present, or there may be small (≤ 1 cm^2) areas of skin loss. The skin margins may be necrotic and retracted, exposing subjacent structures.

Within the first week, desiccation of the exposed dermis and underlying fat occurs, with consolidation into an eschar. If the dermal injury is not extended through a cellulitic process, re-epithelialization and contraction beneath the eschar gradually advance the edges until the wound is healed by secondary intention. Although usually of little consequence, this may result in skin shortening and an easily traumatized scar epithelium. Such scars can interfere with function through restriction of motion or through recurrent ulceration, depending on the location and extent of injury. For example, such an area located over a digital flexion crease can shorten the skin enough to cause a flexion contracture of the joint.

Severe Injury

The skin is open and large portions may be missing. "Large" is, at best, a judgmental matter. Certainly what is termed "large" on the digit may mean an area smaller than 1 to 2 cm^2 if it exposes structures vital to the functioning of the digit or has the potential of restricting motion with scar. On the other hand, a similar area on the forearm or dorsum of the hand may be well tolerated and heal on its own without limiting function due to exposure or skin shortening. If large areas are avulsed, the underlying joints, neurovascular structures, or bones are vulnerable to trauma or desiccation. Such areas will re-epithelialize only after necrotic tissue has been extruded from the wound and the eschar has been cast off. This lengthy process, which may take weeks, results in unserviceable scar epithelium, which is restrictive due to adherence to underlying structures and is also easily injured. There is usually extensive woody fibrosis in the area due to the chronic inflammation and repair process, which ultimately restricts the motion of adjacent tissues as well.

Management

In the *mild injury*, areas of contusion require no specific therapy because they heal well without intervention. Abraded areas should be kept clean, and daily washing is generally all that is required. Crusting, infection, and desiccation can be minimized by the use of a lanolin or petroleum-based antibacterial ointment.

With *moderate or severe injury*, the crush wound edges are conservatively excised and obviously necrotic skin is removed. Skin of doubtful viability may be left *in situ* for later evaluation at the delayed closure, or intravenous fluorescein may be administered and the viability assessed under ultraviolet light.[12] After thorough débridement and irrigation, the wounds are left open and placed in a sterile, elevated, bulky hand dressing for delayed closure in 4 or 5 days. At that time, if the wound has an exudative character, it is left open, and wet-to-dry dressings or homograft are utilized to clean the wound in preparation for closure. If it appears to be "clean," closure is done. The clinical appearance of a "clean" wound correlates well with bacterial counts that allow a safe closure ($\leq 10^5$) organisms/gm of tissue.[1]

Every effort is made to close the wound at the earliest opportunity consistent with safe wound management. However, it is our feeling that traumatic wounds of this nature are best left open for delayed closure. These wounds are often highly contaminated, contain foreign or necrotic debris, and are prone to infectious complications. Thus, primary closure can result in a devastating closed space infection that also jeopardizes the uninjured portions of the extremity. On the other hand, very little collagen has been applied to the wound bed during the short waiting period for delayed closure. Thus, although it requires another procedure, one stands to lose little by delaying the wound closure, and the awesome threat of serious infection is avoided. In our experience, this has offered the safest method of management.

If skin is missing, our preference is to provide closure after the delay, with split-thickness skin grafts, usually meshed 1.5:1 and applied unexpanded. This gives durable coverage, conforms well to irregularities of the recipient bed, and provides drainage to the contaminated area. We feel that skin flaps have no place in the primary closure of this type of wound due to the contamination and unstable condition of the recipient bed. Such surgery may be done at the delayed closure in selected cases, but is generally reserved for reconstruction at a later date when tissue equilibrium has been reached.

VASCULAR COMPLICATIONS

Ischemia is an emergency and must be dealt with on the initial examination. The crush wound, however, is similar to a high-velocity missile wound in that vascular damage is often more extensive than is evident grossly. This is due to avulsion of the vessels that disrupts the intima for relatively great distances along the vessel, predisposing any local repair to thrombosis and failure.

Natural History

Mild Injury

This injury corresponds to disruption at the capillary and venular levels, with minimal loss of blood into the tissues. Due to arteriolar anastomoses, the ischemia is usually very mild and is reversible without intervention. After the edema subsides, full recovery of function can be expected.

Moderate Injury

The major arteries are intact but arterioles are disrupted, with greater quantities of blood lost and greater degrees of muscular and skin ischemia present. Patchy areas of necrosis result, which manifest themselves as fibrosis of muscle and shortening of the skin. Intrinsic muscle tightness and loss of full excursion of the extensor mechanism may be the final outcome. Necrosis of the skin can result in shortening, which also limits range of motion.

Severe Injury

A major artery has been disrupted, with the threat of ischemic necrosis of the hand or of one of its structural units. The blood loss may be life-threatening. In this setting, unless circulation is restored, irreversible ischemia and dry gangrene of the hand or injured portion are inevitable. This injury also predisposes to the systemic coagulopathy (see below).

Management

In the *mild injury* no therapy is warranted, because healing occurs without functional loss. In the *moderate injury*, the bleeding is stopped and non-viable tissue is excised. If doubt exists as to viability, one may return to the operating room in 24 to 72 hours for repeat evaluation, at which time ischemic margins will be more clearly demarcated. Compart-

ments are released to restore as much capillary flow as possible. In the *severe* vascular *injury*, one must quickly assess the feasibility of arterial repair or vein grafting versus amputation of the ischemic digit or portion of the hand. The key decision is whether the injured area is salvageable or beyond hope due to the destructive influence of the crush. If microvascular reconstruction is indicated, the patient should be referred to centers knowledgeable in these judgmental and technical factors. Such considerations are beyond the scope of the present discussion.

If amputation is warranted due to irreversible ischemic changes, an attempt is made to save as much viable tissue as is safely possible. Again, one may elect to wait until the delayed skin closure in 3 to 5 days to make the final assessment on tissue of doubtful viability. One must be mindful of hypercoagulability in patients with the severe vascular injury, as will be discussed. These patients are at increased risk for thrombotic complications.

COMPLICATIONS RELATED TO NERVE INJURY

Several factors influence rehabilitation after a nerve injury to the upper extremity. The type of trauma, level of injury, and the timing and techniques of repair are all extremely important in dealing with this sort of injury. The present discussion is limited to crushing injuries of the hand and forearm, so we have narrowed this truly encyclopedic problem down to a relatively specific set of circumstances. Table 19–1 combines the classifications of nerve injuries currently in use. First- and second-degree injuries heal without intervention in a period of months (neurapraxia and axonotmesis). Third-degree injury results in limited recovery; fourth- and fifth-degree injuries (neurotmesis) offer no opportunity for regeneration on their own.[7, 21]

Natural History

Mild Injury

In this injury the continuity of the endoneural tubes is preserved, but the nerve is contused. Axonal flow may be interrupted or the axon itself separated, which results in wallerian degeneration distal to the point of injury. Because the endoneural sheath remains, however, axonal regeneration is guided into the original end-organ, and full recovery can be expected to occur with time. This injury corresponds to Sunderland's first- and second-degree categories of injury.[21]

Moderate Injury

With more severe crushing the fascicular groups are in order, but there is loss of continuity of the individual nerve fibers (axons and endoneural sheaths). Regeneration of axonal endings is haphazard but may blindly enter a distal tube within the same fascicle, so that only a partial, if any, return of function occurs. However, because the trauma is more severe, there is a greater degree of edema, inflammation, and fibrosis, with formation of a neuroma-in-continuity. In the neuroma, it is impossible to determine grossly the degree of regeneration that has occurred. This represents the so-called third-degree injury.

Severe Injury

In this injury, there is loss of continuity of the nerve fibers and the fasciculus (group of fibers). Although the epineurium may be spared in some cases, the destruction is severe, and all other elements of the trunk are severed (neurotmesis). Regeneration of nerve filaments and fascicles is totally disorganized, and is marked by fibrosis and by the absence of any useful function. This represents the fourth- and fifth-degree injuries.

Management

The goals of treatment are, of course, full return to function. With the *mild injury*, the prospects for attaining this are reasonably good. A complete motor and sensory evaluation is done during the initial examination and, in the closed injury, regeneration is observed by repeated clinical and electrical examinations. If there is no return of function as detectable by the usual clinical and electrical means, and after the tissues have reached equilibrium, exploration is warranted. At that time, the need for neurolysis or resection of the neuroma with repair or grafting is ascertained.

In the open injury, in which a preoperative neurologic deficit is found, the nerve is explored at the initial débridement. If the nerve is found to be damaged, but is in continuity *(moderate injury)*, the condition is carefully documented and no specific treatment for the nerve is done. If the nerve has a partial transection, the groups are aligned and the transected area is repaired with fine epineural sutures. Even this amount of extra trauma is done with some trepidation, because it is likely that the nerve is not simply lacerated but is crushed and severely damaged at that point. Therefore, the efficacy of suturing in this milieu is questionable.

If complete transection has occurred *(severe injury)*, the general rule is to defer the repair. Unfortunately, in the severe crush injury, the tissue bed is far from optimal for early nerve repair or grafting. Likewise, it is difficult to judge the condition of the nerve accurately in such a setting. Accordingly, we have avoided vigorous resection of the damaged area of the nerve and mobilizing (and hence adding more trauma to) the nerve for repair at the initial sitting. A conservative débridement of obviously necrotic nerve is done and, if the bed is favorable at the delayed closure in 4 or 5 days, a repair is done. If the bed is doubtful, as is the usual case, conditions are so documented and the repair is deferred until tissue equilibrium has been attained.

If the threat of compression secondary to swelling is felt to exist at any time, the carpal canal or any other potential constraint is released.

COMPLICATIONS RELATED TO MUSCULAR INJURY; COMPARTMENT SYNDROMES

Direct crushing injury to intrinsic and extrinsic muscles can severely derange the strength and function of the hand and forearm. Muscular injury can also occur secondary to the development of compartment syndromes and, fortunately, this latter complication is often preventable through early diagnosis and treatment.

Natural History

Muscular Injury

In the *mild injury*, the muscle is viable but is contused. The fascicles are disrupted by hematoma, but the swelling is minimal and the muscles within the compartment are not considered to be in danger. This injury, although warranting close observation, heals without intervention.

In the *moderate* to *severe injury*, there is a greater degree of muscular disruption with direct crushing and bleeding into the tissues. In the open injury, there may be loss of muscle substance and contamination within necrotic fascicles. In these deep injuries the threat of anaerobic infection is great—especially clostridial myonecrosis or fasciitis. Barring such life-threatening infections, the absence or fibrosis of muscle can result in loss of motion and weakness. In the closed injury danger also exists from the development of a compartment syndrome.

Compartment Syndromes

In this setting, swelling within certain rigid enclosures can endanger the viability of contained structures secondary to increased pressure. The intrinsic musculature of the hand and the long musculotendinous units of the forearm are enclosed by unyielding fascial barriers that are essentially watertight. Within these compartments, the addition of small increments in volume leads to large increases in intracompartmental pressure.[10, 11, 13–15]

Although this arrangement facilitates the strength and function of the motor unit, it likewise renders it vulnerable to tamponade when injured. With the edema and bleeding secondary to injury, intracompartmental pressure rises, destroying the delicate balance of the Starling equation and closing off the lymphovenous exits from the compartment.[20] Arterial pressure is gradually exceeded, and eventually all circulation stops. Necrosis of the contained myoneural structures is inevitable unless the compartment is opened to restore flow. If necrosis occurs, Volkmann's ischemic contracture of the involved muscles follows, with all of its tragic sequelae.

Figure 19–5. Incisions for intrinsic compartmental releases. The muscles are easily and quickly approached through dorsal incisions.

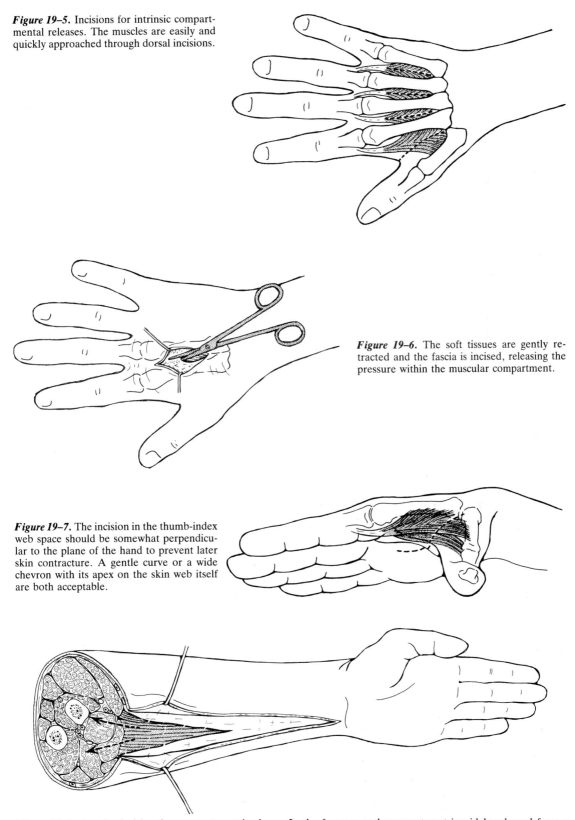

Figure 19–6. The soft tissues are gently retracted and the fascia is incised, releasing the pressure within the muscular compartment.

Figure 19–7. The incision in the thumb-index web space should be somewhat perpendicular to the plane of the hand to prevent later skin contracture. A gentle curve or a wide chevron with its apex on the skin web itself are both acceptable.

Figure 19–8. A volar incision for compartmental release. In the forearm each compartment is widely released from a volar or dorsal approach, as deemed necessary. The wound is left open for delayed closure, with or without skin grafting.

Management

Muscular Injury

The *mild injury* heals without operative intervention. *Moderately* severe and *severe* injuries require an aggressive approach, whether open or closed. In the open injury, tetanus prophylaxis is ensured and necrotic muscle is conservatively excised. Foreign matter is cleared with forceful irrigation. The viability of the muscle is assessed by color, bleeding, and contractility. If the muscle contracts on stroking with a forceps or with electric stimulation, it is viable. The compartments at risk for increased pressure are generously released by incising the fascia. Both intrinsic and extrinsic muscle compartments must be assessed and released if doubt exists.

Compartment Syndromes

In the closed injury, an assessment is made as to the risk of the compartment syndrome developing in those spaces directly involved with the trauma, or in those in close proximity. Unfortunately, this is notoriously difficult. One cannot rely on palpation of the distal arterial pulsation or even pain with passive stretch to establish the diagnosis. Hypesthesia and paresthesias are likewise difficult to assess in the injured patient. Pressure-sensitive (wick) catheters are useful in this regard, and are now available.[14, 15] However, conditions may exist in which the patient cannot be followed closely. For example, the patient may require rapid evacuation to a better equipped facility, or a mass casualty situation may exist that precludes careful sequential examinations by the surgeon. On the other hand, the patient may be unresponsive or unable to cooperate with such examinations. Under such circumstances it is best to proceed with release of the compartments of the hand and forearm that are at risk. Under local or regional anesthesia, the fascia is incised and the muscle assessed for viability (Figs. 19–5 through 19–8). Necrotic muscle is removed, and the wound is left open for delayed closure in 4 or 5 days. If doubt exists as to the viability of the muscle, the area can be reinspected in 24 to 72 hours in the operating room. At this point necrotic muscle will have demarcated, and a more accurate débridement can be performed.

COMPLICATIONS RELATED TO FRACTURES

The criteria for analyzing fractures include stability, alignment, angulation, displacement, rotation, and shortening (see Chaps. 14 and 16). However, a few points pertinent to the crush injury should be mentioned.

First, the general principle is to establish motion as early as possible, within the limits of stability. However, in dealing with crush injuries, this must be modified in certain cases, because the situation may call for both skeletal immobilization due to fracture and for early motion to preserve soft tissue and joint function. In these cases, skeletal stability generally comes first, and the pins are extracted as early as possible to allow dynamic splinting with protected motion. On the other hand, some fractures do not require such rigid fixation. Thus, each case must necessarily be individualized.

Secondly, metacarpal fractures generally differ in functional prognosis from phalangeal fractures. The phalanges have a more intimate relationship with the surrounding tendinous structures, both intrinsic and extrinsic, and adherence to the fracture site can disrupt balance and limit the gliding of these structures. In comparison, metacarpal fractures can sometimes tolerate a greater degree of malposition without significant functional loss.

Finally, in evaluating fractures in this setting, one of the most important criteria is stability. If, under local anesthesia (wound conditions permitting), there is no displacement or malpositioning of the fragments after active range of motion, the fracture is considered to be stable and safe for early motion. If satisfactory reduction is not maintained with active motion, it is unstable.

Natural History

Mild Injury

The fracture is in an acceptable position either after initial injury or after reduction and, after active range of motion, maintains this reduction without external or internal fixation (*i.e.,* it is stable). With appropriate postfracture management, this fracture heals with a good functional return.

Moderate Injury

The fracture is unstable. Left unattended, it will go on to malunion, fibrous union, or nonunion. The long-term complications may include pain, loss of function due to tendon imbalance, instability at the fracture site, skeletal malalignment, or cosmetic problems.

Severe Injury

This category pertains to any fracture in which there is loss of bone. The natural history is nonunion with collapse of the digit, ray, or other structural unit of the hand. Again, there can be chronic pain, loss of function due to malalignment, tendon imbalance, instability at the fracture site, and all the problems of the moderate injury, but to a greater degree.

Management

Mild Injury

In general, it can be helpful in the milder injuries to administer a local anesthetic block to the digit or injured portion and to attempt full active motion. If reduction is maintained without added support, then the fracture is stable. Stable phalangeal fractures can be treated with early active range of motion to prevent stiffness of nearby joints, utilizing a buddy tape to an adjacent digit until the tenderness recedes. Stable metacarpal fractures are splinted to allow full metacarpophalangeal motion, and the splint is maintained only for as long as the tenderness persists. Full active motion is the goal for these injuries.

Moderate and Severe Injuries

The overall goal remains full functional restitution. The means with which to achieve this goal is to regain stability with good external or internal fixation to ensure adequate length, alignment, and rotation. In contrast to mild injuries, local anesthesia usually has little place in this injury. Therefore, at the initial débridement, fractures are reduced and internally fixed with Kirschner wires, which are effective in these injuries.

If bony portions are missing or must be removed, length is maintained with Kirschner wires to preclude collapse and for later reconstruction.

COMPLICATIONS RELATED TO THE JOINTS

The general principal is the prevention of stiffness by early active motion as soon as possible after the crush injury. An important criterion in assessing injured joints is, again, stability. A *stable* joint (open *or* closed injury) is one that possesses normal ligamentous or bony support in all directions. It may be associated with avulsion fractures, which usually involve less than 10 to 15 per cent of the joint surface but do not render it unstable in any direction. Joint surfaces are otherwise normal.

Natural History

Mild Injury

In this injury, the joint is contused but stable. These injuries heal without intervention, and the long-term prognosis is very good if stiffness can be forestalled through early motion.

Moderate Injury

These include injured joints that are unstable in certain positions *or* exhibit subluxation or a tendency to dislocate. They may be associated with fractures that contribute to the instability (*e.g.,* volar lip fractures of the proximal interphalangeal (PIP) joint, which displace on extension). This injury leads to incongruity of the joint and a relatively poor prognosis due to the abnormal forces and long-term wear on the gliding surfaces. Later complications include fibrous ankylosis, early degenerative joint disease, or tendon imbalance.

Severe Injury

In the severe crush injury, there is loss of articular surface with or without ligamentous instability. This injury carries a poor prognosis, and the natural history is one of progressive stiffening and ankylosis. Severe functional loss, with essentially no joint motion, is the final outcome.

Management

Mild Injury

The treatment is aimed at early active motion commensurate with limitations imposed by adjacent injuries. If interim immobilization is required, the hand is splinted in the protective position (see Fig. 19–4) or, preferably, dynamic splinting is utilized.

Moderate Injury

Because instability with motion is the major clinical and functional deficit, treatment is aimed at regaining stability during motion. This may be done through external dynamic splinting. The splint allows protected movement within the stable arcs of motion until the injured areas are stable enough to allow free range of motion. If this cannot be reliably achieved externally, internal fixation is accomplished with Kirschner wires until dynamic splinting can be safely applied.

Severe Injury

In this destructive injury, in which loss of articular and periarticular tissue have occurred, it becomes a value judgment as to the salvability of the joint. Initially, one should try to determine if the joint lends itself mechanically to reconstruction. In other words, under optimal care, what would the end result of this injury be? If it appears that ankylosis will occur due to the extent of the injury, the treatment is to pin the joint in the position of optimal function—a functional arthrodesis. If articular reconstruction is feasible, the fragments are replaced and pinned. Pins are removed when adequate healing has occurred, and motion is then undertaken to regain as much movement as possible. Another alternative is to go for motion early, accepting a degree of malposition and allowing the fragments and healing fibrous tissue to "grind to fit" (functional arthroplasty).

COMPLICATIONS RELATED TO TENDONS

In caring for tendon injuries in the crush wound, several factors must be considered. The goal is a freely gliding tendon with full unrestricted excursion. The optimal bed for a tendon repair or graft is supple, mature, soft tissue with absence of inflammation and full passive joint mobility. Unfortunately, these conditions are rarely met in the acute crush injury, either at initial débridement or at delayed closure. Thus, in general, reconstruction is deferred until these conditions are met.

Natural History

Mild Injury

The tendon is exposed with an intact paratenon. Barring desiccation, and depending on the degree of skin coverage, these wounds heal with good functional recovery.

Moderate Injury

In this injury, the tendon is exposed and the paratenon is lost. The tendon is damaged, but in continuity. Left unattended, the tendon may go on to necrosis due to ischemia and desiccation. Healing by secondary intention occurs, and the tendon remnants are frozen in scar. Unless good skin coverage is provided, functional recovery is poor.

Severe Injury

There is loss of tendon substance. Untreated, the proximal tendon end retracts, with reattachment at another level. Both ends are bound down in the subsequent scar. Secondary complications include joint stiffness due to lack of motion by flexor or extensor forces and loss of articular balance, which may compromise later reconstruction.

Management

Mild Injury

Coverage of the exposed tendon is provided at the delayed closure of the skin in 3 to 5 days. If necessary, split-thickness skin grafts are utilized for coverage.

Moderate Injury

Conservative débridement of the injured tendon is done and coverage is provided at the delayed skin closure. Split-thickness skin grafts can "take" on the tendon but will become adherent, and the "take" is not as reliable as when paratenon is present.

Severe Injury

With tendon transection or loss of substance, repair is deferred until conditions are optimal. It must be remembered that this is not a simple laceration but rather a crush-avulsion injury, and that the damage to the tendon and surrounding structures is often extensive. Repair sometimes requires mobilization beyond the confines of the immediate tendon injury, and this only adds to the trauma in the acute crushing injury. Therefore,

repair or grafting is delayed until tissues are supple and the tendon bed is stable, with good passive joint mobility.

Special Problems

The PIP Joint Central Slip

With crush-avulsion of the extensor surface of the PIP joint, and destruction of the central slip, the potential exists for the development of the chronic boutonnière deformity. An initial assessment is made as to the extent of the soft tissue loss over the joint. Necrotic skin and tendon are débrided, and the joint is pinned in the functional position. At this point, there may be little left in the way of a central slip or of the lateral bands. Delayed closure of the skin or skin grafting is accomplished, and the pins are removed when enough stability has been acquired for protected motion. Dynamic extension splinting with active flexion is utilized to preserve motion and to maintain the joint in extension when not in use. If the flexion deformity ensues despite these measures, consideration for later soft tissue reconstruction is modified by the degree of passive motion attainable at the PIP joint. Other later alternatives include prosthetic joint replacement or fusion. Such reconstruction is beyond the scope of this discussion, but our results with late reconstruction of the chronic boutonnière deformity have not been ideal.

Zone II

Crush injuries to the tendon in this area ("no man's land") are approached with caution. The first priorities are for stable soft tissue coverage and maximum joint mobility. Tendon repair or grafting is deferred until the bed has reached equilibrium and optimal conditions are obtained. Again, it is emphasized that these are not simple lacerations, but represent crushing trauma with all its implications of extensive tissue disruption, inflammation, and fibrous wound healing.

SYSTEMIC CONSEQUENCES

Renal Injury

The renal failure associated with crush injuries has long been appreciated. The most commonly accepted theories implicate myoglobin or hypotension as the cause of this serious complication.[6, 22]

Myoglobin is structurally related to hemoglobin, and is absorbed into the bloodstream secondary to muscular disruption and necrosis. However, unlike hemoglobin, it is freely diffusable into the urine. In an acidic urine, such as that which commonly occurs in the traumatized individual, myoglobin may be precipitated in the collecting tubules and effectively obstruct the kidney. In addition, it seems that

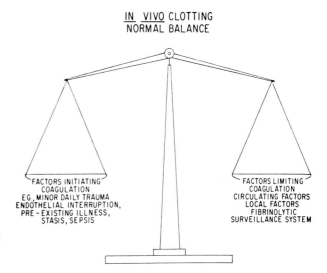

Figure 19–9. Normal balance between the forces that initiate intravascular coagulation and those that prevent it.

myoglobin may be nephrotoxic and can injure the renal parenchyma through direct contact. The extent of injury roughly correlates with the volume of muscle injured.

Hypotension, with its deleterious effects on the renal tubules, has also been implicated. Tubular epithelium is extremely sensitive to ischemic injury, and hypotension, also common in the traumatized patient, may result in necrosis of the tubular epithelium. The overall effect is a pattern resembling that of acute tubular necrosis both clinically and histologically, which usually occurs within the first 48 to 72 hours postinjury.

A brisk diuresis is the key to prevention of this injury. Thus, urinary output is maintained and serum creatinine and urea nitrogen levels are monitored. Bicarbonate may be administered, if deemed necessary, to alkalinize the urine in an effort to avoid myoglobin precipitation. Again, oliguria secondary to a contracted extracellular fluid volume must be avoided, and intravenous fluids are administered to ensure adequate volume. Thus, the initial steps in management include a secure intravenous pathway, baseline urinalysis and electrolyte determinations, and indwelling catheterization. If renal function deteriorates, dialysis may be necessary both to protect the kidneys from further injury and to eliminate metabolic waste.

The Hypercoagulable State

In addition to previously discussed problems, the patient with a severe crushing injury is also at increased risk for intravascular thrombosis. Although the so-called "hypercoagulable state" has been recognized since the days of Virchow, only recently have reliable methods become available for documenting the subtle changes in coagulation that could lead to serious clinical problems.

It is now known that trauma upsets the normal balance between the circulating factors that initiate

coagulation and those that inhibit it (Figs. 19–9 and 19–10).[21] These latter factors are extremely efficient in limiting and localizing intravascular coagulation and, in effect, are responsible for maintaining the fluidity of the blood.[9]

In the patient with upper extremity trauma such as the crush injury, there is a drift toward increased coagulability that seems to be proportional to the magnitude of the injury. In this setting, thrombosis and loss of the hand or arm becomes a real possibility.

In a series of 40 patients, it was found that elective extremity operations slightly increased the risk of thrombosis, whereas severe hand and upper extremity trauma markedly influenced the risk of intravascular clot formation. In a group of 20 patients who had sustained hand and upper extremity trauma, five had thrombotic complications, and three of

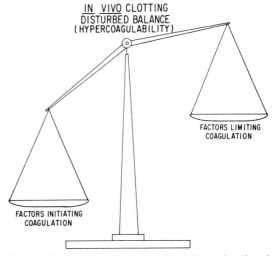

Figure 19–10. The coagulation "scale" can be tipped toward a hypercoagulable state by severe trauma to the extremities.

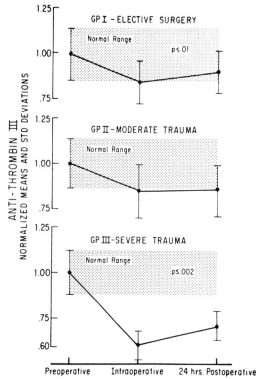

Figure 19–11. Comparison of antithrombin-3 (AT-3) levels in patients undergoing elective surgery and in those sustaining moderate and severe trauma to the extremities. Note the low levels at AT-3 related to severe trauma. This finding correlated with severe complications due to intravascular thrombosis.

these lost the involved hand and arm. The factor which correlated most closely with these findings was abnormally low levels of a circulating protein, antithrombin III (AT-III). This circulating globulin appears to be clinically the most important naturally occurring plasma inhibitor of thrombin.[17]

It appears that, in severe upper extremity trauma, the AT-III level is markedly reduced. In certain individuals, a critical level is reached at which uncontrollable thrombosis is a distinct possibility. At this point loss of the injured limb can occur, as well as other serious thrombotic complications. The critical time period is within the first 72 hours of the trauma (Fig. 19–11).

To manage this condition, the patient is kept well hydrated and, if hypercoagulability is suspected, AT-III activity is measured by any of several commercially available assays. If the AT-III level is low, replenishment with fresh-frozen plasma can be undertaken. The use of heparin is felt to be ineffective without replenishment of antithrombins.[9]

Infection

Soft tissue necrosis, especially in the deep crushing injury with contaminating foreign material, pre-

disposes to infection. Gas gangrene, clostridial myonecrosis, and other anaerobic and aerobic infections are a threat when necrotic muscle, ischemia, and contamination coexist. Septicemia can occur in this setting, especially in the immunosuppressed, diabetic, or debilitated individual, and the consequences can be life-threatening.

The management of infection is incision and drainage of the abscess. It must be emphasized that infection is best prevented in the crush wound by forceful irrigation, removal of devitalized tissue, and not closing the wound with such a high infectious potential. However, prophylactic antibiotics are administered in accordance with the guidelines established by the American College of Surgeons' Committee on Control of Surgical Infections.[2] This is done, as stated by the Committee, as an adjunct and not as a substitute for thorough operative cleansing of the wound. Generally, if the crush injury is open, and is associated with fracture or joint injury, preoperative intravenous broad-spectrum antibiotics are given. This is also done if there is heavy contamination. Tetanus prophylaxis is ensured in each individual.

Electrolyte Abnormalities

With muscle necrosis, intracellular potassium is released and absorbed into the bloodstream. Ordinarily this is well tolerated, but in the patient with renal or cardiac insufficiency, hyperkalemia can result in serious arrhythmias. The critical period lasts as long as necrotic muscle is still present in the body.

Electrolyte abnormalities are corrected by infusion of appropriate intravenous solutions while cautiously avoiding fluid overload.

CASE HISTORY

A 21-year-old soldier sustained a moderately severe crush injury when a bucket loader on an engineering vehicle fell on his left, dominant hand. On initial evaluation, 1 hour postinjury, it was noted that there was already severe swelling over the dorsum. Nerves and major arteries were intact, and flexor tendons were intact. There were lacerations over the dorsum and lateral border, as well as in the first web space. X-rays revealed fractures of the ring and small finger metacarpal bones. These fractures were unstable, and there was collapse of the ulnar mobile unit of the hand (Fig. 19–12).

The patient was taken to the operating room and the wound was débrided. There was dirt and grease within the lacerations, and the wound was vigorously cleansed and irrigated. Intrinsic muscle compartments were released, fractures were internally fixed with Kirschner wires, and small Penrose drains were inserted into the deep spaces (Fig. 19–13). The skin was left open for delayed closure. The

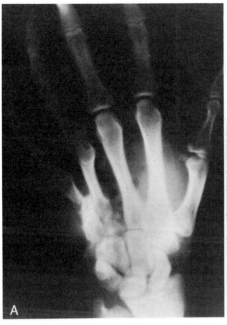
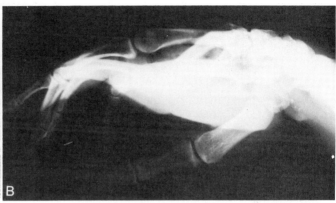

Figure 19–12. *A,* Preoperative x-rays showing fractures of the metacarpals to the ring and small fingers; *B,* lateral x-rays. These fractures were unstable.

hand was elevated (Fig. 19–14). In 5 days a delayed closure was performed, because the wound was "clean" (Fig. 19–15). Dynamic splinting was started immediately, and full motion was gradually restored. The patient was well motivated toward this end. Figure 19–16 shows the condition 1½ years later. There is no limitation of motion nor intrinsic tightness (Fig. 19–16*C*).

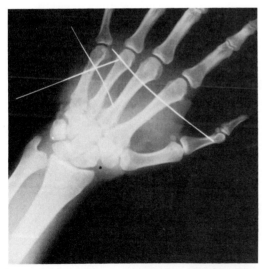

Figure 19–13. Intraoperative x-ray after intrinsic releases, reduction and fixation of the fractures, and a thorough cleansing of the wound. Motion, supported by dynamic splints, was started immediately after removal of the first dressing.

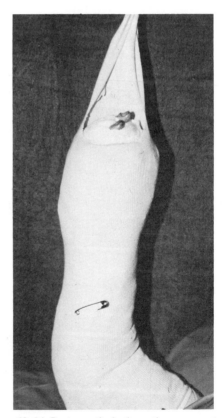

Figure 19–14. Postoperatively the entire upper extremity was placed in a soft conforming elevated dressing, supported by a well-padded posterior plaster splint, similar to the dressing shown here.

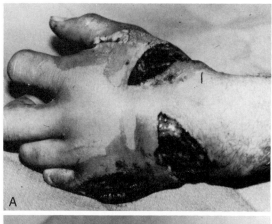
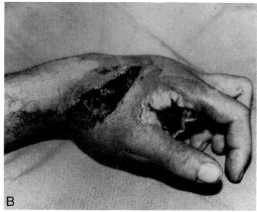
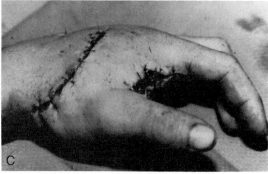

Figure 19–15. *A,* Dorsal view of the skin disruptions at the time of delayed closure; *B,* radial view of the skin lacerations, which communicated freely with each other on digital examination; *C,* final closure of the wound.

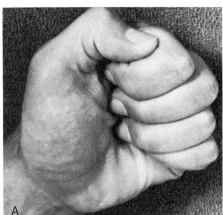
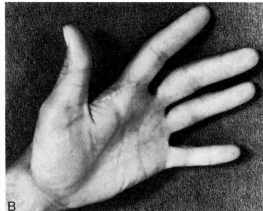
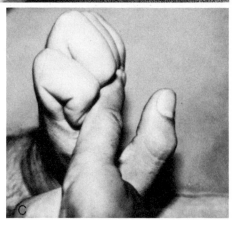

Figure 19–16. *A,* The patient recovered full power in flexion, largely due to his excellent attitude and motivation during the rehabilitation program; *B,* there was no restriction of motion on extension. *C,* There was also no evidence of intrinsic muscle contracture despite an injury in which this is a frequent complication.

References

1. Altemeier, W. A., and Alexander, J. W.: Surgical infections and choice of antibiotics. *In* Sabiston, D. C., Jr. (ed.): Davis-Christopher Textbook of Surgery, Philadelphia, W. B. Saunders, 1977, pp. 340–362.
2. Altemeier, W. A., et al. (eds.): Manual on Control of Infection in Surgical Patients, Philadelphia, J. B. Lippincott, 1976.
3. Arem, A. J.: The stiff hand: An approach to prevention and treatment. Contemp. Orthop., 3:501, 1981.
4. Beasley, R. W.: Principles of managing acute hand injuries. *In* Converse, J. M. (ed.): Reconstructive Plastic Surgery: Principles and Procedures in Correction, Reconstruction, and Transplantation, 2nd ed., Philadelphia, W. B. Saunders, 1977, p. 3000.
5. Brown, P.: Less than ten. Presented at the Annual Meeting of the American Society for Surgery of the Hand, Las Vegas, 1981.
6. DeWardener, H. G.: The Kidney. London, J & A Churchill, 1967, p. 352.
7. Grabb, W. C., and Smith, J. W.: Repair of peripheral nerves. *In* Converse, J. M. (ed.): Reconstructive Plastic Surgery: Principles and Procedures in Correction, Reconstruction, and Transplantation, 2nd ed., Philadelphia, W. B. Saunders, 1977, p. 875.
8. Griffiths, D.: Volkmann's ischemic contracture. Br. J. Surg., 28:239, 1940.
9. Lane, J., and Briggs, R.: The natural inhibitors of coagulation: Anti-thrombin III, heparin co-factor and antifactor Xa. *In* Poller, L. (ed.): Recent Advances in Blood Coagulation, London, Churchill-Livingstone, 1977.
10. Matsen, F. A.: Compartment syndrome: A unified concept. Clin. Orthop. Rel. Res., 113:8, 1975.
11. Matsen, F. A., Winquist, R. A., and Krugmire, R. B.: Diagnosis and management of compartmental syndromes. J. Bone Joint Surg., 62A:286, 1980.
12. McCraw, J. B., Myers, B., and Shanklin, K. D.: The value of fluorescein in predicting the viability of arterialized flaps. Plast. Reconstr. Surg., 60:710, 1977.
13. Mubarak, S. J., and Hargens, A. R.: Compartment Syndromes and Volkmann's Contracture, Philadelphia, W. B. Saunders, 1981.
14. Mubarak, S. J., et al.: The wick catheter technique for measurement of intramuscular pressure. J. Bone Joint Surg., 58A:1016, 1976.
15. Mubarak, S. J., et al.: Acute compartment syndrome: Diagnosis and treatment with the aid of the wick catheter. J. Bone Joint Surg., 60A:1091, 1978.
16. Robbins, S. L.: Pathology, Philadelphia, W. B. Saunders, 1968, p. 10.
17. Seyfer, A. E., et al.: Coagulation changes in elective surgery and trauma. Ann. Surg., 193:210, 1981.
18. Sheridan, G. W., Matsen, F. A., and Krugmire, R. B.: Further investigations on the pathophysiology of the compartmental syndrome. Clin. Orthop., 123:266, 1977.
19. Spinner, M.: Management of nerve compression lesions of the upper extremity. *In* Omer, G. E., and Spinner, M. (eds.): Management of Peripheral Nerve Problems, Philadelphia, W. B. Saunders, 1980, p. 570.
20. Starling, E. H.: On the absorption of fluids from the connective tissue spaces. J. Physiol., 19:312, 1896.
21. Sunderland, S.: Nerves and Nerve Injury, London, Livingston, 1968, p. 127.
22. Weeks, R. S.: The crush syndrome. Surg. Gynecol. Obstet., 127:369, 1968.
23. White, W. L.: Restoration of function and balance of the wrist and hand by tendon transfer. Surg. Clin. North Am., 40:427, 1960.
24. Whitesides, T. E., Harada, H., and Morimoto, K.: Compartment syndromes and the role of fasciotomy, its parameters and techniques. *In* American Academy of Orthopaedic Surgeons: Instructional Course Lectures, Vol. 26, St. Louis, C. V. Mosby, 1977, p. 179.

20

COMPLICATIONS FOLLOWING ACUTE INFECTIONS OF THE HAND

Nashaat Naam
and John A. Boswick, Jr.

Infections of the hand are still very common problems. In one study, 20% of all patients admitted to a hand surgical service had infections.[1] The introduction of antibiotics and early decisive treatment have decreased the incidence of severe disability that may follow hand infections. Antibiotics alone will not be effective in treating hand infections except in selected cases and if the condition is treated very early, in the first 24 to 48 hours after onset.[2]

Adequate drainage, rest, elevation, and proper antibiotics are considered to be the general principles in treating hand infections. Selection of the initial antibiotics is usually empiric until the results of culture and sensitivity tests are available. Two thirds of the patients give a history of injury.[3] The organisms often gain entrance through trivial injuries or scratches of the skin or about the nails, or through lacerations, pricks, crushing injuries, or burns.[4] There has been increasing incidence of severe infection at sites of injections in drug addicts.[5] Most infections of the hand are caused by *Staphylococcus aureus* (47–59%), followed by β-hemolytic streptococci (12–16%), *Enterococcus* (2–10%), *Escherichia coli* (5–8%), and *Aerobacter aerogenes* (3–11%). Multiple organisms are found in 25% of patients.[1, 3, 6] Resistant strains of bacteria, especially *Staphylococcus*, are emerging, particularly in hospital settings.

Most infections start as cellulitis. Incision and drainage have no place in treating this early stage. Later an abscess may form, and this must be treated by adequate surgical drainage. Most complications of hand infections are due to inadequate initial management. One should take into consideration not only adequate drainage of the pus but also the subsequent function of the hand.

Good anesthesia and tourniquet control are essential for adequate surgical drainage. The arm should not be exsanguinated by elastic wrapping, because this may spread the infection proximally. Elevation of the arm for a few minutes before inflating the tourniquet is sufficient.

Incisions should be properly placed to permit extension in any direction, and to avoid injuring vital structures and the formation of contractures or painful scars.

LYMPHANGITIS

Lymphangitis is an inflammation of the lymphatic vessels. There are two systems of lymphatics in the upper extremity. The superficial vessels arise from plexuses in the skin and run in the subcutaneous tissue. They drain in trunks at the sides of the fingers, which run to the dorsum of the hand and wrist. The lymphatic trunks unite, forming a few bundles in the forearm and a single bundle on the external surface of the arm. Most of the lymphatic trunks enter into the humeral chain of axillary lymph nodes. Some lymphatic trunks ascend in the deltopectoral groove to empty in the subclavian lymph nodes. The deep system is composed of lymph vessels that accompany the major blood vessels and that also terminate in the humeral chain of axillary lymph nodes.

Lymphangitis is still seen in patients with hand infections. However, its incidence has decreased compared with that in the preantibiotic era to about

20%.[7] The causative organism is usually *Streptococcus*, and it is sensitive to penicillin. It is important to differentiate between superficial and deep lymphangitis.[7] In superficial lymphangitis, there are red streaks extending from the area of the wound up the forearm and the arm. There is no swelling of the hand or the forearm compared with deep lymphangitis, in which rapid and massive swelling of the hand and forearm occur. General signs of infection, such as fever, leukocytosis, and tachycardia, are more pronounced in deep lymphangitis.

Treatment

General rest, hospitalization if necessary, immobilization of the affected part, and elevation of the hand are essential measures. Antibiotics should be started when indicated. Gram stains and cultures should be obtained, if possible. Otherwise the selection of an antibiotic must be empiric.

Complications

The incidence of complications following lymphangitis has been greatly decreased due to the use of antibiotics. Superficial lymphangitis has been greatly decreased due to the use of antibiotics. Superficial lymphangitis may cause extensive sloughing of subcutaneous tissue, which may require incision and drainage, and often extensive débridement. Abscess formation from the infected epitrochlear, axillary, or supraclavicular lymph nodes may occur, requiring incision and drainage. Infection from axillary lymph nodes may spread under pectoral or subscapular muscles. Abscesses of the shoulder region rarely develop along the course of the lymphatics in the deltopectoral groove. Tenosynovitis may complicate deep lymphangitis because of the close proximity of deep lymphatics to the tendon sheath. Generalized sepsis may occur because of spread of infection from axillary lymph nodes to the general circulation via the thoracic duct.[4, 7]

PARONYCHIA

This is the most common infection of the hand, accounting for approximately 30% of hand infections.[2, 4, 9] It involves the tissues adjacent to and below the nail. The process may start between the nail and eponychium, usually on one side. It may extend beneath the base of the nail between the nail and its bed. The causative organism is usually *S. aureus*, which is often introduced into the paronychial tissue by a sliver of nail or hangnail. Spontaneous rupture of small abscesses may occur but the drainage is often inadequate.

Treatment

In the very early stages, simple elevation, rest, and perhaps antibiotics are sufficient. If an abscess is superficial, it can be drained often without anesthesia by passing the tip of the knife blade into the abscess obliquely away from the nail bed and matrix. If the abscess is deep or extensive, adequate surgical drainage should be done under digital block anesthesia. The incision should be made in the lateral fold with the blade at an oblique angle away from the nail bed and matrix, extending proximally to the base of the nail and exposing the lateral margin of the nail. The subungual space should be inspected to avoid missing any subungual abscess, which can be drained by removing part of the nail to facilitate drainage. A gauze wick is left in place for 48 hours.

Complications

Pulp space infection is the most common complication of infections around the nail. Infection spreads through a sinus at the side of the nail bed. The infected pulp space should be adequately drained through the existing sinus. Osteomyelitis of the distal phalanx can occur, and its presence is suspected if the infection persists despite adequate drainage or by palpation of rough bone denuded of periosteum. Septic arthritis of the distal interphalangeal joint is an unusual complication of paronychia. Rarely, in adolescents, epiphyseal separation by pus may occur. In that case, the finger should be immobilized in plaster similar to that used for mallet finger.[3] Skin necrosis may complicate an extensive paronychia. This is best treated by skin grafting after adequate control of infection.

PULP SPACE INFECTION

Pulp space infection is a difficult problem primarily because it is a closed space infection, which if not treated early and adequately may lead to serious complications.[3, 10–12] The space extends from the distal interphalangeal crease to the fingertip, with many fibrous strands that are attached to the skin and periosteum.

The infection is often preceded by history of injury, or it may follow untreated paronychia or subungual abscess. *S. aureus* is usually the offending organism. The inflammation may start as a cellulitis, which may progress into abscess formation. Due to the unyielding nature of the closed pulp space, skin necrosis, bone necrosis, osteomyelitis, or tenosynovitis may result. The pulp space is swollen, red, and severely tender. Spontaneous decompression through a skin sinus on the volar aspect may occur, but drainage is usually inadequate and surgical drainage is required.

Treatment

The early stages can be treated by antibiotics, splinting, and elevation. However, it is usually advisable to proceed with incision and drainage because it is difficult clinically to assess the presence

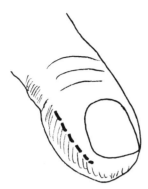

Figure 20–1. Incision for felon.

of an early abscess. There is much debate about the site of incision. It is advisable to use a unilateral longitudinal incision if no skin sinus is present. The incision is made just dorsal to the midlateral line of the finger, about ½ cm distal to the distal interphalangeal joint flexion crease. It is extended distally in a straight line to within ½ cm of the nail edge (Fig. 20–1). The incision is deepened volarly to the distal phalanx, draining the abscess. A gauze pack is left in place until the drainage ceases. In the presence of the skin sinus, longitudinal incision of the sinus with excision of necrotic skin edges is recommended. In cases secondary to subungual abscesses, a hockey stick incision may be used. Fishmouth incisions and through-and-through incisions should not be used. They often result in instability of distal phalangeal skin and the fat pad, and sometimes in necrosis of the fat pad, leaving a deforming, tender scar.[2, 11, 13]

Complications

Osteomyelitis of the distal phalanx is the most important complication of the pulp space infection. This can be suspected by palpating rough bone denuded of periosteum, finding a sequestrum during drainage of the felon, or development of radiologic signs of osteomyelitis. Loose pieces of sequestrum can be removed, and most of the remaining sequestrae will be extruded subsequently if the abscess is adequately drained. In some cases, sequestrectomy may be indicated.

Septic arthritis of the distal interphalangeal joint may develop as a result of direct spread from a proximal abscess or from osteomyelitis. Sloughing of the pulp or skin necrosis may develop, requiring skin grafting after clearing of the infection.

Infection may spread to the middle compartment or to the dorsum underneath the nail bed. Acute tenosynovitis may result from spread of infection from a proximal abscess, but it often results from inadvertent injury of the flexor tendon sheath during incision and drainage of the felon.[12, 14] Occasionally, a pulp space infection of the thumb may spread to the thenar space.

Inappropriately placed incisions may result in serious iatrogenic complications, such as decreased sensitivity of the fingertip secondary to digital nerve injury, unstable fat pad, or deforming, painful, and tender scars.

DEEP SPACE INFECTIONS IN THE PALM

The deep fascial spaces are potential spaces deep to the flexor tendons. There are two deep spaces of clinical importance. The two are separated by a septum attached volarly on the surface of the flexor tendons of the long finger and dorsally to the entire length of the long finger metacarpal. The midpalmar space lies to the ulnar side of the midpalmar septum. It is bounded anteriorly by the flexor tendons of the long, ring, and little fingers, and posteriorly by the fascia covering the long, ring, and little finger metacarpals and the intervening interosseous muscles. Distally, the space is bounded by vertical septae extending from the palmar aponeurosis to the floor of the space about 2 cm proximal to the webs. Proximally, it is limited by a thin fascial septum at the distal end of the transverse carpal ligament. The thenar space, to the radial side of the midpalmar septum, lies volar to the adductor pollicis muscle. Anteriorly lies the flexor tendons of the index finger. The radial boundary of the thenar space is formed by the thin layer of fascia extending over the radial edge of the adductor pollicis muscle.[15]

Midpalmar Infections

Infections of the midpalmar space may result from direct infection by a penetrating wound, flexor tenosynovitis of the long, ring, and little fingers or ulnar bursa, or spread of infection from the long, ring, or little fingers through the lumbrical canals.

There is loss of the normal palmar concavity, with localized tenderness over the midpalmar space. The dorsum of the hand becomes swollen, the long and ring fingers are held in a position of semiflexion, and their motion is painful and limited.

Treatment

The midpalmar space can be drained through a transverse incision parallel to a distal palmar crease (Fig. 20–2A).[7–9, 16] The palmar aponeurosis is opened, and the space is entered to one side of the flexor tendons of the ring finger. A drain is left until the drainage stops. A longitudinal incision parallel to the thenar crease may also be used (Fig. 20–2B).[2, 4, 17]

Instead of putting in a rubber drain and leaving the wound open, a polyethylene catheter can be inserted from the proximal end of the longitudinal incision, a small Penrose drain brought out at the distal end, and the wound in between closed. Continuous saline irrigation with or without antibiotics through the catheter is started and continued for 48 to 72 hours. This method has the advantage of primary wound closure and early return of active motion.[2, 18]

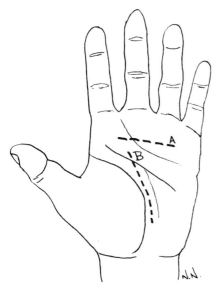

Figure 20-2. Transverse *(A)* and longitudinal *(B)* incisions.

Thenar Space Infections

Thenar space infections can result from penetrating wounds, tenosynovitis of the index finger or the thumb, or spread of infection from the radial bursa or midpalmar space. There is marked swelling of the web space of the thumb with the thumb held in a position of abduction and semiflexion (Fig. 20-3). The index finger is usually held in a position of semiflexion with pain on motion.

Treatment

The thenar space can be drained via dorsal, volar, or combined dorsal and volar incisions. In the dorsal approach, an incision is made in the middle of the dorsum of the first web space and carried down

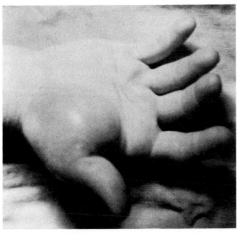

Figure 20-3. Thenar space abscess.

between the first dorsal interosseous and adductor pollicis muscles.[2, 4, 17, 19] The volar approach is through an incision made parallel to the thenar crease, avoiding injury to the motor branch of the median nerve. Dissection is carried down over the distal margin of the adductor pollicis, thereby draining both the adductor and first dorsal interosseous compartments.[4, 16, 20, 21]

Continuous saline irrigation of the abscess cavity through combined dorsal and volar incisions can be performed. The polyethylene catheter is inserted into the volar incision and a small Penrose drain inserted into the dorsal incision, and both incisions are closed. Continuous sterile saline irrigation is started and continued for 2 or more days. This technique has the advantage of thorough mechanical irrigation and primary wound closure.

Complications

Infections from the midpalmar space may extend into the forearm through the carpal canal or may spread to the thenar space. Infection of ulnar bursa or tenosynovitis of the long, ring, and little fingers may occur. Thenar space infection may spread through the lumbrical canal of the index finger, or it may spread to the radial bursa or the flexor tendon sheath of the index and the thumb.[22, 33] Osteomyelitis of the metacarpal bones may result from inadequate treatment of deep space infections.

TENOSYNOVITIS

Pyogenic infection of the flexor tendon sheath is one of the most serious infections of the hand. It rapidly destroys the gliding mechanism, forming dense adhesions that limit the tendon excursion and leading to severe loss of motion. The source of infection is usually secondary to penetrating injury or is caused by spread from an infected neighboring structure. Occasionally, the infection is hematogenous.

The index, long, and ring fingers are the most commonly involved. Most tendon sheath infections are secondary to *S. aureus.* Kanavel mentioned four cardinal signs of purulent tenosynovitis: generalized symmetric swelling of the finger, localized tenderness over the flexor sheath, semiflexed position of the involved finger, and severe pain on passive extension of the finger.[8]

Treatment

Tenosynovitis is a closed space infection. Thus, it has to be diagnosed and treated as early as possible to avoid devastating complications. If the patient is seen very early, conservative treatment in the form of rest, elevation, splinting, and high doses of parenteral antibiotics can be effective in controlling the infection, provided the patient is closely observed. Surgical drainage can be done through a midaxial incision along the whole finger. Dissection

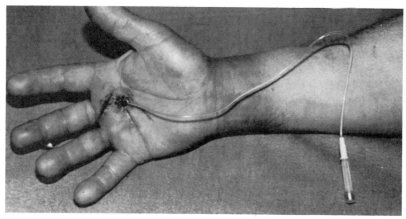

Figure 20–4. Closed tendon sheath irrigation using polyethylene catheter. Note the drain in the ulnar side of distal long finger.

is carried dorsally to the neurovascular bundle to reach the flexor sheath, which is incised between the pulleys. The accumulated cloudy or purulent material is drained and sent to the laboratory for Gram staining and culture and sensitivity tests. Another incision is made in the palm over the involved tendon for adequate drainage. All annular pulleys should be left intact. The wound is left open with drains left in place for 48 hours or more. Besser recommended antibiotic installation in the tendon sheath through a transverse incision in the palm over the infected tendon.[24] A small polyethylene catheter is inserted in the sheath and the wound is then closed. Postoperatively, an installation of antibiotics into the sheath is started and continued for 48 to 72 hours. Active motion is started immediately after removal of the catheter.

Closed tendon sheath irrigation has been described by Neviaser.[2, 25, 26] Exposure of the tendon sheath in the palm is made through a zigzag incision. The sheath is opened proximal to the A1 pulley, and the seropurulent material is drained and sent for culture and sensitivity testing. A 16-gauge pol-

yethylene catheter is inserted in the sheath for a distance of 1.5 to 2 cm. The distal end of the sheath is exposed through another incision on the ulnar midaxial side of the middle and distal phalanges. Part of the sheath distal to the A4 pulley is resected, and a small drain is inserted into the wound and sutured to the skin. The proximal and distal wounds are closed around the catheter and drain (Fig. 20–4).

Postoperatively, the sheath is irrigated by manual injection of 50 ml sterile saline solution every 2 hours. The catheter and drain are removed in 2 or 3 days. This technique has proved effective in thorough mechanical irrigation of the sheath and rapid return of function with primary wound healing (Fig. 20–5).

Complications

Infection in the closed space of the tendon sheath may lead to ischemic necrosis of the tendon, not only because of compromise of vincular circulation secondary to pressure and sepsis, but also because of compromised diffusion of synovial fluid.[27] Tendon

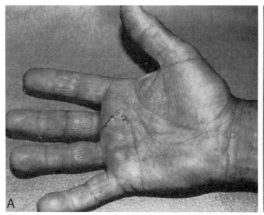
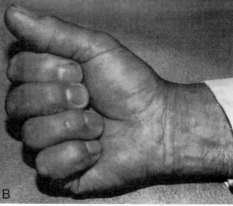

Figure 20–5. *A, B,* Excellent range of motion 10 days after closed tendon sheath irrigation for tenosynovitis of the left long finger.

sheath infection may spread to the deep spaces, forming a thenar or midpalmar space abscess. Tenosynovitis of the thumb may lead to radial bursa infection, and tenosynovitis of the little finger may lead to infection of the ulnar bursa. Infection may extend proximally from the bursae along the intramuscular planes of the forearm.

Compression of the median nerve may occur secondary to infection of radial or ulnar bursa. Immediate decompression of the carpal tunnel should be carried out. Osteomyelitis and septic arthritis may complicate flexor tenosynovitis and, on some occasions, it may lead to amputation of the affected finger.[28]

BITE INJURIES

Human bite injuries of the hand are relatively common, and their inadequate treatment can lead to devastating complications.[29] Many of these injuries are the result of striking another person's mouth with a clenched fist. The metacarpophalangeal joint is the most common site of injury. The proximal interphalangeal or occasionally the flexor tendon sheath may be injured.[27]

Infection is mostly caused by mixed organisms, including *S. aureus*, α-hemolytic streptococci, fusiform bacilli, gram-negative organisms, and anaerobic organisms such as bacteroids.[29–32] *Eikenella corrodens*, a gram-negative bacteria that is part of normal oral flora, has been isolated frequently from infected human bite injuries.

All dorsal wounds in the area of the metacarpophalangeal joint should be suspected as tooth injuries. Radiologically, joint injury can be suspected by the presence of a small intra-articular chip fracture of the metacarpal head or occasionally by the presence of air in the joint. All these injuries should be treated by thorough cleansing, débridement, and exploration of the wound to its depth. Cultures are taken of the wound, and the joint, tendon, and skin are left open.[27, 33] Antibiotics are selected empirically until results of cultures are known.

Exploration of the proximal interphalangeal joint is preferably done through a midaxial incision to avoid damage of the central slip of the extensor mechanism and the subsequent development of a boutonnière deformity.[27]

Complications

Osteomyelitis and septic arthritis are serious complications that may follow human bite injury. Occasionally, amputation of the involved digits is necessary. Infection may spread rapidly to the forearm, causing marked soft tissue damage that requires extensive débridement or, rarely, amputation at a higher level.[31]

Suppurative tenosynovitis of flexor tendons, and rarely of the extensor tendons, may develop.[29] Severe stiffness of the affected finger with loss of

function of the finger and sometimes the hand may complicate this type of infection.

Hand infection following animal bites is commonly caused by *Pasteurella multocida*, a small gram-negative penicillin-sensitive coccobacillus present in the normal oral flora of cats and dogs. Complications of infected animal bites include lymphangitis, septicemia, chronic infection, osteomyelitis, and septic arthritis. Treatment of animal bites should include irrigation and thorough débridement of the wound. The wounds are usually small, and should be left open. Initially, cephalosporin is the prophylactic antibiotic of choice until the results of the cultures are known. If *P. multocida* is cultured and there is clinical evidence of infection, penicillin should be used as the drug of choice.[34]

References

1. Stone, N. H., et al.: Hand infections. J. Bone Joint Surg., 51A:899, 1969.
2. Neviaser, R. J.: Infections. *In* Green, D. (ed.): Operative Hand Surgery, New York, Churchill Livingstone, 1982, pp. 771–791.
3. Robins, R. H. C.: Infections of the hand. A review based on 1000 consecutive cases. J. Bone Joint Surg., 34B:567, 1952.
4. Linscheid, R. L., and Dobyns, J. H.: Common and uncommon infections of the hand. Orthop. Clin. North Am., 6:1063, 1975.
5. Petrie, P. W. R., and Lamb, D. W.: Severe hand problems in drug addicts following self-administered injections. Hand, 5:130, 1973.
6. Eaton, R. G., and Butsch, D. P.: Antibiotic guidelines for hand infections. Surg. Gynecol. Obstet., 130:119, 1970.
7. Flynn, J. E.: The grave infections of the hand. *In* Flynn, J. (ed.): Hand Surgery, 3rd ed., Baltimore, Williams & Wilkins, 1982, pp. 688–706.
8. Kanavel, A. B.: Infections of the Hand. A Guide to the Surgical Treatment of Acute and Chronic Suppurative Processes in the Fingers, Hand, and Forearm, 7th ed., Philadelphia, Lea & Febiger, 1943.
9. Bingham, D. I. C.: Acute infections of the hand. Surg. Clin. North Am., 40:1285, 1960.
10. Crandon, J. H.: Lesser infections of the hand. *In* Flynn, J. (ed.): Hand Surgery, Baltimore, Williams & Wilkins, 1982, pp. 676–688.
11. Kilgore, E. S., Jr., et al.: Treatment of felons. Am. J. Surg., 130:194, 1975.
12. Bolton, H., Fowler, P. J., and Jepson, R. P.: Natural history and treatment of pulp space infection and osteomyelitis of the terminal phalanx. J. Bone Joint Surg., 31B:499, 1949.
13. Boyes, J. H.: Infections. *In* Boyes, J. (ed.): Bunnell's Surgery of the Hand, 5th ed., Philadelphia, J. B. Lippincott, 1970, pp. 613–642.
14. Butler, E. D.: Discussion of paper by Kilgore et al. Am. J. Surg., 130:197, 1975.
15. Kaplan, E. B.: Functional and Surgical Anatomy of the Hand, 2nd ed., Philadelphia, J. B. Lippincott, 1965.
16. Shamblin, W. R.: The diagnosis and treatment of acute infections of the hand. South. Med. J., 62:209, 1969.
17. Milford, L. W.: The hand. *In* Crenshaw, A. (ed.): Campbell's Operative Orthopedics, 6th ed., St. Louis, C. V. Mosby, 1980, pp. 385–393.
18. Flynn, J. E.: Modern consideration of major hand infections. N. Engl. J. Med., 252:605, 1955.
19. Brown, H.: Hand infections. Am. Fam. Physician, 18:79, 1978.
20. Loudon, J. B., Miniero, J. D., and Scott, J. C.: Infections of the hand. J. Bone Joint Surg., 30B:409, 1948.
21. Scott, J. C., and Jones, B. J.: Results of treatment of infections of the hand. J. Bone Joint Surg., 34B:581, 1952.
22. Entin, M. A.: Infections of the hand. Surg. Clin. North Am., 44:981, 1964.

23. Mann, R. J., and Peacock, J. M.: Hand infections in patients with diabetes mellitus. J. Trauma, 17:376, 1977.
24. Besser, M. I. B.: Digital flexor tendon irrigation. Hand, 8:72, 1976.
25. Neviaser, R. J., and Gunther, S. F.; Tenosynovial infections of the hand. Part I. Acute pyogenic tenosynovitis. *In* American Academy of Orthopaedic Surgeons: Instructional Course Lectures, Vol. 29, St. Louis, CV Mosby, 1980.
26. Neviaser, R. J.: Closed tendon sheath irrigation for pyogenic flexor tenosynovitis. J. Hand Surg., 3:462, 1978.
27. Burkhalter, W. E.: Infections. *In* Boswick, J. (ed.): Current Concepts in Hand Surgery, Philadelphia, Lea & Febiger, 1983, pp. 43–50.
28. Michaeli, D.; Osteomyelitis with special reference to the hand. Prog. Surg., 16:38, 1978.
29. Farmer, C. B., and Mann, R. J.: Human bite infections of the hand. South. Med. J., 59:515, 1966.
30. Goldstein, E. J. C., et al.: Infections following clenched-fist injury: A new perspective. J. Hand Surg., 3:455, 1978.
31. Mann, R. J., Hoffeld, T. A., and Farmer, C. B.: Human bites of the hand. Twenty years of experience. J. Hand Surg., 2:97, 1977.
32. Malinowski, R. W., et al.: The management of human bite injuries of the hand. J. Trauma, 19:655, 1979.
33. Boswick, J. A.: Discussion of paper of Malinoswki et al. J. Trauma, 19:655, 1979.
34. Arons, M. S., and Polayes, I. M.: *Pasteurella multocida*, the major cause of hand infections following domestic animal bites. J. Hand Surg., 7:49, 1982.

21

COMPLICATIONS FOLLOWING RHEUMATOID AND DEGENERATIVE JOINT DISEASES

Charley J. Smyth

The term "rheumatoid arthritis" (RA) was first used by Garrod in 1859, but it was not clear whether he distinguished between this polyarthritis and degenerative joint disease (DJD) or osteoarthritis as they are recognized today.[1] The first definite differentiation between these two most common types of rheumatic diseases was made by Nichols and Richardson in 1909[2] in their excellent observations of the pathologic lesions of these two diseases. Their milestone reports introduced a new era in research and understanding of the rapidly expanding field of rheumatic diseases. Today, more than 100 different connective tissue diseases are clearly defined; these constitute the greatest cause for crippling in the United States.

It is important in a book such as this, devoted to the upper extremity, to emphasize that both RA and DJD are widespread joint disorders, and that RA also involves multiple systems having many extra-articular manifestations with associated constitutional symptoms. The following discussion will present the distinguishing clinical, laboratory, and radiographic features of these two most common types of generalized rheumatic disorders.

RHEUMATOID DISEASE

Distinguishing Features

A Multisystem Illness

Rheumatoid arthritis is the most common (1 to 3% of the world population) and most disabling of

the inflammatory arthritides.[3] There is general agreement that it affects women more frequently than men, with a female:male ratio of from 3:1 to 3:2 in most large series. In most patients, the disease starts between the ages of 20 to 50 years, but the onset also occurs in young children of 3 to 5 years and may also begin in those 65 to 70 years of age or older. In most individuals, the disease has an insidious onset in one or two joints, but an abrupt onset can occur in approximately 8 to 15% of patients.[4] When the onset is acute, it may literally start overnight with fever, malaise, myalgias, and polyarthralgias or polyarthritis. It is more characteristic to note a few joints involved slowly with pain, swelling, and stiffness, with a gradual extension to other joints over the next several months. There is a strong tendency to have symmetric involvement of the small joints of the hands, wrists, and feet.

As the disease progresses and additional joints become affected, the patients may report low-grade fever, fatigue, malaise, and prominent early morning stiffness. Restricted range of motion of affected joints is the rule. Although the smaller peripheral joints of the hands and feet are prone to be affected first, large joints may be the original site of the disease; the hip and shoulder girdle joints and the spine, however, are usually spared until much later in the illness. It is well to point out that any diarthrodial joint may become involved. Less frequently, but no less crippling, is the involvement of the temperomandibular, sternoclavicular, and cricoarytenoid joints.

Extra-Articular Manifestations

A striking aspect of the general picture is the degree and often the speed of onset of muscle atrophy, with accompanying weakness.

One of the most typical lesions of rheumatoid disease is the occurrence of rheumatoid nodules; these diagnostic lesions most often develop at points of pressure, such as the extensor surface of the forearms near the elbow (Fig. 21–1), about the knees, Achilles tendons, fingers (Fig. 21–2), and toes; they are occasionally found in the pads of the fingers. About 20 to 25% of patients will manifest these asymptomatic nontender, firm nodules during some stage of their illness. They are rarely seen in the absence of a positive rheumatoid factor in the serum. A few instances of rheumatoid nodules developing in the absence of arthritis have been reported.[5]

Additional clinical features of this systemic disease include enlargement of regional lymph nodes and spleen and circulatory changes, with cold clammy hands and feet and excessive sweating. These vascular changes also produce mottling and dusky cyanosis, numbness, and tingling of the fingers, but the classical series of color changes of Raynaud's phenomenon are rare. Small skin infarcts around the base of the nails are characteristic (Fig. 21–2D). Massive digital vascular occlusion with ulceration and dry gangrene are exceedingly rare.

Other manifestations of the multisystem involvement of rheumatoid disease include the following: dryness of the eyes and mouth (Sjögren's syndrome); pleural and pericardial frictions, effusions with pulmonary fibrosis or both; neurologic symptoms, including dysthesias, paresthesias, and neuritis, and, with rheumatoid arteritis, occlusion of a nutrient artery to a peripheral nerve, and mixed sensory and motor neuropathy—mononeuritis multiplex. Peripheral neuropathy of this degree has a grave prognosis. Joints of a hemiparetic limb remain unaffected.

Myositis associated with RA is a contributing factor to the characteristic morning stiffness and gelling in the joints. Muscle atrophy and wasting is the rule in severe RA, and can be confirmed by tests indicating elevated serum creatine phosphokinase (CPK) levels, electromyography, and muscle biopsy. The clinical picture of myopathy in RA may be extremely difficult to differentiate from that of polymyositis. It is currently thought that the loss of muscle mass is related to direct cell-mediated tissue destruction by lymphocytes, and is not entirely ascribed to disease or inactivity.

Laboratory Tests

Only a few laboratory test results are abnormal in this disease, and none are diagnostic. Mild anemia is common, with the hemoglobin ranging from 10 to 11 g; the erythrocyte sedimentation rate is usually moderately elevated, and hypergammaglobulinemia is often observed in active disease. The serum test for the rheumatoid factors is positive in 80 to 85% of patients, but may not become positive during the first 6 to 9 months of the illness. It is not specific and is found in other diseases, and even in normal subjects. Analysis of the synovial fluid reveals slight turbidity and decreased viscosity; the white cell counts usually are between 10,000 to 35,000/mm^3, with 35 to 50% polymorphonuclear leukocytes.

Radiographs

The radiologic features of rheumatoid disease assist in the diagnosis and reflect the anatomic changes. Soft tissue swelling, due to synovial thickening, effusions, and edema, are some of the earliest radiologic manifestations. X-rays of the hand during

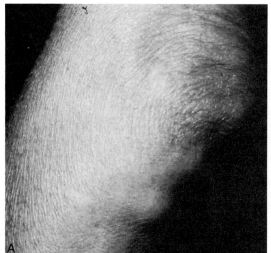
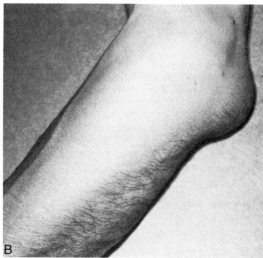

Figure 21–1. *A,* Rheumatoid nodule in typical location below bursa on extensor surface of the forearm; *B,* olecranon RA bursa.

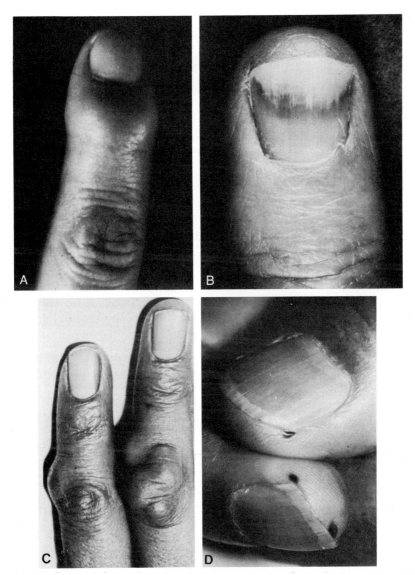

Figure 21–2. *A,* Degenerative joint disease of distal interphalangeal joint of finger (Heberden's nodes); *B,* nail and subjacent distal interphalangeal arthritis of psoriasis; *C,* rheumatoid nodules of the fingers; *D,* periungual skin infarcts of rheumatoid arthritis.

the first 6 to 12 months may show only the characteristic soft tissue swelling, with the production of fusiform enlargement of the proximal interphalangeal joints. At the same time, osteoporosis in the juxta-articular bone occurs.

When the disease persists and progresses the hyaline articular cartilage is absorbed, and a characteristic uniform reduction in the joint spaces results. A fibrous membrane or pannus growing across the surface of the cartilage leads to further cartilage destruction and to joint space narrowing.

As a result of the lytic effects of the fibrous pannus growing inward from the synovial membrane, further cartilage loss occurs, and the subchondral bone is invaded. Also, bony trabeculae become thin or are absorbed, leading to bony

erosions or cystlike subcortical lesions. These pseudocysts are sharply marginated and occur in both large and small joints.

The same destructive inflammatory changes that produce the cartilage loss cause ligamentous laxity and muscle imbalance between groups of flexors and extensors. This combination of changes within and about the joint produce malalignment and subluxation. In the hands, there are volar subluxation at the metacarpophalangeal articulations and the characteristic ulnar drift of the fingers. Similar changes within the radiocarpal joints lead to radial deviation at this level. In advanced disease, additional contributing factors lead to further functional and structural deformities that are reflected in the radiographs. Generalized osteoporosis develops, and microfractures and bone absorption occur. In the hands, this destructive process may lead to shortening of the fingers, corrugation of the overlying skin, and hypermobility of the digital joints—the so-called opera-glass hand (la main en lorgnette).

In weight-bearing joints or in those in constant use, sclerosis may be noted adjacent to areas of bone erosion. This probably represents a reparative process that results in the secondary formation of osteophytes along the bone margins. Thus, the radiographs in late rheumatoid disease may present the changes of osteoarthritis. This has led to the x-ray term "secondary osteoarthritis."

Bony ankylosis may be the result of the sequence of pathologic changes, and is not an uncommon roentgenographic finding in late rheumatoid disease. Such joints are without motion and without function, but also without pain.

Clinical Course and Progress

It is not possible to predict the course that rheumatoid disease will take, but several general patterns are recognized (Fig. 21–1). Many patients nave only one or two brief clinical episodes (clinical course I). Those with this type will usually go into complete and permanent remission within 12 to 18 months after onset of the disease. The majority (50% or more) follow a chronic or progressive course (course II), with either short or prolonged remissions or relapses. It is also well documented in several large series that only 12 to 15% of patients progress without remission and lead to permanent disability (course III).

Factors associated with a poor prognosis include the persistence of symptoms and active synovitis for more than 1 year, age less than 30 years old, the presence of rheumatoid nodules, and a high titer of serum rheumatoid factors.

Certain stress conditions may be associated with increases in the severity of the active disease, including emotional and physical stress, prolonged exposure to cold or dampness, and recurrent bacterial or viral infections. However, there is no direct evidence that these factors contribute to the course of rheumatoid disease. There is strong indirect evidence that hereditary factors combined with immunologic influences, perhaps viral-induced, are responsible for this illness of unknown etiology with its variable and unpredictable course.

Determination of Progression and Functional Capacity: Stage of Disease—Pathologic Damage

Based on clinical features and radiographic changes as shown in Table 21–1, criteria have been accepted that establish the extent of pathologic damage (stage) and the degree of functional limitation (class).[6] Both clinical features and x-ray changes are essential in establishing the "stage" of the disease (Fig. 21–4).

Rheumatoid Disease of the Upper Extremity

Shoulder

Synovitis. This is commonly missed in the early RA, and is incorrectly called "bursitis." Involvement of one or both shoulders occurs in 47% of patients with RA, and is frequently the first joint involved.[3]

A moderate to considerable amount of synovial thickening or fluid must be present in the glenohumeral joint to produce detectable swelling of the articular capsule. A visible bulge usually occurs over the anterior aspect of the joint. In thin patients or

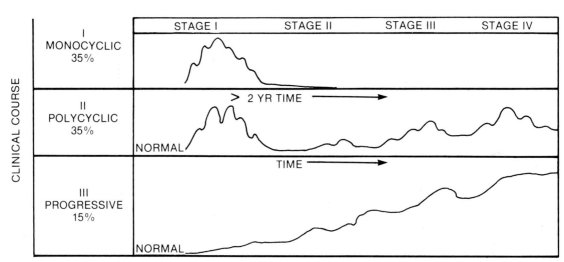

Figure 21–3. Three possible clinical courses of RA, indicating the highly variable and unpredictable activity and the four stages of the disease, as defined by the American Rheumatism Association. (From Ropes, M. W., et al.: Revision of the diagnostic criteria for rheumatoid arthritis. Bull. Rheum. Dis., 9:175, 1958.)

Table 21–1. CRITERIA FOR EVALUATING PROGRESSION AND FUNCTIONAL CAPACITY IN RHEUMATOID DISEASE*

Stage	Class
I (early): soft tissue swelling with no destructive changes, but osteoporosis may be present	I (early): complete ability to perform all usual duties without handicap
II (moderate): osteoporosis with or without slight subchondral bone and cartilage loss; soft tissue swelling or atrophy tenosynovitis and nodules may be present; no joint deformities or bone erosions	II (moderate): ability to conduct normal activities despite handicap of discomfort or limited motion of a few joints
III (severe): joint deformities such as subluxations, ulnar deviation, or hyperextension; extensive muscle atrophy with or without nodules or tenosynovitis; roentgenologic evidence of cartilage destruction, osteoporosis plus bony erosions, but without fibrous or bony ankylosis	III (severe): only able to perform little or none of the duties of the usual occupation or self-care
IV (terminal): criteria of stage III, plus fibrous or bony ankylosis	IV (terminal): largely or wholly incapacitated; confined to wheelchair or bed, with little or no self-care

*Modified from Ropes, M. W., et al.: Revision of the diagnostic criteria for rheumatoid arthritis. Bull. Rheum. Dis., 17:388, 1958.

in those with atrophy from disuse, intra-articular effusion may be detected along the long head of the biceps in the area of the bicipital groove.

Restricted motion, especially in abduction and internal and external rotation, are early signs of synovitis. To measure the range of motion of the shoulder accurately, the scapular motion must be prevented.

Pain caused by intrinsic shoulder disease is aggravated by motion, particularly full elevation in the forward flexed position on abduction to 90°. If the pain is referred from disease of the cervical area of the spine, a cervical rib, or midline mediastinal disease (cardiac, subphrenic inflammatory mass, or Pancoast tumor) motions of the shoulder do not produce or modify the discomfort. The history and examination must be utilized to establish the origin of the pain. Whenever pain in the shoulder or arm is not related to motion of the joint, and the examination is normal, referred pain should be considered as a probable cause.

Adhesive Capsulitis. Synovitis from RA is often associated with adhesive capsulitis (also called frozen shoulder). As a result of pain, the periarticular tissues of the shoulder may be restricted in motion, and it may be impossible to differentiate other shoulder lesions that can also result in a frozen shoulder (degenerative arthritis, tears of the musculoskeletal cuff, reflex sympathetic dystrophy, and posttraumatic conditions).

The Elbow

Rheumatoid Arthritis. Pain in one or both elbows occurs in 21% of patients with adult onset rheumatoid arthritis.[3] The condition is first apparent as pain, with thickening or a bulge in the para-olecranon grooves on each side of the olecranon process. Fluid can be detected by palpation. Local heat or tenderness are reliable signs of joint inflammation; redness is rare. These changes commonly cause restricted extension of the joint.

The bursa overlying the olecranon process is a frequent site of rheumatoid involvement, with swelling, heat, tenderness, and effusion. Firm nodules may be palpated in the lining of the bursa sac (see Fig. 21–1).

A characteristic lesion in rheumatoid disease is the subcutaneous nodule that is usually seen along the extensor surface of the forearm, usually 3 to 4 cm distal to the tip of the elbow. Some can only be detected when the examiner runs a finger along the extensor surface of the ulna. They are raised, firm, nontender, and may be firmly attached to the underlying fascia (see Fig. 21–1).

Wrist and Carpal Joints

Rheumatoid arthritis is a frequent cause of severe wrist disability. Synovitis may affect the radiocarpal, intercarpal, and radioulnar joints singly or in combination. The destructive effects of the rheumatoid inflammation relax the ligaments, lyse the cartilage, and cause erosive changes in the bones, thus disturbing the balance in the wrist. When bony erosions and absorption are severe, loosening of the ligaments and complete dislocation may occur. In some cases, spontaneous fusion of the intercarpal, carpometacarpal, and radiocarpal joints may occur before subluxation. A common deformity results when the ligaments on the radial aspect of the joint loosen and allow ulnar displacement of the proximal row of carpals; radial deviation of the hand or the forearm may then occur. Dislocation of the distal radioulnar articulation may be associated with this deviation, causing an instability on the ulnar side of the wrist.

Destructive rheumatoid synovitis of the radioulnar joint is a common cause for wrist disability. This lesion is characterized by the dorsal dislocation of the ulnar head, pain and weakness of the wrist, and decreased dorsiflexion and rotation. Also, there is increased flexion at the fourth and fifth metacarpophalangeal joints.

If active synovitis persists, the ulnar head, which has been dislocated dorsally, undergoes erosive changes and becomes sharp and irregular. The ulnar styloid may become roughened or absorbed. The extensor tendons passing over this jagged bone may rupture. Ruptures of tendons may also be secondary to direct invasive rheumatoid granulation tissue.

Wrist Tendon and Ligament Lesions

Rheumatoid patients frequently develop cystic and irregular soft swellings on both the dorsal and volar

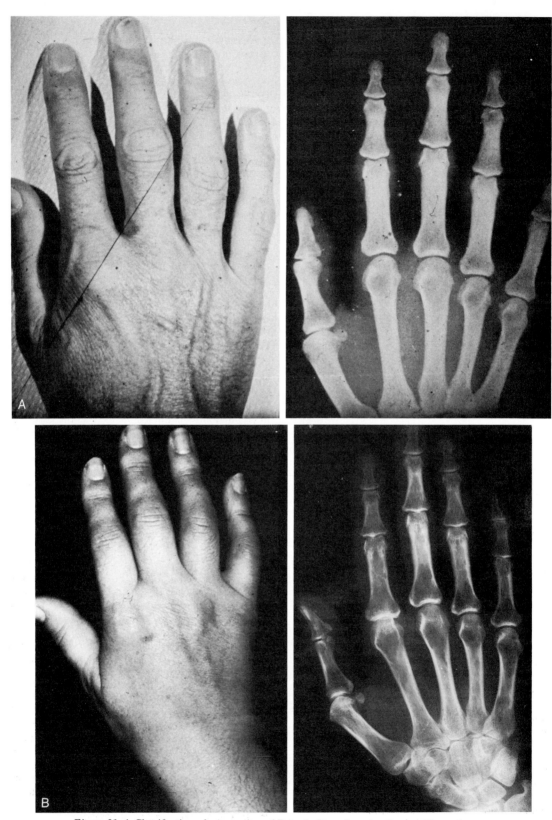

Figure 21–4. Classification of progression of RA. *A,* Stage I: early; *B,* stage II: moderate;

Illustration continued on opposite page

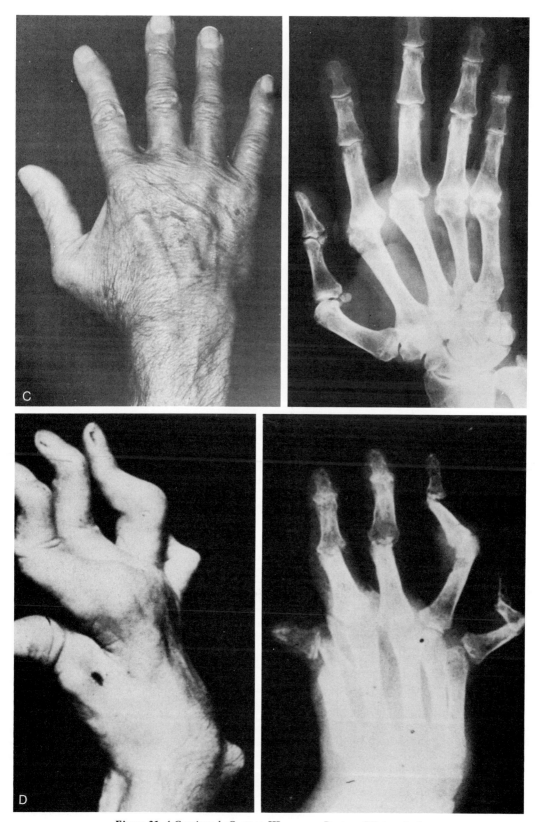

Figure 21–4 Continued. C, stage III: severe; *D,* stage IV: terminal.

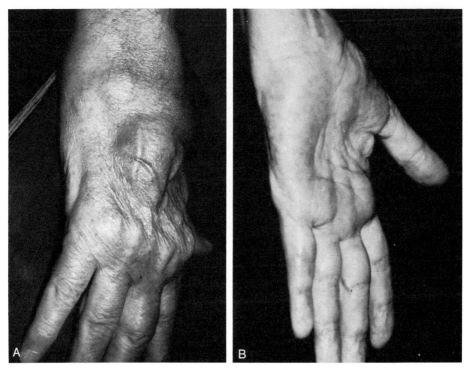

Figure 21–5. *A,* Tenosynovitis of extensor tendons of wrist in RA; *B,* thenar atrophy due to carpal tunnel syndrome.

surfaces of the wrists. These masses extend along the common extensor tendon sheaths. The term "ganglion" has frequently been used to describe these lesions (Fig. 21–5). Similar synovial rheumatoid proliferative changes occur at the base of the dorsal aspect of the wrist on the radial side in the anatomic "snuffbox"; also, there is swelling just distal to the ulna.

Rheumatoid proliferation of the volar tendon sheaths is a common cause for carpal tunnel syndrome. Entrapment of the median nerve with increased pressure causes pain and paresthesias in the hands in the distribution of the median nerve. Atrophy of the thenar muscles may result from these lesions (see Fig. 21–5).

Several tests are used to confirm the carpal tunnel at the wrist. When the wrist is held in acute palmar flexion for 60 seconds, numbness and tingling will occur in the hand and fingers over the distribution of the median nerve (Phalen's sign). These symptoms clear within a few minutes after the wrist is placed in the straight position. Another test is the percussion of the volar surface of the wrist directly over the median or ulnar nerve, with a resulting tingling or prickling sensation in the hand over the distribution of the affected nerve (Tinel's sign). Compression of the median nerve at the wrist level will produce weakness of the flexor pollicis longus, abductor pollicis brevis, and opponens pollicis. The strength of these muscles should be tested when the carpal tunnel syndrome is suspected.

Entrapment of the ulnar nerve at the wrist in the canal of Guyon may occur with RA, but is rare.

Symptoms include weakness of the intrinsic muscles of the hands and numbness in the ulnar nerve distribution. Confirmation of both median and ulnar entrapment at the wrist may be obtained by electromyographic nerve conduction studies.

The Rheumatoid Hand

The small joints of the hands are often the first affected in rheumatoid disease. Stiffness in the early morning lasting for 1 to 2 hours in one or several metacarpophalangeal and proximal interphalangeal joints is a common presenting complaint. It is usually associated with arthralgias, tenderness, synovial thickening, and joint effusions. These soft tissue changes most often involve the index and long fingers, resulting in the characteristic spindle-shaped deformity, but any proximal interphalangeal (PIP) joint may be involved. Paired joints of the opposite hand are commonly involved, producing a symmetric pattern. Soft tissue changes within the capsule of the metacarpophalangeal (MP) joints may obliterate the groove between the metacarpal heads on the dorsal surface of the hand. The second and third joints are most frequently involved, but any of the MP joints may be affected. The distal interphalangeal (DIP) joints are rarely the site of rheumatoid arthritis, except in association with psoriasis with fingernail involvement. This association is designated "psoriatic arthritis" (Fig. 21–6).

Prolonged active rheumatoid inflammation results in hyaline cartilage loss, laxity of the joint capsule, instability, and subluxation with deformities. Flex-

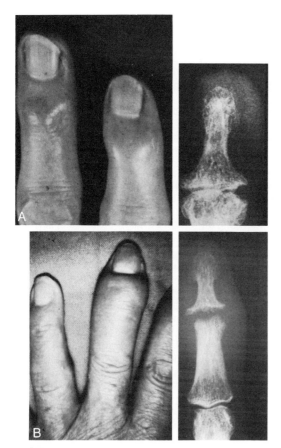

Figure 21–6. A, Heberden's nodes showing DIP enlargement *(left)* and x-ray changes *(right); B,* psoriatic arthritis with distal PIP involvement *(left)* and x-ray changes *(right).*

ion contractures of the MP joints are commonly associated with an ulnar drift of the digits (see Fig. 21–4, stage IV).

Swan-Neck Deformity. The middle interphalangeal joints are commonly subluxed in the volar direction, producing the swan-neck deformity (Fig. 21–7A). This abnormality consists of hyperextension of the PIP joint and flexion of the DIP joints. It results from destruction by the rheumatoid synovitis, allowing the dorsal displacement of the extensor apparatus with contracture of the joint and extensor apparatus.

Boutonnière Deformity. Another common and characteristic deformity of the rheumatoid finger has received the designation "boutonnière" (buttonhole) deformity. It results in flexion of the PIP joint and extension of the DIP joints (Fig. 21–7B). This is not as functionally disabling as the swanneck deformity, because grasp is still possible. The two changes may exist in the same hand.

Tenosynovitis (Trigger Finger). Thickening of the tendon sheaths resulting from rheumatoid proliferative disease is detected as a grating sensation and intermittent pain. Involvement of the volar compartments of individual digits is common. These changes may be detected by putting pressure across the palmar surface of the metacarpal heads and asking the patient to flex the fingers actively. Firm pressure directly over the nodule produces tenderness. Nodular enlargements can frequently be demonstrated on one or more of the fingers at the level of the proximal annular ligament or at the proximal pulley. Such rheumatoid granulomas may cause a temporary locking in the position of flexion or extension, and the patient may experience a clicking sensation as the nodule passes the area of constriction in the tendon sheath. This condition is known as the "snapping" or "trigger" finger. The digits that show this finding most frequently are the thumb and ring fingers, but any digit may be involved.

When the rheumatoid granuloma invades the tendon, it may rupture the involved flexor tendon and cause an episode of knifelike pain; sudden flexion occurs and active extension of the digit will not be possible. Such tendon ruptures may be painless and go unnoticed by the patient.

Thumb Deformities. Rheumatoid arthritis frequently produces disabilities in the thumb, the most important digit of the hand. The boutonnière deformity is due primarily to arthritic involvement of the MP joint, and is found in 57% of hands affected by rheumatoid disease. Synovitis stretches the capsule and extensor apparatus. The extensor pollicis longus tendon and adductor expansion are displaced toward the ulnar side, and the lateral thenar expansions. As a result, there is a flexion deformity of

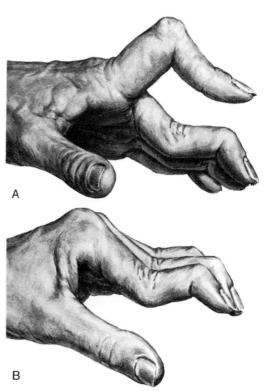

Figure 21–7. Characteristic finger deformities of RA. *A,* Boutonnière; *B,* swan-neck.

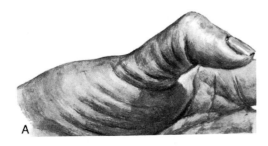

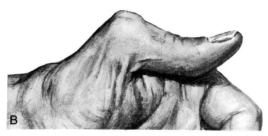

Figure 21–8. *A,* Boutonnière deformity of the thumb with flexion at the metacarpal joint; *B,* swan-neck deformity with subluxation of the carpometacarpal joint and extension of the MCP joint.

the proximal phalanx and hyperextension of the IP joint (Fig. 21–8*A*). Destructive changes in the cartilage with fibrous and bony ankylosis may cause fixed deformities with subluxations. Swan-neck deformities of the thumb occur in 9% of patients with rheumatoid arthritis (Fig. 21–8*B*). It is caused by synovitis, joint capsule stretching, and radial subluxation at the carpometacarpal (CM) joint. Usually there is hyperextension of the MP joint, adduction of the first metacarpal, and flexion of the IP joint, as in a swan-neck deformity of the finger.

Unstable Thumb Deformities. In far advanced rheumatoid disease with bone absorption, instability and painless hypermobility may occur in the IP, MP, and CM joints of the thumb. These changes are usually associated with similar changes in other digits in la main en lorgnette (opera-glass hand).

Tendon Disabilities. Rheumatoid disease may produce similar disabilities in the thumb as in other digits, including muscle contractures, tendon displacements, adhesions, or tendon ruptures. The most common rupture involves the extensor pollicis longus in the area of the distal tubercle of the radius, resulting in a sudden drop of the MP joint of the thumb and in some loss of extensor strength of the distal phalanx. Rupture of the flexor pollicis longus tendon may cause a hyperextension deformity of the thumb IP joint.

Stenosing Tenosynovitis. Thickening of the synovial sheaths of the long abductor and short extensor tendons of the thumb at the radial styloid process may result in localized pain and tenderness (de Quervain's disease). In most instances it is related to trauma. To demonstrate this lesion, the patient is asked to place the thumb in the palm of the hand and to flex the fingers over the thumb. This causes sharply localized pain near the radial styloid process. An increase in the pain will result

if the examiner moves the patient's wrist into ulnar deviation (Finkelstein's sign).

DEGENERATIVE JOINT DISEASE (OSTEOARTHRITIS)

Distinguishing Features

Clinical Findings

Based on radiological evidence, degenerative joint disease (DJD) occurs in 80% of people over 55 years of age, and is the most common type of chronic arthritis affecting the general population.[7] It is classified into primary and secondary forms, depending on whether a pathogenic factor has been identified. Weight-bearing joints (hips, knees, and lower spine) are frequently involved. It is further characterized by the lack of systemic features and inflammatory signs. It affects most older people to some degree and, in many, causes serious crippling. It is a noninflammatory progressive disorder of movable joints that results from deterioration of the articular cartilage and the formation of new bone in the subchondral areas and at the joint margins (osteophytes). Synonymous with the condition are osteoarthritis, osteoarthrosis, hypertrophic arthritis, and senile arthritis. Although it is far more common in individuals over 50 years of age, it may occur in younger people secondary to cartilage loss from repeated trauma, hemorrhage (hemophilia), infections, crystal deposition, and loss of the proprioceptive sense (neurotrophic arthropathies).

In some instances genetic factors are involved with a predisposition to DJD. In population studies by Kellgren and colleagues in 1963, involvement of the DIP joints showed a clear familial aggregation.[8] Simple mendelian inheritance was claimed by Stecher in 1955.[9]

In the skeletal remains of fossil dinosaurs of the Mesozoic period (200,000,000 BC), and of the earliest human (Neanderthal man, 40,000 BC), degenerative disease involving the vertebral joints has been found.

Symptoms

Patients with DJD commonly have dull aching pain involving one or a few joints, especially on motion and in weight-bearing joints. Stiffness after rest and inactivity is frequently noted, and is limited to the specifically involved joints. At first, any motion of an affected joint is slow and pain may be sharp, but, after a few minutes, the joint will "limber up" and, as motion is increased, the intensity of the discomfort decreases or may disappear entirely. Joint motion may cause a grating or creaking sensation.

Physical Findings

On physical examination, there is usually firm enlargement and moderate tenderness but without heat or redness; the range of motion may be restricted, and the surrounding muscles spastic. Later in the disease, malalignment and subluxation may be found. Effusions may occur after injury or vigorous exercise.

Laboratory Tests

The results of the complete blood count, serum electrophoretic pattern, urinalysis, and erythrocyte sedimentation rate are usually normal unless some other disease coexists. The rheumatoid factors are absent from the serum. The synovial fluid white blood cell count ranges between 1000 and 5000/mm^3, with 25% polymorphonuclear leukocytes. The viscosity of the synovial fluid is only slightly reduced. The protein level is usually less than 2.0 g. It is seldom helpful to send synovial fluid from osteoarthritic joints to the laboratory for an analysis.

Radiology

The single most helpful aid in the diagnosis of DJD is the radiologic examination. As the cartilage thins, the joint space on x-ray appearance becomes narrowed. Another early change is the presence of new bone that projects outward around the joint margins (osteophytes). At the same time new bone is laid down in the subchondral bone ends, leading to increased density or sclerosis. Cysts with dense walls appear in the periarticular bone, and vary in size from 1 or 2 mm up to a few centimeters. In the later stages there are deformities, subluxations, and gross bony overgrowths, and loose bodies may occur within the joint cavities.

Degenerative Joint Disease of the Upper Extremity

Shoulder

The acromioclavicular joints are frequent sites of degenerative changes but rarely give rise to symptoms. Because they are superficial they are easily examined and, when involved, a visible prominence and tenderness may be noted. Motion of the arm, especially over the shoulder, may produce discomfort that is sharply limited to this area.

The infrequent involvement of the glenohumoral articulation in primary generalized osteoarthritis contrasts with the great variety of inflammatory and degenerative changes of other structures around this joint. Lesions of these periarticular structures in the region of the shoulder joint are discussed below.

Secondary osteoarthritis of the shoulder is common in a number of inherited disorders that produce cartilage damage, including developmental disorders such as chondrodystrophy (Morquio-Brailsford) and Marfan's syndrome. Also, inherited metabolic diseases may affect articular cartilage and render it more vulnerable to wear and tear (*e.g.*, homogentisic acid metabolites in ochronosis, or urate or calcium pyrophosphate crystals in gout and pseudogout). Such inherited illnesses may damage any diarthrodial joint of the upper extremity and render it vulnerable to secondary osteoarthritis. Other causes of secondary DJD include trauma, bleeding dyscrasias, aseptic necrosis, prior infections, neuropathic joint disease, and RA.

Elbow

Osteoarthritis of this joint is seldom severe unless there has been a predisposing cause, such as a fracture or repeated trauma. Osteophytes may cause a blocking of this joint and reduce flexion, extension, range of motion, and rotation of the radial head. Another important result may be an "entrapment neuropathy," with a neurologic deficit in the areas innervated by the ulnar nerve.

Wrist

Primary osteoarthritis rarely involves the wrist. However, secondary osteoarthritis may develop following a fracture of the navicular, an inadequately reduced Colles' fracture, aseptic necrosis, or a previous septic or inflammatory process.

Hand

Heberden's and Bouchard's Nodes. Knobby enlargements with tenderness on the dorsal surface of the DIP finger joints are commonly associated with flexion and angular dislocations of the distal phalanges (Heberden's nodes; see Fig. 21–6A). These highly characteristic lesions usually develop slowly and produce varying degrees of pain, but become symptomless after maximum growth. Rarely, they enlarge rapidly and are acutely tender and red, with development of gelatinous cysts. These lesions are most common in middle-aged women, and have been shown to be determined by a single autosomal gene that is dominant in the female and recessive in the male.

Similar degenerative changes involving the PIP joints were described by Bouchard in 1887, and are often given his name.

First Carpometacarpal Joint. A highly characteristic and frequent site of DJD is the joint between the base of the first metacarpal and the trapezium. Actions such as pinching may be difficult or impossible, and rotary motions are particularly painful. Bony swelling, tenderness, and a typical deformity occur, in which the thumb is adducted and the base of the metacarpal becomes subluxed laterally to produce a prominence at the base of the thumb with a "shoulder," or square, hand. With abduction of the first metacarpal, the MP joint becomes hyperextended.

Erosive Osteoarthritis. This syndrome is characterized by intermittent, severe, and painful inflammatory episodes, and is confined to the DIP and PIP joints. The test for rheumatoid factors is negative and the sedimentation rate is normal. Ultimately marked deformity, bony erosions, and ankylosis may occur. This syndrome resembles that of

Heberden's nodes, but the severe inflammation, marked synovitis, and bony erosions followed by bony fusion are changes that rarely occur with Heberden's nodes. This syndrome is considered to be a distinct entity, and is clinically separable from both rheumatoid arthritis and classic DJD.[10, 11]

References

1. Garrod, A. B.: The Nature and Treatment of Gout and Rheumatic Gout, 1st ed., London, Walton and Maberly, 1859.
2. Nichols, E. H., and Richardson, F. L.: Arthritis deformans. J. Med. Res., 21:149, 1909.
3. Harris, E. D., Jr.: Rheumatoid arthritis: The clinical spectrum. *In* Kelley, W. N., et al. (eds.): Textbook of Rheumatology, Philadelphia, W. B. Saunders, 1981, p. 928.
4. Geschwend, N.: Surgical Treatment of Rheumatoid Arthritis, Philadelphia, W. B. Saunders, 1980.
5. Gelberman, R. A., Aronson, D., and Weisman, M. H.: Carpal-tunnel syndrome. J. Bone Joint Surg., 62A:1181, 1980.
6. Ropes, M. W., et al.: Revision of the diagnostic criteria for rheumatoid arthritis. Bull. Rheum. Dis., 9:175, 1958.
7. Kellgren, H. J., and Lawrence, J. S.: Osteoarthritis and disc degeneration in an urban population. Ann. Rheum. Dis., 17:388, 1958.
8. Kellgren, H. J., Lawrence, J. S., and Bier, F.: Genetic factors in generalized osteoarthritis. Ann. Rheum. Dis., 22:237, 1963.
9. Stecher, R. M.: Heberden's nodes: A clinical description of osteoarthritis of the finger joints. Arthritis Rheum., 14:1, 1955.
10. Crain, D. C.: Interphalangeal osteoarthritis characterized by painful inflammatory episodes resulting in deformity of the proximal and distal articulations. J.A.M.A., 175:1049, 1961.
11. Peter, J. B., Pearson, C. M., and Marmor, L.: Erosive osteoarthritis of the hands. Arthritis Rheum., 9:365, 1966.

22

JUVENILE CHRONIC ARTHRITIS

Stewart H. Harrison*

It has been estimated that the incidence of juvenile arthritis in the United Kingdom, in those under the age of 16 years, is 1 in 1000 births. There are 10,000 children in the United Kingdom who have juvenile arthritis. Early diagnosis and treatment will save many of them from crippling deformity.

The classification has been subject to considerable discussion. Juvenile chronic polyarthritis has been categorized as follows:[1]

1. Adult-type rheumatoid arthritis with IgM rheumatoid factor (RF)

2. Polyarthritis, with ankylosing spondylitis-type sacroiliitis

*I would like to express my sincere thanks to Dr. Barbara Ansell, Consultant Rheumatologist at the Juvenile Rheumatism Unit, Canadian Red Cross Memorial Hospital, Taplow, Bucks, England, and Northwick Park Hospital, Middlesex. Dr. Ansell is recognized as an international authority in Juvenile Polyarthritis and, over the years, she has advised and instructed me on the medical problems associated with this condition, for which I am most grateful.

3. Still's disease (includes three variants): systemic manifestation, polyarticular disease, or pauciarticular disease (with or without chronic iridocyclitis)

4. Psoriatic arthropathy

5. Arthritis associated with ulcerative colitis or regional enteritis

6. Polyarthropathies associated with other disorders, such as systemic lupus erythematosus and familial Mediterranean fever

More recently the classification has been simplified to systemic onset-type of juvenile arthritis (Still's), polyarticular (resembles adult rheumatoid arthritis), and pauciarticular, in which four joints or fewer or affected. The classification of Dodd and colleagues is shown in Table 22–1.[2]

Clinically, the manifestations in the hand are fairly well defined. Still described more than one variant of polyarthritis, but the type that is more commonly associated with his name is the RF-positive variety, affecting many joints (polyarticular) or four or fewer (pauciarticular).[3] In the RF-

Table 22–1. CLASSIFICATION OF JUVENILE CHRONIC POLYARTHRITIS*

Type	Juveniles Affected	Laboratory Results†	Features
Polyarticular, systemic	60% boys	ANA, negative; RF, negative	25% severe arthritis
RF-negative polyarticular	90% girls	ANA, negative; RF, negative	10–15%, severe arthritis
RF-positive polyarticular	80% girls	ANA, 75%; RF, 100%	50%, severe arthritis
Pauciarticular disease with chronic uveitis	80% girls	ANA, 50%; RF, 100%	Severe arthritis uncommon; 10–20%, ocular damage
Pauciarticular disease with sacroiliitis	90% boys	ANA, negative; RF, negative; HLA-B27, 75%	Some have ankylosing spondylitis

*Based on the classification of Dodd, M. J., et al.[2]
†ANA: antinuclear antibody; RF: rheumatoid factor.

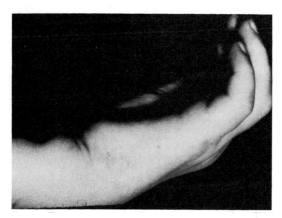

Figure 22–1. (From Harrison, S. H.: Juvenile chronic polyarthritis. *In* Arden, G. P., and Ansell, B. M. [eds.]: Surgical Management of Juvenile Chronic Polyarthritis. London, Academic Press, 1978; Courtesy of Academic Press.)

negative form of juvenile arthritis, wrist involvement affects more than half of patients seen within 1 year of onset, and this may be associated with joint and tendon sheath involvement. In the pauciarticular type, it is rare for the tendon sheath to be involved. Flexion deformity of the wrist is the earliest sign, and this could be due to flexor spasm (Fig. 22–1). Early recognition is important if permanent flexion deformity is to be avoided. Early treatment is by adequate splintage and good supervision.

An adult type of RF-negative polyarthritis can occur, as will be described later. One patient had a progressive deformity of the thumb, and the other ruptured the extensor tendons.

Adult-type rheumatoid arthritis, or RF-positive juvenile arthritis, is less common than RF-negative juvenile arthritis, but is much more destructive, and, like the adult type, requires more surgical interference. Growth defects are common, particularly in the region of the wrist. Rapid destruction of the joint can lead to instability and deformity.

Psoriatic arthritis affects mainly the terminal joints, often causing severe destruction, with loss of bone. The proximal interphalangeal joints can also be affected, and there can be a synovial proliferation of tissue around the tendon, similar to that in rheumatoid arthritis. Roberts and associates reviewed 227 cases with psoriasis, and 168 had arthritis.[4] In most cases skin lesions preceded the arthritis, but in 16% the arthritis appeared first. The majority were RF negative. In two of our cases, it has been necessary to do an ulnar styloidectomy for severe destructive change and the hypermobility of the ulnar head. The destructive nature of the disease, associated with RF negativity, separates the condition from its counterpart of rheumatoid arthritis.

Incidence. RF-negative juvenile arthritis cases constitute about 70% of the total referrals, and about 30% of these are pauciarticular. Of the total,

10% are RF-positive juveniles and, although this is a much smaller group, it provides a greater percentage of surgical problems. Psoriatic arthritis cases constitute about 5% of the total.[5]

RF-NEGATIVE JUVENILE POLYARTHRITIS

The systemic onset occurs in 60% of boys (see Table 22–1), and is associated with high fever, and in 90% of girls, in whom it is associated with low-grade fever, mild anemia, and growth retardation.[2]

Although this is a synovial disease, early flexor spasm is common, and often the initial manifestation is in the wrist. There is a flexion deformity of the wrist that, if not corrected by splintage, will lead to permanent deformity. Figure 22–2 shows the hand and arm of a 12-year-old girl who developed RF-negative juvenile polyarthritis at the age of 11 years. There is a flexion of the wrist, and swelling in the palm extending into the flexor aspect of the fingers is due to synovial proliferation around the flexor tendons. This patient had hyperemic decalcification seen on radiographs, with associated periostitis of the proximal phalanges. Clinically, there is evidence of early flexor spasm in the wrist and fingers.

One characteristic feature of RF-negative polyarthritis is the presence of fibrosing synovitis around the flexor tendons. The long flexors can become adherent in the palm, and cause limited flexion of the fingers, or they may produce a nodule due to the differing excursion of the two tendons. The disease, however, is synovial, and it is not uncommon to find fibrosing synovitis in the palm and proliferative synovitis in the joints. Proliferative synovial tissue can also occur around the extensor tendons, but less commonly than in the adult type.

The young patient shown in Figure 22–3, with

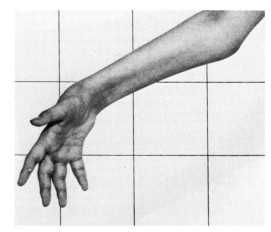

Figure 22–2. (From Harrison, S. H.: Juvenile chronic polyarthritis. *In* Arden, G. P., and Ansell, B. M. [eds.]: Surgical Management of Juvenile Chronic Polyarthritis. London, Academic Press, 1978; Courtesy of Academic Press.)

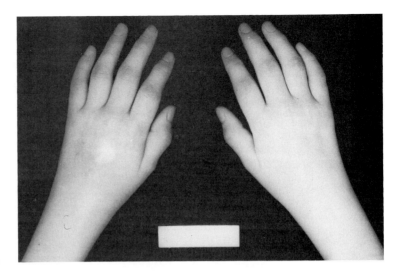

Figure 22–3.

RF-negative juvenile polyarthritis, had a flexion deformity of the wrist with synovial proliferation around the extensor tendons. Fusiform swelling of the proximal interphalangeal joints can be seen, and this is consistent with an acute synovitis rather than the proliferative type. There is also a flexion contracture of the fingers, which in this case is associated with synovial proliferation around the flexor tendons. Flexor spasm is a feature of this disease, and is probably toxic in origin from its effect at the neuromuscular junction.

Figure 22–4 shows a 17-year-old boy, with RF-negative juvenile arthritis of 9 years' duration, who developed acute flexion of the proximal interphalangeal joints and a compensatory hyperextension of the metacarpophalangeal joints. There was some flexion of the terminal joints, which became slightly more obvious after correction of the proximal joints. The serial linkage of joints is reversed here. By this it is meant that normally wrist extension is associated with finger flexion, but in this case there is a flexion deformity of the wrist associated with hy-

perextension of the metacarpophalangeal joints and flexion of the interphalangeal joints. The appearance of the fingers is not consistent either with fibrosing or proliferative synovitis. There is no massive synovial swelling of the palm and fingers to suggest synovial proliferation, and the extension of the metacarpophalangeal joints precludes a fibrosing synovitis.

The patient in Figure 22–5 had bilateral and symmetric deformity, which seriously interfered with function in that both grip and precision pinch were inhibited. The illustration shows the right hand after correction by surgery, in which the contracted tissue around the metacarpophalangeal joints was released, the sublimis tendons were divided, and the interphalangeal joints were stabilized with intramedullary pegs in a position of function. An improvement in the position of the wrist naturally follows restoration of the serial linkage of joints, which arises from correction of the extension at the metacarpophalangeal joints to a more normal position of flexion. The radiograph in Figure 22–6

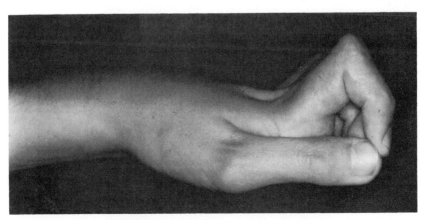

Figure 22–4. (From Harrison, S. H.: Juvenile chronic polyarthritis. *In* Arden, G. P., and Ansell, B. M. [eds.]: Surgical Management of Juvenile Chronic Polyarthritis. London, Academic Press, 1978; Courtesy of Academic Press.)

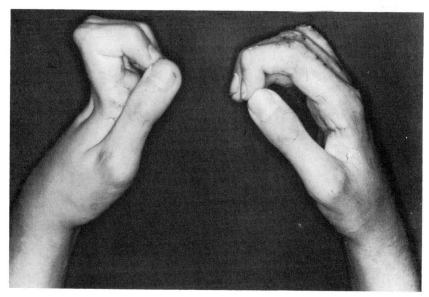

Figure 22–5. (From Harrison, S. H.: Juvenile chronic polyarthritis. *In* Arden, G. P., and Ansell, B. M. [eds.]: Surgical Management of Juvenile Chronic Polyarthritis. London, Academic Press, 1978; Courtesy of Academic Press.)

shows that there has been a hyperemic decalcification with periostitis, and there is evidence of epiphyseal deformity.

The 15-year-old girl shown in Figure 22–7 developed RF-negative juvenile arthritis at the age of 3 years. A bizarre pattern of deformity can be seen, in which in the right hand there is an acute flexion deformity of the proximal interphalangeal joints of the middle, ring, and little fingers, but full extension of the index finger. The thumb showed deviation of the terminal interphalangeal joint toward the radial side, which was tending to a state of instability. In

the left hand there is a flexion contracture of the metacarpophalangeal joint of the thumb and of the proximal interphalangeal joints of the index and little fingers.

Figure 22–8 shows a close-up picture of the right hand prior to surgery. This girl was going blind from iridocyclitis, and it was necessary to correct her finger deformities so that she could learn Braille. At surgery fibrosing synovitis was found, involving the flexor tendons, and the tendons were freed by removal of this tissue (Fig. 22–9). The joints were excised and stabilization was obtained by the inser-

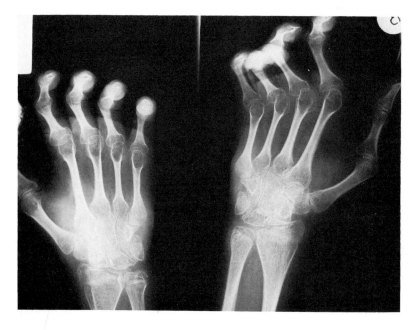

Figure 22–6.

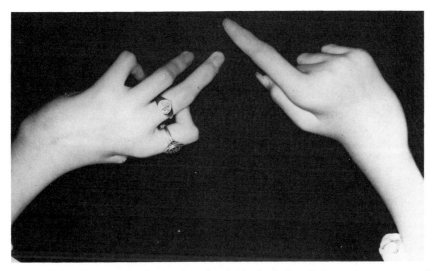

Figure 22–7. (From Harrison, S. H.: Juvenile chronic polyarthritis. *In* Arden, G. P., and Ansell, B. M. [eds.]: Surgical Management of Juvenile Chronic Polyarthritis. London, Academic Press, 1978; Courtesy of Academic Press.)

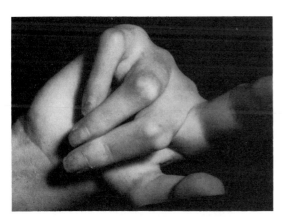

Figure 22–8.

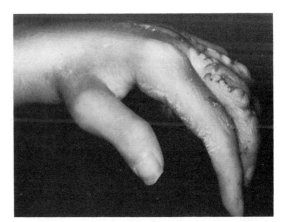

Figure 22–9.

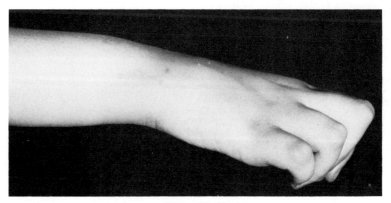

Figure 22–10.

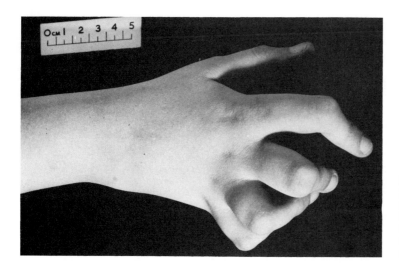

Figure 22–11. (From Harrison, S. H.: Juvenile chronic polyarthritis. *In* Arden, G. P., and Ansell, B. M. [eds.]: Surgical Management of Juvenile Chronic Polyarthritis. London, Academic Press, 1978; Courtesy of Academic Press.)

tion of angle pegs, after division of the sublimis tendons. Capsulotomy of the metacarpophalangeal joints, supplemented by dynamic splintage, produced a correction that enabled her to function more normally, and to utilize her fingertips to learn Braille.

The 16-year-old girl shown in Figure 22–10 developed RF-negative arthritis at the age of 10 years. This picture, taken from the medial side, shows the acute flexion of the fingers at the proximal interphalangeal joint. Figure 22–11 shows the dorsal view of the hand of the same patient. The index finger deviates medially, and shows a compensatory hyperextension of the terminal joint, suggestive of intrinsic shortening. Hyperextension at the metacarpophalangeal joints of the middle, ring, and little fingers is similar to that shown in Figure 22–4.

This radiograph of the same patient shows that the metacarpals are tapered, and the heads deformed (Fig. 22–12). Epiphyseal involvement is characteristic of this condition, and in this case not only caused deformation of the epiphysis but also retardation of growth, as can be seen in the short ulna. Ligamentous structures become detached from bone by erosion, leading to abnormal mobility. In this case, the ulnar head shows evidence of mobility from the scalloping that can be seen to

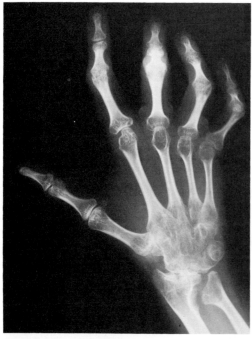

Figure 22–12. (From Harrison, S. H.: Juvenile chronic polyarthritis. *In* Arden, G. P., and Ansell, B. M. [eds.]: Surgical Management of Juvenile Chronic Polyarthritis. London, Academic Press, 1978; Courstey of Academic Press.)

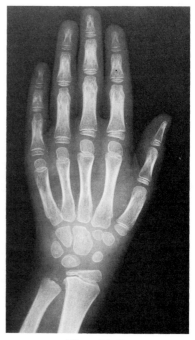

Figure 22–13.

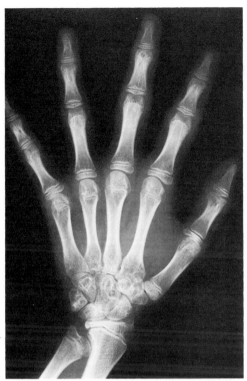

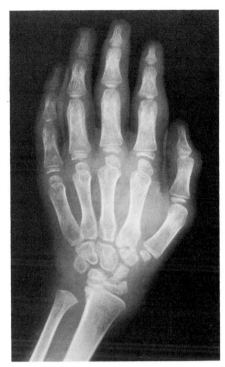

Figure 22–15.

Figure 22–14. (From Harrison, S. H.: Juvenile chronic polyarthritis. *In* Arden, G. P., and Ansell, B. M. (eds.): Surgical Management of Juvenile Chronic Polyarthritis. London, Academic Press, 1978; Courtesy of Academic Press.)

have occurred in the medial side of the radius. The short ulna and the apparent ligamentous disruption have allowed the hand and carpus to slide medially off the end of the radius and ulna. This is called "glissement carpien."

As the hand shifts medially, it also deviates radially. When radial deviation occurs in the adult, it alters the angle of incidence of the extensor

tendons and, in the presence of synovial involvement of the metacarpophalangeal joints, associated with laxity of the periarticular structures, the extensor tendons will tend to shift medially off the dorsum of the joints and initiate ulnar drift of the fingers. In children, however, with a medial shift of the hand, the extensor tendons alter their course medially and not laterally, and thus tend to cause a radial deviation of the fingers, accentuated by radial deviation of the wrist.

The 10-year-old girl shown in Figure 22–13 developed RF-negative arthritis at the age of 4 years, when this radiograph was taken. A further radio-

Figure 22–16.

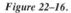

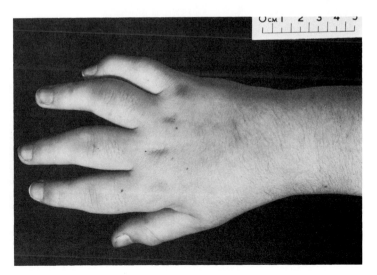

graph, taken 6 years later, shows evidence of widening of the metacarpal metaphysis (Fig. 22–14). A growth defect in the ulna with some scalloping of the radius can be seen. The radial epiphysis is deformed, and cystic changes can be seen in the epiphysis and in the carpus. There is a deformity of the metacarpal head of the little finger.

This 8-year-old patient developed RF-negative polyarthritis at the age of 3 years (Fig. 22–15). The short ulna and epiphyseal deformities are clearly evident on the radiograph. The systemic response associated with high fever is reflected in the hyperemic decalcification that occurs in the fingers and subsequently leads to periosteal new bone formation, which affects the proximal phalanges.

The 15-year-old girl shown in Figure 22–16 developed RF-negative polyarthritis at the age of 18 months, and the growth defects can be seen in the short fingers. There is angulation at the proximal interphalangeal joints, and noticeable thickening of the proximal phalanges. Destructive changes have occurred in the metacarpal and interphalangeal joints, with a tendency toward the formation of cup arthroplasty of the second metacarpophalangeal joint (Fig. 22–17). There is a growth deformity of the radius, and early fusion of the carpus. It is interesting to note the manifestation of deformity affecting the terminal joints.

Joint destruction can lead to instability and this is particularly disabling when it affects the terminal joint of the thumb, because the capacity to pinch becomes difficult. At the same time it is not unusual

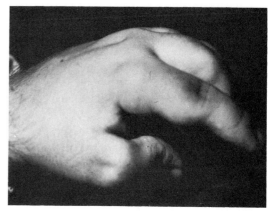

Figure 22–18.

to have a flexion deformity of the first metacarpophalangeal joint, so that both thumbs come to be clasped into the palm.

The 32-year-old man in Figure 22–18 developed RF-negative arthritis in childhood. He shows the characteristic appearance of clasped thumbs. The terminal joints of the thumb were flail, and pinch was very inadequate. To restore function, it was necessary to stabilize both the metacarpophalangeal and terminal joints, and to bring the thumb into opposable relationship to the index finger. This correction was obtained by the use of intramedullary pegs, and there is a greatly improved functional relationship between the thumb and index finger (Fig. 22–19).

This 14-year-old girl developed RF-negative arthritis at the age of 8 years (Fig. 22–20). The proximal interphalangeal joints have fused, which is an unusual feature. It can occur as a single joint fusion, without any other evidence of joint involvement in the hand (Fig. 22–21). Because these joints tend to fuse in either the extended or the acutely flexed position, the angle may have to be corrected to a more functional one.

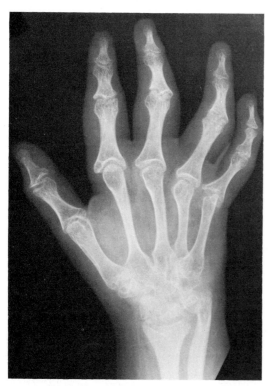

Figure 22–17.

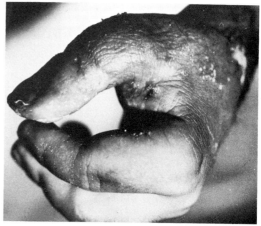

Figure 22–19.

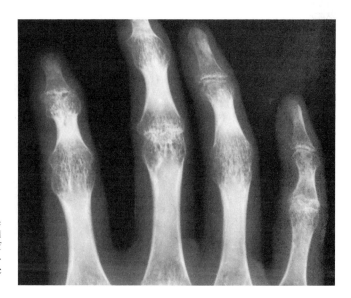

Figure 22–20. (From Harrison, S. H.: Juvenile chronic polyarthritis. *In* Arden, G. P., and Ansell, B. M. [eds.]: Surgical Management of Juvenile Chronic Polyarthritis. London, Academic Press, 1978; Courtesy of Academic Press.)

Late complications of RF-negative arthritis present problems in treatment. Some require wrist fusion or the stabilization of joints that have become deformed or unstable. This 50-year-old woman developed RF-negative arthritis at the age of 6 years (Fig. 22–22). She ruptured her extensor tendons at the age of 50 years. She was a pianist by profession, and it was necessary to repair a rupture of the tendons of the middle, ring, and little fingers. The radiographs showed a deformity of the head of the ulna and scalloping of the radius (Fig. 22–23).

The 45-year-old woman in Figure 22–24 developed RF-negative juvenile arthritis in childhood. From the radiograph, it would appear that she had a bilateral and selective involvement of the epiphysis

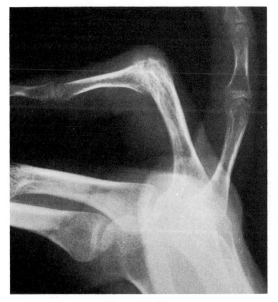

Figure 22–21.

at the base of the first metacarpals. A progressive adduction of the thumb occurred, which caused an interference with the pinch mechanism that was sufficiently disabling to warrant surgical correction. It is typical of this type of case that the adduction deformity is associated with a secondary hyperextension of the metacarpophalangeal joint, similar to that seen in osteoarthritis and in contrast to that in RF-positive juvenile arthritis, in which carpometacarpal joint destruction leads to an adduction deformity and is associated with a secondary radial deviation of the first metacarpophalangeal joint.

The correction was obtained by inserting a bone strut from the olecranon into the bases of the first and second metacarpals to correct the adduction deformity. The patient was satisfied enough to request a similar procedure on the opposite hand. Figure 22–25 shows the difference between the left side after grafting and the right side prior to grafting.

Operative Procedures

In RF-negative arthritis, synovectomy of joints and tendons may be necessary but the indications are much less frequent than in the more florid RF-positive types. Trigger fingers are relatively common, however, and this may be due to the much higher incidence of fibrosing synovitis. The constricting effect of fibrosing synovitis on the flexor tendons presents an indication for surgery, and the release of the tendons often produces a considerable improvement when supplemented by intensive physiotherapy.

This type of arthritis is more surgically oriented to the correction of joint deformities and instability of joints. As already described, the stabilization of finger joints and the correction of deformities have been achieved by the use of intramedullary pegs.[6, 7]

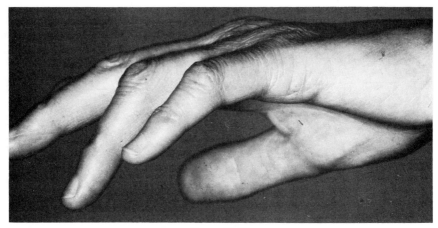

Figure 22–22.

The wrist is frequently involved in juvenile arthritis, and Nalebuff and co-workers stated that 90% of juvenile wrists studied showed destructive changes.[8] They also drew attention to the frequency of involvement of the distal epiphysis of the radius and ulna, in which growth deformities are commonly seen. It is indeed fortunate that spontaneous fusion does occur, because further growth may be jeopardized by early surgical fusion of the wrist.

In conclusion then, the surgery for RF-negative juvenile arthritis is primarily the correction of deformity, and secondarily the stabilization of the unstable joints.

Complications

In RF-negative juvenile chronic polyarthritis, the complications are related to muscle spasm. If not

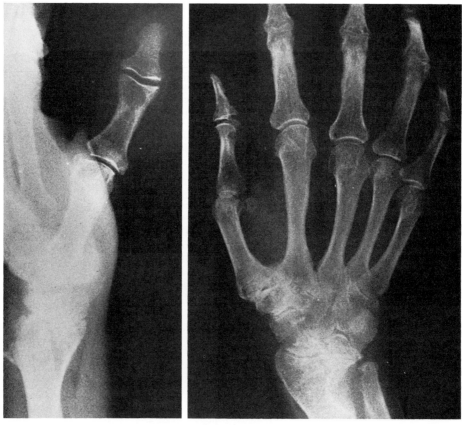

Figure 22–23.

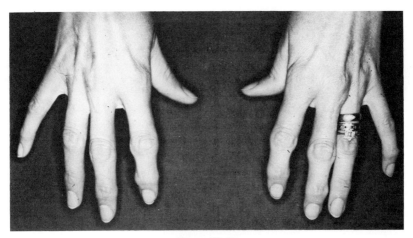

Figure 22–24.

relieved, this will cause permanent deformity of the wrist, claw hand, and other bizarre deformities.

Epiphyseal involvement leads to stunted growth and to deformities of the interphalangeal joint. Fibrosing synovitis is characteristic of juvenile chronic polyarthritis, and the palm can be relieved by synovectomy, releasing the adherence of the flexor tendons. Failure is inevitable, however, unless the patient will cooperate with immediate and intensive active exercises.

Destructive joint changes necessitate fusion and are often seen affecting the terminal joint of the thumb. A small 25°-angle peg is used, but can be difficult to insert because of the absence of an adequate medullary cavity and attenuation of the cortex. Crossed K-wires can also be used, but using either method there can be problems in obtaining bony fusion.

RF-POSITIVE JUVENILE ARTHRITIS

Ansell has stated that 10% of those with juvenile arthritis carry IgM rheumatoid factor, and these tend to be girls with an older age group of onset of 10 to 11 years.[5] There are features very similar to those of the adult disease, with a particular tendency to rapid joint destruction. These patients require more surgical intervention than the RF-negative cases, and the type of surgery resembles that for adult rheumatoid disease. The 18-year-old girl in Figure 22–26 developed RF-positive juvenile rheumatoid arthritis at the age of 11 years. The illustration shows radial deviation of the wrist and fingers. There were gross destructive changes in the interphalangeal joints, with severe instability. The radiograph shows that the outstanding deformity is the destruction of the proximal interphalangeal joints

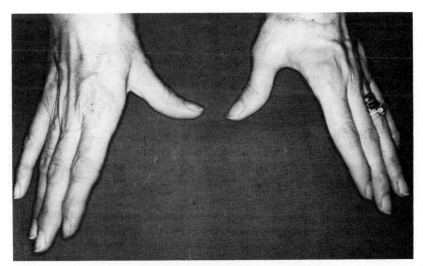

Figure 22–25. (From Harrison, S. H.: Juvenile chronic polyarthritis. *In* Arden, G. P., and Ansell, B. M. [eds.]: Surgical Management of Juvenile Chronic Polyarthritis. London, Academic Press, 1978; Courtesy of Academic Press.)

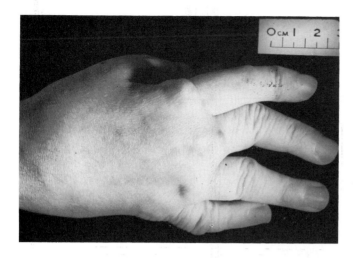

Figure 22–26. (From Harrison, S. H.: Juvenile chronic polyarthritis. *In* Arden, G. P., and Ansell, B. M. [eds.]: Surgical Management of Juvenile Chronic Polyarthritis. London, Academic Press, 1978; Courtesy of Academic Press.)

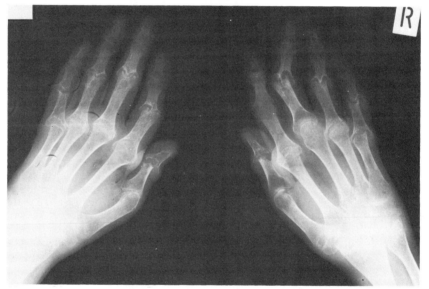

Figure 22–27.

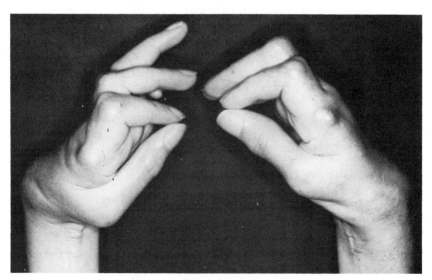

Figure 22–28.

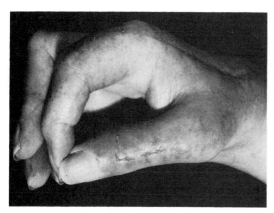

Figure 22–29.

and the subluxation of the metacarpophalangeal joints.

A 32-year-old woman contracted RF-positive juvenile rheumatoid arthritis at the age of 14 years. She had a right lobectomy, and had cutaneous vasculitis. In 1960 she had an extensor tendon repair of the thumb by an extensor pollicis brevis transplant. In 1963 she had a repair of the long flexor tendon of the left little finger. In 1966 she had a repair of the extensor tendons of the right ring and little fingers. In 1974 pegs were inserted into the first metacarpophalangeal and terminal joints of the left thumb to correct the "Z" deformity and to provide stability. In 1975 a straight peg was inserted

between the first and second metacarpals to correct the adduction of the thumb. The proximal phalanx of the index finger had retracted into the palm by 2 to 3 cm and the subluxation could be reduced only by inserting a combination of an angled peg into the joint and a K-wire into the second metacarpophalangeal joint. The immediate result was good alignment and subsequently a good functional recovery (Fig. 22–29). The radiograph shows the gross deformity and destruction of the wrist joint that necessitated arthrodesis (Fig. 22–30).

There are many techniques for providing an arthrodesis of the wrist. One method involves a polypropylene peg, which is inserted into the distal end of the radius and into the third metacarpal (Fig. 22–31). This peg is 10 cm in length. The cavity around the peg is packed with cancellous bone from the iliac crest, and the hand is immobilized in plaster of Paris for 3 months. This is followed by immobilization in a Futuro splint for 3 months more. An alternative method is that recommended by Nicolle.[9] This involves the insertion of a Steinmann pin or Rush nail along the third metacarpal into the radius.

This radiograph of a young female patient with RF-positive rheumatoid arthritis shows the extent of destruction that can occur in the joints of the hand (Fig. 22–32). There are extensive destructive changes in the wrist, progressing to fusion. All the digital joints are involved, and it is interesting to note that the terminal joints also show evidence of destructive change, a feature that is not normally

Figure 22–30.

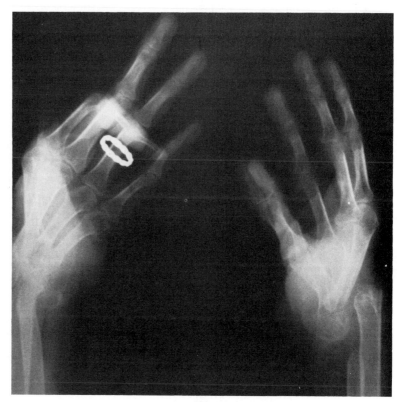

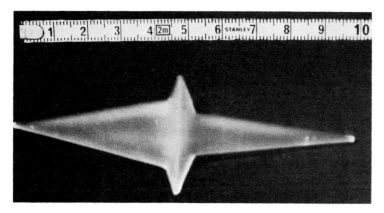

Figure 22–31.

seen in adult rheumatoid arthritis but that is characteristic of psoriatic and degenerative arthritis.

In RF-positive juvenile arthritis, there is a much greater degree of synovial proliferation both in the joints and around the tendons, causing swelling of the joints and distortion of the anatomy and often requiring synovectomy. The cartilage is eroded and there is bone absorption. This is in contrast to RF-negative juvenile arthritis, in which disappearance of the articular cartilage associated with fibrosing synovitis is more commonly seen than the destructive variety.

Destructive changes in the wrist joint not only lead to wrist deformity but also to involvement of the first carpometacarpal joint, and there can be an adduction deformity of the first metacarpal. The secondary result of the deformity is a radial angulation at the first metacarpophalangeal joint. Note that the trapezium has been completely destroyed (Fig. 22–33).

A straight peg or bone graft may be required between the first and second metacarpals to correct the adduction deformity. The deformity of the first metacarpophalangeal joint will require stabilization by excision of the joint and by insertion of a straight peg.

Deformities due to joint destruction of the first metacarpophalangeal joint are common in both juvenile and adult rheumatoid arthritis, and these can readily be corrected by the use of a straight polypropylene peg (Fig. 22–34). Follow-up studies show that in most cases bone union occurs around the peg.[6]

Flexor or extensor tendon ruptures do occur in young people, but less often than in adults. The long extensor of the thumb is the most common extensor to rupture, and is normally repaired by using an extensor pollicis brevis transplant.[10] Stabilization of the first metacarpophalangeal joint with a straight peg may be necessary at the same time if there is evidence of bone destruction in the first metacarpophalangeal joint.

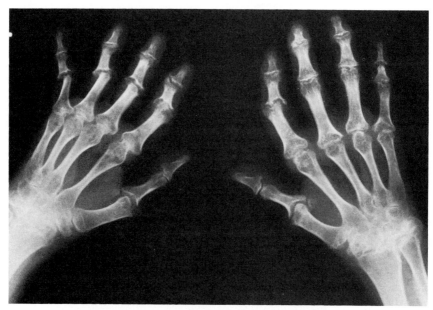

Figure 22–32.

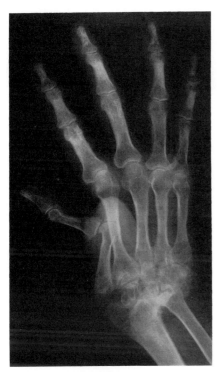

Figure 22–33.

In the palm, massive proliferation of synovial tissue can occur, extending from the carpal tunnel to involve the flexor tendon sheath into the digit, and this mass of proliferating tissue can extend up above the carpal tunnel into the lower forearm. The mass of tissue may have to be removed by synovectomy to allow recovery of full flexion in the fingers; otherwise, permanent limitation of flexion may occur. It has frequently been stated that the mass of proliferating tissue is a cause of carpal tunnel syndrome, but this tissue is readily compressible and the syndrome does not occur in children. It is doubtful that the tissue is responsible for this syndrome in adults, because it tends to appear in a similar age group to that of otherwise normal patients.

Nodules can occur in the flexor tendon and can cause trigger finger. This disabling condition is readily corrected by removal of the nodule or of half of the tendon.

Flexor tendon rupture can also occur, and will require repair either by a tendon graft or a tendon transplant. The most common flexor tendon to

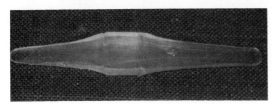

Figure 22–34.

rupture is the long flexor tendon of the thumb. The results of flexor tendon repair in the thumb are consistently better than repair of the flexor tendons of a digit.

Thus, in RF-positive juvenile arthritis, many more procedures are required, similar to those for adult rheumatoid arthritis. Unstable joints require stability, deformities need correction, and a chain-reaction deformity needs to be interrupted early before one deformity leads to another. Surgery, however, should be conservative, and emphasis should be on the prevention of deformity by splintage. There is no place for destructive surgical procedures, and the use of prostheses other than those required to provide stability should be avoided.

Complications

In RF-positive juvenile rheumatoid arthritis, the complications of the disease are severe joint destruction, and the problems of treatment involve the wrist and interphalangeal joints. Destructive changes in the wrist lead to instability and deformity. Standard methods of fusion, using metal, wrist pegs, bone grafts, or a combination of these may fail to establish bony union. The timing of such procedures in relation to the fusion of the wrist and digital joints is influenced by the presence of the epiphysis and its effect on growth.

Ulnar styloidectomy is occasionally necessary, but care should be taken to avoid removing too much of the ulnar or the proximal end may cut through all the extensor tendons. Erosion of the ulnar head is a causative factor in rupture of the extensor tendons of the little and ring fingers, and repair of the tendons then becomes necessary. If the tendons rupture when there are destructive changes in the metacarpophalangeal joints, there will be subsequent subluxation of the joints unless the accident was dealt with as an emergency, or, alternatively, unless the fingers were held in full extension at the metacarphophalangeal joints pending repair. If subluxation of these joints has occurred, it may be necessary to correct the subluxation at the same time as the repair of the tendons, or the repair will fail to effect full active extension of the involved metacarpophalangeal joints.

Instability and deformities in extension and flexion of the proximal interphalangeal joints necessitate fusion at angles of 30 to 50°. The intramedullary peg, which is graded in different angles, is easy to insert properly but is difficult to maintain against the extension strain of the flat hand pending fusion. It is therefore desirable to supplement the peg with a K-wire, which can be removed, if necessary, at a later date.

Proliferative synovitis often requires treatment by synovectomy and, if this operation is performed on the dorsum of the hand, it may be advisable to immobilize it for 10 days after operation because ischemia of the tendons can occur, which could lead

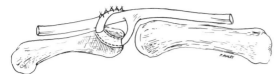

Figure 22–35.

to rupture. In the palm of the hand, flexor synovectomy should not be performed if there is evidence of subluxation of the metacarpophalangeal joints; otherwise, the ensuing fibrosis might cause a flexion deformity, which would be difficult or impossible to correct in this area.

ADDITIONAL CONSIDERATIONS

Metacarpophalangeal Joints

Proliferative synovitis of the metacarpophalangeal joints causes distention of the capsule, and may result in dislocation of the extensor tendon. Although the recurrence rate is high after synovectomy, it is justifiable under such circumstances to do a synovectomy and to centralize the extensor tendon. This is done by using an extensor loop, taking half the extensor tendon, and inserting it through a hole in the dorsum of the phalanx (Fig. 22–35).[11] A more recent method involves taking the

loop through a hole in the anterior part of the base of the phalanx; this is an improvement on the original method.

Evidence of medial shift at the base of the proximal phalanx on the head of the metacarpal implies that there has been a partial collateral ligament detachment (Fig. 22–36). Furthermore, there will be a progressive subluxation toward an irreversible state, in which only salvage procedures can be applied. In such cases, the ulnar intrinsic of the affected finger is divided, and the ulnar intrinsic of the adjacent finger on the radial side is used as an intrinsic transfer. This transfer will only be effective if it is passed through a separate drill hole in the base of the proximal phalanx, and not into the dorsal expansion. Following surgery, a training splint will be necessary (Fig. 22–37).

This 29-year-old woman developed severe RF-positive arthritis at the age of 6 years. The Z deformity was corrected by the insertion of a straight peg after excision of the joint surfaces. The dislocated extensor tendon, and the middle, ring, and little fingers were realigned by using an extensor loop and an intrinsic transfer (Fig. 22–39). This woman also had angle pegs inserted into the proximal interphalangeal joint areas of the middle and ring fingers.

Prosthetic replacement should be avoided in children, as stated by Flatt.[12]

The more serious problems at the metacarpophalangeal joint level arise from subluxation in the

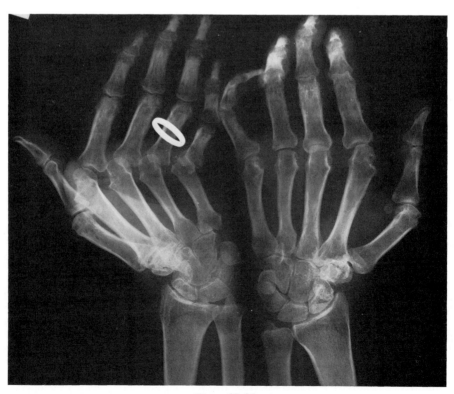

Figure 22–36.

Figure 22–37.

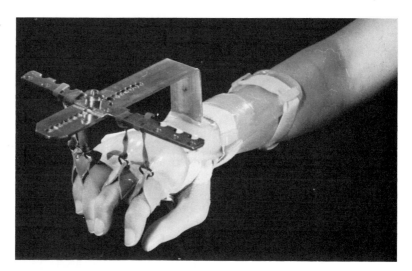

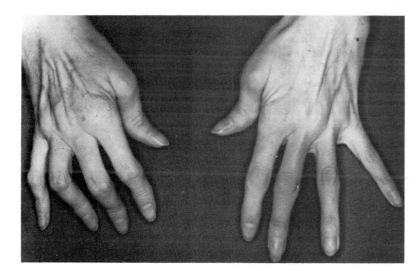

Figure 22–38.

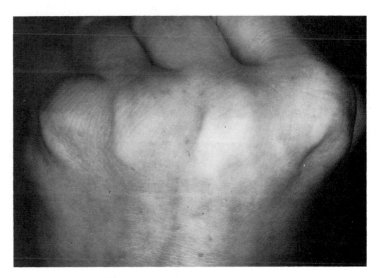

Figure 22–39.

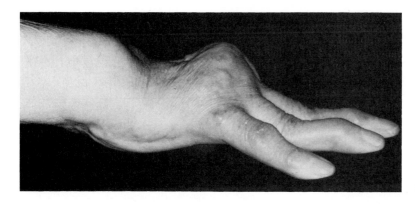

Figure 22–40.

anteroposterior plane. In this situation, swan's-neck deformity of the interphalangeal joints will occur from the inability to hyperextend at the metacarpophalangeal level, and the extension force will be transferred to the proximal interphalangeal joint, with the inevitable complication of swan-neck deformity (Fig. 22–40).

Proximal Interphalangeal Joints

There are four conditions that affect the proximal interphalangeal joints: proliferative synovitis, swan-neck deformity, flexion deformity, and instability caused by loss of ligament stability.

In 1969, Chaplin and colleagues reviewed patients with juvenile arthritis.[13] They noted that the wrist is the most commonly affected joint and, in the younger patients, the most common finger deformity is at the terminal and proximal interphalangeal joints. Of these patients, 30% were boys and 70% were girls. In 414 children below the age of 15 years, boutonnière deformity occurred in 27%, and swan-neck deformity in 3.7%.

Pulkki stated that the incidence of swan-neck deformity in adult rheumatoid arthritis patients was 14%.[14] In a review of 500 cases, he found boutonnière in 32%, swan-neck in 14%, and mallet deformity in 2%.

It is apparent that boutonnière deformity is more common in the 0- to 4-year-old group, and swan-neck deformity is more common in the older group. This is probably due to the high incidence of flexor tendon involvement, or flexor tendon spasm, that occurs in the RF-negative cases. In the older groups, subluxation of the metacarpophalangeal joints is more often associated with secondary hyperextension of the proximal interphalangeal joint due to the transmission of extension strain from the proximal to the distal joint.

It was postulated at one time that fibrosis of the intrinsic muscles occurred, and produced an intrinsic-plus deformity of the proximal interphalangeal joint.[15] This, however, was disproved by biopsy of the intrinsic tendons.

Edmunds and associates recorded the presence of abnormal autonomic function, and suggested that autonomic neuropathy occurred more frequently in rheumatoid arthritis than hitherto suspected. This was probably caused by vasculitis.

It would be reasonable to suggest that flexor spasm can occur in juveniles, especially in the RF-negative cases. This could be the causative factor, if not a contributory cause, in the predominant deformity of flexor contracture. In the older groups, the wasting that occurs in the intrinsic muscles, which is ultimately responsible for the imbalance between the intrinsic and extrinsic muscles, could be the result of a peripheral neuropathy.

References

1. Bywaters, E. G.: The management of juvenile chronic polyarthritis. Bull. Rheum. Dis., 27:882, 1976–1977.
2. Dodd, M. J., Dick, W., and Carson, M. J.: Recent advances in rheumatology. Hosp. Update, 6:655, 1980.
3. Still, G. F.: Med. Shir. Trans., 80:47, 1897.
4. Roberts, M. E. T., Wright, V., Hill, A. G., and Mehra, A. C.: Psoriatic arthritis. Follow-up study. Ann. Rheum. Dis., 35:206, 1976.
5. Ansell, B.: Personal Communication.
6. Harrison, S. H.: The Harrison-Nicolle Intramedullary Peg, Follow-up study of 100 cases. Hand, 6:304, 1974.
7. Harrison, S. H., Smith, P., and Maxwell, D.: Stabilization of the first metacarpophalangeal and terminal joints of the thumb. Hand, 9:242, 1977.
8. Nalebuff, E. A., Yerid, G., and Millender, L.: The incidence and severity of wrist involvement in juvenile rheumatoid arthritis. J. Bone and Joint Surg., 54A:905, 1972.
9. Nicolle, F. V.: In Nicolle, F. V., and Dickson, R. A. (eds.): Surgery of the Rheumatoid Hand. London, William Heineman Medical Books, 1979, p. 68.
10. Harrison, S., Swannell, A. J., and Ansell, B. M.: Repair of extensor pollicis longus, using extensor pollicis brevis in rheumatoid arthritis. Ann. Rheum. Dis., 31:490, 1972.
11. Harrison, S. H.: Reconstructive arthroplasty of the metacarpophalangeal joint, using the extensor loop operation. Br. J. Plast. Surg., 24:307, 1971.
12. Flatt, A.: The Care of the Rheumatoid Hand. St. Louis, C. V. Mosby, 1974.
13. Chaplin, D., Pulkki, T., Saarimaa, A., and Vainio, K.: Wrist and finger deformities in juvenile rheumatoid arthritis. Acta Rheum. Scand., 15:206, 1969.
14. Pulkki, T.: Acta Rheum. Scand., 7:85, 1961.
15. Riley, M., and Harrison, S. H.: Interosseous muscle biopsy during hand surgery for rheumatoid arthritis. Br. J. Plast. Surg., 21:342, 1968.
16. Edmunds, M. E., Jones, T. C., Saunders, W. A., and Sturrock, R. D.: Autonomic neuropathy in rheumatoid arthritis. Br. Med. J., 21:173, 1979.

23

COMPLICATIONS FOLLOWING SURGERY FOR RHEUMATOID AND ARTHRITIC CONDITIONS

Donald C. Ferlic
and Mack L. Clayton

When discussing surgical complications and results in the rheumatoid patient, one must consider that this is a systemic, often progressive, disease. The results of treating a specific joint depend not only on the condition of the adjacent joints but on the progression of disease in the lower extremities as well, because crutch walking may be required for ambulation. Surgery in the rheumatoid patient is fraught with many more complications than comparable surgery for osteoarthritis—specifically, problems with wound healing—but we ran a study that compared wound healing to that in similar operative procedures in patients with rheumatoid and osteoarthritis (OA), and found no difference between patients who were and were not on steroid therapy.

In this chapter we will discuss all the joints of the shoulder and upper extremity. In addition to prosthetic arthroplasty, there are few surgical procedures done for the rheumatoid arthritic shoulder. Occasionally, synovectomy, resection of the distal clavicle, or anterior acromioplasty will be indicated, but usually shoulder problems are treated by nonsurgical methods until there has been destruction of the articular surfaces, at which time replacement arthroplasty is initiated.[13]

SHOULDER

Basically, shoulder replacements are divided into constrained and nonconstrained types; both have their complications. There have been many types of constrained shoulders that have subsequently been modified or abandoned because of loosening or failure of the components. The Michael Reese shoulder, however, has been an exception. Post and colleagues reported on 43 shoulder replacements, of which three were for rheumatoid arthritis (RA) and one for juvenile rheumatoid arthritis.[40] Of these three, one was a failure due to infection (this RA patient was the only case of infection). Of the entire series, there were 14 major complications related to the design of the prosthesis. Subsequently, the design was changed partway through the series. There were four dislocations, and six broken and two bent prosthetic humeral necks.

The nonconstrained resurfacing Neer procedure has had other types of complications. Neer and associates reported 61 patients with RA in a total of 153 procedures with minimal complications.[36] Of 28 done for RA and followed for over 1 year, 11 were excellent and 8 were unsatisfactory. In 1981, Neer and Watson reported 300 shoulder arthroplasties, of which 216 were total shoulder replacements.[37] They reported excellent results, with 30% having a radiologic line around the implant but no clinical loosening.

In 1977, Cofield reported on the status of total shoulder replacement at the Mayo Clinic, at which various types of shoulders were used.[14] The Stanmore constrained total shoulder was used in nine patients, of whom four had RA. Of these nine, three had significant pain, and one of these three was infected. This was subsequently converted to a resectional arthroplasty. The other two painful

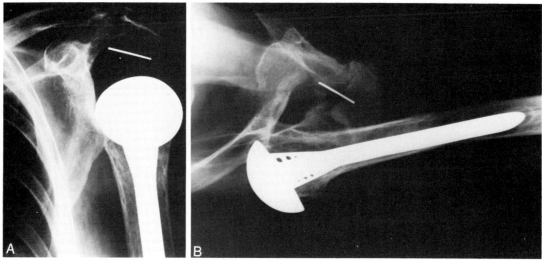

Figure 23–1. A, AP x-ray demonstrating inferior subluxation; *B,* lateral x-ray demonstrating posterior dislocation.

shoulders loosened their glenoid component. One patient dislocated. Two patients (one RA, one OA) underwent satisfactory results with the Michael Reese constrained shoulder, and 25 patients underwent replacement with the Neer resurfacing prosthesis. Nine of these were done for RA, and satisfactory pain relief and stability were achieved in all cases. There was one axillary nerve paralysis and one with no motion after heterotrophic bone formation. Neither of these were done for RA.

We have performed 30 shoulder arthroplasties for both RA and OA, and have used the Neer humeral endoprosthesis alone in the earlier cases, but have added the glenoid replacement more re-cently. In patients in whom there was an irreparable rotator cuff tear, we used a polyethylene subacromial spacer. Pain has generally been relieved by these procedures, but there have been complications. Of the first 22 procedures, all of which were followed over 2 years, there was one case of recurrent dislocation. This patient was the only poor result in this group (Fig. 23–1*A* and *B*). There were no infections, nerve problems, nor cases of clinical loosening, even though some humeral components were not cemented in place. Two patients with only the humeral head replaced showed erosion of the glenoid 5 years after the procedure. One of these developed arthritic-type pain (Fig. 23–2*A* and *B*).

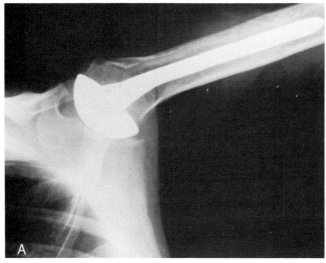
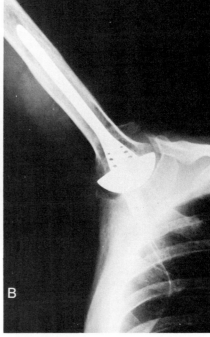

Figure 23–2. A, Shoulder x-ray shortly after surgery; *B,* shoulder x-ray 5 years after surgery demonstrating glenoid erosion. (Photograph of x-ray is reversed.)

Complications with shoulder surgery are best prevented by paying close attention to detail. Particular emphasis should be placed on resecting the humeral head with 35° of retroversion. This enables the surgeon to place the implant in a stable position, thus limiting the possibility of subluxation. Axillary nerve paralysis is an uncommon problem, and is best prevented by avoiding excessive traction on the deltoid muscle.

ELBOW

The elbow is different from the shoulder in that less radical surgery is frequently performed with good results. Synovectomy and radial head resection have consistently given good results for stage II or III disease. Complications resulting from this procedure have been minimal, although some elbows have not gained the expected motion nor achieved the desired level of pain relief. There is, of course, a certain number of patients who will experience progressive disease in the elbow, as in any joint that has had a rheumatoid synovectomy. We previously reported on 34 of 56 such procedures performed at the Denver Orthopedic Clinic with no other complications.[23] Ulnar neuropathy is the one complication that should be mentioned specifically. Although we did not see this in our first 34 procedures, we have had one since then. We routinely use only the lateral incision unless there is an ulnar neuropathy preoperatively.

Ingles and co-workers, using the transolecranon approach, reported on 28 procedures.[31] They had one infection, one radial nerve palsy, and two with separation of the olecranon osteotomy. Wilson and colleagues reported on 57 elbows, with only one case of superficial infection, one with delayed healing, and three developing ulnar nerve symptoms for the first time after surgery.[48] Porter and associates studied 154 procedures and found 17 with ulnar sensory disturbance after surgery, although 10 had symptoms preoperatively.[39]

For more advanced disease, interpositional arthroplasty has been performed using fascia, dermis, Gelfoam, or silicone. Few RA cases have been reported, but the same type of complications can be expected with synovectomy and radial head resection. Instability can also be expected occasionally, but data cannot be found to substantiate the occurrence of this complication. We have not seen instability following fascial arthroplasty in our clinic. The silicone hinge did not hold up, and is not recommended.

For the elbow with more advanced disease, total joint arthroplasty is indicated. The first replacements employed were constrained hinges, which were later modified to semiconstrained hinges. Nonconstrained resurfacing procedures have also been developed. There have been numerous complications with the total elbow devices, and this joint suffers from more serious problems, than with any of the other upper extremity replacements.

In 1974, Street and Stevens reported on their use of a metallic distal humeral resurfacing in ten patients.[42] Only three were for RA; in two of these three, the results were unsatisfactory. One of the two experienced complete ankylosis of the elbow and a transient ulnar neuropathy. The other unsatisfactory case resulted from dislocation of the elbow with erosion of the skin on the medial side; this necessitated removal of the prosthesis. Ankylosis resulted.

Results with the rigid hinges have also been disappointing. Cooney and Bryans tabulated results of a combination of 111 Shiers, Dee, McKee/Dee, GSB, and Coonrad elbows.[16] Poor results were seen in 24%. Cofield and co-workers tabulated the complications in 346 hinge total elbow replacements of both constrained and semiconstrained types and found the following: loosening (13%); fracture (9%); wound (8%); infection (5%); ankylosis (4%); neuropathy (6%)—transient (4%), permanent (2%); triceps rupture (2%); and revision (12%).[15]

The semiconstrained elbow was introduced as a result of rigid hinge failure. These are fixed hinges with a few degrees of "slop," which theoretically absorb some of the force exerted on the prosthesis-cement-bone interfaces. Coonrad reported on 150 elbows done in a multicenter study with 95% good results for rheumatoid arthritis.[17] Of the 150, there were only six failures, four because of loosening and two for infection, although 12% loosened their humeral stems. He concluded that this was a good procedure in RA but not in trauma.

Of the semiconstrained type, Ingles and Pellicci reported 36 elbow replacements followed for a minimum of 2 years.[30] They found a 53% complication rate, but only 25% of the complications affected the outcome. The first 17 in this series were done with the semiconstrained Pritchard-Walker elbow, and the rest with the triaxial prosthesis. Twenty-two patients had RA, and did generally better than the post-traumatic group. The following enumerates the 19 complications found in this group of 36 patients: wound hematoma (4); loosening (2); Fx humerus (2); ulnar neuropathy (2); triceps rupture (2); skin slough (2); broken component (2); Fx olecranon (1); infection (1); and cementophyte (1).

Workers at the Mayo Clinic found satisfactory results in 75% of cases of total elbow replacement in RA patients, again showing better results in the rheumatoid than in the patient with posttraumatic arthritis.

There have been four hinge total elbows for RA (three GSB and one Coonrad) performed at the Denver Orthopedic Clinic. All four resulted in greater than 90° of motion with no pain. We observed no complications in this small group.

The nonconstrained elbow, characterized by the London and Ewald or Japanese type, should not have loosening as a major problem, but other complications have been evident. Kudo and colleagues reported on 24 elbow replacements done for RA using a hingeless surface replacement similar to that of Ewald and London, and found excellent

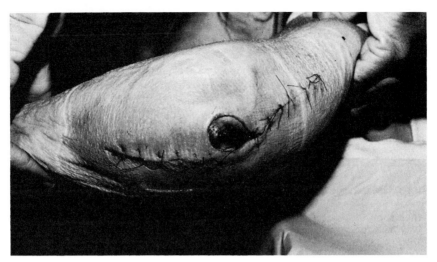

Figure 23–3. Skin slough after Ewald total elbow, leading to failure.

results in 14 and poor results in 3.[32] Complications observed were two elbows that failed to regain useful motion—one had proximal migration of the humeral component and one had persistent subluxation with pain and instability.

Ewald and associates reported 60 prosthetic replacements for RA, and found 87% good or excellent results; however, there was a 39% complication rate, with eight requiring revision of the arthroplasty (four for dislocation, two for sepsis, one for loosening, and one for fracture).[19] Overall, the results included recurrent dislocation in five patients, five permanent and six transient ulnar nerve palsies, and three fractures (two of the olecranon and one humeral shaft). Three elbows demonstrated some degree of wound breakdown and skin loss.

Clark and Weiland reported 17 Ewald elbows for RA, with pain relief in all 17.[10] Complications included one patient who required additional surgery because of subluxation, and one patient with ulnar neuropathy.

Our clinic has performed nine Ewald elbows for stage IV RA. There was one failure due to sepsis following gram-negative septicemia secondary to cholecystitis. This patient also developed a skin slough. (Fig. 23–3). She was converted to a resectional arthroplasty with ultimately 100° of motion and no pain. Other complications included two painless subluxations (Fig. 23–4). These two patients could control this, and expressed a high degree of satisfaction with their results. There was one case of ulnar neuropathy, involving only the sensory component. In replacement arthroplasty the nerve should be exposed and protected and, if indicated, transposed.

How does one avoid these numerous complications? Dislocation of the nonconstrained elbow may be prevented by approaching the elbow laterally instead of posteriorly. This leaves a hinge of medial ligaments intact. It is also necessary to reconstruct the lateral ligaments to obtain stability.

The incidence of ulnar neuropathy may also be reduced by approaching the elbow laterally but, in our series, the only patient who developed an ulnar nerve problem was the only patient we did with the lateral approach. This neuropathy involved only the sensory components of the nerve, and cleared after surgical decompression. Anterior transposition of the nerve is the best method to avoid ulnar neuropathy.

The incidence of component loosening will be

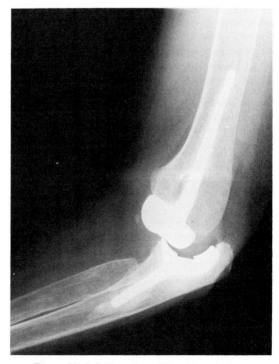

Figure 23–4. Subluxation of Ewald total elbow.

reduced by redesign of the prosthesis. The hinge elbows in use now are "sloppy" hinges with several degrees of laxity, and a new design feature should produce less incidence of loosening. Fracture on insertion of the prosthesis is prevented by careful resection of bone and by avoiding too large a prosthesis without adequate reaming of the medullary canals.

Skin slough is always a potential problem with rheumatoid skin. Careful handling of the skin, avoiding excessive undermining and retraction, will minimize this complication. A straight-line incision should be made, which should not be placed directly over the olecranon or some other bony prominence. Lowering the tourniquet, obtaining hemostasis, and draining the wounds will minimize hematoma formation.

WRIST

The wrist is the key joint of the upper extremity. Surgery is frequently indicated to prevent progression of the disease and rupture of the extensor tendons. After tenosynovectomy, resection of the distal ulna, and transposition of the dorsal carpal ligament, tendon rupture is rare. We reported on 174 such procedures in 1975, and found only one patient who had intact extensor tendons before surgery to rupture a tendon subsequently.[12] This was due to a technical error that resulted in dorsal instability of the distal ulna.

Another complication with dorsal wrist surgery is wound breakdown. We have seen this in about 5% of our cases, and find that this problem can be minimized by the following: making a straight longitudinal incision; not undermining the skin; leaving all the fat on the skin flaps; preserving all possible dorsal veins; avoiding strong retraction; lowering the tourniquet and obtaining hemostasis; drainage of wound; dressing to fingertips with much padding (preferably Dacron batting); using only light compression and splinting.

The complication endemic to this procedure is supination of the carpus, which will then slide off the ulnar side. The incidence of this is lower when the ulnar side of the wrist is carefully reconstructed. The proximal end of the carpal ulnar ligament is attached to the dorsal aspect of the ulnar side of the radius, and the extensor carpi ulnaris is relocated on the dorsum of the wrist using a loop of extensor retinaculum to keep it stabilized. We do not feel that using an ulnar silicone cap will significantly prevent this complication. We have no data available as to the incidence of this; some cases are inevitable because of the natural destruction of the carpus with the rheumatoid disease. Many cases can be prevented by reconstructing the distal radioulnar carpal complex by suturing the lateral volar capsule and retinaculum to the distal radius and splinting postoperatively.

Recurrent dorsal tenosynovitis after tenosynovectomy is rare. On the volar side, carpal tunnel release and flexor tenosynovectomy is commonly performed at the wrist level. Decrease in tendon motion can be prevented by early active and passive motion of the fingers.

Joint replacement at the wrist level has taken two forms: silicone interpositional arthroplasty, and total joint replacement. There have been significant contributions made by Swanson in the field of rheumatoid surgery with his flexible hinges, one of which is used in the wrist. Swanson and Swanson reported on 76 wrists with an adequate pain-free motion, averaging from 21° of extension to 41° of flexion.[45] No complications were recorded.

Goodman and co-workers reviewed 37 silicone wrist arthroplasties in patients with RA.[26] Of these, 16% displayed residual discomfort, 5% had recurrent deformity, and 8% experienced prosthetic fractures. These patients were followed for a minimum of 6 months, and further collapse of the carpus over the implant with more loss of motion and a higher rate of implant breakage would be expected as time passes. We have similarly used the silicon prosthesis in the rheumatoid wrist, with about the same results.

Fracture of the silicone prosthesis is minimized by avoiding sharp edges of bone impinging on the prosthesis, careful handling of the prosthesis (avoiding the use of sharp instruments) and, instead of using the prosthesis for correction of the deformities, using soft tissue reconstruction to balance the wrist.

Total wrist arthroplasty has gained in popularity as total replacement in other joints has progressed. Two joints, the Meuli and the Volz, have gained the widest acceptance. Beckenbaugh and Linscheid reported their experience at the Mayo Clinic in 1977 with 26 Meuli arthroplasties, 21 done for RA.[4] Pain was relieved in 92% of the cases. Postoperative motion averaged 32° dorsiflexion, 27° palmar flexion, 2° radial deviation, and 23° ulnar deviation. Complications requiring reoperation occurred in 35% of the wrists. Six reoperations resulted from abnormal resting stance of flexion or ulnar deviation, three from technical errors that resulted in dislocation in one wrist, one from malpositioned stem, and one from retained radial styloid. Additional complications included temporary subluxation in two patients, delayed wound healing in two, ulnar nerve paresthesia in one, and extensor tenosynovitis in one.

Wrist imbalance is the most common complication after wrist replacement. This can be avoided by making certain that the center of motion of the prosthesis is inserted at the normal center of motion of the wrist, which is at the base of the capitate. Choosing the prosthesis that best allows this will automatically lessen the incidence of this complication. In addition, the tendons may need to be balanced. Adequate bone resection and soft tissue release are necessary to obtain this goal properly. Occasionally, it is necessary to release the flexor carpi ulnaris.

It is often necessary to obtain an x-ray in the operating room to demonstrate proper placement

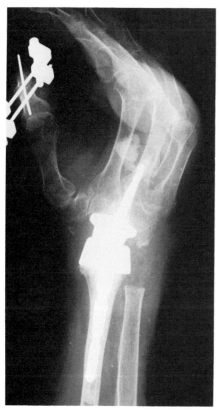

Figure 23–5. Methylmethacrylate extruded through false passage in metacarpal.

of the prosthesis and proper bone resection. Dislocation may occur when applying the dressings. The assistant should not suspend the hand by the fingers during this process. Wound healing is always a potential problem, and the preventative measures for skin incision and handling of the dorsal wrist skin covered earlier should be observed.

Volz reported on the first 100 wrists done from 1974 to 1978 by 15 collaborating surgeons; 83 patients had rheumatoid arthritis.[47] The overall results were 86% good or excellent and 6% failure. The most frequent postoperative problem was wrist motor imbalance, which amounted to 21%, with 13% exhibiting an ulnar deformity. In addition, 6% demonstrated wound healing problems—all rheumatoid patients. Four patients experienced a single episode of subluxation, three in the immediate postoperative period. Two patients developed a wound infection, requiring removal of the prosthesis. One patient demonstrated loosening of the distal component. Of the six failures, five have had their prosthesis removed, leaving solid ankylosis in three and two with fibrous ankylosis.

We have performed 40 Volz wrists and have previously reported on the first 20.[33] Our complications were similar to those of Volz, with balance being the greatest problem. We had 70% excellent or good results. There was one loosening after 3 years in one patient who had osteoarthritis. This wrist required reoperation to recement the distal component. She now has impingement of one of the remaining carpal bones. There were two cases of carpal tunnel syndrome after surgery in the original 20 patients, and one other case subsequent to that group. Of these three, two required surgery. One postoperative hematoma resolved without surgery, even though the wound was drained and hemastosis was obtained after the tourniquet was lowered before wound closure. In one case, the radius was perforated and cement leaked into the interosseous membrane (Fig. 23–5). This could have been avoided by plugging the bone perforation before the cement was injected into the radius. Two patients dislocated immediately after surgery; they were reduced, and had no subsequent problems (Fig. 23–6). One patient had inadequate wrist extensors and was reoperated on in an attempt to balance these motors.

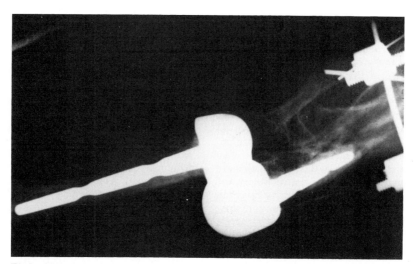

Figure 23–6. Immediate postoperative x-ray showing dislocation of the Volz total wrist.

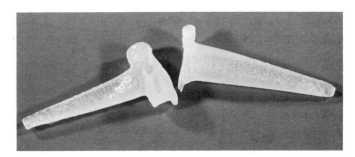

Figure 23–7. Fractured silicone finger prosthesis.

HAND

In the hand, results of soft tissue procedures, such as synovectomy, have been difficult to assess because the variable pattern and course of the disease and uniform condition of involvement are not available in most hand centers.[43] Therefore, is recurrence of ulnar drift after synovectomy or recurrent synovitis a complication? We prefer not to think of it in that way. Flexor tenosynovectomy in the fingers is another matter, however, in that limited motion may follow this procedure. Limitation of motion can best be lessened by starting early motion on the third or fourth postoperative day. Out of 54 flexor tenosynovectomies in the fingers, we found that only one patient needed a tenolysis because of stiffness. He did not start early motion. One other patient required repeat tenosynovectomy.[21]

Much has been written on replacement arthroplasties of the joints of the hand, and complications and expectations are known. There is certainly occasional recurrence of ulnar drift, but is this due to other forces acting on the hand—or is it due to a complication of the implant surgery?[11, 26, 43] To minimize recurrence of ulnar drift, the capsular contracture must be released. Adequate bone must be resected, and the radial collateral ligament should be reattached to the metacarpal through drill holes. The joint should be in neutral when the procedure is completed because the postoperative splinting will not correct a deformity that has not been corrected with the surgery. Care is also necessary to centralize the extensor mechanism over the joint from its subluxed position on the ulnar side of the metacarpal head. The implant itself should not be counted on to align the joint; it is necessary to correct the malalignment by soft tissue reconstruction.

Complications generally fall into three categories: fracture of the prosthesis, infection, and recurrence of deformity. Swanson reported 96 complications in a series of 3915 metacarpophalangeal (MP) replacements, with a 0.94% fracture rate, 0.69% infection, and 0.81% dislocation.[43] Niebauer reported a 2.2% infection rate and 1.1% subluxation in 178 joints.[38] Urbaniak and colleagues reported that, out of a total of 26 patients, there was one hematoma and subsequent infection, and six patients with some recurrence of ulnar deviation.[46] Millender and associates reported on 2105 silicone prosthetic arthroplasties of the hands in 631 patients, with infection occurring in 10.[35] The prostheses were removed in seven patients. Prosthesis fracture can be delayed by avoiding sharp edges of bone abutting on the prosthesis, and by correcting any angular forces on the joint.

Beckenbaugh and co-workers reported a 26.2% fracture rate of the Swanson prostheses and an 11.3% recurrence of clinical deformity.[3] For the Niebauer prostheses, fracture rate was 38.2%, with a 44.17% recurrence of clinical deformity. This study involved a total of 530 arthroplasties done on 119 patients.

We analyzed 173 silicone rubber Swanson prostheses in 45 patients.[22] In this group, 9% of the prostheses showed definite fracture (Fig. 23–7). There were two infections, and one case of skin necrosis. Three prostheses had to be removed, one for fracture and two for infection. The recurrence of ulnar drift ranged from 25 to 45° in four patients.

One other complication with silicone arthroplasty has occasionally been recorded; a foreign body reaction to the silicone (Fig. 23–8).[1, 9, 22] In one of our cases, the prosthesis had not broken.[22]

Since these reports have been published, the high-performance elastomer has been introduced. This more resilient rubber is expected to cut down on the fracture rate, although we still see an occasional fracture with this newer material; at least the time to fracture is prolonged.

With regard to other types of prostheses, Flatt introduced a metal hinge.[25] Over the years, most have ended up as failures due to infection, wound breakdown, erosion, or implant failure. We reviewed the use of this prosthesis in nine thumb MP joints in patients with RA, with eight having good-to-excellent results and only one requiring removal because of infection.[24] This prosthesis is no longer in use (Fig. 23–9).

Methylmethacrylate-cemented metal-polyethylene prostheses in the finger joints seem to vary in popularity. In 1979, Beckenbaugh and Steffee presented a preliminary report on 42 prostheses inserted into the MP joint of thumbs.[5] Follow-up for 12 to 40 months revealed an average motion of 16°. There were no infections and no reoperations were necessary. Two patients had radiologic evidence of loosening, but both were asymptomatic. Although a number of these types of prostheses have been

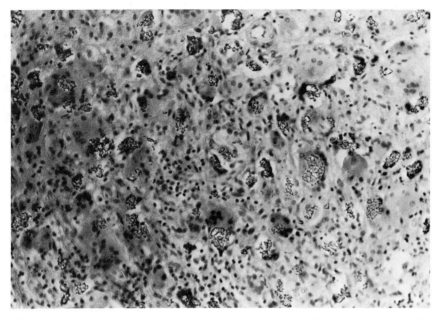

Figure 23–8. Microscopic section of synovium removed after re-exploration of fractured trapezium silicone prosthesis. This shows foreign body giant cells and intracellular silicone.

introduced, usage was decreased because range of motion has deteriorated with time, and there seemed to be no advantage over the use of the more easily inserted silicone prostheses.

Replacement arthroplasty of the trapezium-metacarpal joint is occasionally done for RA, but usually for OA or traumatic arthritis. The most frequent complication after replacement arthroplasty is subluxation of the implant (Fig. 23–10). The incidence of subluxation can be minimized by tight capsular closure, resecting the radialmost portion of the trapezoid, reinforcing the capsule with a

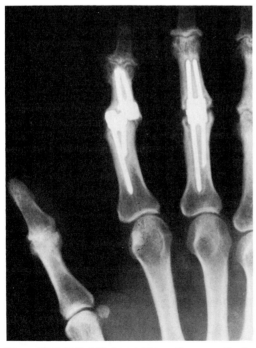

Figure 23–9. Failed Flatt metal hinge finger prosthesis.

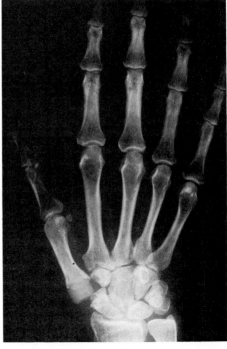

Figure 23–10. Dislocated silicone trapezium implant.

tendon graft utilizing a portion of the distal end of the flexor carpi radialis, weaving this in and out of the capsule and suturing this to the extensor carpi radialis longus, advancing the abductor pollicis longus, and correcting a hyperextension deformity of the MP joint. Complications with other types of therapy have included lack of stability after resectional arthroplasty.

Our series of 11 prosthetic arthroplasties did not reveal any subluxations after a tendon graft was used to reinforce the capsule.[20] Swanson and Swanson reviewed 46 thumbs treated with replacement arthroplasty.[45] Follow-up 6 months to 5½ years after arthroplasty revealed no evidence of bone absorption or reactive bone formation, and no evidence of change in the contour of the implant. Radial subluxation of the implant emerged in eight patients. There were no cases of infection and no fractures.

Total joint replacement at the basal joint is now being advocated. Braun presented 21 cases with complications in two cases of loosening;[6] Hamlin and colleagues reported 35 cases of the "Caffiniere" prosthesis with no infection.[27] There were two failures, and two components necessitated recementing.

The interphalangeal (IP) joints of the fingers become stiff and deformed in the rheumatoid patient. Boutonnière, swan-neck, and flexion and extension contractures may occur. Postoperative splinting is very important to prevent recurrence after the deformity has been surgically corrected. When the joint itself is destroyed, implant arthroplasty or arthrodesis is indicated. Nonunion is the only significant complication after arthrodesis of the IP joints; the incidence varies from 0 to 20% using various techniques.[8, 28, 34, 41] Only good fixation and adequate bony opposition will minimize nonunion. The other alternative is replacement arthroplasty. Complications of this procedure include all those listed for implant arthroplasty of the MP joints. Again, these can best be avoided by correcting the deformity with soft tissue reconstruction, and not by relying on the prosthesis to correct the deformity.

In 1972, Swanson reported no infections, fractures, or dislocations after 148 PIP silicone arthroplasties.[43] For the deformities at the IP and MP joints of the thumb, arthrodesis is the most commonly performed operation. Complications of this procedure are pin tract drainage and nonunion, which is reported at 0 to 20%.[2, 7, 29]

In our series of 82 thumb fusions with a compression clamp, only three joints went into nonunion. Two of these were reoperated on and obtained solid bony fusion. We also had eight patients with pin tract drainage. This complication could be avoided by using a different method of fixation utilizing buried pins.

References

1. Aptekar, R. G., Davie, J. M., and Cattell, H. S.: Foreign body reaction to silicone rubber. Complication of a finger joint implant. Clin. Orthop., 98:231, 1974.
2. Beckenbaugh, R. D.: Arthrodesis of the metacarpophalangeal joint of the thumb. Orthop. Trans., 4:291, 1980.
3. Beckenbaugh, R. D., Dobyns, J. H., and Bryon, R. S.: Review and analysis of silicone-rubber metacarpophalangeal implants. J. Bone Joint Surg., 58A:483, 1976.
4. Beckenbaugh, R. D., and Linscheid, R. L.: Total wrist arthroplasty: A preliminary report. J. Hand Surg., 2:339, 1977.
5. Beckenbaugh, R. D., and Steffee, A. D.: Total joint arthroplasty for the metacarpophalangeal joint of the thumb. A preliminary report. Orthop. Trans., 3:268, 1979.
6. Braun, R. D.; Total joint replacement for arthritis at the base of the thumb. Orthop. Trans., 4:315, 1980.
7. Brumfield, R. H.: Reconstructive surgery of the thumb in rheumatoid arthritis. Orthop. Trans., 2:242, 1978.
8. Carrol, R. E., and Hill, N. A.: Small joint arthrodesis in hand reconstruction. J. Bone Joint Surg., 51A:1219, 1969.
9. Christe, A. J., Weinberger, K. A., and Dietrich, M.: Silicone lymphadenopathy and synovitis complications of silicone elastomer finger joint prosthesis. J.A.M.A., 237:1463, 1977.
10. Clark, G., and Weiland, A.: Total elbow arthroplasty of the Ewald Type. Presented to the Midyear Meeting of the American Society for Surgery of the Hand, Boyne Mountain Michigan, July, 1979.
11. Clayton, M. L., and Ferlic, D. C.: Tendon transfer for radial rotation of the wrist in R.A. Clin. Orthop. Rel. Res., 100:176, 1974.
12. Clayton, M. L., and Ferlic, D. C.: The wrist in rheumatoid arthritis. Clin. Orthop. Rel. Res., 106:192, 1975.
13. Clayton, M. L., and Ferlic, D. C.: Surgery of the shoulder in rheumatoid arthritis. Clin. Orthop. Rel. Res., 106:166, 1975.
14. Cofield, R. H.: Status of total shoulder arthroplasty, Arch. Surg., 112:1088, 1977.
15. Cofield, R. H., Morrey, B. F., and Bryans, R. S.: Total shoulder and total elbow arthroplasties: The current state of development. Part II. J.C.E. Orthop., 7:17, 1979.
16. Cooney, W. P., III, and Bryans, R. S.: Rheumatoid arthritis in the upper extremity: Treatment of the elbow and shoulder joints. In American Academy of Orthopaedic Surgeons: Instructional Course Lectures, Vol. 28, St. Louis, C. V. Mosby, 1972, pp. 247–262.
17. Coonrad, R. P.: Results with the Coonrad total elbow arthroplasty. Presented to the Piedmont Orthopaedic Society, Boca Raton, Florida, May 8, 1980.
18. Entin, M. A.: Cruess, R. L., and Mitchel, N. (eds.): Surgery of Rheumatoid Arthritis, Philadelphia, J. B. Lippincott, 1971.
19. Ewald, F. C., et al.: Capitello-condylar total elbow arthroplasty, J. Bone Joint Surg., 62A:1259, 1980.
20. Ferlic, D. C., Busbee, G. A., and Clayton, M. L.: Degenerative arthritis of the carpometacarpal joint of the thumb: A clinical follow-up of eleven Niebauer prostheses. J. Hand Surg., 2:212, 1977.
21. Ferlic, D. C., and Clayton, M. L.: Flexor tenosynovectomy in the rheumatoid finger. J. Hand Surg., 3:364, 1978.
22. Ferlic, D. C., Clayton, M. L., and Holloway, M.: Complications of silicone implant surgery in the metacarpophalangeal joint. J. Bone Joint Surg., 57A:991, 1975.
23. Ferlic, D. C., Clayton, M. L., and Parr, P. L.: Synovectomy and arthroplasties of the elbow in rheumatoid arthritis. Orthop. Dig., 5:11, 1977.
24. Ferlic, D. C., Serat, D. I., and Clayton, M. L.: The use of the Flatt hinge prosthesis in the rheumatoid thumb, Hand, 10:94, 1978.
25. Flatt, A. E.: The Care of the Rheumatoid Hand, St. Louis, C. V. Mosby, 1963.
26. Goodman, M. J., et al.: Arthroplasty of the rheumatoid wrist with silicone rubber; An early evaluation. J. Hand Surg., 5:114, 1980.
27. Hamlin, C.: Total joint replacement of the thumb carpometacarpal joint. Proceedings of the American Society of Surgery of the Hand, Annual Meeting, Las Vegas, February 1981.
28. Harrison, S. H.: The Harrison-Nicolle intramedullary peg: follow-up study of 100 cases, The Hand, 6:304–307, 1974.
29. Harrison, S., Smith, P., and Maxwell, D.: Stabilization of the first metacarpophalangeal and terminal joints of the thumb. Hand, 9:242, 1977.
30. Ingles, A. E., and Pellicci, P. N.: Total elbow replacements. J. Bone Joint Surg., 62A:1252, 1980.
31. Ingles, A. E., Ronavat, C. S., and Straub, L. R.: Synovectomy and débridement of the elbow in rheumatoid arthritis. J. Bone Joint Surg., 53A:652, 1971.

32. Kudo, H., Iware, K., and Watanabe, S.: Total replacement of the rheumatoid elbow with a hingeless prosthesis, J. Bone Joint Surg., 62A:277, 1980.
33. Lamberta, F. J., Ferlic, D. C., and Clayton, M. L.: Volz total wrist arthroplasty and rheumatoid arthritis. A preliminary report. J. Hand Surg., 5:245, 1980.
34. Leonard, H., and Capen, D. A.: Compression arthrodesis of finger joints. Clin. Orthop. Rel. Res., 145:193, 1979.
35. Millender, L. H., et al.: Infection after silicone prosthetic arthroplasty in the hand. J. Bone Joint Surg., 57A:825, 1975.
36. Neer, C. S., II, et al.: Total shoulder replacement: A preliminary report. Orthop. Trans., 1:244, 1977.
37. Neer, C. S., II, and Watson, K.: Seven-year experiences in total shoulder replacement. Presented to the American Academy of Orthopaedic Surgeons, Annual Meeting, Las Vegas, 1981.
38. Niebauer, J. J.: Dacron-silicone prostheses for the metacarpophalangeal and interphalangeal joints. *In* Cramer, L. M., and Chase, R. A. (eds.): Symposium on the Hand, St. Louis, C. V. Mosby, 1971, pp. 96–105.
39. Porter, B. B., Richardson, P. C., and Vainio, K.: Rheumatoid arthritis of the elbow: The results of synovectomy. J. Bone Joint Surg., 56B:427, 1974.
40. Post, M., Haskell, S. S., and Jablon, M.: Total shoulder replacement with a constrained prosthesis. J. Bone Joint Surg., 62A:327–335, 1980.
41. Potenza, A. D.: A technique for arthrodesis of finger joints. J. Bone Joint Surg., 55A:1534, 1973.
42. Street, D. M., and Stevens, P. S.: A humeral replacement prosthesis for the elbow: Results in ten elbows. J. Bone Joint Surg., 56A:1147, 1974.
43. Swanson, A. B.: Flexible implant arthroplasties for arthritic finger joints. J. Bone Joint Surg., 54A:435, 1972.
44. Swanson, A. B.: Disabling arthritis at the base of the thumb. J. Bone Joint Surg., 54A:456, 1972.
45. Swanson, A. B., and Swanson, G.: Flexible implant resection arthroplasty: A method for reconstruction of small joints in the extremities. *In* American Academy of Orthopaedic Surgeons: Instructional Course Lectures, St. Louis, C. V. Mosby, 1978, pp. 27–60.
46. Urbaniak, J. R., McCollum, D. E., and Goldner, J. L.: Metacarpophalangeal and interphalangeal joint reconstruction. South. Med. J., 63:1281, 1970.
47. Volz, R. G.: Total wrist arthroplasty. A review of 100 patients. Orthop. Trans., 3:268, 1979.
48. Wilson, D. W., Arden, G. P., and Ansell, B. B.: Synovectomy of the elbow in rheumatoid arthritis. J. Bone Joint Surg., 55B:106, 1973.

24

RESULTS OF INSENSITIVITY IN PATIENTS WITH NERVE INJURY, LEPROSY, AND OTHER NEUROPATHIES

Paul W. Brand

INHIBITED AND UNINHIBITED SENSORY LOSS

The complications that result from sensory loss in the hand may be conveniently divided into two groups: sensory loss that results in uninhibited use of the hand; and sensory loss that results in inhibition of use of the hand.

To understand the difference one needs to realize that the use of muscle power is constantly controlled by sensory feedback. Most of the time we do not watch our hands to see what they are doing, or to ensure that we have firm hold of the hammer that we are using to drive in some nails. Despite popular belief, neither do we rely on the sensory nerve endings in the musculoskeletal chain. These are available, but they are far from being the primary source of sensory feedback. What we use is sensory feedback from the touch and pressure systems of sensory endings in the surface of the hand. Moberg has shown that these are also the endings responsible for the perception of joint sense and position sense.[1] Thus, the nerve endings in the skin—involving touch, pressure, temperature, and pain—dominate the interaction between the brain and the hand, modifying muscular action until the appropriate sensory feedback from the skin is perceived. Compare the way a hand holds an ax and the way it holds a cactus or a hot potato. In holding an ax, the flexor digitorum muscles contract until the skin gives a pressure feedback that says that the handle of the ax is secure. In swinging the ax vigorously to cut down a tree, there may be a momentary tendency for the ax to slip away from the hand, but this is prevented by a tightening of the muscles in response to the perception by the skin that the ax handle is slipping, or that it is about to slip. The muscles contract just strongly enough so that they do not waste a 50-lb grip if a 40-lb grip will do. Grasping a cactus or a hot potato, the action is dominated by sensations of pain or temperature, and the hand is quite likely to abandon the task and let go at the behest of unpleasant sensory feedback. The grasp is *inhibited* by the sensation.

In most sensory neuropathies, such as leprosy, diabetes, and the various toxic neuropathies, all sensations at the level of the skin gradually diminish as the disease progresses. There may be a stage at which perhaps only 10% of the nerve endings are responding. In most cases, there is a simple diminution of sensation. There is no rearrangement of modalities, and no new sensations are brought into the picture. Thus, the person swinging an ax may know that he is holding an ax but may be getting feedback that tells him he is holding it insecurely. To get the feeling that he is exerting a 40-lb grip he may have to contract his muscles strongly enough to produce an 80-lb grip. In holding a hot potato or a cactus, he will be less inhibited by the painful reactions and may hold the hot potato for twice as long before he realizes that he is in danger of a burn.

A person whose nerve has been divided and then repaired is in a different situation. During the stage of recovery, not only does he have a diminished number of effective nerve endings but their orientation has been changed, both from the skin and from the nerve fibers trapped in the neuroma. The patient gets a feedback of "pins and needles." He has a constant sensation that something about the hand is wrong, and it may give him the feeling that he is holding a cactus when he is actually holding the handle of an ax. He responds to the inhibition of the pricking paresthesias, and either lets go or holds the ax reluctantly and with inadequate strength.

I have used the terms "inhibited" and "uninhibited" because they represent a sharp contrast in matters of management. There are some patients who need to be encouraged to use their hands more than they do, and to discount or ignore their paresthetic sensations, while there are others for whom the chief thrust of re-education must be to restrain them from excessive and improper use of the hand. For most of this chapter I will be discussing the complications of insensitivity as if we were dealing only with the uninhibited hand, and I will then add just a few remarks about the problems of inhibition of activity.

AUTONOMIC DENERVATION

Loss of Vasomotor Control

When a hand is freshly denervated, it is usually hot. If a single nerve is divided, that part of the hand will be palpably hotter than the other part. This is because with the loss of vasoconstrictor control all the vessels will be dilated. In the ensuing few weeks the vessels become sensitized to circulating vasoconstrictors, and become more constricted than the normally innervated parts of the hand. Thus, the long-term results of denervation will usually be that the hand has a diminished circulation and feels cold to the touch. However, this does not mean that the blood supply is inadequate nor that the capability of the circulation is diminished. If a denervated hand becomes injured or infected, or if repetitive stress results in some traumatic inflammation, this previously cool part of the hand will become significantly warmer than the normally warm innervated part of the hand, which has been protected from injury by its sensitivity.

An uninhibited hand, therefore, which tends to use its insensitive part excessively, will often be warmer and have a richer blood supply in the denervated than in the normal part. A quick assessment of temperature distribution is consequently one of the most reliable ways of determining the pattern of use and misuse of an insensitive hand.

Dryness

Because sweating is under the control of the autonomic nerves, a denervated hand is usually dry, although there are some forms of sensory neuropathy in which the autonomic system is preserved. Dryness of the hand is a problem for two reasons. First, dry skin is slippery. For precision grip and for holding small articles between the thumb and fin-

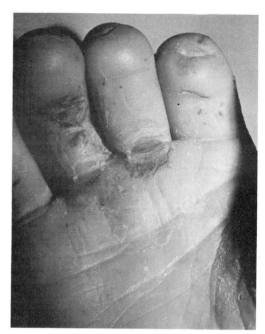

Figure 24–1. Dry skin in a denervated hand. Cracks in flexion creases develop into wounds and then into severe infections. The final results may be loss of a digit.

gertips, moist skin is far more secure than dry skin. Secondly, dry skin is liable to crack. The cuticular layer of skin is composed of keratin, a protein that changes dramatically between the hydrated and dehydrated states. Hydrated keratin is soft, pliable, and compliant; dry keratin is hard and brittle. Denervated skin has a tendency to develop cracks along the flexion creases and cracks across parts of the palmar skin where calluses have developed (Fig. 24–1). Denervated skin is not without some moisture content, but this is so slight that it is quickly lost by evaporation. I advise patients with insensitive dry skin to soak their hands for 15 minutes or so at least once a day, and then to prevent evaporation by rubbing petroleum jelly or lanolin over their hands. It is a mistake for such patients to use detergents and harsh soaps, because the sebaceous secretions need to be preserved and natural oils should not be extracted from the skin. Whenever soap is used, the hand should again be moisturized with an appropriate cream or lanolin.

Healing of Insensitive Tissues

Denervation does not significantly affect the healing time of soft tissues. I usually allow an extra day or two before the removal of stitches from the skin after surgery, and I generally keep postoperative plaster casts in place longer after tendon repairs. This is not because the healing is significantly slower, but because patients are likely to use their hands more freely and forcefully if they are denervated than if they are inhibited by postoperative pain. In cases of long-standing sensory loss in which the hand has been subjected over many years to improper use, resulting in a succession of wounds and ulcerations, the tissues may be infiltrated with scar, and at this stage the blood supply may be poor and healing substantially delayed. This, however, is not a direct result of the denervation but rather of the subsequent misuse.

Bones actually do take longer to heal in the denervated hand following fractures and arthrodesis. It can be shown on x-ray that there is a smaller cloud of callus after fracture and this, in addition to the expectation of immediate use when the cast is removed, should force the surgeon to maintain immobilization for much longer than would be done in the normal limb. This is particularly true of digital arthrodesis. Hand surgeons are accustomed to fixing an arthrodesed interphalangeal joint with two crossed K-wires, and then allowing the patient substantial freedom as soon as the skin has healed. This is totally unacceptable in an insensitive hand. In a normal hand, this type of immobilization is successful entirely because any strong attempt to move the finger is inhibited by the sensitive feedback from the wounded area. Pressure and bending stress on the pins and wires result in a feedback, which inhibits further stress. If I release my leprosy patients from a plaster cast after their arthrodesis has been fixed by K-wires, they proceed to use their full force. The pins quickly become bent or loose, and the result is disastrous.

I am sure that this is why surgeons have long thought that neuropathic joints cannot be successfully arthrodesed. Arthrodesis can be successful only if immobilization is prolonged. When the external cast is finally removed, the surgeon or therapist should monitor the temperature of the arthrodesed joint. The plaster cast should be reapplied if use of the hands results in an increase in the temperature of the joint.

Stretching of Ligaments and Capsules

Following paralysis, if skin sensation remains normal, it is possible to depend a good deal on the firm support of ligaments, palmar plates, and the restraints of skin and fascia to maintain the stability of a joint that is no longer supported adequately by muscles. In the presence of denervation, however, every joint must be supported by appropriate muscle-tendon units, or should be arthrodesed if it is going to be placed under stress.

A good example of this is the metacarpophalangeal joint of the thumb in cases of low median and ulnar paralysis. If there is adequate sensation, surgeons will obtain an apparently successful result by restoring opposition of the thumb by an abductor opponens replacement, and then allowing the patient to pinch. In such cases the index finger will usually approach the thumb at an angle between the palmar and ulnar sides of the thumb. If the tip of the thumb now flexes uncontrollably (Froment's sign), the distal interphalangeal joint is often arthrodesed in a straight position. The index finger will then tend to thrust the thumb into abduction at the metacarpophalangeal joint, at which it is supported only by the medial collateral ligament, because the adductor is paralyzed. In an insensitive hand, I have often seen the ulnar collateral ligament of the thumb become gradually stretched over a period of years, until finally the thumb can be pushed out from the hand and be at right angles to the metacarpal, useless for the purposes of pinch (Fig. 24–2). In a sensitive hand this does not happen, because the sensitivity of the ulnar collateral

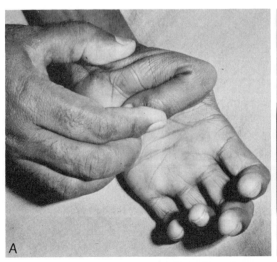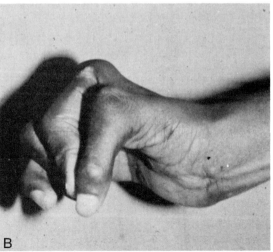

Figure 24–2. A, The ulnar collateral ligament at the metacarpophalangeal joint of this thumb has become progressively stretched following paralysis of the adduction and short flexor muscles; *B,* in a sensitive thumb this paralysis would have resulted in a weak pinch. In this insensitive thumb the pinch was strong but stretched the ligaments.

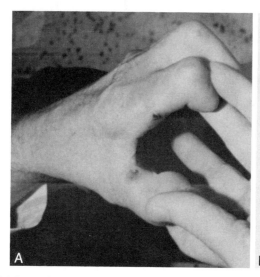 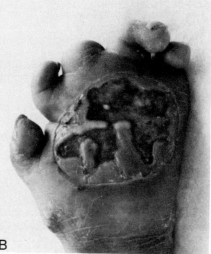

Figure 24–3. *A,* These two burns were found after a patient had forgotten that he had a cigarette in his hand—it burned right through; *B,* with no usable fingers remaining, this patient lifted a cooking pot between his two palms. The burn was noticed only afterward.

ligament results in an inhibition of pinch. The insensitive person pinches firmly and develops deformity, whereas the sensitive person with the same paralysis pinches gently and inadequately but avoids the deformity. In either case it is proper to provide a substitute for the abductor muscle, or to arthrodese the metacarpophalangeal joint and leave the interphalangeal joint free.

Wounds and Injuries

The overwhelming problem with uninhibited insensitive hands is that they are constantly being injured and, having injured them, the patients do not take care of the resulting wound and infection. Burns and mechanical force are frequent causes of injury in certain occupations.

Burns

In our own institution, in which most patients have insensitive hands, the largest number of wounds comes from cigarettes—the patient forgets that he is holding a cigarette and it burns between his fingers (Fig. 24–3). There are other causes of burns: from patients' attempts at cooking, from adjusting the steam heating system, and from drinking hot cups of coffee. These problems have been considerably diminished in recent years by careful attention to a burn prevention program. Occupational therapists have analyzed the causes of many of these burns. There are now special handles for controlling steam radiators, and there are thermally insulated cups. Unnecessary cooking by individual patients is discouraged, and there are appropriate utensils for those who feel the need to cook.

Injury from Mechanical Causes

Mechanical forces can result in injury of the hand in three different ways: direct damage; ischemia; and repetitive stress.

Direct Damage. It is almost impossible to control and anticipate every type of activity of the hand. It is only through forethought, anticipation, and constant vigilance that someone with insensitive hands may remain free from injury. Both the surgeon and therapist need to consider the range of activities of the hand in terms of pressure and sheer stress. We are accustomed to thinking in terms of force but, for the protection of the skin, it is not the amount of *force* that matters but the amount of *pressure*. Because pressure is equal to force divided by area, it is obviously proper to double the force providing one doubles the area through which the force acts. The real problem arises when a relatively moderate amount of force is used, but it is applied through an extremely small area. One of the most common problems involves small metal handles on furniture, such as on doors and on the drawers of filing cabinets (Fig. 24–4).

The door to a room will usually have a doorknob about 5 cm in diameter, or it may have a lever handle perhaps 10 cm long and up to 2 cm wide. In either case, the greater part of the surface skin of the hand may be applied to the door handle. Even if it requires a lot of force to turn the handle, it will almost never damage the hand. For some reason, furniture manufacturers seem to like small ornate metal handles perhaps 1 cm in diameter, with narrow edges that can only be effectively grasped by the rim. Cupboard doors are often hard to open, and the drawers of filing cabinets may be extremely stiff or may have been locked without the knowl-

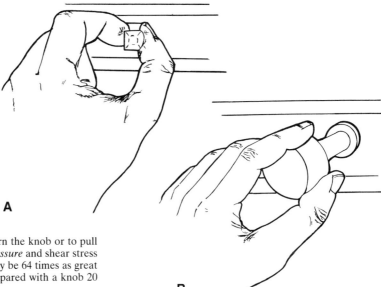

A

Figure 24–4. The *force* needed to turn the knob or to pull on it is the same in *A* and *B*. The *pressure* and shear stress that is needed to apply that force may be 64 times as great for a knob 5 mm in diameter as compared with a knob 20 mm in diameter.

B

edge of the person trying to open them. A normal inidividual will struggle to use these small handles and will give up, while a person with insensitive hands will apply much larger amounts of force on extremely small areas of metal, and will tear a flap of skin from the side of the finger. The same is true of small keys (Fig. 24–5). I have known leprosy patients to put a key into the ignition of their automobile and then to turn their hand firmly, thinking that they were turning the key. The key remains stationary, and gouges a piece of skin from their finger.

Inexperienced physicians find it difficult to believe that such a gross wound can be caused by such a simple act. Every insensitive patient and every treating physician must remember that "small means danger." Occupational therapists should in-spect the workbenches and houses of patients who have insensitive hands, and should arrange for every small handle to be removed and replaced with a good bulky handle. Every key should be fitted with a large handle that can be slipped over the original handle to make it safe. Finally, patients must be drilled to recognize the inherent danger of small handles and of objects that could be hot. The occupational therapist should go around the work-bench, kitchen, and living room with the patient, who should point out all the potential dangers and the way in which they might cause injuries.

Then, again, the patient who actually develops an injury must never be allowed to assume or to say that "it came by itself." The patient may not remember how it happened that a finger was bleed-ing or blister has developed, but the therapist and

Figure 24–5. The metal edge of a small key is a constant danger to insensitive fingers. Keys are safer if enclosed in a leather sandwich riveted over the key.

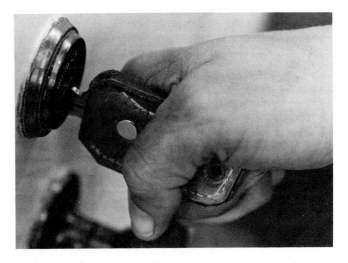

patient together must sit down and review all the activities of the previous few hours, and find out what article was being held and what activity was being done that would have caused the problem.

It is these time-consuming exercises that will help the patient to develop the consciousness of danger that will finally protect him from the succession of injuries that would otherwise destroy his hands.

Pressure Sore or Ischemic Necrosis. This type of damage, caused by the continuous application of a small pressure, is quite unusual in the hand. It occurs on insensitive buttocks in patients who sit still for a long time, or in an insensitive foot trapped inside a tight shoe. A hand, however, will very rarely remain absolutely still for long enough to suffer any ill effects from prolonged pressure that produces ischemia. It sometimes occurs when a person who has been wearing a ring develops swelling in that finger. The part of the finger distal to the ring is deprived of blood supply, and this will sometimes require cutting the ring off. The only difference in the insensitive hand is that it may not be noticed as early as it would in a sensitive hand.

Perhaps the greatest cause of damage from ischemia of the insensitive hand is caused by splints or appliances applied by the surgeon or therapist in an attempt to correct deformity. We so often depend on the patient to tell us if a splint is too tight, or is "uncomfortable," that we may forget that an insensitive person will accept a splint for long-term application that is applying too much pressure through a sling or under a reaction bar. No splint or plaster cast should be applied to an insensitive hand without carefully calculating the pressures that might result from it, and taking extraordinary care to mold it precisely to body contours so that no local point of pressure is allowed to persist. For long-term splinting, the maximum pressure should not exceed 40 mm Hg, (50 g/cm^2, or 8 oz/inch^2).

Repetitive Stress. Whereas it takes several hundred pounds per square inch to result in the actual breaking or crushing of the skin, very much smaller pressures and stresses will result in damage if repeated many thousands of times over a period of a few days. People with normal hands who undertake activities involving repetitive stress, such as digging the garden or twisting a screw-driver to tighten hundreds of screws, often find that their hands begin to be sore and uncomfortable. They will change their grip or perhaps change their tool or even their occupation for a time. If this is not done, they will find that after 1 or 2 days of such activity a blister is produced in the palm.

A person without sensation doing the same type of activity will not feel the discomfort, will not notice the blister, and will go on until the skin breaks down and develops ulcerations. An additional factor is that many people with insensitivity also have some muscular weakness or deformity, so that they are limited in the number of different ways in which they can hold a given object. When a normal person would change grip, a person with deformity may be trapped into a single way in which

he can hold an instrument. For example, a person who cannot oppose the thumb will often hold things between the side of the thumb and the side of the index finger. This may be the most useful type of grasp, and it will be used for everything. Such patients quite often may have ulcers on the side of the thumb and on the side of the index finger (see Fig. 24–3A).

A person who has paralysis of the intrinsic muscles and clawing of the fingers may be unable to hold any object without the main force of the grasp coming down through the fingertips. A person may exert 50 lb of grip through a normal hand, and this 50 lb may be spread over 10 inches^2 or more of the palmar surface of the fingers. Thus, the average pressure would be only 5 lb/inch^2. A person with clawed fingers, using the same amount of force on the same object, will concentrate all the force on four fingertips, which together may have an area of 1 inch^2. The pressure, therefore, will be ten times as great. Even this is not harmful for a single application of force, or perhaps even 10 or 20 applications, but if a person is working all day or for several days, and is using this type of grip, there will probably be a breakdown of the skin of the fingertips directly over the distal end of each phalanx (Fig. 24–6).

To avoid this type of damage, the surgeon and therapist should study the way a patient uses the hands and note the distribution of calluses and the points of high stress. It may be possible to reconstruct the hand so that larger areas of skin are involved in simple types of grasp and pinch, or the patient may be provided with protective gloves selectively padded at points of stress. Most importantly the patient should be helped to understand the problem, and warned not to undertake repetitive activity without changing the instrument or tool being used or the type of handle by which it is held. Also, the patient should be warned to look at the hands carefully occasionally, and to have somebody feel his fingers so that if one finger or part of the skin is becoming hot it will be noticed. This may be a signal to discontinue such work before the skin breaks down.

Care of the Wound

The most serious cause of damage to the insensitive hand is continued use of the hand after it has become wounded and after the skin has been broken. The most important single measure for preserving insensitive hands is to insist that patients regard every wound as an emergency, and not to use the wounded part of the hand until it heals.

No matter how much care is taken, people with insensitive hands will sometimes suffer wounds. This is not very serious, because the wound will heal quite satisfactorily if that part of the hand is immobilized. What is serious, though, is that patients do not notice their wound, or may feel that it is adequate to treat the wound with a Band-Aid or

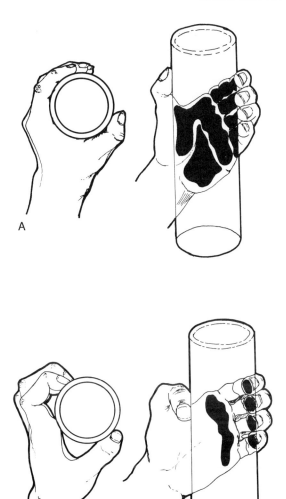

with some antiseptic or antibiotic dressing held on by adhesive strapping or bandages. When I examine the hands of those who are doing productive work even though they have a disease such as leprosy, it is not uncommon to find five or six places where they have covered a small wound with an adhesive dressing. Such a habit will result inevitably in one or more wounds becoming more deeply infected, and the infection being spread by the recurrent pressure until it involves bone and joint and tendon sheaths and finally destroys the hand. The progressive absorption of the fingers of leprosy patients, which was formerly thought to be due to tissues "rotting away," is nothing more than the effects of secondary infection and osteomyelitis that result from the continued use of wounded fingers. Such patients, once they are taught to take care of their hands, find that they can keep their remaining fingers for the rest of their lives.

People who have loss of sensation should be provided with various small gutter-shaped plastic finger splints (Fig. 24–7). They may keep these splints at home or at the work place, so that if they should wound themselves or break the skin in any way, they can find a splint to fit the finger, put it into position, and strap it there with adhesive. Depending on the availability of medical services, they may then go to their physician, or continue their work with the affected finger kept out of action and protected by the splints. Those with insensitive hands are often reluctant to seek medical help for every trivial injury, and this ability to use a simple splint that they can apply themselves is much more acceptable and allows most wounds to heal very well. Patients may be instructed about how to monitor the finger and the circumstances in which they do need to seek help.

THE INHIBITED HAND

Many patients, after nerve injury, are quite unwilling to use the denervated finger. They have a sense of inhibition, particularly if the rest of the hand is sensitive and only one finger is insensitive or has paresthesia.

Figure 24–6. *A, A normal hand uses all the palmar skin to hold a cylindric object; B, a clawed hand uses only the fingertips and metacarpal head areas. If the force used is the same, and the area involved is only one tenth, the pressure is multiplied by ten. However, even the force is often increased because of the sense of insecurity of grasp.*

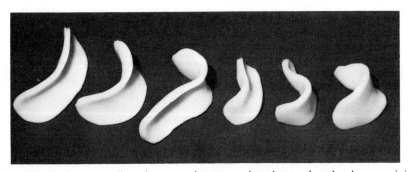

Figure 24–7. Simple plastic gutter splints given to patients to apply at home when they have any injury or burn.

It is important for these patients to undergo sensory re-education; this involves training programs supervised by hand therapists, in which the patient is given tasks involving all the digits. Patients have to learn to relate to the sensations they feel with the denervated finger, and to compare them with what they feel with their normal fingers. I find that it is helpful to expose the fingers to fine sand, coarse sand, small rounded pebbles, and various textures of cloth or sandpaper, as well as to different temperatures, warm and cool water, and warm wax. Also, having patients use the fingers in an alternating fashion—tapping on the keys of a typewriter or a musical instrument—does not allow them to spare the affected finger.

Inhibited fingers will sometimes become injured, particularly from burns, even though a patient is trying to keep the finger out of danger. Whether the finger is inhibited or uninhibited, once a finger is injured it is equally important not to use it and to treat it with a splint.

THE UNWANTED FINGER

Occasionally, when a single finger has become denervated or perhaps has been severed and reattached, the quality of sensation is imperfect and may be accompanied by cold intolerance and by numbness or paresthesia. Under such circumstances, a patient may come to dislike the finger and it will undergo a form of psychological rejection. This is particularly true of index fingers, which can rather easily be kept out of activity. The thumb bypasses the index finger and pinches against the middle finger. Even when grasping a large object, the index finger may be kept hyperextended and not be used.

Once this rejection begins, it is quite important to insist on continuing active occupational therapy, which is supervised to ensure that the finger is used equally with other fingers and is coordinated in the activity of the whole hand. We have devised a glove that can be impregnated with a dust of fine microcapsules, and that leaks a dye when subjected to pressure or shear stress. Patients wearing this glove can see whether they are using their hand equally, because uninhibited fingers will stain blue, while lesser used inhibited fingers remain pale yellow (Fig. 24–8).[2, 3] With proper sensory education, particularly in younger patients, the finger will again become accepted and coordinate with the rest of the hand. In older patients, however, especially in those who have developed an active dislike for an insensitive or malsensitive finger, it may be advisable at some point to accept the patient's own evaluation and to amputate the digit. A single insensitive finger may actually hinder the use of the hand, and frequently may cripple it by incurring repeated injuries and infections. The possibility of rejection should be taken into account in deciding whether to reattach a single amputated finger, or to allow the patient to re-educate the hand and body image to

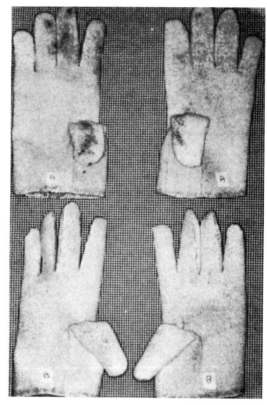

Figure 24–8. Pressure-sensing gloves are made with microcapsules that contain dye. High pressure and shear stress result in the fracture of the capsules and in the release of dye. Shown here are a pair of pressure-sensing gloves worn by a person with insensitive hands, holding a broom for 15 minutes while sweeping a corridor *(A)* and similar gloves on normal hands, holding the same broom for 15 minutes while sweeping the same corridor *(B)*. Note the excessive localized stress used only by the uninhibited insensitive hand.

accept a good three-fingered hand rather than spend frustrating months or even years trying to adapt to a finger that does not feel as if it belongs.

I would very rarely amputate an insensitive finger in disease conditions involving many fingers. In the case of leprosy, I usually preserve all the fingers that can be saved, because in 10 years a damaged and shortened finger may turn out to be the best remaining digit when the other fingers have been even more seriously damaged.

ACCEPTANCE BY THE MIND

The hand is an instrument of the brain. If someone is determined to make good use of the hand, it is amazing how effectively a totally insensitive and partially paralyzed or deformed extremity will be used. I had a blind patient whose hand was totally insensitive and who had lost, through repeated injury and infection, at least half of every finger, yet his zest for life and his determination to succeed were such that he could play the piano and organ with his remaining insensitive stumps, controlling his fingers by ear. Others in a similar situation have been able to play the violin. I have also known those who retained their sight, but had no sensation, who were skillful dressmakers and craftsmen in many fields demanding manual dexterity. If the mind is determined to succeed, it will find a way. Therefore, both the surgeon and therapist must begin by being attuned to the patient's desires and ambitions, and must help them to believe that their

damaged and insensitive hand can do great things. Once awakened, the patient's faith may be translated into great achievement. No one needs to be crippled by loss of sensation alone.

References

1. Moberg, E.: Personal communication, 1983.
2. Brand, P. W., and Ebner, J. D.: Pressure-sensitive devices for denervated hands and feet, a preliminary communication. J. Bone Joint Surg. 51A:109, 1969.
3. Brand, P. W., and Ebner, J. D.: A pain substitute; Pressure assessment in the insensitive limb. Am. J. Occup. Ther., 23:1, 1969.

25

COMPLICATIONS OF SURGICAL TREATMENT OF TUMORS OF THE HAND

Richard J. Smith

By training, practice, and disposition, the hand surgeon is a reconstructive surgeon who tries to save all viable tissue, replacing what is injured and restoring what is lost. Hours will be spent repairing a digital artery or grafting small nerves. To excise normal, healthy, and functioning tissues is contrary to his usual practice; his primary goal is generally to improve function. However, in managing patients with tumors of the hand, priorities change. With benign tumors, the primary goal of surgical treatment is to excise the tumor so that it does not recur. When treating aggressive tumors, whether they are frankly malignant or locally invasive, the most important criterion of success is whether or not the tumor reappears elsewhere.

Recurrence or metastasis of a tumor after surgery is not always a "complication" of treatment. Recurrence and metastasis should be considered as complications only if they are caused by methods of biopsy and treatment that are inappropriate according to generally accepted standards of care. Occasionally, acceptable and appropriate methods of surgical excision may prove inadequate. With some lesions, the surgeon is justified in risking recurrence in an effort to preserve function. For example, aggressive fibromatosis is locally invasive but does not become malignant or metastasize. If this tumor is located in the distal volar forearm, it may be appropriate to excise it so as to spare the median and ulnar nerves. In this case, recurrence should not be considered a complication of surgery. However, local resection of a rhabdomyosarcoma of the palm is not a generally accepted method of treatment. If there is subsequent recurrence and metastasis after local resection, these problems may

well be considered as complications of inadequate tumor treatment.

Unlike most reconstructive hand surgery, surgery for tumors of the hand should often be combined with other forms of treatment. Radiotherapy and chemotherapy may be indicated preceding or following tumor excision or amputation. Lymph node dissection may be an important adjuvant to hand surgery in treating many malignant tumors. If a hand surgeon ignores these other methods of treatment, a recurrence or metastasis may be considered a complication of treatment.

Although preserving function and reconstructing an esthetic hand are only secondary goals in tumor surgery, surgeons should not squander normal tissue needlessly in the treatment of tumors of the hand. The distinction between inadequate excision and excessively radical surgery is often difficult to determine. It is based on a thorough understanding of the nature and location of the tumor, its expected biologic behavior, alternative methods of treatment, and the potential for structural and functional restoration of the hand after excision.

PROBLEMS OF DIAGNOSIS

Occasionally, a tumor of the hand may remain undiagnosed despite localizing symptoms. For example, a young woman with a red tender swelling at the base of the thumb was treated with anti-inflammatory medicines for 6 months before the correct diagnosis of epithelioid sarcoma was made. A man with malignant schwannoma in the palm received several local steroid injections before the correct diagnosis was made. In both cases, delay in providing appropriate care and multiple needle punctures through the lesion may have contributed to the tumor spread and metastasis. Recurrence in these patients may be considered complications because of the delay in tumor diagnosis. Although such examples are infrequent, the potential dangers of permitting aggressive tumors to remain undiagnosed can be tragic.

Appropriate noninvasive diagnostic procedures are indicated for lesions of the hand in which pain, swelling, and deformity are persistent and the cause is not apparent. The most important diagnostic procedure is a careful history and physical examination. Most neoplasms enlarge slowly. Symptoms usually develop gradually and are not directly related to trauma. By contrast, an infectious granuloma, neuroma, false aneurysm, epidermal inclusion cyst, or infection usually develop soon after injury. Most tumors do not subside spontaneously. A mucous or ganglion cyst, or inflammatory synovitis, however, often undergo remissions and exacerbations that may be related to activity, weather, or time of day. In most cases, careful palpation should permit the surgeon to differentiate the resilience of a ganglion cyst, the soft fluctuance of an extensor tenosynovitis, or the tender hot swelling of a subcutaneous abscess from the irregular firmness of a pseudoencapsulated sarcoma.

But even the experienced surgeon may be misled. Except in the most obvious cases, history and physical examination should be supplemented by multiple plane x-rays and laboratory studies. Routine blood tests usually include determination of sedimentation rate, complete blood count, rheumatoid screen, and uric acid and acid and alkaline phosphatase levels. Xerograms may help to locate and diagnose many soft tissue tumors. Arthrograms, tomograms, and angiograms may define the size of a mass. Technetium-99m or gallium scans are useful in finding "hot spots" of increased blood supply that deserve further study.

Occasionally, needle biopsy may provide sufficient tissue for the pathologist to diagnose soft tissue tumors and bone tumors. Most pathologists, however, believe that they can better diagnose a lesion if an open biopsy is performed. Open biopsy usually allows the surgeon to obtain more tissue from the most representative part of the tumor with less distortion than with needle biopsy. Needle aspiration may be of great value to the surgeon in the differential diagnosis of cystic lesions. If there is fluid in the aspirate, the diagnosis of a cyst is confirmed. Often, the appearance of the aspirate suggests the precise diagnosis before the fluid is formally analyzed. For example, one can usually differentiate the clear jellylike fluid of a ganglion from the yellow cloudy fluid of a synovial cyst.

If a serious doubt remains about the nature of a lesion despite the most meticulous examination and nonoperative studies, exploration and open biopsy are mandatory.

PROBLEMS WITH BIOPSY

Complications often follow open biopsy of suspected tumors. These complications may be related to the operative technique, the incision used, the type of biopsy, and the location of biopsy.

Operative Technique

To provide a bloodless field for other types of hand surgery, the usual technique is to exsanguinate the limb with a rubber (Esmarch) bandage and to inflate a pneumatic tourniquet on the upper arm. If the biopsied tumor is malignant, this procedure may increase the risk of metastasis. When a compressive bandage is tightly wrapped about the lesion, tumor cells may dislodge and be forced into the lymphatics or veins that drain the tumor, or into the normal tissues that border it. Tumor cells entering the circulation are blocked distal to the tourniquet throughout the operation. During this time, they may aggregate into small clumps that are showered into the general circulation when the tourniquet is deflated. Thus, it has been suggested (but not proven) that the risk of metastasis may be increased with the use of a tourniquet. Some surgeons, however, believe that the bloodless field provided by a tourniquet requires less sponging, retraction, and clamping. Therefore, they argue, fewer tumor cells are dislodged. I do not use an Esmarch bandage for tumor surgery. I elevate the limb for 2 or 3 minutes after the appropriate prep and drape, and then inflate the pneumatic arm tourniquet. Throughout the operation, I manipulate the wound as little and as gently as possible.

The tourniquet should be released prior to closure to prevent a hematoma from developing. This precaution is particularly important with tumor surgery, because there is a risk that tumor cells may pool in a hematoma and increase the risk of local seeding. If a drain is used, it should exit from the incision so as not to risk contaminating remote areas with tumor cells.

Some surgeons feel that the risk of metastasis from incisional biopsy may be minimized by allowing the biopsy wound to remain open until secondary surgery. They reason that, with an open wound, cells from the cut edge of the biopsied tumor will be less likely to spread locally or to enter the circulation. I believe that the retraction of wound edges, edema, and bacterial contamination of an open wound may complicate secondary surgery. Therefore, I usually close the biopsy incision.

Incisions

With all hand surgery incisions must be planned so that relevant structures are properly visualized. The scar should be esthetic and should cause neither contracture nor pain. When planning biopsy of a potentially malignant tumor, there is one further consideration: the biopsy incision should not contaminate the proposed borders of a definitive secondary procedure—the biopsy incision should not extend into the field of possible tumor excision. Two examples may illustrate this point.

First, if a mass lies between the fourth and fifth metacarpal heads, one may be tempted to consider biopsy through a transverse incision in the distal palmar crease. Although a transverse incision would provide adequate exposure and would be esthetic when healed, such an approach would be unwise, because if the tumor proves to be malignant the entire wound would have to be considered potentially contaminated with tumor cells. En bloc excision probably would require amputation of the ulnar three or four rays. However, if the biopsy were to be performed through a short dorsal longitudinal incision between the fourth and fifth metacarpals, en bloc excision would include only the ulnar two rays.

Second, for reconstructive surgery, many surgeons are reluctant to use an incision at the ulnar side of the hand because of fear of producing a tender scar in an area frequently subjected to pressure. However, if the hypothenar region is to be biopsied, a more palmar incision would contaminate a much larger area if the lesion proves to be malignant. The ulnar incision would be preferred.

In planning a biopsy of a potentially malignant tumor, the surgeon should assume the worst. An incision should be selected that is adequate for the biopsy and that would be acceptable esthetically and functionally if no other operation will be necessary. Whenever possible, the incision should be vertical and should be placed within the area to be excised if the tumor proves malignant (Fig. 25–1).

To help plan the biopsy incision, the surgeon should do the following:

1. Determine the incision that would be used to excise the tumor if it proves malignant.

2. Use a longitudinal biopsy incision at least 2 cm from the potential excision borders.

Type of Biopsy

Open biopsies may be excisional or incisional. An *excisional biopsy* has both advantages and disadvantages. Among the major *advantages* of excisional biopsy are that all the clinically apparent tissue is available for histologic examination and, if the lesion is benign, no further treatment will be necessary.

The major *disadvantage* with larger tumors is that, if the tumor is malignant, excisional biopsy will transect the pseudopods of tumor cells that emanate from the apparent borders of the lesion. After biopsy, the entire tumor bed will be grossly contaminated with malignant cells. In the few days that are

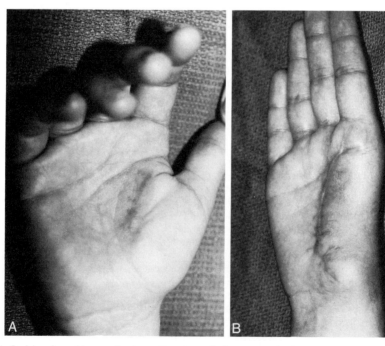

Figure 25–1. A, Incision for a biopsy of a 4-cm diameter soft tissue mass in the thenar eminence. The incision is short and vertical. Biopsy revealed malignant histiocytoma. *B,* En bloc excision of the tumor 2 cm from the tumor and from the biopsy incision required amputation of the thumb only. Dorsal thumb skin is used to close the palmar defect. If the biopsy incision had been transverse or more extensive, greater dissection and more radical amputation would have been necessary.

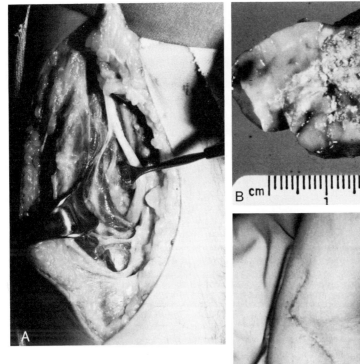

Figure 25–2. *A,* Exploration of the upper forearm for median nerve compression revealed a large soft tissue tumor deep to the pronator teres; *B,* uncertain of the diagnosis, the surgeon performed excisional biopsy. The tumor was an extraosseous chondrosarcoma and was incompletely excised. *C,* The entire biopsy wound was contaminated with sarcoma cells. Above-elbow amputation was necessary.

necessary to examine the tumor, confirm the diagnosis, and reoperate, these cells may readily metastasize through the opened veins and lymphatics. En bloc excision will require dissection at least 2 cm from the borders of the tumor and biopsy incision, (Fig. 25–2).

Example. A 12-year-old girl has a tumor at the base of her thumb. Excisional biopsy requires a longitudinal incision over the thenar eminence to the radial side of the wrist flexion crease. The histologic diagnosis is "clear cell sarcoma." En bloc excision now requires resection of the first and second rays and a large segment of the distal radius. If incisional biopsy had been performed, first ray resection alone would probably be sufficient.

I usually perform excisional biopsy only for deep soft tissue lesions smaller than 2 cm in diameter and for skin lesions that are not attached to the underlying structures. Excisional biopsy of relatively large benign soft tissue tumor may also be justified if the surgeon is confident of the diagnosis preoperatively on the basis of history and tumor size, shape, and location. The gross appearance of the tumor at operation must also correspond to the preoperative diagnosis. No patient will be displeased if the biopsy shows a benign tumor that can be safely excised at a subsequent operation.

Example. A slowly growing, painless, multilocular soft tissue mass at the volar side of the finger is diagnosed on the basis of history and physical examination as "giant cell tumor of tendon sheath." X-rays show no calcification or bone involvement. The surgeon is justified in performing an excisional biopsy if, at operation, an encapsulated yellow brown firm lesion is found in the flexor tendon sheath. However, if at operation the lesion appears unusual in any way, an incisional biopsy should be performed.

Location of Biopsied Tissues

Some tumors are difficult to diagnose even with ample representative tissue. Occasionally, the tissue that the pathologist receives is either unrepresentative of the tumor or insufficient for appropriate diagnostic studies. Some surgeons suggest that the adequacy of the biopsy may be judged by frozen section examination of the tissue specimen while the patient is still in the operating room. At this time, the pathologist need only report whether tumor tissue is present and if the tissue appears adequate for diagnosis. Definitive diagnosis may await paraffin section. The pathologist may be helped in making a diagnosis if the tissue can be studied by electron microscopy or by special staining techniques. The surgeon and pathologist should discuss the manner by which the specimens should be handled to facilitate such studies.

An incisional biopsy of soft tissue tumors should include the capsule (or pseudocapsule), the tumor-normal tissue interface, and the soft tissues at the center of the lesion. However, it is the more peripheral tissue that is usually most representative of the tumor. If a bone tumor has broken through the cortex, incisional biopsy need not include the bone cortex. To minimize the risk of pathologic fracture, the corners of any cortical bone window should be rounded.

PROBLEMS WITH TUMOR EXCISION

Benign tumors such as lipoma, enchondroma, and osteoid osteoma may be excised by local resection without exicising wide borders of normal tissue. These lesions rarely recur. Resection of normal adjacent nerve or tendon or removal of one of the bones of the hand to lessen the chance of recurrence of these benign tumors is not justified.

Aggressive or frankly malignant tumors that arise in the hand must be treated differently. Once the diagnosis is confirmed by biopsy, the surgeon should consult with the oncologist and radiotherapist regarding the value of adjuvant chemotherapy or radiotherapy. If surgery is to be performed, usually radical or wide (en bloc) excision is necessary. For soft tissue tumors, radical excision refers to removing the tumor and all soft tissues within its fascial compartment. Thus, radical excision of a deep malignant tumor at the proximal flexion crease of the thumb would include all tissues within the fascial compartment of the synovial sheath of the flexor pollicis longus. The surgeon would remove all soft tissues at the volar side of the thumb, fingers, palm, and forearm up to the elbow. Such radical excision of the upper limb would preserve very little function—the patient might be better off with an amputation.

Fortunately, most malignant deep soft tissue tumors of the hand can be excised successfully if a 2-cm border of apparently normal tissue is excised with it. This is considered a wide or en bloc excision. For malignant deep tumors in the distal two segments of the finger, metacarpophalangeal disarticulation or ray amputation is indicated. If the malig-

nant tumor is located more proximally, however, a border of normal tissue must be excised with it. The pathologist should perform frozen section studies of the borders of the excised tissue to be certain that the margins are clear of tumor cells. The patient and surgeon must be prepared to proceed at once with amputation if there is extensive involvement of the tumor about the operative site. Failure to remove malignant tumors en bloc with tumor-free margins will risk recurrence and metastases—the two most serious complications of tumor surgery (Fig. 25–3). With tumor excision, as with incisional biopsy, an Esmarch bandage must never be applied prior to inflating the tourniquet.

Aggressive nonmalignant or locally malignant tumors are lesions that do not metastasize but that are not encapsulated and have a high incidence of local recurrence. Local excision is rarely adequate, and en bloc excision is usually indicated. For example, although an enchondroma (benign) may be treated by curettage, a "benign" giant cell tumor of the bones of the hand is aggressive, and there is a high incidence of recurrence after curettage. Therefore, for giant cell tumors of the bones of the hand that have not broken through the bone, I advise en bloc excision—resection of the entire bone. For some aggressive nonmalignant lesions, I prefer local resection despite the fact that the tumor may recur. For example, villonodular synovitis is a locally aggressive lesion that never metastasizes. With villonodular synovitis of the palm, I would prefer to perform local excision and reoperate every few years rather than do an en bloc excision that would sacrifice adjacent tendons and nerves.

The treatment of a patient with a malignant tumor that has metastasized to the hand would be palliative. Such tumors usually originate in the lung, kidney, breast, or thyroid. If the primary lesion can be treated successfully, one may perform en bloc excision of the hand tumor. Unfortunately, most of these patients die within a year of metastasis to the hand. Because of this poor prognosis, it is probably best to perform the least surgery compatible with relief of pain and continued hand function.

RECONSTRUCTIVE SURGERY
AFTER EXCISION OF TUMORS
OF THE HAND

The most serious complication of reconstructive surgery after excision of tumors of the hand is seeding tumor cells to remote sites of donor tissues. A curetted metacarpal or phalanx should be bone grafted to promote rapid healing. If the same curettes that removed the tumor are used to obtain the iliac bone graft, the surgeon may transplant the tumor to the ilium. Forceps or gloves contaminated with fibrosarcoma of the hand may deposit these cells on the donor site of a skin graft, such as the buttock or thigh. After en bloc excision of the fourth and fifth rays for malignant histocytoma, the

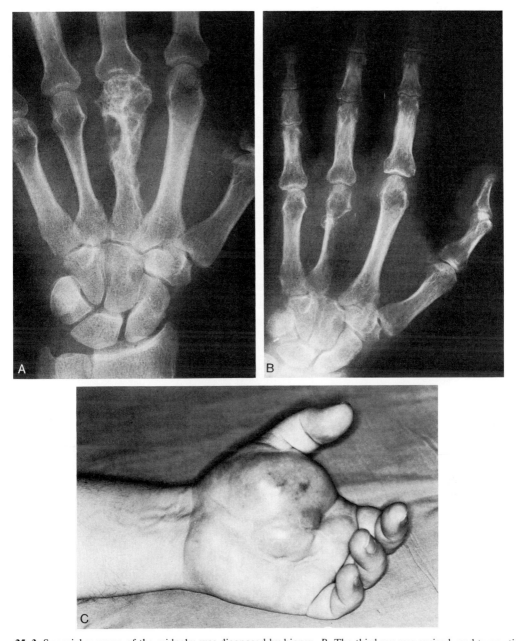

Figure 25–3. Synovial sarcoma of the midpalm was diagnosed by biopsy. *B,* The third ray was excised, and tumor tissue was removed from the second and third interosseous spaces. The fourth metacarpal was curetted. The surgeon had performed a local excision—not an en bloc excision—of a malignant tumor. The wound still harbors malignant cells. *C,* Recurrence and metastasis developed within 2 years.

surgeon may be tempted to cover the large defect with a groin flap or abdominal pedicle flap. If tumor cells should remain at the borders of the excised tumor, not only will the patient develop a local recurrence but tumor may appear in the abdomen or groin. In reconstructing defects after excision of tumors of the hand, several rules should be observed:

1. The gloves, gowns, drapes, and instruments used in obtaining donor tissue from remote sites must not have been used in excising the tumor.

2. Whenever possible, remote flaps should not be used to cover defects caused by excision of aggressive or frankly malignant lesions.

3. Local flaps such as filet and rotation flaps are usually preferred to cover soft tissue defects.

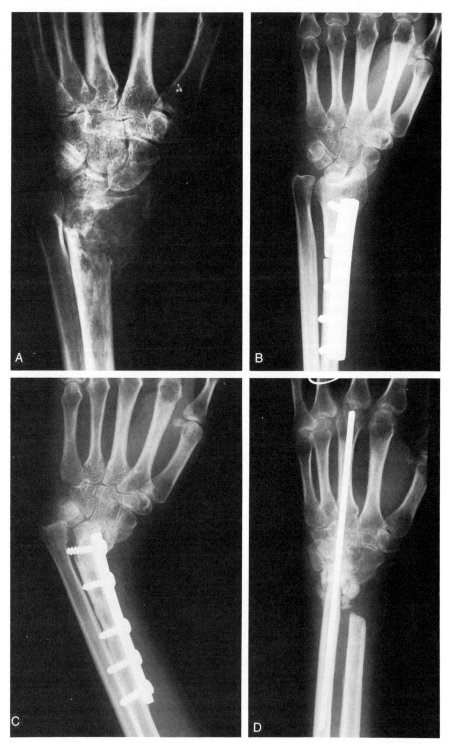

Figure 25–4. Benign giant-cell tumor of the distal radius; *B,* The distal radius was removed and replaced with an allograft; *C,* Pain and deformity 2 years later. There has been a fracture distal to the plate. Was this due to injury? Biopsy showed recurrent giant cell tumor. *D,* The allograft was removed with an en bloc excision of local tissues. The carpus was arthrodesed to the ulna, restoring wrist stability.

OTHER PROBLEMS AFTER TUMOR SURGERY

This chapter has stressed the unique complications of tumor surgery: recurrence and metastasis. Of course, the potential complications of reconstructive hand surgery such as infection, hematoma, neuroma, and scarring may also develop after tumor surgery. These complications are as troublesome after tumor surgery as after reconstructive surgery. At times they may be even more distressing and confusing. For example, 2 months after an en bloc excision of a malignant tumor, the wound becomes swollen, warm, and tender. Is this recurrence or infection? Should it be drained or biopsied? Three years after replacement of the distal radius with an allograft because of recurrent giant cell tumor, the patient fractures the allograft distal to the fixation plate. Is this due to osteoporosis, stress fracture, or tumor recurrence (Fig. 25–4)? A hematoma develops in a biopsy site. Will it spread the tumor?

With tumor surgery, serious concerns are added to the interpretation of any complication. Was the complication caused by tumor recurrence? Will it increase the risk of recurrence? As with the diagnosis of the tumor itself, all complications must be carefully evaluated. If there is serious doubt as to its nature, biopsy may be helpful. Ideally, the treatment will correct the complication and eradicate the tumor. With serious complications after surgery for malignant lesions, one must always consider amputation. Such radical treatment would rarely be warranted after reconstructive surgery, but in dealing with malignant tumors, the priority must always be to prevent recurrence and metastatic disease.

Bibliography

Averill, R. M., Smith, R. J., and Campbell, C. J.: Giant-cell tumors of the bones of the hand. J. Hand Surg., 5:39, 1980.

Bowden, L., and Booher, R. J.: The principles and techniques of resection of soft parts for sarcoma. Surgery, 44:963, 1958.

Cantin, J., et al.: The problem of local recurrence after treatment of soft tissue sarcoma. Ann. Surg., 168:47, 1968.

Dahlin, D. C.: Bone Tumors. General Aspects and Data on 6221 Cases, 3rd ed., Springfield, IL, Charles C Thomas, 1978.

Enneking, W. F., Spanier, S. S., and Goodman, M. A.: Current concepts review. The surgical staging of musculoskeletal sarcoma. J. Bone Joint Surg., 62A:1027, 1980.

Hajdu, S. I.: Pathology of Soft Tissue Tumors, Philadelphia, Lea & Febiger, 1979.

Mankin, H. J., Lange, T. A., and Spanier, S. S.: Hazards of biopsy in patients with malignant primary bone and soft-tissue tumors. J. Bone Joint Surg., 64A:1121, 1982.

Peimer, C. A., Schiller, A. L., Mankin, H. J., and Smith, R. J.: Epithelioid sarcoma of the hand and wrist: Patterns of extension. J. Hand Surg., 2:275, 1977.

Peimer, C. A., Smith, R. J., Sirota, R. L., and Cohen, B. E.: Multicentric giant-cell tumor of bone. J. Bone Joint Surg., 62A:651, 1980.

Russell, W. O., et al.: A clinical and pathological staging system for soft tissue sarcomas. Cancer, 40:1562, 1977.

Schajowicz, F., and Derqui, J. C.: Puncture biopsy in lesions of the locomotor system. Review of results in 4050 cases including 941 vertebral punctures. Cancer, 21:531, 1968.

Simon, M. A.: Current concepts review. Biopsy of musculoskeletal tumors. J. Bone Joint Surg., 64A:1253, 1982.

Simon, M. A., Spanier, S. S., and Enneking, W. F.: Soft tissue sarcomas of the extremities. Surg. Annu., 11:363, 1979.

26

COMPLICATIONS OF DUPUYTREN'S DISEASE

Robert M. McFarlane

CONDITIONS ASSOCIATED WITH DUPUYTREN'S DISEASE

If Dupuytren's disease (DD) is defined as a pathologic change in the palmar and digital fascia that results in flexion contraction of the digital joints, other changes that occur in association with or because of these fascial changes may be considered to be complications. Often it is difficult to know if some of these changes occur because of a similar process—for example, carpal tunnel syndrome and trigger finger—or because of the contracting effect of the fascia—for example joint changes. The following discussion presents some of the conditions frequently associated with DD.

Within the Hand

Skin Involvement and Knuckle Pads

DD is a disease of fascia. However, the fascia in the palm and digits attaches to the dermis to prevent shearing of the skin on the underlying tissue, so the skin becomes involved. In fact, the extent of involvement is an indication for operation. The skin may be thinned by pressure atrophy of an underlying nodule, or it may be drawn into pits and folds as the underlying fascia foreshortens. Skin involvement is almost always present, but, when severe, it makes adequate excision of fascia and preservation of the overlying skin difficult, if not impossible. When operating on recurrent disease, in particular, it may be necessary to excise skin because it no longer has an adequate blood supply. Fortunately, in most cases that come to operation, the skin can be dissected from the underlying fascia and preserved.

Knuckle pads are not a complication as much as a manifestation of the disease. They appear infrequently, usually over the dorsum of the proximal interphalangeal joint, but may be anywhere on the dorsum of the finger. They do not "complicate" the course of the disease or the treatment per se but represent a component of Dupuytren's Diathesis (see below).

Joint Changes

The metacarpophalangeal joint is most often contracted in DD. However, joint changes do not occur even though the joint has been flexed for many years. Full extension is the rule following incision or excision of the offending fascia. The opposite is true of the proximal interphalangeal joint—even a few months of flexion contracture may not be corrected by operation. Thus, it is wise to operate early when the proximal interphalangeal joint is contracted. Only surgical judgment will determine if a surgical procedure should be performed on the joint. An operation on the joint should not replace complete excision of the offending fascia, however. Only after the surgeon is satisfied that all the fascia has been removed should a joint procedure be considered.

Several procedures have been described. Often, simple incision of the flexor tendon sheath and manipulation of the joint are sufficient. Both Curtis and Watson and colleagues, have described incision and excision of portions of the capsular ligament.[1, 2] Fusion and joint replacement with a silicone prosthesis have both been described. The difficulty in gaining lasting correction increases with the duration of the contracture and with the age of the patient. An arthroplasty may gain a few degrees of extension, but at the expense of loss of full flexion. Therefore, in severe long-standing proximal interphalangeal joint contracture in older patients, if the joint can be straightened to about 40°, no joint procedure is recommended. This position can usually be maintained by splinting and therapy. The finger is placed in a useful position, and flexion is not compromised.

294

Vessel Disease

Vascular disease has been implicated as both the cause and result of DD. Disease within the distribution of the ulnar artery has been suggested by Davis in addition to a sympathetic effect.[3] Examination of the vessels will show a high incidence of atherosclerosis, but this may coincide with the age group affected. Cold intolerance may be more common than appreciated in DD. In our study 40% of patients complained (in retrospect) of cold intolerance. However, most of these patients had cold intolerance postoperatively as well.

Nerve Displacement and Compression

Although the neurovascular bundle can be encased in the diseased fascia, there is always a plane of dissection between the bundle and the fascia. Symptoms of nerve compression, such as tingling and numbness, are uncommon. Displacement of the nerve and vessel are common but occur only in the finger (Fig. 26–1). Displacement by a spiral cord is most severe, because the neurovascular bundle can be displaced to the midline of the finger.[4] This mechanism of displacement places the neurovascular bundle in an exposed position, just deep to the

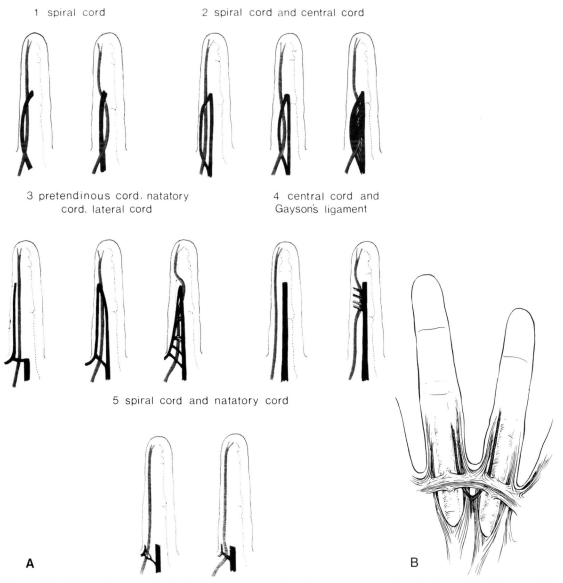

1 spiral cord   2 spiral cord and central cord

3 pretendinous cord, natatory cord, lateral cord   4 central cord and Gayson's ligament

5 spiral cord and natatory cord

A   B

Figure 26–1. The various ways in which the neurovascular bundle can be displaced in the finger. In addition, a thick lateral cord on the ulnar side of the little finger can displace the neurovascular bundle to the midline of the finger. It is not possible to predict accurately when the neurovascular bundle has been displaced and, therefore, the bundle must be visualized before the fascia is removed. (From McFarlane, R. M.: Patterns of the diseased fascia in the fingers in Dupuytren's contracture. Plast. Reconstr. Surg., 54:31, 1974.)

skin, so it is easily cut during dissection, if not during skin incision.

Associated Diseases

Penile (Peyronie's) and Plantar (Ledderhose's) Fibromatosis

Both these conditions are seen alone or in combination with DD.[5, 6] Histologically, the three diseases are similar but the clinical course is different. Characteristically, DD is progressive, leading to finger joint contracture. Peyronie's disease may persist or regress, and may regress with treatment with vitamin E. Ledderhose's disease results in a subcutaneous mass in the foot that may reach a large size; it may be multiple but it does not develop the typical cords of DD nor associated toe contracture.

Dupuytren's Diathesis

This term was suggested by Hueston to describe an especially aggressive state of Dupuytren's disease.[7] There is a strong family history, the onset is at an early age, both hands are extensively involved, and there is a marked tendency to recurrence after excision of the diseased fascia. These patients usually have knuckle pads, and may have either Peyronie's or Ledderhose's disease. Dupuytren's diathesis is uncommon but, if recognized, the patient should be warned about the likelihood of continuing problems with the hands.

Epilepsy, Alcoholism, and Diabetes

For many years there has been controversy about whether the disease epilepsy or the drug phenobarbital was the factor in the relationship between DD and epilepsy. According to Critchley and associates, the incidence of DD is similar in congenital and acquired epilepsy, and is clearly related to the duration of phenobarbital therapy.[8]

In the same way, the relationship between alcoholism and DD has been known for many years, but the causative relationship is unclear. Does alcohol produce a change in the palmar fascia, or is the presence of cirrhosis of the liver the causative factor? It has even been suggested that alcoholism is a genetic disease, perhaps sharing some of the genes responsible for DD, and therefore the two diseases are frequently seen together. According to Su and Patek, it is the alcohol and not the cirrhosis that is the cause of the relationship between these disease.[9]

The relationship between diabetes and DD is not as obvious. Those in diabetic clinics who have studied this association are convinced that there is an increased incidence of DD in diabetic patients.[10] Many surgeons, including myself, have not seen an increased incidence of diabetes in patients with DD. According to Ravid and co-workers, the presence of DD is not related to the type of treatment (diet, oral, or injected insulin) or to the severity of hyperglycemia.[11] The presence of DD is a nonhyperglycemic manifestation of diabetes.

Trigger Finger

Many years ago, Mason mentioned that patients with trigger finger sometimes developed DD later. I have noted this on several occasions, and in particular I have a group of diabetic patients with DD, mostly women, whose presenting complaint was trigger finger or thumb. Interestingly, these patients do not have progressive disease that causes finger contracture. Parker reported that the cause of the triggering was involvement of the A1 pulley by the overlying nodule of DD.[12] I have not noted this, but it is a reasonable explanation because some fibers of the pretendinous band of the palmar aponeurosis attach to the fibrous tendon sheath.

Trauma

Not enough has been written about the association of trauma and DD, probably because it is difficult to collect statistical data. It is unlikely that repetitive trauma to the hand is a causative factor. To date, no group of people who subject their hands to repeated trauma, such as handball players and those who use vibrating tools, have shown a causative relationship in the development of DD.

However, one cannot ignore the patient who has had a single traumatic episode to the hand who then develops DD in that area (Fig. 26–2). This patient may have a family history of the disease and evidence of DD in the other hand, but disease in the injured hand is more aggressive. A single episode of trauma must be a cofactor in the development of DD, but the mechanism is unknown.

The above diseases or conditions represent a fascinating aspect of the study of DD. An understanding of their causative relationship should help to solve the riddle of DD.

COMPLICATIONS FOLLOWING OPERATION FOR DUPUYTREN'S DISEASE

The frequency and severity of complications following operation for DD can be lessened by minimal surgery. However, this approach may not produce a satisfactory or a lasting result. The operation should be done within the limits of the surgeon's ability and should strive to achieve not only correction of the joint contracture but also prevention of recurrent contracture.

Tourniquet Paralysis

This complication is considered in detail elsewhere, but should be mentioned in relation to DD.

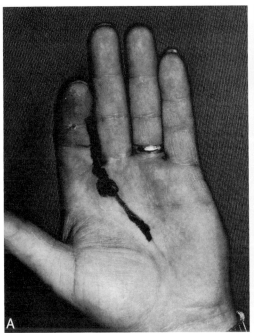 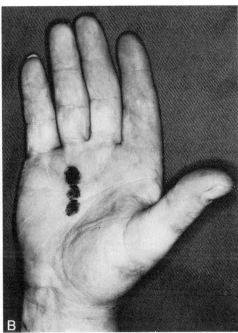

Figure 26–2. *A,* The left hand of a 40-year-old farmer who suffered a chain saw laceration of the palm of the hand and the web space between the index and middle fingers 20 years ago. A nodule and cord have appeared gradually in the area over many years, so that he now has 60° of contracture at the metacarpophalangeal joint and 55° of flexion at the proximal interphalangeal joint. There is no other disease in this hand, but he has nodules in the palm of the right hand *(B)* and 25° of contracture at the metacarpophalangeal joint of the ring finger. Pathologically, the specimen was typical of Dupuytren's disease. Although the patient has bilateral disease, the distribution in the injured hand is atypical, and is clearly related to the single episode of trauma.

Many patients have a degree of peripheral neuropathy such as that associated with alcoholism or diabetes.[13] Tourniquet pressure that could be tolerated by normal nerves may damage these susceptible nerves. Often the dissection can be completed within an hour, and the tourniquet can then be released. If the dissection will take longer, it is best to release the tourniquet for about 15 minutes each hour.

Nerve and Arterial Injury, and Gangrene of the Finger

In the palm the nerve and artery are separate, and therefore would be cut separately. However, they are both deep to the diseased fascia, so they are not likely to be cut. At the web space the nerve and artery form the neurovascular bundle. From this level distally, if one is cut, it is likely that the other will also be cut. At the web space the neurovascular bundle is involved in a three-dimensional scheme of diseased fascia that involves the natatory cord and the central, lateral, and spiral cords (see Fig. 26–1). Also, there is abundant fat that covers the nerve and artery. Exposure of the nerve and artery before dissection of the diseased fascia is essential. This exposure is facilitated by spreading the adjacent fingers, thereby stretching the vessels

and nerves. If the metacarpophalangeal joint is severely contracted, the dissection is made easier if this joint is straightened by incising the pretendinous cord. Damage to the neurovascular bundle is unlikely in the finger if the neurovascular bundle is exposed to its full length before any fascia is incised or excised. There is always a plane of dissection between the fascia and the bundle. It is difficult to develop this plane at the level of the proximal interphalangeal joint when a severe flexion contracture is present.

The ulnar digital nerve and artery to the little finger are difficult to find in the distal part of the hypothenar eminence because they are surrounded by fat. They should be identified before any fascia is removed.

When operating for recurrent disease, the nerve and artery are more susceptible to injury because they are surrounded not only by Dupuytren's fascia but also by scar tissue. Preoperatively, if one or both sides of the fingertip are numb, one can assume that the corresponding neurovascular bundle has been cut. If one neurovascular bundle was cut at the first operation, and the other is cut at the second operation, gangrene of the finger is likely to occur. Great care must be taken to protect the digital arteries when operating for recurrent disease, and some degree of flexion contracture may have to be accepted to prevent arterial injury.

Injury to the neurovascular bundle can be minimized if the surgeon's vision is aided by loupe magnification (4.5× is ideal). If a digital nerve is cut, it should be repaired when the dissection has been completed. If both arteries have been cut, they should be repaired.

Hematoma, Skin Necrosis, and Infection

These three complications are considered together because one often follows the other. Some degree of hematoma is inevitable after an extensive dissection of the palm. The most reliable method of preventing further complications is to leave the palmar wound open, after the method of McCash.[14] If a hematoma is not recognized and properly drained, some degree of skin necrosis at the suture line is likely, and this will be followed by infection.

Skin necrosis commonly occurs in the finger where the diseased fascia and skin are intimately attached, and where the skin is often very thin following excision of the fascia. Inappropriate Z-plasties or small flaps often result in necrosis of one or other flap. If the blood supply to the skin is precarious, the application of a bolus dressing similar to that used with a free skin graft, often prevents necrosis. If the skin obviously has no blood supply, it is best removed and replaced by a free graft.

Infection alone, without hematoma or skin necrosis, is unusual. If may occur in patients who have long-standing and severe contractures, in which the skin is macerated and difficult to clean preoperatively. On occasion it is wise to perform a fasciotomy in these patients to straighten the metacarpophalangeal joint so that the skin can be properly prepared for a more extensive procedure.

Failure to Gain Full Extension at Operation

The aim of operation is to gain full extension of the involved digit. Usually this can be achieved but, under certain circumstances, the surgeon should be prepared to accept some residual flexion contracture. In this regard it is unlikely that postoperative therapy will increase the correction obtained at operation.

Contracture at the metacarpophalangeal joint can always be fully corrected, regardless of the duration or severity of contracture. The same is not true at the proximal interphalangeal joint.[15] Some residual contracture is the rule when the joint has been flexed for a long time (*e.g.*, 2 or 3 years).

Nevertheless, many patients fail to gain full extension simply because of inadequate excision of diseased fascia. The only fascia that contracts the metacarpophalangeal joint is the pretendinous cord of the palmar aponeurosis. Therefore, incision or excision of this cord results in full correction at this joint. However, at the proximal interphalangeal joint there are four cords that cause contracture,

alone or in combination, and each should be identified and removed. These are the central, lateral, spiral, and retrovascular cords.[4] Although one or another may be obviously diseased in a finger, there may some change in the others, so all the diseased and potentially diseased tissue should be removed.

Sympathetic Dystrophy and Loss of Flexion

Sympathetic dystrophy, although fortunately uncommon following operation for DD, can prolong morbidity and result in permanent disability—in particular, loss of digital flexion. Patients almost always have full flexion, even with severe and long-standing contractures. To lose full flexion is usually more disabling than lack of full extension.

Sympathetic dystrophy generally follows one of the complications discussed above. Undue postoperative pain and swelling of the hand are ominous signs, and should be attended to immediately. Although the surgical procedure may well qualify for an outpatient procedure, it is prudent to hospitalize the patient so that the hand can be elevated and the immediate postoperative pain controlled. If pain and swelling persist, a sympathetic block is indicated, and blocks should be repeated for as long as the pain and swelling persist. For this reason alone, a brachial or axillary nerve block is the anesthetic of choice and, furthermore, a long-acting anesthetic agent is recommended because the sympathetic block may last for 24 hours.

Recurrence and Extension of Disease

The cause of recurrent contracture is inadequate removal of the disease, and it usually affects the proximal interphalangeal joint. Frequently, the retrovascular cord was not removed at the first operation. Recurrence is frequent in the little finger and is generally due to failure to remove a lateral or spiral cord that arises from the tendon of the abductor digiti minimi muscle. Occasionally, one encounters a patient who develops recurrent disease in spite of adequate surgical excision. These patients usually have the other features of Dupuytren's diathesis. Hueston recommends excision of the overlying skin and the application of a full-thickness skin graft as a reliable method of preventing recurrence.[7]

Attempts to remove diseased fascia in the hand and digits, in which the blood supply is so profuse and the fascia is attached to the skin, invites postoperative problems. Various types of fasciotomy procedures have therefore been described. However, the best long-term results occur following removal of all the diseased fascia. At present a compromise seems best to prevent the complications discussed. The surgeon should attempt to remove the disease but should modify the operation according to experience, the severity of the disease, and the condition of the patient.

References

1. Curtis, R. M.: Capsulectomy of the interphalangeal joints of the fingers. J. Bone Joint Surg., 36A:1219, 1954.
2. Watson, H. K., Light, T. R., and Johnson, T. R.; Checkrein resection for flexion contracture of the middle joint. J. Hand Surg., 4:67, 1979.
3. Davis, J. E.: On surgery of Dupuytren's contracture. Plast. Reconstr. Surg., 36:277, 1965.
4. McFarlane, R. M.: Patterns on the diseased fascia in the fingers in Dupuytren's contracture. Plast. Reconstr. Surg., 54:31, 1974.
5. Williams, J. L., and Thomas, G. G.: The natural history of Peyronie's disease. J. Urol., 103:75, 1970.
6. Demetrakopoulos, N. J., and Mason, M. L.: Ledderhose's disease. Q. Northwest. Univ. Med. School, 31:1, 1957.
7. Hueston, J. T.: Dupuytren's contracture, Edinburgh and London, E. & S. Livingstone, 1963.
8. Critchley, E. M. R., et al.: Dupuytren's disease in epilepsy. J. Neurol. Neurosurg. Psychiatry, 39:498, 1976.
9. Su, C. K., and Patek, H. J.: Dupuytren's contracture. Its association with alcoholism and cirrhosis. Arch. Intern. Med., 126:278, 1979.
10. Spring, M., Fleck, H., and Cohen, B.: Dupuytren's contracture. Warning of diabetes? N. Y. State Med. J., 70:1037, 1970.
11. Ravid, M., Dinai, Y., and Sohar, E.: Dupuytren's disease in diabetes mellitus. Acta Diabetol. Lat., 14:170, 1977.
12. Parker, H. G.: Dupuytren's contracture as a cause of stenosing tenosynovitis. J. Maine Med. Assoc., 70:147, 1979.
13. Bolton, C. F., and McFarlane, R. M.: Human tourniquet paralysis. Neurology, 28:787, 1978.
14. McCash, C. R.: The open palm technique in Dupuytren's contracture. Br. J. Plast. Surg., 17:271, 1964.
15. Legge, J. W. H., and McFarlane, R. M.: Prediction of results of treatment of Dupuytren's disease. J. Hand Surg., 5:608, 1980.

27

COMPLICATIONS FOLLOWING SECONDARY RECONSTRUCTIVE PROCEDURES OF SKIN AND SUBCUTANEOUS TISSUE

Ian Winspur

WOUND HEALING

When there is close apposition of the edges, wounds heal by primary intention to form linear scars. This happens whether the wound is closed by primary or delayed primary means. Wounds in which there is a tissue defect heal by secondary intention. This process consists of the progression across the wound of granulation tissue, composed of capillaries, fibroblasts, and collagen fibers, with progressive shrinkage of the wound (wound contracture) caused by chemical and cellular factors. There is progressive spread of epithelial elements from the edges of the wound over the granulation tissue until the process is complete and the wound has been completely closed, or "epithelialized."

Healed scars, both linear and nonlinear, continue to contract (scar contracture) due to the maturing and rearrangement of the collagen fibers and to the action of the fibroblasts and myofibroblasts in the wound.[1] All tissues involved in the wound—mobile and nonmobile—heal en block, and elective skin incisions involving mobile structures should therefore be located at a distance from these structures.

The ultimate maturing of a wound, which takes 6 to 8 months, should allow freeing of the underlying mobile structures and slight resolution of the contracted scars. Scar contracture is only acceptable to a degree insufficient to cause limitation of joint motion. In the hand, there is little tissue to spare, and secondary revision of scars is occasionally needed.

Factors Causing Increased Scar Formation

There are a number of factors that lead to increased formation of scars. The mechanism of injury is important; for example, scars from burns and severe crushing injuries contract much more severely than those from incised wounds. The presence of foreign bodies in the wound, severely crushed tissues, or infection in the early course of healing will increase scar formation, as will the presence of unrecognized or uncompensated skin loss, which leads to increased tension in the scar. The location of the injury is significant; for example, injuries on the trunk and flexor aspect of limbs show a strong propensity to hypertrophy.

Lastly, the genetic make-up of the patient is an influential factor. Blacks, redheads, and blonds tend to develop hypertrophic scars readily.[2] Children also tend to develop thickened troublesome scars more frequently than do the elderly. Patients of Anglo-Saxon heritage with hand injuries, particularly those in the northern European countries, show a particularly strong tendency to develop dense scar, swelling, hypersensitivity, and joint stiffness in the injured hand.

Complications of a Linear Scar

These include scar contracture and hypertrophy and keloid formation.

Scar Contracture. The contracture that occurs in a healed linear scar over the first 3- to 4-month

300

period is particularly troublesome in injuries of the hand, especially in linear wounds on the volar aspect of the hand or digits that cross joint creases. The process of scar contracture can be overcome with splintage, provided this is started early and maintained continuously for over 3 to 4 months.[3] Splintage and immobilization in themselves, however, may be deleterious to other structures in the hand and may, in fact, be unacceptable. Therefore, in certain situations, or when established soft tissue contracture has taken place, surgical correction is sometimes necessary. This requires the addition of skin, either by split skin grafting, full-thickness grafting, flap coverage, or Z-plasty (discussed below).

Scar Hypertrophy and Keloid Formation. As mentioned above, certain types of wounds in certain areas or on certain people of a given age or genetic make-up do, in fact form more scar tissue than one would normally expect. When a scar, seen 3 to 4 months after injury, is raised, red, thickened, feels like wood, and itches, it is said to be "hypertrophic" (Fig. 27–1). Hypertrophy implies an increase in the number of both chemical and cellular elements in the scar. Hypertrophic scars will usually settle with time, although constant compression will speed the resolution.[4] Occasionally, the scar will remain reddened and thickened, and may progressively increase in size. If this process persists after 9 to 12 months, it is referred to as a "keloid." Keloids can be particularly troublesome in certain areas of the body or in certain races, particularly in blacks. Unfortunately, keloids tend to recur following excision. Sometimes intradermal or intralesional steroid injection will promote resolution of the keloid. Continuous pressure, either in the form of compression dressings or elastic support, may reduce the volume of a keloid. Excision accompanied by low-dose radiation of no more than 800 rad postoperatively may also prevent the recurrence of a keloid.[2]

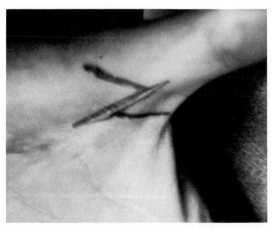

Figure 27–1. Hypertrophic scar. This posttraumatic linear scar at the base of the thumb, about 6 months after injury, crosses the joint creases at a right angle and is ideal for Z-plasty release.

Complications of Nonlinear Scars

These include the following: wound and scar contracture; scar instability; scar adherence to underlying structures; unsuitability for underlying reconstruction; and insensibility.

Scar Instability. In nonlinear scars, particularly in those that have closed either by natural epithelialization or by the application of a very thin split skin graft, the resulting surface has little resistance to abrading forces or to motion, and frequently splits and bleeds. This leads to further scar formation and contracture. Healed areas such as these are unsatisfactory; if left over many years squamous cancers may develop within the unstable scar.[5] It is therefore undesirable to leave this type of coverage permanently. If the instability in the skin graft or wound remains longer than 6 to 12 months, resurfacing should be performed, either with better quality (thicker) skin graft or with a flap.

Adherence of Scar to Underlying Tissues. As mentioned above, all scars heal en bloc. Healthy linear scars, however, will soften over a period of months to allow independent gliding of the various elements of the wound. Wounds healed by granulation tissue or skin grafting, by definition and by observation of simple wound physiology, heal by deriving their blood supply from the vascularized structures at the base of the wound. Therefore, it is physiologically impossible for the scar or graft to become detached from its supportive base, which may totally prevent the gliding of mobile structures under the scar. It may also prevent the surgeon from elevating the scar to allow the deeper reconstruction of gliding or longitudinal structures, particularly tendons. When adherence of a scar presents these problems, the scar must be replaced by tissue that will remain mobile and allow gliding. This is normally achieved by providing flap coverage, with a flap being a peninsula of tissue that retains its own blood supply and subcutaneous tissue, and is therefore not dependent on nor adherent to the wound base.

Insensibility. In areas of critical sensibility, particularly fingertips and the volar aspect of the thumb, an anesthetic scar or graft may cause considerable functional deficit. Given time, even split grafts will acquire some form of deep perception secondary to sympathetic ingrowth, but this will seldom provide satisfactory two-point discrimination.[6] If the two-point discrimination is over 20 mm in one of these critical areas, resurfacing of the area by innervated tissue might be considered. The techniques are discussed below.

RECONSTRUCTIVE PROCEDURES

The reconstructive procedures available for dealing with a problem scar can be divided into two groups: skin grafting procedures and flap procedures.

The following is a brief but comprehensive review

of fundamental techniques and their complications available for the management and reconstruction of unsatisfactory cutaneous and subcutaneous scars. It should be stressed that wounds proceed through a maturing process and that many scars, which at 3 months appear red, thickened, and contracted, if given time (provided no joint contraction is present), will mature and will require no secondary revision.

Skin Grafting

Split Skin Grafting. Split skin grafting is the workhorse of the reconstructive surgeon. Split skin may be cut anywhere from 0.012 to 0.025 inch thick, depending on the donor site, and leaving a dermal bed that will re-epithelialize in 10 to 12 days. It is readily available for resurfacing large areas. A split skin graft, however, requires a healthy vascularized base on which to live and, unless splinted, will contract up to 50% of its original size. Loss of a split skin graft may be due to the unsuitable nature or poor quality of the bed, improper hemostasis and the development of hematoma, or the effect of traction forces in the early postoperative period. Late contracture of the graft may be prevented by splinting. If contracture does occur, it can be released by further skin grafting and splintage.

Full-Thickness Skin Grafting. Full-thickness skin grafts contain all the elements of skin without subcutaneous tissue. The secondary defect becomes a problem, because it will not heal spontaneously and it either has to be sutured or split skin-grafted itself. This limits the availability of the full-thickness skin graft. A full-thickness skin graft has a great advantage in that it does not shrink as much as a split-thickness graft. On the other hand, it will only "take" on an extremely healthy bed, and it is much less reliable in this regard than split-thickness skin. However, in an area with a healthy bed, and in

which the contracture of a split graft would cause deformity, full-thickness skin may be used, particularly in the secondary release of scars over joints.

Flap and Z-Plasty Procedures

A flap is a peninsula of living tissue raised on a pedicle or base through which the blood supply of the flap courses. Living tissue was not designed to be elevated and moved on small vascular pedicles and, unless the flap is properly constructed and handled with care and experience, it will certainly die, leaving a defect twice the original size.[7] Therefore, one should not embark on flap procedures without having excluded all possibilities of providing coverage by simpler means. A flap procedure should not generally be performed primarily, unless one is extremely experienced with the use of flaps. Flaps may be classified on the basis of their composition, geometry, or vascular pattern, but the classification important in their consideration in upper extremity surgery is the differentiation between a local flap (created from tissues adjacent to the defect) and a distant flap (created from tissues on other parts of the body).[8]

Z-Plasty

Z-plasty is a fundamental technique in the management of linear and contracted linear scars.[9] The procedure basically consists of the elevation of two equilateral triangular flaps of equal size. By transposing these triangular flaps, the length of the contracted scar may be increased by approximately 50%. Also, the line of the scar can be redirected to lie in a much more satisfactory direction. For example, in web space release, the transverse limb is constructed to lie in a neutral line so as to minimize the forces on the scar when it is stretched and to allow the scar to settle much more rapidly without

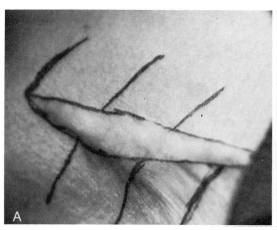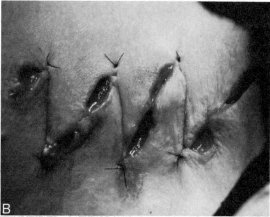

Figure 27–2. Multiple Z-plasty. *A,* Hypertrophic scar on the volar aspects of the wrist; *B,* this was excised, lengthened, and converted to lie within the skin lines of tension by multiple Z-plasties.

contracture (see Fig. 27–6). Z-plasties may be arranged in combination, in which case the gain in length is cumulative and the direction of the scar is radically altered (Fig. 27–2). The technique of Z-plasty is sophisticated. The design is complex, because there are obviously at least two possible combinations of triangles. The local triangular flap shows a propensity to necrose at its tip, particularly if the pedicle is not well designed, or has scar in its base. Triangular flaps must be constructed in healthy tissue, and will not survive in irradiated or devascularized tissue. The gain in length is at the expense of tissue on the lateral margins of the wound, and therefore redundant tissue must be present in this area for the procedure to have application. Thus, it is often not adequate in providing release for contracted burn scars.

Flaps

Local Flaps. Local flaps have a considerable place in hand surgery, particularly when utilizing the skin of the dorsum of the hand or fingers, which is extremely mobile and to a certain degree redundant (Fig. 27–3). Local transposition flaps are often frequently used on the arms to release burn scars (Fig. 27–4). The breadth of the flap increases the distance between the ends of the scar and, as the scar continues to contract, the transposed flap tissue stretches and the scar contracture does not cause additional skeletal contracture or scar hypertrophy.[10] Local flaps on the palmar aspect are poorly mobile. There is also little tissue to spare, and therefore they are seldom used. Local flaps do not provide a large area of coverage, so to resurface

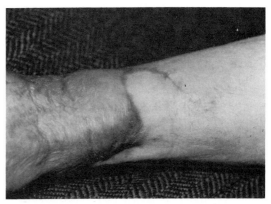

Figure 27–4. This local transposition flap has been interposed into a longitudinal, contracted burn scar of forearm, "decompressing" the hypertrophic scar and thus allowing it to settle.

larger defects either a free skin graft or distant flap must be utilized.

Distant Flaps. Distant flaps are readily available from many parts of the body to cover even the largest defects on the hand or upper extremity.[11] The most commonly employed flaps are random flaps (flaps without a specific arterial supply) from the thorax, or axial flaps (flaps with a specific arterial supply) from the infraclavicular area or the groin (Fig. 27–5).[12–14] The problems of distant flap coverage are multiple and serious, and generally these procedures should not be performed as a primary procedure unless there is in-depth consultation with both the patient and family, and a thorough consideration of all the reconstructive requirements involved. Specific problems include the following:

1. The limb must be held in an unnatural stiffened position for 3 weeks.

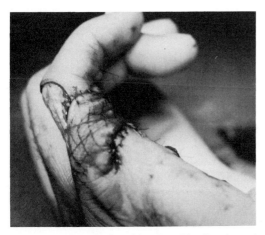

Figure 27–3. Local transposition flap. The flap from the dorsum of the little finger has been used to close a full-thickness volar defect from a gunshot wound with exposed joint, tendon, and interruption of the digital nerves; this also allows simultaneous nerve grafting of the digital nerves. Note the dorsal defect, and also that a full-thickness graft will be used to minimize the graft contracture in the closure of the dorsal defect.

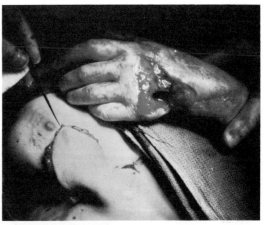

Figure 27–5. Random chest flap. The careful location and geometry of this flap was used to resurface the dorsum of the hand prior to secondary extensive tendon reconstruction. The flap was placed in such a position to allow the hand to be comfortable and to minimize donor defect.

2. The hand must be immobilized in this position for up to 3 weeks, with potentially deleterious effects on joints and tendons.

3. The procedures are multistaged.

4. The secondary defect may be significant; for instance, a large, unsightly infraclavicular scar in the female.

5. The coverage may be unsuitable for reasons of bulk, color-match, or hair.

Skin from different parts of the torso has different characteristics. Skin from the thorax is generally fine textured and hair-free, and with only a small amount of subcutaneous fat. Flaps from the thorax provide a good match for dorsal coverage of the hand. The groin provides very large flaps with minimal cosmetic defect from the donor site. However, the skin is coarse and may be pigmented. In most nonorientals it is hairy and also includes excessive subcutaneous fat, which cannot be thinned without real chance of damage to the vascular supply of the flap.

The commonly used distant flaps within the hand are the cross-finger flap for resurfacing of volar skin defects of digits, and thenar and hypothenar flaps for the resurfacing of fingertip injuries. These flaps have all the problems detailed above, not only in the affected digit but also in the donor digit, particularly when using them in patients over 40 years of age. In general terms, both these flaps should be avoided unless used for very limited and very specific indications, such as a full-thickness defect on the volar aspect if the middle segment of the finger with bare tendon exposed, unsuitable for coverage by a split-thickness skin graft.

Neurovascular Flaps. Insensible scars or grafts on fingertips cause considerable functional disability. However, the patient should be allowed time to rehabilitate completely with a mature graft before embarking on revision. If functionally significant areas of anesthesia are present, resurfacing by a neurovascular flap is indicated. These flaps may be either local or distant and, in general, local flaps are preferable.

Neurovascular flaps are flaps that, in addition to carrying their own blood supply, contain and carry their own functioning nerve supply. Examples of local neurovascular flaps are the volar V-Y advancement flap for fingertip injuries, which is satisfactory for revising insensible fingertips, and the oblique volar flaps for fingers or thumb (Fig. 27–6).[15, 16] Distant neurovascular flaps, classically the island neurovascular flap based on the digital artery and nerve from the less important ulnar side of the long and ring fingers, may be used to resurface the radial border of the index finger or the volar aspect of the thumb.[16] These flap procedures are tricky to perform and are extremely delicate. The two-point discrimination deteriorates with transfer.[17] When contemplating use of these flaps, one must also realize the possibility of damage to an otherwise undamaged digit. An additional source of neurovascular island flaps is the dorsum of the hand, utilizing intact radial nerve elements. These flaps have been well described for covering radial defects on the fingers or volar and tip defects on the thumb.[18]

Flap Loss: The Ultimate Disaster

When a skin flap is raised, one always "robs Peter to pay Paul." In planning the procedure, the loss

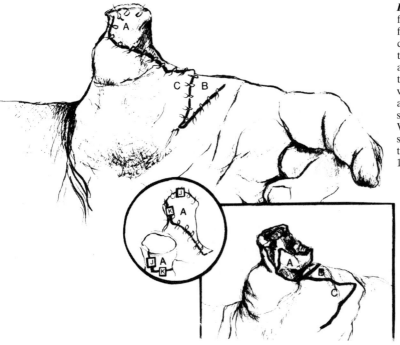

Figure 27–6. Local neurovascular flap. This oblique "Hueston"-type flap, including both digital bundles, provides sensory coverage to the tip of the thumb stump. Note also the deep Z-plasty in the web that deepens the web, allows advancement of the thumb flap, and also changes the direction of the surgical scar in the web. (From Winspur, I.: Single-stage reconstruction of the subtotally amputated thumb. J Hand. Surg., 6:70, 1981.)

to Peter must never outweigh the benefits to Paul. If the flap is lost, however, the resultant double loss will be disastrous. Flaps may be lost in all three phases of the surgical procedure.

Preoperative Phase. There are a number of local and systemic contraindications to flaps, including diabetes, chronic arterial or venous disease, irradiated tissues, electrical burns, scar within the proposed pedicle or old injury to the axial vessels, and psychosis. Design problems include an inadequate pedicle, inadequate size of the flap, and inappropriate positioning and location of the flap.

Obviously, any condition that compromises the vascularity of the tissues being utilized for flap transfer must affect the viability of the proposed flap. Hence, it is imperative to assess carefully the quality of the local tissue and to determine the presence or absence of any generalized disease. The psychotic patient will not tolerate the immobilization required when the transfer of the distant flap is proposed, and the presence of mental illness is an absolute contraindication to the transfer of distant flaps. In planning the design and geometry of the flap, the vascularity of flap proposed, whether random or axial, should be clearly delineated, and the geometry of the proposed flap should be determined beforehand. In general, random flaps on the abdomen can be raised at a length-to-breadth ratio of 2:1, on the chest of 3:1, and on the hand of 3:1. Axial flaps can be raised to a much greater length, although many axial flaps contain a random distal portion and this must be taken into account. Skin is elastic, and flaps shrink on elevation. When raising a local transposition flap, it should also be remembered that the point of rotation of the flap is that point furthest away from the defect, not the point adjacent to the defect, so a much larger flap is required than one would have initially imagined. The details of flap construction are found in many standard texts of plastic surgery, but the most common cause of misplanning of local transposition flaps remains ignorance of the geometry of flap transfer.

Operative Phase. Causes of tissue loss here include excessive tissue crushing and injury, direct injury to the vascular pedicle or to the vascular plexus of the flap, and suture of the flap under tension, particularly over convex surfaces. Skin and subcutaneous tissues were not designed to be moved over a distance, and any additional factor causing tissue injury will magnify the insult to the transferred tissue. The techniques and principles of atraumatic tissue handling have been well delineated in the literature. These techniques must be used compulsively when any flap transfer is performed.

During transfer, the vascular basis of the flap, even though it may be the random subdermal plexus or a direct axial vessel, must be very carefully preserved. Direct dissection of axial vessels, unless absolutely indicated, is not recommended, and the vessels should be maintained within a healthy supporting sheath of subcutaneous fat. The blood supply in a random flap, carried on a subdermal plexus, will not be violated if sufficient subcutaneous tissue is left on the underside of the flap, and if there are no additional random skin incisions that could disturb the subdermal plexus. When the flap is sutured into place very accurate apposition of the skin edges should be attained, classically using a half-buried vertical mattress suture. The suture should never be of greater diameter than 4–0 nylon and, if suture of greater strength is required, then tension is too great, the flap is too small, or the geometry of the flap is unsatisfactory. When suturing a flap over a convex surface, one must allow for swelling within the flap during the first 24 or 48 hours. The flap must be of liberal proportions. If a raised flap proves to be under too much tension, (1) the flap may be sutured over only part of the defect and the additional defect split skin-grafted, (2) the flap may be returned to its bed for use in a few days after delay, or (3) another flap should be utilized.

Postoperative Phase. Causes of flap failure during this period involve hematoma, use of tight dressings, and postoperative swelling. Hemostasis should be secured meticulously during surgery on the recipient defect. If satisfactory hemostasis cannot be secured, drainage should be provided either by simple rubber drains or suction drains. These should be maintained until all drainage has ceased. If an early postoperative hematoma develops one should, under full surgical conditions, re-evaluate the flap, irrigate and remove the hematoma, secure hemostasis, and resuture the flap. Hematoma is the most common cause of flap loss. Postoperative dressings should be kept to a minimum, and there should be no pressure on either the flap or the pedicle. The dressings should always include a window so that continuous inspection of the flap can be made, particularly during the first 48 hours. When a flap is sutured over a convex surface ample allowance should be made for swelling, and the flap should be created of liberal size.

Aids in Minimizing Compromise to a Flap. These include the following:

1. Careful preoperative design of the procedure, with the patient awake and in a comfortable position
2. Design that allows a 10 to 20% overestimate in the flap size
3. Provision of delay
4. Use of the "crane" principle

When planning a flap procedure, particularly a distant flap transfer, the planning and design should be made with the patient awake so that the anatomic feasibility and comfort can be carefully checked. Positions can be obtained under general anesthesia that may be impossible or intolerable when patient is awake. The phenomenon of delay is clearly discussed in the plastic surgical literature. It is a surgical maneuver to encourage the blood supply to a given area of skin to localize from a given specific point—that is, along the line of the pedicle of a flap. Delay can be encouraged when a portion of tissue is elevated from its bed on a pedicle but is not transferred at that time. It is subject to the insults of ischemia with elevation but not to further injury with transfer, and so is encouraged to regain a healthy blood supply only from the pedicle. The maximum effect of the delaying procedure is seen between the 10th and 14th days. Only randomly supplied tissue benefits from delay. If the proportions of a flap are questionable, a formal delaying procedure should always be performed prior to transfer.

The crane principle allows a distant flap to be transferred and to remain attached to the recipient defect for a number of days; then, if the flap appears to be marginal or dying, it can be transferred back to its original defect and saved. By this time a healthy granulating wound will have been obtained at the base of the recipient defect, which will then take split skin grafting. This should not be a planned maneuver but may save the distant flap from total loss and provide a sufficiently healthy wound for coverage.

It should be again emphasized that the techniques for flap surgery are fundamental in themselves and have been clearly delineated over the years. Such procedures are described in many plastic surgery texts. This brief review is an attempt to highlight the areas of danger and perhaps to provide an escape route should an unfortunate end be anticipated.

References

1. Madden, J. W.: Wound healing: The biological basis of hand surgery. Clin. Plast. Surg., 3:3, 1976.
2. Gillies, H. G., and Millard, R. D.: The Principles and Art of Plastic Surgery, Boston, Little, Brown & Company, 1957, pp. 85–88.
3. Wynn-Parry, C. B.: The Stiff Hand in Rehabilitation of the Hand, 3rd ed., London, Butterworth, 1973, pp. 210–217.
4. Linares, H. A., Larson, D. L., and Bauer, P. S.: Influence of mechanical forces upon burn scar contracture and hypertrophy. In Krizek, T., and Hoopes, J., (eds.): Symposium on Basic Science in Plastic Surgery, St. Louis, C. V. Mosby, 1976, p. 101.
5. Marjolin, J. N.: Dictionnaire de Médecine, Paris, Chez Béchet Jeune, 1828, pp. 21–31.
6. Mannerfeldt, L.: Evaluation of functional sensation of skin grafts in the hand area. Br. J. Plast. Surg., 15:136, 1962.
7. Gillies, H. G., and Millard, R. D.: The Principles and Art of Plastic Surgery, Boston, Little, Brown & Company, 1957, p. 112.
8. Grabb, W. C.: Classification of skin flaps. In Grabb, W. C., and Meyers, M. B. (eds.): Skin Flaps, Boston, Little, Brown & Company, pp. 145–154.
9. McGregor, I. A.: The theoretical basis of the Z-plasty. Br. J. Plast. Surg., 9:256, 1957.
10. Larson, D. L., et al.: Prevention and treatment of scar contracture. In Artz, C. P., Moncrief, J. A., and Pruitt, B. A., Jr. (eds.): Burns: A Team Approach, Philadelphia, W. B. Saunders, 1979, pp. 486–488.
11. Cannon, B.: Flaps old and new. J. Hand Surg., 6:1, 1981.
12. McGregor, I. A., and Morgan, R. G.: Axial and random pattern flaps. Br. J. Plast. Surg., 26:202, 1973.
13. McGregor, I. A., and Jackson, I. T.: The groin flap. Br. J. Plast. Surg., 25:3, 1972.
14. Bekamjian, V. Y.: A two-stage method of pharyngo-esophageal reconstruction with a primary pectoral skin flap. Plast. Reconstr. Surg., 36:173, 1965.
15. Winspur, I.: Single-stage reconstruction of the sub-totally amputated thumb: A synchronous neurovascular flap and Z-plasty. J. Hand Surg., 6:70, 1981.
16. Littler, J. W.: Neurovascular skin island transfer in reconstructive hand surgery. In Transactions of the Second Congress of the International Society for Plastic Surgery, London, E & S Livingstone, 1959, pp. 175–179.
17. Murray, J. F., Ord, J. V. R., and Gavelin, G. E.: The neurovascular island pedicle flap, J. Bone Joint Surg., 49A:1285, 1967.
18. Holevitch, J.: A new method of restoring sensibility to the thumb. J. Bone Joint Surg., 45B:496, 1963.

28

COMPLICATIONS FOLLOWING INJURY TO THE SKIN AND TO THE SUBCUTANEOUS TISSUE

Ian Winspur

Skin is living tissue, with many functions vital to homeostasis. Two of these functions are of paramount importance in the hand and upper extremity—protection and sensibility. Skin protects the underlying vital structures in the hand from mechanical injury, drying, desquamation, and bacterial invasion, with the subsequent problems of inflammation and swelling. The unique sensibility of the palmar skin provides the ability of the hand and digits not only to feel but also to "see and discern"—"tactile gnosis" as recognized by Moberg.[1] Without this ability the digit, the whole hand, and indeed the whole upper extremity may become an insensitive, useless appendage. Hence, in the consideration of injuries to the skin, prime importance must be given to the following:

1. Achieving early, safe, and complete skin closure
2. Preserving to the maximum degree all viable, innervated skin
3. Providing sensible coverage in areas critical to touch

PRIMARY CLOSURE VERSUS DELAYED PRIMARY AND SECONDARY CLOSURE

Under ideal circumstances, the most satisfactory management of the simple open wound is primary closure followed, hopefully, by primary healing. Wounds, left open, will heal very satisfactorily, however, by secondary intention. Wounds left open may be sutured after a period of 4 or 5 days, a technique termed "delayed primary closure."

Wound closure with revision or grafting at the time of closure, usually between the fifth and seventh days, or possibly later, is referred to as "secondary closure."[2] The open wound techniques are very acceptable and well proven in hand injuries. The ultimate resulting scar from that of primary closure, delayed primary closure, or secondary closure of an equivalent wound is virtually identical, although wounds closed by delay tend to be thicker and more indurated for a longer period, and the period of swelling is also prolonged. This is not significant enough, though, to warrant primary closure when a safer approach would be one of delayed or secondary closure.

TIDY WOUNDS AND UNTIDY WOUNDS

Wounds may be divided into two categories, tidy and untidy. Tidy wounds are basically sharply incised wounds without any additional crushing or damaging component (Fig. 28–1). Untidy wounds, which are either crushed or avulsed, are ragged and may include multiple avulsion flaps, degloved areas, or areas of frank tissue and skin loss (Fig. 28–2).

Tidy Wounds

The desired treatment of a tidy uncontaminated wound seen early is, after adequate cleansing of the wound, primary suture. However, a number of complicating factors may exist:

1. Damage to important underlying structures

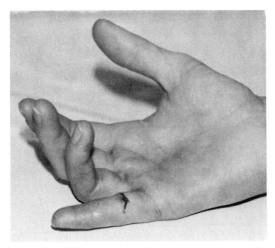

Figure 28–1. Tidy wound. There is an abnormal extended position of the digit; both flexor tendons and the ulnar digital nerve have been severed. Delayed primary repair of all structures was performed.

2. Delay between the time of injury and repair
3. Obvious or suspected excessive bacterial or chemical contamination
4. Unfavorable direction or location of the wound

Damage to Underlying Important Structures

On examining the injured digit or hand with an open wound, it is important to check completely for damage to underlying important structures. This requires a fundamental knowledge of the anatomy of the hand, and also detailed knowledge of the anatomy of the area in which the laceration lies,

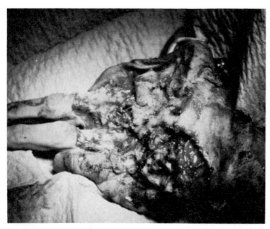

Figure 28–2. Untidy wound. There is a severely crushed and avulsed nonviable dorsal skinflap, loss of two digits, multiple compound fractures, and tendon and nerve injury.

and the distal manifestations of injury to underlying structures.[3] A very detailed, accurate, and anatomically related examination should be performed on any open wound in the hand (see Fig. 28–1). The details of the hand examination can be found elsewhere, but one important observation should be made at this point. It is extremely difficult and unusual to cut the digital arteries without cutting the digital nerves; when both digital nerves are cut in the finger, one should also be highly suspicious that both digital arteries have also been cut. This is important, because the only injuries that demand immediate reconstruction are those causing a loss of blood supply distally. This is very much in contradistinction to damage to underlying tendons and nerves, which can very acceptably be repaired by a delayed primary or secondary procedure. Having noted that underlying structures are damaged, the wound can usually be managed in the emergency room by simple skin closure, and arrangements can be made for definitive and skilled care of the underlying damage.

Delay

Open wounds in the preantibiotic era were notorious for developing significant and deep infections if not properly cared for within 2 to 3 hours of injury; this safe period was termed the "Golden Period." It is true that, with modern antibiotics, the Golden Period can safely be extended. However, it is potentially dangerous to extend it beyond 8 to 12 hours after hand injuries and, in general, if wounds are seen beyond this time limit, or if there is doubt, the wound is better left open for either delayed primary or secondary closure. Also, if doubt exists about the nature of the wound, or there is a possibility of bacterial contamination, (as in agricultural wounds or dog bites) or of significant chemical contamination (as in meat-cutting injuries) then, indeed, it is better not to close the wound formally but to dress the hand firmly and plan either delayed primary or secondary closure.[4]

Wounds in Unfavorable Locations or Directions

It is known that longitudinal wounds on the volar aspect of the hand or digits, crossing the joint creases at right angles, heal and contract and subsequently cause both soft tissue and joint contracture (Fig. 28–3). Elective incisions on the digit should never be made in this direction, or tissue adjustment should be made so that they come to lie in more favorable positions.[5] Traumatic wounds, recognized as being in an unfavorable line, will generally require revisional surgery to minimize the scar contracture. The timing of the revisional surgery, however, unless one is extremely experienced in reconstructive techniques, particularly in the use of multiple Z-plasties, should be delayed. Furthermore, unless one is absolutely sure of the benign nature of the wound, no revisional surgery should

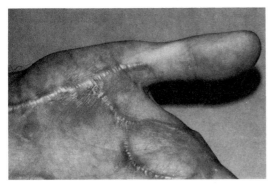

Figure 28–3. Unfavorable scar. This thickened contracted scar, 6 months following injury, crosses the volar aspect of the thumb base at right angles to the joint creases. Release was effected by multiple Z-plasties.

be performed until complete wound healing has occurred. Z-plasty procedures are, by definition, flap procedures, and the healing of flaps is much less satisfactory than that of a simple incised wound. The risk of infection and wound necrosis is much higher and, if the primary Z-plasty fails, one is left with a defect larger than that of the original wound. A simple revisional Z-plasty can always be performed 2 or 3 months after the original injury without significant risk either to the digit or the patient, and without significant delay in rehabilitation.

Untidy Wounds

Complicating factors in the management of this type of wound are multiple, small, marginally viable flaps, distally based flaps, massive degloving and devascularized flaps, and skin loss.

Multiple Small Marginally Viable Flaps

All dead tissue must always be meticulously excised at the time of primary wound care. The tissues of the hand are extraordinarily well vascularized, however, and multiple small flaps, which appear only marginally viable at the time of primary surgery, will survive if cleansed and loosely tacked in place. Often the small flaps are of sensible palmar skin over important areas, and are therefore of considerable importance. Every effort should be made to conserve them. Fluorescein dye, injected intravenously, is sometimes useful in assessing the viability of larger flaps.[6]

Distally Based Flaps

Distally based flaps with adequate pedicles are viable, but the venous return of the distally based flap is certainly compromised. During the first 24 to 48 hours of the flap's life, swelling further compromises venous return and, unless allowance has been

made for this, the flap will, in fact, proceed first to venous strangulation and then to arterial death. Correct management of the distally based flap with adequate initial vascularity involves very loosely suturing the flap into the position in which the flap naturally lies (not stretched back over the original defect), and to apply either a wet dressing or split skin graft to the residual defect. Distally based flaps should not be excised and grafted as a matter of course.

Degloved Tissue

Degloved tissue, as seen in the classic "wringer injury," differs from the distally based avulsed flap in that, although the tissues may appear viable, most of the avulsed skin and subcutaneous tissue is, in fact, dead. This can be ascertained very easily by incising the flap from its distal edge to its base 1 cm at a time and observing that there is no fresh bleeding from the cut edge until one is virtually at the base of the flap. The degloved flap should therefore be resected back to a fresh bleeding edge, the viable tissue treated as a distally based flap and sutured lightly into place, and the remaining defect covered with split-thickness skin grafts harvested either from the avulsed tissues, if they are not too contused or, more satisfactorily, from a fresh donor area.

Skin Loss

Full-thickness skin defects, when allowed to heal spontaneously, demonstrate rapid and dramatic wound shrinkage and active wound contracture. A given wound will contract to 70 to 80% of its original size in 2 or 3 weeks.[7] In areas of skin excess and laxity, this produces no functional deficit. However, in the hand, such a process causes disastrous joint contracture and stiffness. The process of wound contracture is markedly reduced by providing additional skin coverage by skin graft or flap; therefore, the appreciation of skin loss is important in the assessment and management of the untidy wounds. It is surprising to see, in many untidy and mangled hand wounds, when all the small viable flaps are carefully preserved, how little tissue has actually been lost.

If, however, after preservation of all existing and viable flaps, tissue is seen to be lost or, due to gross swelling of the hand, there is a relative skin loss, provision must be made for early skin coverage, preferably by split skin grafting. All areas of full-thickness loss can be managed temporarily by application of wet saline dressings, kept moist, and changed every 6 hours. This may well be the primary treatment of choice; it allows a period for the resuscitation of the patient, deliberation by the surgeon, and perhaps for skilled consultation. Often definitive coverage by split skin is all that is required to provide coverage for large open wounds. Full-thickness grafts have no place in providing primary coverage because the survivability of this type of

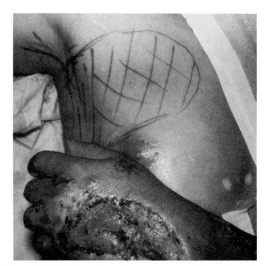

Figure 28–4. Secondary flap coverage. There is a full-thickness defect of the dorsum of the hand, with loss of extensor tendons. Primary coverage has been obtained, despite the fact that bare metacarpals without periosteum lay at the base, by split skin graft. Secondary flap coverage was provided on the tenth postinjury day to facilitate later reconstruction of the extensor tendons.

graft is much lower than that of split-thickness skin grafts. Also, the full-thickness donor defect limits the availability of full-thickness skin. The presence of denuded bone, open joint, and bare tendon theoretically necessitates coverage by a skin flap, a peninsula of the skin with its own blood supply that will provide coverage over a nonvascularized bed. Split skin grafts, however, applied primarily will take over the most surprising areas, and should be utilized (Fig. 28–4).

THE TIMING OF FLAP COVERAGE

All open wounds of the extremity can be managed for a period of days by the application of wet dressings without significant deterioration. Additional coverage can usually be obtained by split skin grafting. However, in certain circumstances, flap coverage may be necessary due to the nature of the defect or to the unsuitability of the bed for skin graft. It may also be recognized that flap coverage will be required over a defect to allow subsequent underlying reconstruction by bone, nerve, or tendon graft, or to minimize flexion contracture of an underlying joint (see Fig. 28–4).

Under these circumstances, it is reasonable to consider flap coverage at an early point. The provision of flap coverage is a formal procedure, only to be performed after all other methods have been excluded, and only after the patient has been fully assessed and informed about the extent of the procedure and its dangers and risks. It should only be done after the primary surgeon and all consult-

ants involved have thoroughly explored all the possibilities of flap coverage, and have ascertained that the flap that is ultimately chosen provides not only the skin coverage required, but also meets all other reconstructive requirements of that particular damaged hand. Unless one is extremely experienced or there is an unusual but overriding reason, primary coverage (i.e., at the time of injury), is seldom indicated. It *has* been performed and proved successful at times, and the major argument is that the patient is projected along the reconstructive road rapidly. However, the 5-day difference between a primary and a delayed primary flap is of little consequence in the reconstructive effort, which may sometimes take up to 18 months. An ill-conceived flap that fails to provide all the elements of coverage required and renders the patient helplessly immobile with the hand hanging in a dependent, nonphysiologic, and unfavorable position, inaccessible to both the nurse and the therapist, uncomfortable throughout the early hospital course, and leaves him contemplating a hideous scar of which he was not informed, is to be avoided at all costs.

FINGERTIP INJURIES

Fingertip injuries are extremely common and represent the most common, complex hand injury seen in the emergency room. The type of surgical care required for a given injury is determined primarily by the anatomy of the injury itself. The injuries can be divided into two basic types: those with bone exposed, and those without bone exposed.

The basic treatment for injuries without bone exposed and a healthy vascular subcutaneous bed is simple coverage by a split skin graft. The basic treatment for injuries with bone exposed consists of coverage of the wound by some form of local flap.

The complications following adult fingertip injuries include the following: (1) painful adherent scar; (2) an area of anesthesia at the site of reconstruction; (3) persisting joint stiffness; (4) neuroma formation; (5) cold intolerance; (6) distortion of the nail bed; and (7) sympathetic dystrophy (Table 28–1).

Adherent Painful Scar

The prevention of this complication requires the provision of well-vascularized, full-thickness skin coverage supported on a mobile base. When subcutaneous tissue is present, a split-thickness skin graft will fulfill these criteria. It will ultimately shrink in size, leaving a small mobile scar, and satisfactory coverage will be obtained. A full-thickness graft is not nearly as satisfactory in this regard, and should seldom be used.[8] When bone is exposed a graft may still survive, but it remains adherent and cannot shrink. Coverage is more satisfactorily

Table 28–1. COMPLICATIONS IN ADULT FINGERTIP INJURIES*

Type of Repair	Number of Repairs (%)	Complications						
		Infection (%)	Nail Bed (%)	Loss of Flap (%)	Cold Intolerance (%)	Neuroma: 3 months	Neuroma: 6 months (%)	Revision (%)
Bone shortening and existing local flap	41 (40)	4 (10)	3 (7)	1 (2)	1 (2)	5	0	5 (12)
Split-thickness skin graft	16 (16)		1 (6)			2	1 (6)	2 (12)
Full-thickness skin graft (from amputated part)	7 (6)							
V-Y flap	30 (30)	1 (3)	2 (7)			1	0	
"Hueston-type" flap	7 (7)					1	1 (14)	
X finger flap	1 (1)							
Total:	101 (100)	5 (5)	6 (6)	1 (1)	1 (1)	9 (9)	1 (1)	7 (7)
Total complications	14 (14)							
Total revisions	7 (50% of complications)							

*101 consecutive fingertip injuries treated with a minimum follow-up of 6 months and a maximum follow-up of 2½ years. The type of repair was dictated by the anatomy of the injury. Full-thickness grafts were only used when the injury was a clean cut, and when the amputated part could provide a satisfactory full-thickness graft. (From Winspur, I.: Fingertip injuries. *In* Boswick, J. A., Jr. [ed.]: Current Concepts in Hand Surgery. Philadelphia, Lea & Febiger, 1983.)

provided by a local flap, with two types being commonly used: the V-Y volar advancement flap, as popularized by Kleinert, and local rotation flaps of the type described by Hueston (Figs. 28–5 and 28–6).[9, 10] These are formal procedures requiring experience and a good anatomic knowledge. If the patient is elderly, or has peripheral vascular disease or diabetes, these procedures are contraindicated. If there is extensive local crushing, potential contamination, either bacterial or chemical, or delay, the procedure should be performed on a delayed primary or secondary basis. The flaps are only suitable for guillotine-type amputations and, when the amputation is oblique or additional lacerations exist, modifications to the standard procedures must be made. Often coverage can be obtained with a small degree of bone shortening, and with the use of an existing volar (or local) flap. The insertions of flexor tendons should never be sacrificed and the thumb should never be shortened to facilitate closure.

Area of Anesthesia at the Site of Reconstruction

Fingertip sensibility is of the ultimate importance in performing fine work. It may not be critical in a manual laborer, but may be extremely critical to a musician. Split skin grafts and full-thickness grafts will develop a degree of sensibility over 12 to 18 months, probably as a result of sympathetic ingrowth.[11] Split-thickness skin grafts have the advantage of contracting and thus minimizing the area of sensory loss. They are much preferred over full-thickness grafts, which provide little better sensibility or durability but do not contract, and leave larger areas of numbness. When appropriate, as in guillotine amputations, coverage by a local neurovascular flap of the volar triangular advancement type will provide coverage with tissue that retains its innervation. This is the choice coverage in areas

Figure 28–5. VY-plasty. The triangular neurovascular island is raised on a vertical subcutaneous pedicle (no undermining), and the flap is also secured by the minimum number of sutures to allow for swelling in the first 48 hours. (From Winspur, I.: Fingertip injuries. *In* Boswick, J. A., Jr. [ed.]: Current Concepts in Hand Surgery. Philadelphia, Lea & Febiger, 1983.)

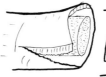

Figure 28–6. "Hueston"-type local flap. The existing laceration and the type of wound make it unsuitable for VY-closure. The laceration is utilized to create a neurovascular transposition flap containing both digital bundles. (From Winspur, I.: Fingertip injuries. *In* Boswick, J. A., Jr. [ed.]: Current Concepts in Hand Surgery. Philadelphia, Lea & Febiger, 1983.)

of prime tactile importance, particularly of the distal thumb or radial border of the index fingertip.

Joint Stiffness

All damaged digits are liable to swelling and stiffness, unless the wounds are closed at the earliest safe moment and posttraumatic swelling is rigidly controlled by dressings and elevation. Generally, with adequate primary care, wounds are sealed in 7 to 10 days from repair and, at that point, an aggressive program of mobilization can be initiated. Long-term stiffness, when closure has been effected by skin graft or local flap, is not a problem provided early mobilization is performed. However, in patients over 40 years of age, joint stiffness can be a particularly dangerous and troublesome phenomenon, and any procedure that requires excessive mobilization of the digit in this older age group is potentially dangerous. A technique described for fingertip injuries, which uses a distant thenar flap or a distant random flap from the dorsum of the thumb, is particularly dangerous in the older patient.[12] In younger patients these flaps do provide satisfactory coverage, although the same quality of coverage can usually be obtained by much simpler means.

Neuroma

Neuroma on the stumps of the terminal branches of the digital nerve in fingertip injuries can be particularly troublesome. In the recently injured fingertip, even with excellent skin coverage, neuromas will be present, and do irritate and cause pain. Instituting early motion and encouraging early use of the hand, early desensitizing exercises, and early return to normal function will minimize the trouble from these neuromas. In most patients in whom satisfactory, well-vascularized mobile coverage has been provided, neuromas will settle after 3 months. However, 1 to 2% of patients may remain with persisting severe neuroma problems, usually caused by a large adherent neuroma under an adherent unstable scar.[16] Under these circumstances surgical resection of the neuroma and provision of more satisfactory coverage by an additional local flap will usually provide relief.

Cold Intolerance

All digits can be expected to be intolerant of cold during the first winter after injury. It is unusual for troublesome cold intolerance to persist, however, beyond two winters. If cold intolerance does persist, a search should be made for local aggravating factors such as persisting neuroma, tender, adherent, or unstable scar, or for a cause of reduced vascularity to the finger elsewhere. If the problem appears to be related to the digital arterial supply,

appropriate steps should be taken, either by microvascular reconstruction at the required level or, if this is not appropriate, by digital sympathectomy to provide some degree of relief.[14]

Sympathetic Dystrophy

This is the complex phenomenon in which a patient develops, from what appeared to be a simple and uncomplicated but painful finger injury, severe symptoms and signs involving the whole limb with pain, sweating, erythema or cyanosis, swelling and stiffness, and disuse atrophy of the arm.[15] Extensive research over many years has produced a number of theories regarding causation. However, it is well known that, in situations of simple distal injury (i.e., fingertip injuries as opposed to more complex proximal nerve lesions), using simple analgesics, providing firm supportive care and early active and passive therapy and desensitizing exercises, and firmly controlling the compensation elements of the injury, most of the dystrophic-type phenomena can be avoided. For the patient with the established sympathetic dystrophy, conventional methods of care—such as analgesics, physiotherapy, desensitization, stellate ganglion blocks, and the more recently described intravenous reserpine blocks—may be of value.[16]

In conclusion, the maltreated cutaneous injury to the hand may cause serious disruption to the function of the whole hand, and disability and economic ruin to the patient. Properly cared for, most cutaneous injuries will heal or can be closed rapidly to allow rapid healing or reconstruction of underlying deeper and complex structures. In the more massive untidy injuries, loss of skin may be a limiting factor in the ultimate reconstruction of the hand. Therefore, timely, conservative, accurate, and sometimes extremely sophisticated techniques are needed in the management of skin and subcutaneous problems in hand injuries.

References

1. Moberg, E.: Aspects of sensation in reconstructive surgery of the upper limb. J. Bone Joint Surg., 46A:817, 1964.
2. Rank, B. K., Wakefield, A. R., and Hueston, J. T.: Surgery of repair as applied to hand injuries, 4th ed., Edinburgh, Churchill Livingstone, 1973, pp. 83–115.
3. Lister, G.: The Hand: Diagnosis and Indications, Edinburgh, Churchill Livingstone, 1977, pp. 4–10.
4. Krizek, T. J., and Rohsen, M. C.: Biology of Surgical Infections. Surg. Clin. North Am., 55:1261, 1975.
5. Littler, J. W.: Hand, wrist, and forearm incisions. In Littler, J. W., Cramer, L. M., and Smith, J. W. (eds.): Symposium on Reconstructive Hand Surgery, St. Louis, C. V. Mosby, 1974, pp. 87–97.
6. Creech, B. J., and Miller, S. H.: Evaluation of circulation in skin flaps. In Grubb, W. C., and Myers, M. B. (eds.): Skin Flaps, Boston, Little Brown & Company, 1975, pp. 26–27.
7. Madden, J. W.: Wound healing: The biological basics of hand surgery. Clin. Plast. Surg., 3:3, 1976.
8. Glikenstein, J.: Fingertip injuries. In Campbell-Reed, D. I. A., and Gesset, J. (eds.): Mutilating Injuries of the Hand,

G.E.M. Monograph 3, Edinburgh, Churchill Livingstone, 1979, pp. 30–35.

9. Atasoy, E., et al.: Reconstruction of the amputated fingertip with a triangular volar flap. J. Bone Joint Surg., 52A:921, 1970.

10. Hueston, J. T.: Local flap repair in fingertip injuries. Plast. Reconstr. Surg., 37:349, 1966.

11. Ponten, B.: Grafted skin. Acta Chir. Scand. (Suppl.), 257:1–78, 1960.

12. Flatt, A. E.: The thenar flap. J. Bone Joint Surg., 39B:80, 1957.

13. Eaton, R.: Painful neuromas. *In* Omer, G. E., and Spinner, M. (eds.): Management of Peripheral Nerve Problems, Philadelphia, W. B. Saunders, 1980, pp. 195–202.

14. Flatt, A. E.: Digital artery sympathectomy. J. Hand Surg., 5:550, 1980.

15. Lankford, L. L.: Reflex sympathetic dystrophy. *In* Omer, G. E., and Spinner, M. (eds.): Management of Peripheral Nerve Problems, Philadelphia, W. B. Saunders, 1980, pp. 216–244.

16. Chuinard, R. G., et al.: Intravenous reserpine for the treatment of reflex sympathetic dystrophy (A.S.S.H. Proceedings). J. Hand Surg., 5:289, 1980.

29

COMPLICATIONS FOLLOWING WOUND CARE

Paul W. Brown

GENERAL CONSIDERATIONS

To speak of complications following treatment of a wound of the hand implies that things have not gone well, that they have not proceeded according to expectations, that healing has not progressed comparably with other wounds of a similar nature, or that the end results have not been as good as they should be. To use the term "complication" is to pass retrospective judgment on the course of healing and on the ultimate result: complication is equated with unsatisfactory results, not up to the usual standard.

Complications are viewed differently, even defined differently, by the physician and the patient. Certainly, the definition of complication as used by the physician and by the attorney are very different. The physician tends to explain complications as unavoidable acts or, sometimes, as problems that are the fault of the patient, whereas the patient more often sees the complication as the result of the physician's fallibility. The patient's attorney will usually define the complication as the direct result of poor management.

Thus, the definition of complication is imprecise depending on whose complication it is, what one's expectations were, and what standards of normal or usual are used. Neither the physician nor the patient can be expected to agree on the matter: they are too close to it, and objectivity is denied them. One need only attend a complications conference at any hospital to realize that there is even little agreement among physicians as to the definition of complication, let alone its cause.

In simplest terms, complication means that healing has been delayed beyond normal expectations or that, following a wound, matters have gotten worse rather than better—for the wound, for the hand, or for the patient. The key to the definition lies in the words "expectations" and "usual."

Unavoidable complications are those beyond a surgeon's control: failure of wound healing due to damage of tissue beyond its capability of repair, irreversible systemic disease, malignancy, or other such conditions. Again, recognition of the complication is retrospective, and it is usually then realized that the unavoidable complication was not really a complication at all but a normal (if such term can be used with disease) progression of events and unrealistic expectations.

The *avoidable complication* interests us more, because these are the poor results from which one can learn, the knowledge gained thereby helping us to avoid the same complication in the future. Avoidable complications are of two types, *errors of omission* and *errors of commission*. Those of omission are those in which the surgeon has failed to recognize or to do something. The patient may also contribute to this type of complication by neglecting to supply information or by failing to follow instructions. Errors of commission are complications arising as the result of poor judgment, faulty technique, or failure to utilize data readily available in a way consistent with accepted standards of practice. It can readily be seen that the classification is often inexact, particularly so when the patient contributes to a poor result through failure to understand or unwillingness to cooperate. The categorization of complications can only be inexact but, nevertheless, can be of some practical value.

ERRORS OF OMISSION

Inadequate History

Most common is the missed or erroneous diagnosis in which the physician has failed to gather the necessary data for a proper diagnosis and has proceeded to treat for the wrong condition, or has treated only one aspect of the patient's pathology. Traditionally, and properly, the initial approach to any wound is through a detailed history of the cause, time, and circumstances of the wound.

Wounds of the hand are often very deceptive in this regard, because the apparent damage done to tissue may seem very obvious but the true significance may only be understood by knowing how, where, and when the wound was incurred. A wound sustained several hours earlier may appear similar to a very recent wound but, if the two are treated similarly, the older wound may well develop complications that the recent wound will not. The environment in which the wound occurred is of equal importance. The wound of the barnyard is far more likely to contain clostridial spores than that of the kitchen; primary closure of the former entails a much higher risk of the complications of anaerobic

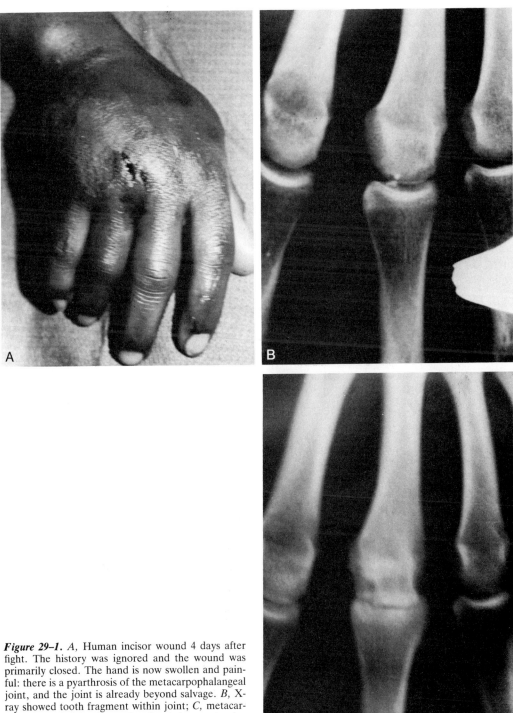

Figure 29–1. *A,* Human incisor wound 4 days after fight. The history was ignored and the wound was primarily closed. The hand is now swollen and painful: there is a pyarthrosis of the metacarpophalangeal joint, and the joint is already beyond salvage. *B,* X-ray showed tooth fragment within joint; *C,* metacarpophalangeal joint 6 months after injury: extensive degenerative arthritis.

infection than does primary closure of the household wound. The "how" is also important; because understanding forces and mechanics of wounding will allow the surgeon to avoid complications—a hand that has been damaged by great crushing force may not show the results of that force for several hours. The complications of increasing edema and nerve pressure can often be avoided by ice applications, compression dressings, and elevation soon after injury, measures that would not be employed for similar appearing wounds in which crush was not a factor.

A common error of omission due to an inadequate history is the hand wound caused by human teeth (Fig. 29–1). The knuckle punctured by someone's incisors is usually rather inconsequential in appearance for the first few hours. If the treating physician is unaware of the cause of injury because an adequate history has not been obtained, or is unaware of its significance, such a wound may be treated lightly—it may not be cleansed thoroughly, antibiotics may not be prescribed and, worst of all, the wound may be closed. Typically, the patient with such a poorly treated wound will reappear a few days later with a badly swollen hand and great pain and may, by then, have already developed a full-blown pyarthrosis with dissolution of articular cartilage and a destroyed joint.

Less common, but even more damaging, are mixed infections of the hand caused by human bites. Human teeth, in contrast to those of dogs and cats, act not as simple penetrators of tissue but as lacerators, crushers, and grinders. As they create the wound, they inflict a combination of tearing and crushing on the tissues and, at the same time, deposit great numbers of mixed and potentially virulent bacteria. The crushed tissue is locally ischemic, its defense mechanisms are thereby sparse, and an excellent medium is created for these bacteria, which often support each other synergistically and progressively. This type of infection contributes further to ischemia and necrosis, and the stage is set for a mixed infection of oral flora. Once started, such an infection may be impossible to control without sacrifice of large parts of the hand or even of the entire extremity (Fig. 29–2). This type of complication is dire, it can be life-threatening and, saddest of all, it is usually quite avoidable by early and simple measures of wound care.

Inadequate Physical Examination

A complete physical examination of the hand is quite simple; if done in an orderly and organized manner, it takes but a few minutes. It requires

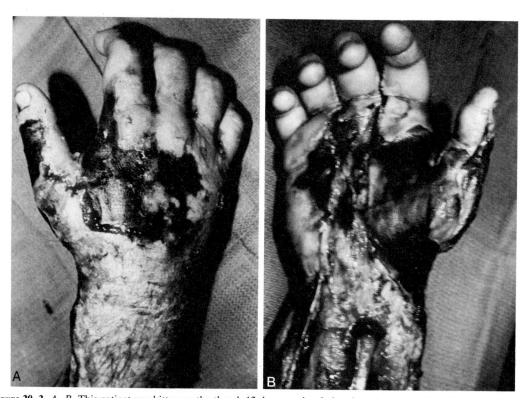

Figure 29–2. A, B, This patient was bitten on the thumb 12 days previously in a barroom brawl. The history was ignored, the wound was irrigated and sutured, and antibiotics were started. There was progressive pain, edema, and tissue necrosis extending into the forearm, as a mixed anaerobic-aerobic life-threatening infection ensued. The final result is loss of the thumb and all intrinsic flexors in the hand and forearm.

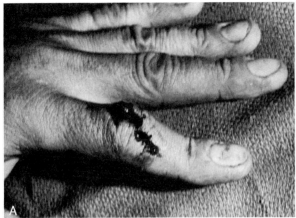

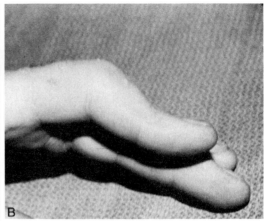

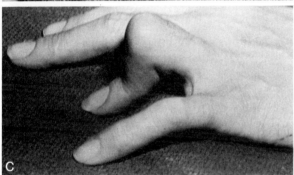

Figure 29–3. A, Small laceration over proximal inter-phalangeal joint. There is normal active flexion but active extension lacks 30°. The wound was sutured but no splint was used. B, The wound healed 2 months later. The proximal interphalangeal joint is painless, with full extension but lacks 45° of extension. Hyper-extension of the distal interphalangeal joint is begin-ning, and there is an early boutonnière deformity; this can still be salvaged by extensor reconstruction. C, This boutonnière deformity developed from an injury similar to that shown in 3A; the joint is now beyond reconstruction.

patient cooperation, and this requires the patient to have confidence in the examiner. Gentleness and reassurance are better tools for a good examination in a freshly wounded patient than is anesthesia or analgesia. Pain is not great with most hand wounds for the first hour or two, unless potentiated by anxiety. Perform the examination with the patient supine and the arm and hand outstretched on an arm board. Reassure the patient that the examina-tion will not cause pain. Assess the wound visually. Wash or wipe away blood; if bleeding continues, control it with finger pressure on the artery proximal to the wound or with a blood pressure cuff on the upper arm. Pump the cuff pressure to approximately 250 mm Hg. This is easily tolerated for at least 15 minutes by most patients.

In inspecting the wound, one should determine the degree of tissue damage and the degree of contamination. Are the skin edges lacerated or are they torn or bruised? Is exposed muscle torn, dis-colored, or ischemic? Is there gross distortion of the hand? Any hint of fracture or dislocation re-quires x-ray examinations in the anteroposterior, lateral, and oblique planes. Lastly, and with a minimum of manipulation and probing, determine if deeper structures such as tendons and nerves are involved.

After this search, active participation of the pa-tient in the examination is necessary. Severed flex-ors or extensor tendons are missed, not because they are difficult to diagnose, but because they are not looked for. Frequently missed are a severed flexor pollicis longus and severance of any of the flexor digitorum profundi and the two extensors of the thumb. Easy to overlook is the severed or ruptured central slip of the extensor digitorum com-munis over the proximal interphalangeal joint of a finger, which can lead to development of a bouton-nière deformity. The tendon may be avulsed by forcible flexion of the joint while it is held rigidly in extension or, more commonly, by a blow by a sharp or blunt object directly on the dorsum of the joint. There may or may not be an open wound. The only hint as to tendon involvement is inability of the patient to extend the proximal interphalan-geal joint actively the last 30°. Flexion will be normal, and the joint will have normal passive range of motion. If such an injury is left unsplinted, boutonnière deformity will gradually develop during the next few weeks; and what was originally an injury easy to treat will have progressed to a serious deformity impossible to correct completely (Fig. 29–3).

Severed nerve trunks and motor and sensory branches of nerves go unnoticed if not specifically examined for, and the place to look is generally not in the wound itself but distal to the wound, where a simple motor and sensory examination will tell the story. Obviously, it is important to perform such an examination before any anesthetic, either local or regional, is given. Tiny lacerations caused by glass slivers, knife points, or woodworking tools

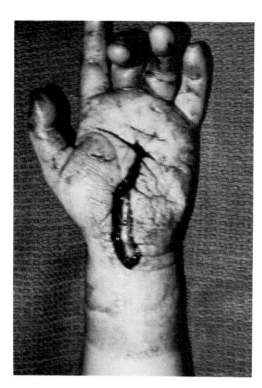

Figure 29–4. Glass laceration of child's hand. The wound was not explored; lack of index finger flexion was noted, but no sensory examination was done. The wound was primarily closed, and the child was referred to a hand surgeon "for a simple tendon repair." Later surgery revealed a glass sliver in the palm overlying the arborization of the median nerve; all sensory branches of the median nerve had been severed. The parents claimed that the nerve had been injured after the accident, and the jury agreed, because the emergency room physician had made no notation of a sensory examination of the hand.

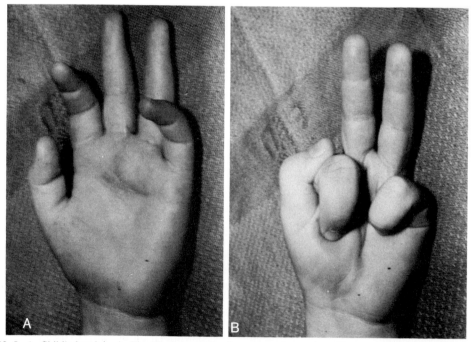

Figure 29–5. *A,* Child's hand (as in Fig. 29–4) 1 month after palmar laceration. The wound was primarily closed. The emergency room physician claimed that adequate examination of hand could not be done as the "child was frightened and crying." *B,* Subsequent surgery revealed transection of flexors of middle and ring fingers, as well as of common digital nerves to second and third clefts.

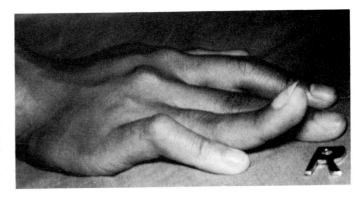

Figure 29–6. Ring finger injured while playing basketball. The emergency room note stated that "patient can make a fist and x-rays are negative." The rupture of the flexor digitorum profundus was missed, and resulted in this deformity.

may look inconsequential but may overlay combined tendon and nerve damage, which is obvious only if one specifically examines for such damage.

The dilemma of the delayed tendon rupture is typified by the patient who has lacerated the volar aspect of the base of the finger or thumb, has had the wound sutured in the local emergency room, and then discovers a day or two (or occasionally a week or more) later that some or all interphalangeal flexion in that digit has been lost. Quite understandably, the patient believes that the treating physician missed the diagnosis, whereas the physician will claim that the tendon had normal function at the time of examination and subsequently ruptured. The latter explanation is occasionally valid, due to unrecognized hemisection of the tendon followed by rupture under stress, but valid only if the examining physician has made a note to the effect that the function of the tendon(s) in question has been examined. Lacking that documentation, the jury will find for the patient (Figs. 29–4 and 29–5).

Most acute hand wounds are seen in hospital emergency rooms. Unless they are obviously very severe wounds, they are treated by emergency room physicians or by junior house staff who are often unskilled, untrained, or disinterested in accurate examination of the hand. Undetected tendon and nerve injuries are commonplace, and what might have been simple to treat becomes complex, leading to other complications, both medical and legal. A precise though simple examination, which takes only a few minutes, could prevent most of them (Figs. 29–6, 29–7, 29–8, and 29–9).

Inadequate Wound Care

The most common and most serious complication of wounds of the hand is infection. Most infections result from poor wound management, although a few may develop regardless of the treatment given. If, however, our understanding of wound healing is sound, our examination thorough, and our treatment meticulous, serious infections will be less frequent.

All wounds are contaminated. The challenge is to decontaminate them as much as possible, to remove anything that will foster the proliferation of bacteria, and to support all that contributes to wound healing. The bacteria introduced to the wound are opportunistic; they will cause infection if the environment and the tissues of the wound are conducive to their multiplication. All healing is dependent on good circulation. Blood must bring in the defense mechanisms—primarily the polymorphonuclear leukocytes without which bacteria cannot be controlled—and blood is required to nourish the surrounding tissues that will supply the fibroblasts, which are the building blocks of wound healing.

It follows that removing all damaged tissue, for-

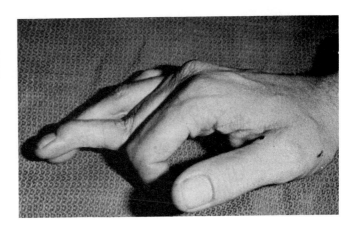

Figure 29–7. Middle finger forcibly hyperextended in football. The emergency room physician noted that "patient can make a complete fist and x-rays are negative." The rupture of the flexor digitorum sublimis was missed, and resulted in this swan-neck deformity.

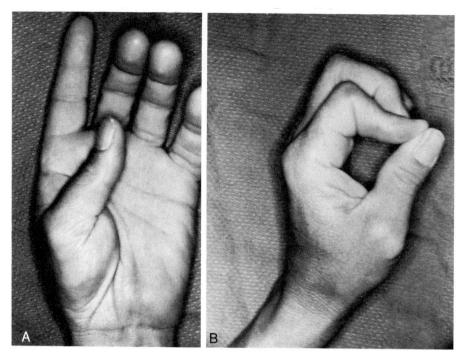

Figure 29–8. A, B, The patient lacerated the thumb 1 month previously in proximal flexion crease with paring knife. The wound was primarily sutured in the emergency room but no note was made regarding active motion of the thumb. The patient claims she was unable to bend the tip of the thumb at that time; the physician said she could. The patient has obvious severance of flexor pollicis longus but, due to inadequate physical examination or inadequate documentation, it is impossible to tell whether the tendon was severed by the knife or hemisected and later ruptured.

eign material, and debris that interfere with good blood supply and harbor and nurture bacteria will promote orderly healing. *Débridement* is the key to this. Many infections that develop in wounds of the hand are caused by omission of this most important part of treatment, probably the *most* important. It is done in two ways, instrumental and hydraulic.

Both may be necessary, depending on the nature of the wound. Instruments are used to remove all foreign material that harbors bacteria, or anything conducive to their multiplication, specifically tissue deprived of circulation and for which circulation cannot be re-established. Foreign material is removed by forceps and devitalized tissue by scalpel

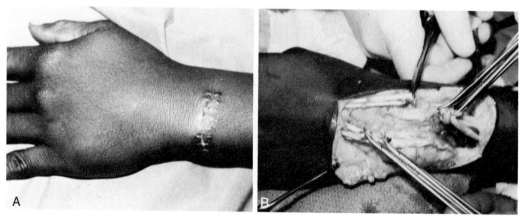

Figure 29–9. A, This patient was lacerated 6 weeks previously by a razor. "Bleeding was profuse." *B,* The treating physician concentrated on suturing the wound but neglected to do a simple motor examination of the hand. All extensor tendons to the index, middle, ring and small fingers have been severed.

and scissors. The hydraulic method uses lavage. A jet of fluid, preferably pulsating, is used to flush out debris and the unseen bacteria from nooks and crannies in the wound. It has been clearly shown that copious lavage effectively delivered can decrease the number of bacteria in a badly contaminated wound to well below the number of bacteria necessary to cause infection.

Failure to remove *devascularized tissue* from a wound (usually muscle and fascia), or allowing fluids to collect, will furnish the bacteria a medium in which to multiply. Failure to reduce the number of bacteria to less than $10^5/mm^3$ of tissue will allow them to proliferate, even in healthy tissue. Antibiotics are a poor substitute for inadequately cleaned wounds. Most patients with well-débrided wounds that have been copiously lavaged and properly managed subsequently don't need treatment with antibiotics. In fact, the unnecessary use of antibiotics produces other complications, such as drug sensitivities, changes in gastrointestinal flora, and the invitation to development of gram-negative infections.

Dead spaces and potential spaces will fill with fluids—exudates, transudates, and blood. These fluid accumulations are avascular and thereby devoid of body defenses, specifically white blood cells, and are thus excellent breeding media for bacteria. Dead spaces should be drained or left open, preferably the latter. Failure to do so is a serious error of omission, leading to infection and failure of wound healing. If great force has been applied to the hand in the wounding process, a crushing injury, it must be anticipated that edema will follow. Weeping tissues, the build-up of extracellular fluid and transudates, will cause both early and late trouble. Early problems stem from a mounting pressure head in unyielding closed spaces, which in turn impair venous drainage and lead to venous stasis, more pressure, and more edema, to the point at which arterial input may be jeopardized. The resulting dysvascularity then leads to tissue necrosis and bacterial proliferation. Furthermore, increasing pressure in confined tissues may lead to compartment syndromes, peripheral nerve degeneration and, ultimately, an irreversible situation, such as that which occurs with local ischemic contracture in the hand or Volkmann's ischemic contracture of the forearm.

Two steps must be taken to prevent such a vicious cycle. The first is to foresee such a chain of events in hands that have been crushed and to allow for expansion by opening all closed compartments by incisions, which includes splitting of all fascial boundaries of spaces. The second is to dress the hand properly with a fluff or sponge compression dressing applied from fingertip to elbow. The compression is mild—the dressing is barely snug—and must be applied uniformly without constricting bands. Lastly, the extremity should be suspended, with the hand held higher than the heart continuously until the threat of edema has subsided.

Poor Fracture Reduction

Open fractures of the hand offer both hazard and opportunity. The danger is that fractures will be neglected, that so much attention will be directed to the wound that the opportunity for accurate reduction will be lost. Fractures of metacarpals or phalanges left unreduced will quickly stabilize permanently in their position of deformity as muscles shorten, tendons and ligaments adhere, and fibrosis and scar form. They are usually easily reduced at the time of débridement, and can then be stabilized with Kirschner wires. The wires may be used to tranfix the fracture in a criss-cross fashion, may be placed through the intramedullary space, or may buttress the fracture fragments to adjacent solid bones. Traction is seldom required; it is difficult to maintain, prevents early motion, and may result in stiffening of the hand.

The opportunity for realigning a mangled hand is brief. After a day or two accurate reduction becomes increasingly difficult and, by the end of the first week, it may be impossible. The complications thus created in the case of metacarpal fractures are shortened metacarpals, which cause a relative lengthening of intrinsic and extrinsic muscle tendon units, loss of motion of metacarpophalangeal and interphalangeal joints, and fixed edema of the hand, which then progresses to permanent fibrosis (Fig. 29–10). Phalangeal fractures are relatively easy to reduce when associated wounds are treated. Their reduction is best retained with Kirschner wires, because splinting or traction will interfere with return to early motion. Once healing has started, reduction of the fracture and the deformity becomes increasingly difficult; for example, joints stiffen, or tendons don't glide. Although the wound may heal, the net result is a stiff finger that acts as an impediment to the rest of the hand.

ERRORS OF COMMISSION

Delayed Healing Due to Premature Closure

A wound from which all foreign material and devitalized tissue has been removed, in which a less than significant amount of bacteria have been left, that will not bleed, and that is in a hand that will not develop swelling, may be sutured and, with a bit of luck, will proceed to orderly healing by primary intention. If the surgeon cannot be confident that all these conditions are met, it would be prudent to use no sutures and to defer closure or coverage until they are fulfilled. Suture of hand wounds before these conditions are met represents *premature closure* and invites the development of infection (Fig. 29–11).

Closure of wounds in which the bacterial concentration is great (generally greater than $10^5/mm^3$) enhances bacterial proliferation. The contaminants

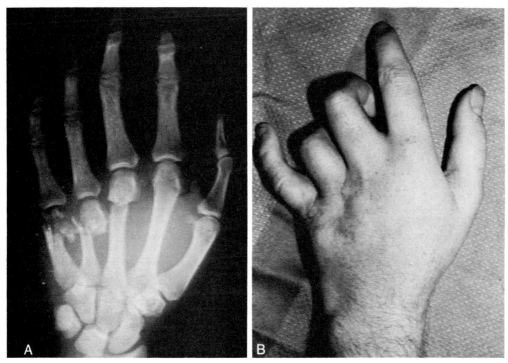

Figure 29-10. *A,* X-ray of punch press injury to hand, with bone loss and metacarpal shortening. "Loose fragments of bone" were discarded during debridement, and bony deformity and metacarpal shortening were accepted. *B,* The ulnar half of the hand is deformed, stiff, and functionless. Function could have been preserved if bone fragments had been retained and metacarpal length had been maintained with Kirschner wires.

then become pathogens, and the cardinal signs of infection will appear within the next week or so. The classic signs of infection are pain, swelling, redness, and heat, followed by pus. Such a chain of events stops the orderly progression of healing. The first phase, that of inflammation, becomes protracted, and does not progress to that of proliferation, in which fibroblasts should begin to form granulation tissue.

Closure of wounds under tension, increasing edema, the development of hematoma, and the pooling of undrained exudates can all halt the progression of healing, because each contributes to infection and to the overwhelming of body defense mechanisms in and around the wound. Occasionally, mixed anaerobic-aerobic organisms, once allowed to start their proliferation, become synergistic, and progressively defeat defense mechanisms as they march proximally up the extremity. Such vicious infections may start from small, poorly treated wounds, usually undébrided and primarily closed, and can cause irreparable damage to the entire extremity, or may even be fatal. Attempts to control them with antibiotics are often not only futile but may lead, in turn, to other complications. They must be dealt with by drastic débridement of all

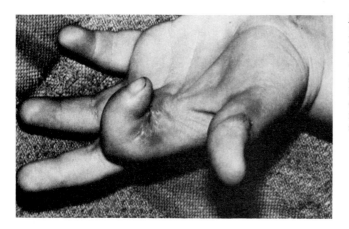

Figure 29-11. The hand of this child sustained jagged laceration and crush of fingers in a conveyor belt. The nerves and tendons were intact. The surgeon primarily closed skin flaps and "dressed finger in flexion to relieve tension on sutures." The wound did not accept closure and became infected, and volar skin and flexor tendons sloughed. The error was compounded by failure to débride the necrotic tissues and to splint the finger in extension.

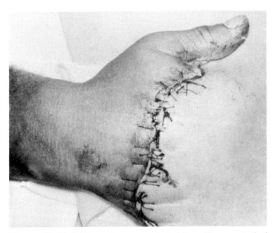

Figure 29–12. This patient amputated four fingers at their metacarpophalangeal joints with a chain saw. The surgeon, in his compulsion to cover the wound, buried it in the patient's stomach, doing neither the hand nor the stomach any good.

compromised tissue. This is not to say that antibiotics are not useful, but they must be carefully selected on the basis of sensitivity studies, which require accurate identification of the causative organisms. Antibiotics are dangerous if the physician depends on them to the exclusion of sound surgical principles.

There is a compulsion to suture among some surgeons and most emergency room physicians. Closing a wound to hide the nasty mess underneath may be tempting, but primary closure calls for both judgment and restraint (Fig. 29–12). If there is doubt as to whether the wound will accept closure safely, it is better to defer it. Any wound of the hand can safely be left open until such time as closure will be accepted. Granulation tissue does not start to form before the seventh day. If closure is done within this period—that is, delayed primary closure—healing by primary intention will still take place, the end result will be every bit as good as with primary closure, and some ugly complications may be avoided.

Some wounds, such as human bite wounds, should *never* be closed but should be allowed to heal by secondary intention. The scar may not be as attractive but that can always be revised; better the scar than loss of an underlying joint.

Premature Reconstruction

Wounds of the hand in which tendons, nerves, joints, and other functional structures are disrupted offer a multiple challenge: to heal the wound (remembering, of course, Paré's credo, "I dressed the wound and God healed it") and to repair or reconstruct damaged parts. "Tidy" wounds are those with relatively little contamination or tissue damage; they will often allow safe primary repair of severed tendons or nerves and primary closure of the

wound. When such wounds progress to uncomplicated healing by primary intention and satisfactory function of the repaired parts, the patient has, indeed, been well served.

If, however, the surgeon has compromised sound principle for the sake of convenience or compulsion, and has attempted to do too much surgery in a wound not receptive to it, the result will usually be a failure. Tendons that have been inexpertly repaired or that have been sutured in an unreceptive tissue bed will not glide, and will become bound down with adhesions along their entire length. This is particularly true of flexor tendons in the distal half of the palm and in the fingers. Primary neurorrhaphy done under less than ideal circumstances will fail more often than deferred nerve repairs. Furthermore, the secondary neurorrhaphy that must follow a failed primary repair has less chance of succeeding than if no primary attempt had been made. Primary nerve or tendon repair should only be attempted under ideal circumstances—for example, minimal contamination, slight tissue damage, "clean" lacerations—and only by experts.

The nature of the wound and the manner in which it is treated are the factors that determine whether or not reconstruction of deeper structures should be undertaken initially (primary) or should be staged for later surgery (secondary). The complications resulting from too much surgery done too soon are as bad or worse than those of too little surgery done too late. An example of this is primary skin flap coverage of wounds of the hand, such as an avulsion and loss of the skin covering the dorsum of the hand. After thorough débridement and restitution of skeletal alignment, the surgeon must decide whether to replace the missing skin immediately or to defer coverage. If the wound has been well débrided, if the element of crush is not great, if the surgeon has the technical competence to plan expertly and to execute a skin flap, and if adequate assistance and equipment, for example, are available, there is great advantage to doing as much as possible at the first operation and to establish a closed system promptly. If healing then proceeds uneventfully the surgeon's judgment will have been vindicated. However, if the skin transfer is done solely because "the wound must be covered," if the surgeon is not expert in such surgery, or if the wound is not conducive to uncomplicated healing, the complications can be dire, both in the hand and at the donor site.

Primary healing is ideal, but this ideal is unattainable in some wounds. In these the end result will be more satisfactory and complications fewer if surgical realism dictates a slower, if less dramatic, approach, in which primary attention is directed to wound management and reconstructive measures are postponed.

Immobilization

Wounded hands that have been allowed to stiffen represent both errors of omission and commission.

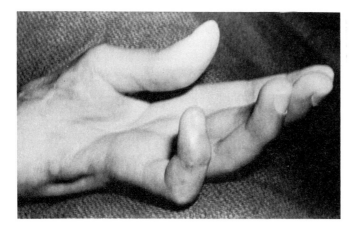

Figure 29–13. High-velocity missile injury to forearm resulted in ulnar nerve injury and to impaired circulation in hand, which led, in turn, to local ischemic contracture of the thenar muscles. The patient now has a flexion adduction contracture of thumb. He cannot abduct, extend, or oppose the first metacarpal and, therefore, cannot make a fist and lacks prehension. This fixed deformity could have been prevented by initially splinting the hand in the position of function.

Hands that have been well débrided, with fractures stabilized by internal fixation and properly dressed, will generally allow some active motion. The compression dressing should not be so snug as to prevent a few degrees of individual finger motion. A comfortable dressing, confidence by the surgeon, and reassurance to the patient will allow the patient to become involved in self-rehabilitation within a day or two of injury. Rehabilitation should start early, as soon as the wounds are treated. It is both naive and fruitless to defer active motion until the wounds are healed. By then the opportunity will have been lost, the hand will have begun to stiffen, and the road back will be long, and sometimes hopeless.

It is usually possible to effect a working compromise between adequate support of damaged parts and early motion. If joints must be immobilized, their position should be a physiologic one compatible with future function, a position that will not allow shortening of ligaments (Fig. 29–13). Perhaps the most common error in this regard is immobilization of metacarpophalangeal joints in extension, which allows shortening of the collateral ligaments and thereby prevents future flexion.

Experienced hand surgeons avoid most of the complications I have described. Their experiences with their own complications and with those of others have impressed on them that hand wounds must be appraised in an orderly and logical manner. This approach, coupled with sound surgical principles and an understanding of the physiologic mechanisms of wound healing, provides a clear picture of what should be done and what can be done, of what is possible and what is not. Healing of the wounded hand cannot be imposed by the surgeon; it must be cultivated.

Bibliography

Ariyan, S., and Krizek, T. J.: In defense of the open wound. Arch. Surg., 111:293, 1976.

Boyes, J. H.: A philosophy of care of the injured hand. Bull. Am. Coll. Surg., 50:341, 1965.

Brown, L. L., et al.: Evaluation of wound irrigation by pulsatile jet and conventional methods. Ann. Surg., 187:170, 1978.

Brown, P. W.: The prevention of infection in open wounds. Clin. Orthop., 96:42, 1973.

Brown, P. W.: The hand. *In* Hill, G. J. II (ed.): Outpatient Surgery, 2nd ed., Philadelphia, W. B. Saunders, 1980.

Brown, P. W.: Open injuries of the hand. *In* Green, D. P. (ed.): Operative Hand Surgery, New York, Churchill Livingstone, 1983, pp. 1129–1160.

Bunnell, S.: The early treatment of hand injuries. J. Bone Joint Surg., 33A:807, 1951.

Burkhalter, W. E., et al.: Experience with delayed primary closure of war wounds of the hand in Vietnam. J. Bone Joint Surg., 50A:945, 1968.

Butler, B., Jr.: Initial management of hand wounds. Milit. Med., 134:1, 1969.

Chuinard, R. G., and D'Ambrosia, R. D.: Treatment of human bite infections. Orthop. Trans., 1:158, 1977.

Conolly, W. B.: Spontaneous healing and wound contraction of soft tissue wounds of the hand. Hand, 6:26, 1974.

Edgerton, M. T.: Immediate reconstruction of the injured hand. Surgery, 36:329, 1954.

Elton, R. C., and Bouzard, W. C.: Management of gunshot and fragment wounds of the metacarpus (abstract). J. Bone Joint Surg., 55A:887, 1973.

Gross, A., Cutright, D. E., and Bhaskar, S. N.: Effectiveness of pulsating water jet lavage in treatment of contaminated crushed wounds. Am. J. Surg., 124:373, 1972.

Hamer, M. L., et al.: Quantitative bacterial analysis of comparative wound irrigations. Ann. Surg., 181:819, 1975.

Hampton, O. P., Jr.: The indications for débridement of gunshot (bullet) wounds of the extremities in civilian practice. J. Trauma, 1:368, 1961.

Iselin, M.: Emergency with delayed operation for wounds of the limbs. J. Int. Coll. Surg., 36:374, 1961.

Jabaley, M. E., and Peterson, H. D.: Early treatment of war wounds of the hand and forearm in Vietnam. Ann. Surg. 177:163, 1973.

James, J. I. P.: The assessment and management of the injured hand. Hand, 2:97, 1970.

Krizek, T. J., and Robson, M. C.: Evolution of quantitative bacteriology in wound management. Am. J. Surg., 130:579, 1975.

Louis, D. S., Palmer, A. K., and Burney, R. E.: Open treatment of digital tip injuries. Orthop. Trans., 3:332, 1979.

McCormack, R. M.: Acute injuries of the hand. Reconstr. Plast. Surg., 4:1574, 1974.

Rank, B. K., and Wakefield, A. R.: Surgery of Repair as Applied to Hand Injuries, 2nd ed., Edinburgh, E & S Livingstone, 1970.

Robson, M. C., Duke, W. F., and Krizek, T. J.: Rapid bacterial screening in the treatment of civilian wounds. J. Surg. Res., 14:426, 1973.

Smith, R. J., and Leffert, R. D.: Open Wounds in Hand Surgery, 2nd ed., Baltimore, Williams & Wilkins, 1975.

Tophoj, K., and Madsen, E.: Delayed primary operation for open injuries of the extremities, especially the hand (two-stage treatment). Injury, 2:51, 1970.

Trueta, J.: The Principles and Practice of War Surgery: With Reference to the Biological Method of the Treatment of War Wounds and Fractures, St. Louis, C. V. Mosby, 1943.

30

CONGENITAL ANOMALIES

Virchel E. Wood

Congenital hand anomalies comprise a very broad spectrum of deformity, the precise classification of which poses a major problem and is still widely disputed among surgeons. The most generally accepted classification is that adopted by the American Society for Surgery of the Hand.[44] Even with this system, however, not all congenital hand deformities fall neatly into one category, and often the traditional term is still the best. In this chapter the sequence of topics will follow a modified version of the international classification.

Only the unusual complications of the congenital anomaly or unusual problems inherited by the anomaly itself will be described. It will be assumed that infection, hemorrhage, hematoma, and anesthetic complications may occur in every operated case.

FAILURE OF FORMATION OF PARTS: ARRESTED DEVELOPMENT

Transverse Deficiencies

Amputations

Most congenital amputations have small remnants of tissue on the end of the stump. Obviously, the more severe the handicap, the greater the value of any functional capacity of a part. Thus, in severe bilateral deformity, the malformed parts are evaluated with a totally different attitude than are unilateral deformities. Great efforts should be made to convert rudimentary parts to functional units in severe bilaterally handicapped patients, even if the results are aesthetically poor.[3]

The little nubbins frequently associated with most unilateral amputations, however, serve only to signal to most observers the stigmata of a congenital deformity, which some societies consider to be a curse (Fig. 30–1). This, of course, can be very damaging psychologically to a young child. Remov-

ing a totally nonfunctional rudimentary part will improve the aesthetics and suggest a surgical or traumatic loss to the callous observer.

Hypoplastic Digits

An appealing method for gaining length for short stubby digits is to insert bone into the nubbins and thereby to push the skin distally (Fig. 30–2). The greatest danger is overzealous stretching of the tube when the bone is implanted. The shorter the insert, the better the circulation, but the functional gain is correspondingly reduced. Many lengthened digits end up with necrosis at the tip or with dead bone protruding from a red, granulating ring of skin.[20] Iliac crest bone tends to be absorbed with time. Toe phalanges make good donor bone, but good judgment is vital in establishing the length of graft to be inserted.

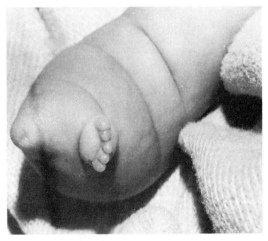

Figure 30–1. This child with an amputation through the midforearm has little nubbins present, which look almost like a foot.

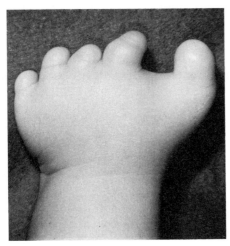

Figure 30–2. No bone is present in the little nubbins that remain as this child's fingers.

Lengthening of digits by slowly stretching the part with some type of device has become popular in recent years, especially for the thumb. The lengthening procedure is an alternative to pollicization or to toe-to-thumb transfer, both of which are fraught with many complications. However, because the procedure is slow and tedious, pin tract infections are almost inevitable, making immediate bone grafting dangerous. Other complications include reabsorption of the graft, fracture of the graft, nonunion secondary to infection, and loss of length in the stretched digit. An unusual complication is the development of an ulcer secondary to a tight-fitting stretching device (Fig. 30–3).

Central Longitudinal Deficiency: Cleft Hand

One should avoid the temptation to operate on an adult patient with a cleft hand that has been neglected during childhood, because these patients have usually acquired good function with their deformity. The worst treatment for someone with almost normal function with a wide deep cleft would be to close the cleft for aesthetic reasons. As Flatt has stated, "The typical cleft hand is a functional triumph, and a social disaster."[20] Cosmetic surgery usually has no place in the treatment of an adult with a cleft hand.

A prosthesis to cover the defect is also seldom indicated, because it usually inhibits function and in most people does not hide but draws attention to the deformity.[22]

Closure of the cleft is not simple. The original skin commissure caused by the cleft should be excised, because it is too far proximal to be rotated, transferred, or transposed distally. Some type of flap has to be fashioned distally, based on one or the other of the two digits, to form a good commissure closure.[2] The dorsal and palmar skin should be closed with interdigitating flaps to avoid the risk of contracture inherent in a straight line closure. Proper closure creates a zigzag line. It is wrong to

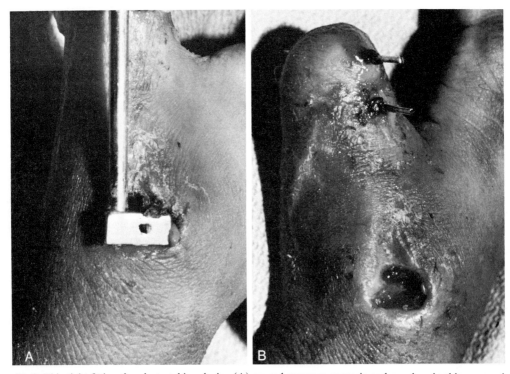

Figure 30–3. This tight-fitting thumb-stretching device (A) caused pressure necrosis and an ulcer in this uncomplaining child (B).

plan the incision so that the distal adjacent edges lie in the new commissure site, because subsequent healing will draw this junction into a very narrow V.

Many cases present with a marked thumb web contracture. Snow and Littler advocated transposition of the second ray to the third metacarpal after an osteotomy of both bones and removal of the remnant of the third metacarpal.[43] They described broadening the first web space by transferring the palmar pedicle skin of the cleft, with prior release of any syndactyly between thumb and index finger. The procedure is difficult, however, and may compromise some part of the skin edges. Furthermore, this procedure should not be attempted in a hand that has already had a standard thumb-index syndactyly release.

The skin flap is developed from the dorsum. The dorsal veins in the incisions must be carefully tied and not dissected off the flap, because the flap will be compromised without good venous drainage. These flaps should never be placed under tension, and one should always err on the side of putting in extra skin, if necessary, usually over the index finger.

How one tackles the problem of the metacarpals during a cleft closure is important. First, all excess bone must be excised. Then, some method must be devised for holding the metacarpals together. Barsky recommended drilling holes through the metacarpals and passing heavy chromic catgut sutures through the drill holes to bring the bones together.[2] He also advised that, if the remnants of the third metacarpal are removed, the origins of the adductor pollicis should be transferred to the fourth metacarpal to preserve motor function for the thumb. Simply putting sutures in the metacarpals, however, is generally inadequate, and there is still a tendency for them to spring apart. Carpometacarpal joint capsulotomies on the outer side may be sufficient to relieve some of the tension. Occasionally, an incomplete metacarpal osteotomy on the outer side of both of the metacarpals is needed. In some cases, a complete metacarpal osteotomy may be required to bring the two bones together. Some surgeons feel that one should try to create an intermetacarpal ligament with tendon or fascia, while others advocate putting a plug of bone between the two metacarpals to create a synostosis. In my experience, transferring the index ray to the long finger metacarpal remnant has proven to be the best way of stabilizing the metacarpals.[35]

If the ring and index metacarpals can be approximated satisfactorily so that there is not too great a divergence of digits, with a resultant central "hole," the long metacarpal should be preserved, because it tends to maintain a strong palm. It has been reported that, when the long metacarpal is preserved, there is not as great a problem with objects dropping through the gap between the index and ring fingers, as there is when the central metacarpal is excised to close the cleft.[36] Moreover, patients who have had cleft closure often have deep webs in the previous cleft area, even though the web may

have appeared normal after surgery. Evidently, these structures cannot keep pace with the growth of adjacent structures during the teenage growth spurt.

It is important to determine if the thumb can reach the ulnar digits before excising any central structures. Often, the only pinch possible is between the thumb and central remnant if the fifth ray is hypoplastic.

Crossbones or phalanges lying transversely should be excised, because they often block motion of adjacent digits and may keep the digits divergent from each other. Often these transverse bones are in fact the proximal phalanx of a deficient ray that is fused to the proximal phalanx of the adjacent ray.

There are several inherent anatomic problems in the cleft hand. The joints may be stiff and the digits may be improperly aligned. Although the digit may appear to be basically normal, the remaining longitudinal phalanx is not normal. It may later develop into a crooked phalanx, which requires an osteotomy to straighten the finger. The joints may have flexion contractures that are most difficult to overcome because of soft tissue defects. Capsulotomies are usually not helpful. If the collateral ligament structures are deficient, they can be reinforced or advanced to overcome the laxity, but results of these procedures are usually poor.

The lobster claw hand may have only one digit. There are two major ways to handle this problem. The first method, transferring a toe to the hand, can now be accomplished by many surgeons with the use of microvascular techniques.[39] The second technique involves creating a composite pedicle tube to provide an oppositional strut.[2] However, the tube pedicle post is a poor alternative, because the bone tends to reabsorb, and there is marginal feeling in the post. Both these factors lead to poor function.

Ulnar Longitudinal Deficiency: Ulnar Club Hand

Any result with the ulnar club hand may be poor because of inherent deformities in the elbow. The elbow may be rigidly fixed in either extension or flexion by a radiohumeral synostosis; even if it is functional, there is usually some limitation of motion. The elbow may be unstable due to a deficiency of the ulna and interosseous membrane, or to dislocation with proximal migration of the radius. Improved function of the elbow can sometimes be obtained by releasing contractures or by resecting the radial head.

Rotational deformity of the forearm may occur with growth. The wrist usually deviates toward the absent ulna. The ulnar fibrocartilaginous remnant, or anlage, has been blamed for wrist deviation secondary to its tethering effect. With growth, the anlage may cause radial bowing and a differential radial epiphyseal growth. Wrist deformity may then require resection of the ulnar remnant and a wedge osteotomy of the radius.

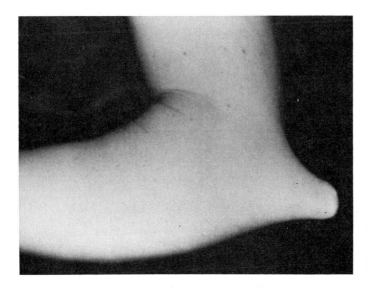

Figure 30–4. If radial head dislocation is not relieved by resection of the anlage and sometimes by removal of the radial head, the radial head may actually erode through the skin.

There has been considerable controversy regarding whether or not the anlage causes complications.[6] Most authors agree that the anlage should be resected if there is progressive bowing of the radius, dislocation of the radial head, or increasing ulnar deviation of the hand.[7] However, bowing of the radius may reflect asymmetric growth of its distal epiphysis unrelated to the presence or absence of an ulnar anlage. Thus, a routine exploration of the forearm of all children with distal ulnar deficiencies to remove the fibrocartilaginous anlage does not appear to be indicated.[6]

On the other hand, early resection of the fibrocartilaginous remnant can prevent shortening, radial bowing, and malrotation of the forearm. If radial head dislocation is not relieved by resection of the anlage, and sometimes even by removal of the radial head, the radial head dislocation becomes unsightly and interferes with elbow extension, supination, and pronation (Fig. 30–4). If there is enough ulna present to give the forearm stability the radial head may be resected, although this is rarely done in children.

However, if there is considerable forearm insta-

bility, elbow motion restriction, and marked shortening of the radius due to bowing, creating a one-boned forearm is one way of solving this problem. Because of vascular anomalies and insufficiency this should be done very cautiously. Volkmann's ischemia has been reported following this surgical procedure.[37]

Finally, because the ulnar artery and nerve are very closely associated with the anlage distally, injury to the artery and nerve is always possible during surgical removal of the anlage. This complication will further cripple an already severely compromised arm.

FAILURE OF DIFFERENTIATION (SEPARATION) OF PARTS

Symphalangism

Occasionally one sees adults who have grown up with this condition. In comparison with their normal peers, there is no doubt that they have impaired function (Fig. 30–5). Most have adapted so well, however, that they often will not admit to being

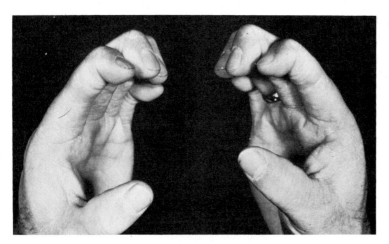

Figure 30–5. This adult with symphalangism has compensated for his lack of proximal interphalangeal flexion with increased flexion of his distal interphalangeal joints.

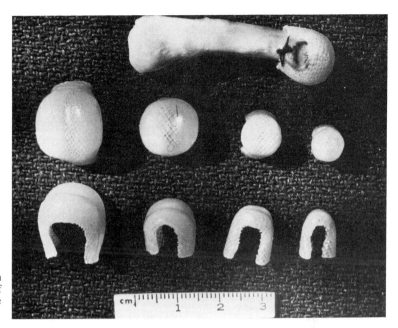

Figure 30–6. Attempts have been made to cap the fused joints of small children. These are some designs created by Flatt.

greatly handicapped, although most cannot grasp many objects in the normal single-handed manner. One report described a woman who had learned to milk cows effectively with her rigid digits, while another paper commented adversely that these patients appear to be engaged in less skilled or less remunerative occupations than their nonafflicted contemporaries.[13, 23]

Although several forms of therapy such as fusion, manipulation, and arthroplasty are available, I have never attempted to restore motion surgically to the stiff digits of an adult.[21] Stiffness of the distal interphalangeal joint is not a significant functional handicap, and none of my patients have been interested in attempts to improve function by fusing the proximal interphalangeal joint into a so-called functional position. One of my patients had a fusion of the proximal interphalangeal joints elsewhere, and was extremely dissatisfied with his resulting "hook."[21] He had been much happier and had better function with his proximal interphalangeal joints straight.

In patients with a single stiff proximal interphalangeal joint in an otherwise normal hand, attempts to restore motion by substitution with an articulated metal or silicone prosthesis have been uniformly unsatisfactory. These prostheses can withstand the relatively weak forces passing through a rheumatoid hand, but should not be expected to resist the major stresses within a normal adult hand.

I believe, therefore, that adults who have adapted to their deformity should not be offered surgery, and great caution is urged in recommending surgery for those who do seek advice.

In children, the problem of movement for stiff digits cannot be solved by a prosthesis with intermedullary prongs or a silicone stem because of the risk of damage to growing epiphyses. Although the radiographs appear to show a joint space, at surgery

one encounters a solid bar of cartilage connecting the two phalanges, and no joint space can be found. In such cases, it is not feasible to expect restored joint movement after a portion of cartilage has been excised. Hematoma fills the space, becomes rapidly organized, and the digit stiffens once again. Repeated failures have also resulted from attempts at various types of excisional arthroplasty, with or without the use of interpositional autogenous tissue. Despite the fact that both flexor and extensor tendons are found in these digits, patients treated in this way cannot maintain their early voluntary postoperative motion. Within 6 months the steadily increasing fibrosis will prevent even passive motion.

Because of the repeated dissatisfaction with conventional arthroplasty procedures, Flatt inserted a variety of differently shaped inert materials between the bone ends (Fig. 30–6). Preliminary reports,

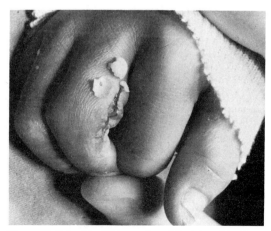

Figure 30–7. In this child, capping of the joint with silicone resulted in failure and breakage of the cap.

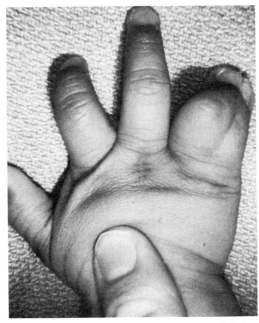

Figure 30–8. This child developed an irreversible bony deformity because the syndactyly was not separated early in life.

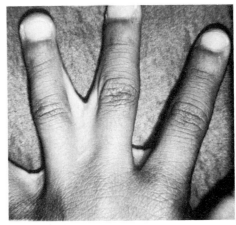

Figure 30–10. A plastic surgeon had repaired this child's syndactyly 7 years ago, but the deformity has recurred.

however, showed that many technical problems remain to be overcome, and that the functional results of this type of surgery when compared with that of a normal hand are poor (Fig. 30–7).[15, 16, 18]

Syndactyly

There are three forms of syndactyly: simple, complex, and syndrome-associated. In the treat-

ment of syndactyly in which the bony elements are fused, it is imperative that the border digits be established early in life. The differential growth between the little and ring fingers, and between the thumb and index finger, can be so great that irreversible deformities of the bones and joints may occur if the syndactyly is not separated in the first 6 months of life (Fig. 30–8). On the other hand, previous review of syndactyly repair by Kettlekamp and Flatt has shown that more postoperative complications and less satisfactory results are obtained in children operated on under 18 months of age.[27] Therefore, if the complexity of the condition allows, surgery should be postponed until after this age.

In the early 1800s, syndactyly was treated by simply cutting the webbing between the fingers with a pair of scissors, thereby separating the digits. It

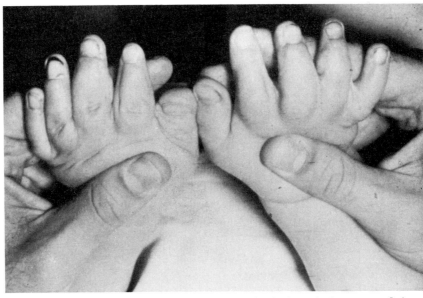

Figure 30–9. This child had a separation of all of his digits with a pair of scissors in the nursery. Only a poor result can occur from this barbaric treatment.

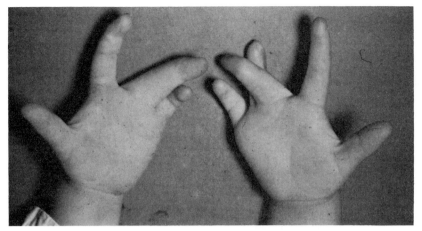

Figure 30–11. Contracture of the skin and bone in this child led to crooked fingers.

became apparent 10 or 15 years later that it was necessary to establish a commissure or web between the two fingers. This led to the first attempts to interpose a flap between the proximal ends of the fingers. Unfortunately, 175 years later one still sees patients in whom this concept of simply cutting between the fingers with scissors has been perpetuated. The young child shown in Figure 30–9 had a separation of a simple syndactylism of all the fingers by the scissor technique. One can see the usual result of this procedure: longitudinal scars and inevitable flexion contractures in all the fingers.

The most frequent long-term complication, even after the most careful and appropriate surgical separation of syndactyly involving skin only, is distal migration of the web or recurrence of the syndactyly (Fig. 30–10).[19] This complication occurs frequently regardless of the operative technique used, and switching from a dorsal flap to two triangular flaps or to some other method is not likely to help. The surgeon must keep to one particular operative technique until proficiency has been attained.

Skin contractures resulting in crooked fingers is another common complication of syndactyly surgery (Fig. 30–11). One immediate cause is the considerable amount of fat present in children's fingers. If this is not removed the flap may become very tight with postoperative edema, producing great complications in healing through necrosis and loss of tissue.

Scars on the digits must not be in straight lines, which can produce contractures (Fig. 30–12). The skin supplied must be thick and supple. There is no place for the secondary healing of granulation tissue that will lead to scar.

The type of skin graft used is important for the end result. Flatt has shown that full-thickness skin grafts give an infinitely better long-term result than split-thickness skin grafts.[20] Ninety percent of skin grafts will develop pigmentation, and heavy pigmentation will develop in blacks. Pedicle flap grafts have no place in syndactyly surgery, because the flap will look like a biscuit sitting on the finger (Fig. 30–13).

Parents of children operated for syndactyly must

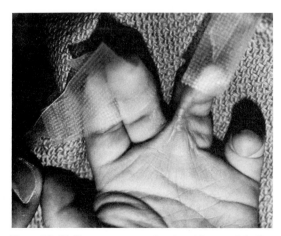

Figure 30–12. Scars must never be placed in a straight line because a skin contracture is the inevitable result.

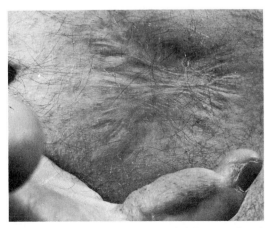

Figure 30–13. This pedicle flap applied for a syndactyly release looks like a biscuit sitting on the finger.

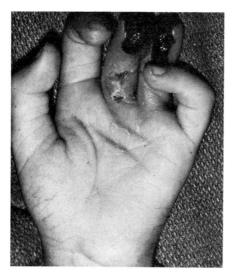

Figure 30–14. Because of a poor blood supply, this child developed gangrene following a syndactyly release and eventually ended up with stiff fingers and the loss of two fingertips.

be warned that during the teenage growth spurt the phalanges may grow faster than some of the postoperative scars, and contractures may result many years later. Because these scars will not stretch, secondary corrective surgery may be necessary.

Infection and poor blood supply may result in loss of the web flap and in excessive scarring. One axiom that most surgeons know well is that both sides of one finger should never be operated on at the same time, because two or three digits may receive their blood supply from only one artery. Also, it is easy to cut an artery in a very young child, even with operative magnification. In a child

with an aberrant arterial supply one may be horrified to discover necrosis and gangrene of one or two digits only a few hours after surgery (Fig. 30–14).

There is one other pitfall that is often seen when attempting to separate out and make two digits from two very hypoplastic parts. It is often better to realize one's limitations, and to strive for function in a part as a whole, than to make two nonfunctioning appendages (Fig. 30–15).

More extensive treatment is required to correct the jumbled skeleton of a very complicated syndactyly, such as is often encountered in Apert's syndrome or acrosyndactyly. It is unrealistic to try to obtain four fingers and a thumb from this sort of a problem. I feel strongly that one can do a disservice to patients if regular attempts are made to preserve four fingers rather than, on occasion, producing three satisfactory functioning fingers. In complicated syndactylism, such as in Apert's syndrome, it is important to establish early in life a skeleton that is as normal as possible to allow the development of a properly shaped and hopefully normally functioning hand. This means, in most cases, using the good judgment to create a three-fingered hand (Fig. 30–16).

Soft Tissue Contracture

Pterygium Cubitale

Very little is recorded in the literature about treatment of this anomaly. Schramm has described a case in which the range of extension was bettered by only 15° with surgery because the blood vessels and nerves prevented further opening of the web.[40] He recommended that, because one can

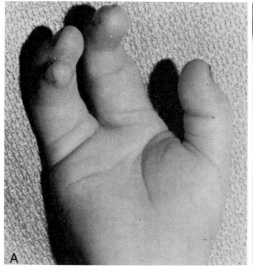
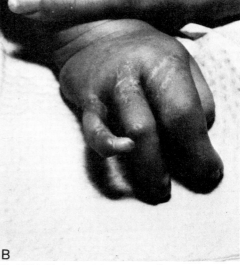

Figure 30–15. A, The little finger in this child is extremely atrophic. There are no functioning tendons. It is best to realize the limitation and to allow these two fingers to function together as one. B, This poor result occurred because someone tried to make something good out of almost nothing.

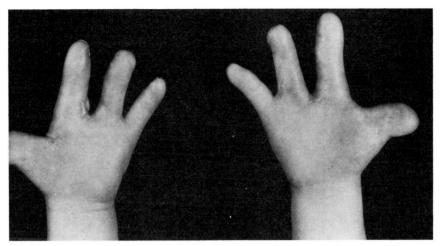

Figure 30–16, This child with a complicated syndactyly in Apert's syndrome had an immediate planned series of operations to make a three-fingered hand.

expect very little functional gain, surgery should not be done. It seems tempting to suggest a Z-plasty and skin graft operation for such a large skin web (Fig. 30–17). However, I have seen several cases of Z-plasties and skin grafts applied to the elbow webbing, with very little gain in function, motion or cosmesis. Surgery is probably not indicated in this syndrome, and with it one can only hope for a minimal cosmetic improvement at best.

Trigger Digit

Of the trigger thumbs discovered at birth, 30% recover spontaneously in 1 year. Of the trigger thumbs discovered between the ages of 6 and 30 months, 12% recover in 6 months. If a trigger thumb develops in a child over 3 years of age, however, it almost never improves spontaneously, so it is wise to operate as soon as acceptable in this age group. Of the trigger thumb release surgeries delayed be-

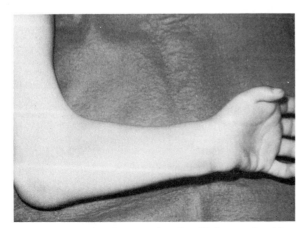

Figure 30–17. One is tempted to do a Z-plasty and a skin graft to such an elbow contracture, but such a procedure would be futile.

yond the age of 4 years, 50% have a residual flexion contracture.[12]

The only real complication in this anomaly is the severing of one of the digital nerves. The reason for this complication is anatomic, because both nerves hug the flexor tendon and one or both can be easily cut by a slight deviation of the knife or scissors in either direction.

Thumb-Clutched Hand and Thumb Web Contracture

In the thumb-clutched hand, the extensor pollicis longus or brevis, or both, are either absent or are weak and attenuated.[9, 48] Although the extensor indicis proprius would be ideal for a tendon transfer, the thumb deformity may be accompanied by affected fingers, with the involvement diminishing from radial to ulnar. Therefore, the extensor indicis proprius may be abnormal and unavailable for transfer (Fig. 30–18). For the same reason the flexed thumb, resulting from the absence or weakness of the extensor pollicis longus and the extensor pollicis brevis, is usually associated with a characteristic droop of the index finger because the muscles originate at almost the same anatomic site. Flatt recommended using the brachioradialis prolonged with a graft for restoration of extensor pollicis longus function.[20]

The contracted thumb web space is an important component of many congenital thumb anomalies.[5] It can be handled with a Z-plasty, a four-flap Z-plasty, a dorsal rotation flap, or a pedicle flap from a distance. Releasing the skin alone, however, may not be enough. At the same surgery one may need to release the adductor and flexor brevis muscles from their insertions, as well as releasing the first dorsal interosseous from the thumb metacarpal. The flexor pollicis longus may also need to be lengthened.

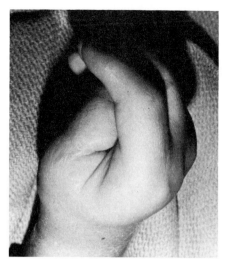

Figure 30–18. This child has had a tendon transfer using the extensor indicis proprius for the extensor pollicis longus, with no success. One must remember that the extensor indicis proprius may also be abnormal if the thumb extensors do not function.

Usually a simple Z-plasty is not enough, because skin is seldom the only structure contracted. A four-flap Z-plasty is often better because the skin is lengthened and the web space is also deepened.[55] A distant flap is a poor choice because it always leaves an unsightly and unyielding blob of skin around which the thumb must work. A dorsal rotation flap works well in most cases, although extra skin graft is always needed. An unsightly scar may be left on the dorsum of the hand, but this may be the only solution for the contracted thumb

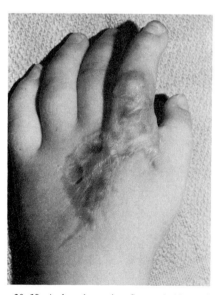

Figure 30–19. A dorsal rotation flap and skin graft left a very unsightly scar in this child. An infection in the graft site added thick scar.

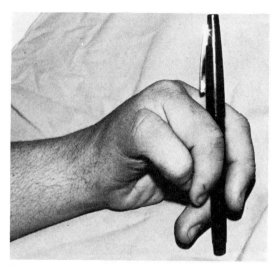

Figure 30–20. This adult has learned to function well with his hypoplastic thumb and contracted thumb web space. Surgery should be avoided.

web (Fig. 30–19). All constricted soft tissue must be released at the same operation. Following complete release of the soft tissues and good mobility of the thumb, tendon transfers may be performed. A tendon transfer will never work unless the thumb is free and mobile.

If a contracted thumb web space is allowed to remain throughout childhood, the index finger will function as a thumb in adult life. In these patients, with well-formed habit patterns, reconstructive surgery of the thumb becomes impractical and should be avoided (Fig. 30–20).

Finally, a real disaster is to lose a dorsal rotation flap because of tension, poor blood supply, or infection (Fig. 30–21). At this point many bridges have been burned, and a pedicle flap from a distance may be the only remaining solution.

Camptodactyly

If left untreated, camptodactyly will progressively worsen in 80% of the cases.[14] Camptodactyly seems to accelerate during the growth spurts, first between the ages of 1 and 4 years, and then during the pubertal growth spurt occurring between the ages of 10 and 14 years. It usually does not progress beyond 18 or 20 years of age.

The anatomic pathology has been summed up by Smith and Kaplan: ". . . virtually every structure at the base of the finger has been implicated as a deforming factor" in camptodactyly.[42] Consequently, the results of treatment are very unpredictable. There can be no single standard successful treatment because there is no single cause for the condition. Flatt noted that with conservative therapy improvement occurred in less than 20% of patients treated nonoperatively, but operative procedures resulted in improvement in only 35%.[14]

It appears that the natural history of this deform-

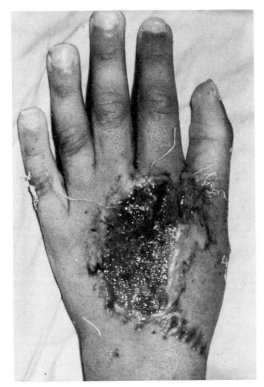

Figure 30–21. This dorsal flap was lost secondarily to infection and tension at the suture line, which is a disastrous complication.

ity is progression or no improvement in 80% of the patients, despite nonoperative or operative therapy, and the results of surgical intervention are usually unsatisfying. Berger and Millesi stated that "a successful result will be obtained only in children and adolescents. Corrective operations in adults should be no longer recommended."[4]

Thus, it is reasonable to advise most patients to live with their deformity. However, the young child with a strong family history and a marked contrac-ture, or the teenager who is going through a growth spurt and suddenly develops increased contracture, may need further treatment. Splinting can be tried first, especially if there are no obvious radiographic bony changes. The distal phalanx must not be used as one of the points of pressure during splinting, because this will force the distal interphalangeal joint into extreme hyperextension.

Division of the fibrous tissue on the palmar side of the hand has been most successful when performed before the age of 4 years. If the skin or capsule are contracted, and prevent passive extension when the wrist is flexed, soft tissue release surgery is contraindicated. Patients with bony changes at the proximal interphalangeal joint are not good candidates for attempts to decompress and remodel the articular surface. Increasing irregularity of the head of the proximal phalanx leads to increasingly poor results.

Numerous operative procedures have been attempted throughout the ages, including such senseless methods as cervical thoracic sympathectomy.[10] Frequent success has been obtained with simple release of the superficialis tendon, but this operation should be used only in early cases, before pericapsular fibrosis develops or before bony deformity is seen on the lateral x-ray.

If there is passive but not active correction of the proximal interphalangeal joint, and the proximal interphalangeal joint extension is weak, the surgery of choice in a young adult is transfer of the flexor superficialis tendon to the extensor apparatus, as advocated by Millesi and Lankford.[29, 33] Unfortunately, after many surgeries and much splinting, the end result is often as shown in Figure 30–22.

Skeletal Contracture: Delta Phalanx

This abnormality occurs in tubular bones, with a C-shaped rather than a straight proximal epiphysis. This arrangement of the epiphysis makes normal longitudinal growth of the digit impossible, and progressive angulation inevitable.

Figure 30–22. This lady has had several surgical procedures; the last one was completed when she was 19 years old. The end result is often unsatisfactory.

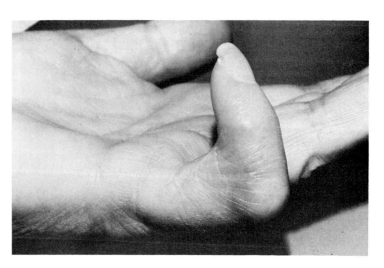

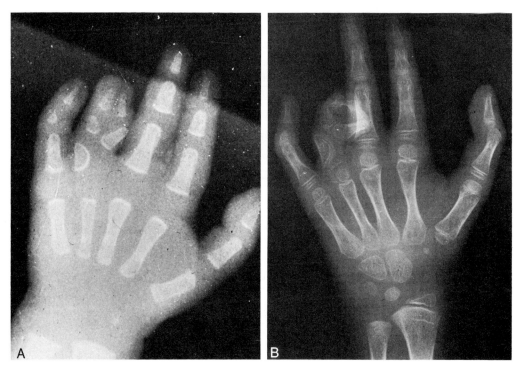

Figure 30–23. A, This child demonstrates a delta phalanx in association with central polysyndactyly. B, At the age of 16 years, the results of no treatment are clearly demonstrated. (From Flatt, A. E.: Problems in polydactyly. *In* Cramer, L. M., and Chase, R. A., (eds.): Symposium on the Hand, Vol. 3, St. Louis, C. V. Mosby, 1971, p. 160.

In central polydactyly associated with a delta phalanx, early removal of the accessory digit is indicated to prevent displacement of the normal phalanx from the longitudinal axis. The continued growth disturbance may necessitate further operation if not treated at an early age, or the finger with the delta phalanx may become useless and hypoplastic (Fig. 30–23). Sometimes treatment of central polydactyly requires sorting out the jumbled bones of a polydactyly within a complicated syndactyly. Creating a three-fingered hand may be the superior approach, and may lead to fewer surgical procedures.

Most authors recommend osteotomies for the delta phalanx, but the phalanx may be small and hard to handle.[8, 24, 25] With osteotomies there is a risk of destroying the terminal epiphysis and of arresting the growth of an already short digit. Power tool fragmentation may cause further shortening of these tiny bones.

Flatt has described the extreme difficulty of creating an osteotomy in infant bones and recommends patiently picking away with a small sharp bone cutter along the line of the cut.[22] However, an opening wedge osteotomy is difficult at best, and may have to be repeated during the growth period of the child. Very small bites must be taken between the jaws of the bone cutter, with care taken not to crush the bone, because it can easily splinter and shatter to powder. I have found that holding the wedge of bone in the proper place with a K-wire is

very difficult. The fragment is difficult to spear properly and is hard to hold (Fig. 30–24). Often, even though the procedure has been done under direct vision, one is horrified to see on radiograph the fragment sitting free and the correction lost.

DUPLICATION

Hyperphalangism

Hyperphalangism is characterized by an extra phalanx between the phalanges of a finger, usually excluding the thumb. Unlike polydactyly and polyphalangism, there are more phalanges in a finger but no more than the normal number of digits in the hand.[52]

Occasionally, the supernumerary bones in the index or middle fingers are confused with an old ununited fracture of one of the phalanges, sometimes resulting in unnecessary treatment.[11, 41]

Triphalangeal Thumb

The abnormal phalanx in the triphalangeal thumb is deviated and excessive in length (Fig. 30–25). It is better to have a short thumb than one that is too long. Most adults report that the extra long thumb significantly alters precision handling abilities and is a gross cosmetic defect.

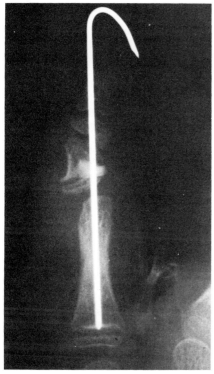

Figure 30–24. An opening wedge osteotomy of a delta phalanx with insertion of bone graft is a difficult procedure to accomplish. (From Wood, V. E., and Flatt, A. E.: Congenital triangular bones in the hand. J. Hand Surg., 2:190, 1977.)

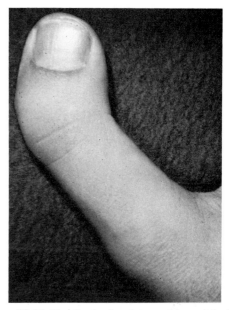

Figure 30–25. Usually the thumb is too long and deviates ulnarly. (From Wood, V. E.: Congenital anomalies. *In* Green, D. P. (ed.): Operative Hand Surgery, New York, Churchill Livingstone, 1982.)

Over 60% of triphalangeal thumbs have a narrow web space, which is a major deterrent to function, limiting dexterity and interfering with large object grasp with one hand (Fig. 30–26). Unfortunately, most children with triphalangeal thumbs become two-handed in most of their activities.

For a minimal thumb web contracture, a four-flap Z-plasty, as described by Woolf and Broadbent, is an excellent procedure to deepen the thumb web and to allow the thumb to drop away from the plane of the finger.[55] In most five-fingered hands with nonopposable thumbs, it is best to fill the thumb web with a large rotation flap from the dorsum of the hand or to do a formal pollicization of the thumb.

Of all patients with a triphalangeal thumb, 50% have thumbs that look like a finger, lying on the same plane as the fingers. With fingerlike thumbs, children cannot develop precision grip, and tend to

Figure 30–26. This man with a triphalangeal thumb has had several attempts to deepen the thumb web, but still remains with a narrow web contracture. (From Wood, V. E.: Polydactyly and the triphalangeal thumb. J. Hand Surg., 3:443, 1978.)

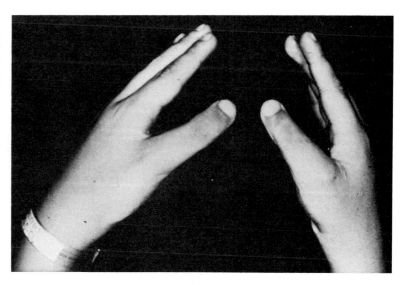

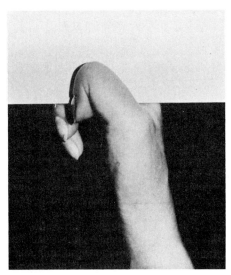

Figure 30–27. Children with a triphalangeal thumb have a side lateral pinch that prevents fine precision work. (From Wood, V. E.: Treatment of the triphalangeal thumb, Clin. Orthop., 120:193, 1976.)

grip things side to side between their index and long fingers. Most patients have a side-to-lateral pinch (Fig. 30–27). Spherical and cylindric grip is very difficult. There is really no true palmar pinch. The average pinch is extremely weak in these children. A pollicization of a finger for the thumb usually becomes necessary. For thenar muscle deficiency, the transfer of the abductor digiti quinti proprius to the position of an abductor pollicis brevis works beautifully.

All nonoperative treatments to straighten the triphalangeal thumb have failed. In fact, any type of corrective force applied to the distal phalanx tends to cause more pronounced retardation of the growth of the epiphysis.

Barsky popularized the technique of migrating the radial digit to the thenar region for the five-fingered hand.[1] This digit is migrated on a neurovascular pedicle in which the metacarpal is shortened and rotated. This is a difficult operation, with two frequent complications. First, there is usually insufficient skin, restricting the thumb from proper positioning in palmar abduction. This can usually be successfully overcome by using a very large dorsal rotation flap. The second complication is instability, with excess motion at the metacarpophalangeal joint. This can be partly alleviated by rotating the metacarpal head.

Even though complete removal has been advocated by several authors, I have frequently encountered instability of the thumb joint and lateral deviation following complete removal of the abnormal phalanx.[31] Total removal of the abnormal phalanx is better done as a subtotal removal, leaving any joint systems intact or even snugged to each other. It is simple and more reliable to wait until

there is enough bone with which to work, and then to fuse the delta phalanx either to the distal phalanx or to the proximal phalanx of the thumb.[51]

In children, if instability results with a retained abnormal phalanx, one must fuse the distal phalanx to the head of the abnormal phalanx or the abnormal phalanx to the proximal phalanx of the thumb (Fig. 30–28). The choice is made by determining the better joint (usually the one with better skin crease patterns), and by fusing the other to it. An osteotomy may be necessary, if deviation persists. In adults, when the extra phalanx is removed, it is necessary to fuse one joint of the thumb, because operations done to reconstruct ligaments from soft tissues have almost always failed.

Preaxial (Thumb) Polydactyly

Crooked digits and unsightly scars are a frequent complication after surgical correction of preaxial polydactyly (Fig. 30–29).[32] When removing an accessory digit it is best to leave a zigzag scar, because a linear scar does not stretch with growth, and the part distal to the scar deviates. All straight lines must be broken with at least a Z-plasty or, if a Z-plasty is not sufficient, with a rotation flap such as that described by Miura.[34] This is a dorsally based triangular flap from the dorsum of the thumb. The flap is transferred to the radial or ulnar side of the

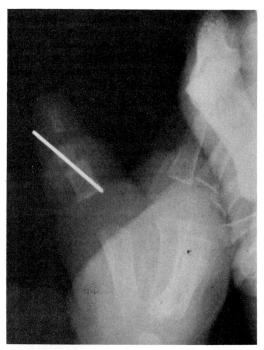

Figure 30–28. The best treatment of the triphalangeal thumb is to fuse the delta phalanx either to the distal or proximal phalanx of the thumb to make two stable joints. (From Wood, V. E.: Congenital anomalies. In Green, D. P. (ed.): Operative Hand Surgery, New York, Churchill Livingstone, 1982.)

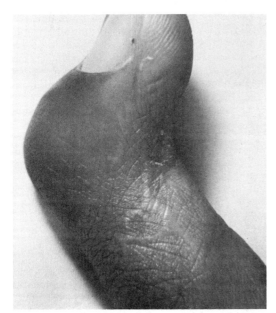

Figure 30–29. This boy had one digit of a polydactyly removed without regard for function or scarring, with this result.

interphalangeal joint, depending on which digit has been removed. A split-thickness skin graft covers the remaining dorsal defect. A rectangular type of flap may also be used as a secondary procedure for a contracted soft tissue scar following removal of the accessory digit.

In type 4 polydactyly, persistent angulation of the remaining digit is a frequent complication. If epiphyseal destruction has occurred in the remaining thumb, shortening or radial deviation of the thumb may occur rapidly during surgery.[17] Normally, in type 4 polydactyly, the duplicated phalanx diverges from the longitudinal axis. Early excision is important, because delay increases the displacement of each component. Osteotomy of the phalanx or fusion of the joint may also be necessary to retain normal alignment.

The operations for removal of the accessory digit are not simple. It is important to know which thumb the patient is using. Adequate function may require a transfer of structures from the accessory digit or from another part of the hand.

If both thumbs are equal in size, appearance, and function it is best to remove the radially placed digit, because the ulnar collateral ligament will remain intact on the ulnar digit, which is preferable to reconstructing a ligament. The transfer of extrinsic or intrinsic tendons into the retained thumb from the deleted thumb is often necessary to obtain the best possible composite thumb. When there is doubt about which thumb to remove, the thumb with greater flexion power should be retained, because good flexion is seldom obtained by tendon transfer while good extension may be.

If both duplicated thumbs are triphalangeal, am-

putation of the lesser thumb followed by removal of the extra phalanx in the remaining thumb, or by fusion of one of the interphalangeal joints to the extra phalanx, is the treatment of choice.[53]

Retention of a two-phalangeal normal thumb accompanying a triphalangeal thumb is obvious, but retention of a hypoplastic two-phalangeal thumb is a difficult decision. Stability of the joints is most important. If the extra phalanx is relatively large and if hypoplasia of the normal thumb is mild, one should retain the two-phalangeal thumb because of potential instability at the site of excision of the accessory phalanx. If a triphalangeal thumb is well aligned, well positioned, and stable, it may be wise to retain it, especially if the two-phalangeal thumb is badly deviated.

Ligament instability is a very frequent complication of preaxial polydactyly (Fig. 30–30).[45] Ligament reconstruction often does not work, even with the best of surgeons under optimal conditions. Because a reconstructed ligament will often stretch, it is extremely important to preserve the ulnar collateral ligament, if at all possible (Fig. 30–31). An intact radial collateral ligament is not as important for function, but even this ligament should undergo attempts at reconstruction using available tissue.

Lack of opposition may follow surgical excision of an accessory thumb, possibly because of abnormal muscle origins or of insertions in duplicated thumbs. The intrinsic thenar muscles, such as the abductor pollicis brevis and adductor pollicis, may be found inserting on one of the abnormal phalanges that is removed. Therefore, these muscles should always be transferred from the amputated digit into the remaining thumb for power and movement.

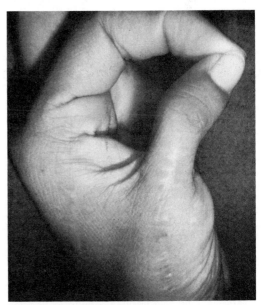

Figure 30–30. Even though a ligament reconstruction was attempted in this girl, the powerful forces generated in pinch soon destroyed and stretched her recreated ligament structures.

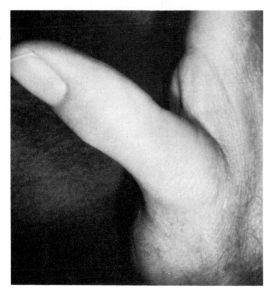

Figure 30–31. At birth this man had the ulnar-placed thumb removed. The end results of not maintaining an ulnar collateral ligament are readily apparent.

All of a complete or incomplete duplicated metacarpal head should be removed at birth, because the protuberance of an accessory metacarpal left behind from surgery may become a distressing problem in adult life. A large head may be reduced in size easily, as described by Miura.[34] A large thumb is cosmetically distressing. This is usually due to the presence of a remaining abnormal metacarpal head, extra bone, or excessively large metacarpal. If the metacarpal is wide at its distal portion, or has an accessory head, it should be narrowed.[30]

Early deviation and late Z-deformity may result from abnormal insertion of the tendons.[28] The Z-deformity is characterized by ulnar deviation at the metacarpophalangeal joint and by radial deviation at the interphalangeal joint of the thumb (Fig. 30–32). Multiple factors may cause this deformity, related to several different problems inherent in polydactyly. A contracted scar may contribute to this deformity. The Z-deformity may also be the result of insufficient function of the thenar muscles, especially the abductor pollicis brevis. Particularly important are the commonly found abnormal insertions of the flexor pollicis longus and extensor pollicis longus tendons. The flexor tendon usually abnormally inserts at the radial margin of the distal phalanx, and the insertion of the extensor tendon may also be slightly radial.

Miura brought our attention to the Z-deformity complication and its simple treatment.[34] He found that splitting the extensor tendon and translocating it to the ulnar side was unsatisfactory, because the flexor tendon was still left in an abnormal position. To correct this, the part of the extensor that is responsible for the deformation should be removed, and the flexor pollicis longus should be reinserted

to the ulnar side in one surgical procedure (Fig. 30–33). It is therefore important to look for these abnormal tendon insertions at the time of the original surgery, even though they are sometimes difficult to visualize. The flexor and extensor tendons should be identified, examined, and moved, if necessary. If not, they may have to be corrected with a secondary operation after removal of the accessory digit. Other abnormalities, such as connections of flexors to other flexors or extensors, connections between the flexors or extensors to each duplicate, and other anomalies, may be found at the same time.

If the Bilhaut-Cloquet operation is used, one should expect at least a line deformity in the fingernail. This is only a minor cosmetic complication, but must be fully explained to the parents before surgery.

Parents must be warned that the remaining thumb of a duplicated digit will never be normal.[47] Most often the joints remain stiff, and the thumb is usually smaller than the thumb on the other side.

Central Polydactyly

Central polydactyly is most often associated with a complex form of syndactyly. Therefore, this anomaly has all the complications of complex syndactyly plus a few of its own. The extra digit hidden in the polysyndactyly is usually very atypical in form. The nerves and blood vessels are anomalous,

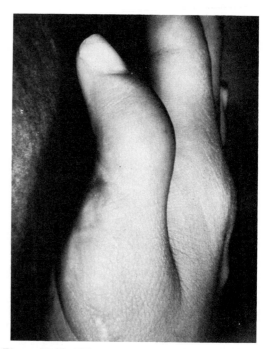

Figure 30–32. This preaxial polydactyly developed the classic Z-deformity of the thumb, with ulnar deviation of the proximal phalanx and radial deviation of the distal phalanx.

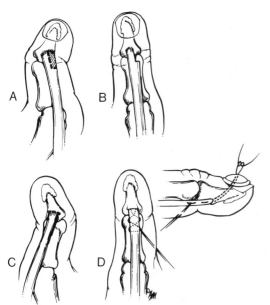

Figure 30–33. Treatment of the Z-deformity of the thumb is accomplished by removing half of the extensor pollicis longus *(A, B)* by reinserting the flexor pollicis longus into a slightly ulnar position *(C, D)*. (From Wood, V. E.: Congenital Anomalies. *In* Operative Hand Surgery, Green, D. P. (ed.): New York, Churchill Livingstone, 1982.)

and the tendon attachments may also show a great deal of variation. Most instances of polysyndactyly consist of a type 2 polydactyly, associated with a complicated syndactylism. The normal-appearing fingers may be atypical, with deformed joints. The metacarpal may be enlarged, distorted, bifurcated distally, or even fused. In many cases there are split tendons, or a central tendon with a wide split for two segments.

It is impossible to determine the full extent of any neurovascular anomaly until the area has been thoroughly exposed at surgery. Early surgical removal of the accessory digit is therefore recommended in type 2 central polydactyly. Early surgery is especially recommended in those cases in which both the normal and the duplicated digits articulate with the same phalanx, because displacement of the normal phalanx from the longitudinal axis often occurs, and the continued growth disturbance may necessitate additional surgery. The extra digit may have its own epiphysis, but these epiphyses do not necessarily lie in normal alignment.

When surgery is delayed, the supernumerary component and abnormal epiphysis tend to displace the normal components into a marked radial or ulnar deviation, and growth will continue in that abnormal direction.

Limitation of movement of the interphalangeal joints that are enclosed in the polysyndactyly may also occur following surgery. The decreased motion may be due to the presence of the accessory digit, incongruent joint surfaces, or abnormal motor elements. However, it is more often caused by inherent stiffness or occasionally symphalangism in apparently normal fingers. When all fingers are retained, there is often a tendency for a lack of longitudinal growth in one of the involved digits, particularly in the ring finger (Fig. 30–34).

After many disappointing attempts to maintain four fingers, Flatt recommended that the more complex central polysyndactyly be reconstructed to a three-fingered hand.[50] It might seem paradoxic to produce a functional three-fingered hand from a five-fingered hand, but I feel that this is often justified. A three-fingered hand would have been functional as well as socially acceptable in many patients whose rigid and useless reconstructed fingers were finally amputated. Creating a three-fin-

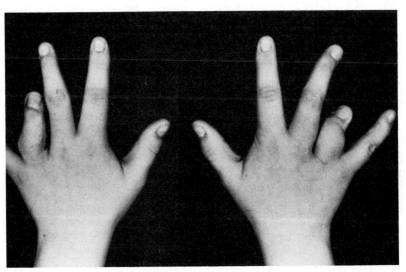

Figure 30–34. The ring finger in central polydactyly may show deformity, limitation of movement, and lack of longitudinal growth. (From Wood, V. E.: Treatment of central polydactyly. Clin. Orthop. 74:204, 1971.)

gered hand by sorting out the jumble of bones in a polysyndactyly may often be a superior method of treatment, requiring far fewer surgical procedures.[49]

Postaxial Polydactyly (Little)

For the type B postaxial polydactyly that consists of only a tag of tissue attached to the finger, surgery should be uncomplicated. Simply tying a suture at the base of the extra digit produces a blackened stump, which will drop off and may leave an almost invisible scar. However, it has been recorded that infants have bled to death following simple ligation of a digit.[20] If the extra tag has a somewhat enlarged bone, or if the knot was tied loosely, or has become untied, I have encountered some minor bleeding from a congested digit that did not necrose.

In type A postaxial polydactyly, or in the older child or adult with type B, formal surgical excision is preferred to remove the extra digit, particularly if there are bony connections.

The most common complication seen in follow-up is a large protuberance of the fifth metacarpal head on the ulnar border of the hand. Many postaxial duplications have a partial or complete reproduction of the fifth metacarpal. The bulging is usually caused by the excessive width of the double metacarpal head (Fig. 30–35). If the head of the

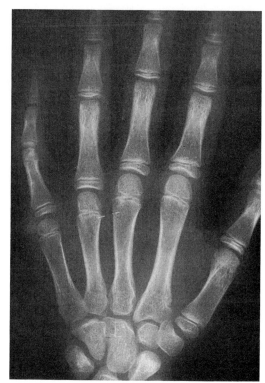

Figure 30–36. When a suture is used to remove a digit in the nursery, often the bony portion of the accessory digit is left behind.

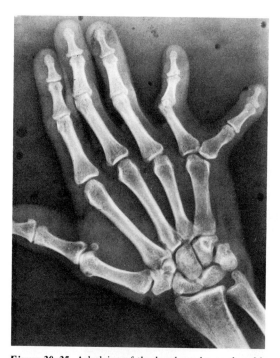

Figure 30–35. A bulging of the hand can be produced by the excessive width of the metacarpal head. The protuberance is often left behind unless the widest portion of the metacarpal is removed. (From Wood, V. E.: Congenital anomalies. *In* Green, D. P. (ed.): Operative Hand Surgery, New York, Churchill Livingstone, 1982.)

accessory digit articulates with the head of the fifth metacarpal, the protuberance will be left behind unless the metacarpal is excised and removed in its widest portion.

To remove this unsightly lump, the periosteum must be elevated and, assuming that the usual removal of the ulnar accessory digit has been performed, the ulnar collateral ligament and other tissues on the ulnar side of the extra digits must then be moved out of the way by sharp or blunt dissection. This allows oblique trimming of the metacarpal head. Following bone removal, it is very easy to reattach and tighten the elevated ligament and periosteal tissues, thus giving good support to the ulnar side of the remaining little finger.

Not infrequently, a portion of an accessory digit will be left behind at the original surgery (Fig. 30–36). In later life the protrusion becomes a troublesome cosmetic complication. Repeat surgery then becomes necessary to remove the excess bone.

Crooked fingers and digit rotation are further complications of incomplete removal of a polydactyly (Fig. 30–37). Particularly in a type 3 polydactyly, when the extra ulnar digit is removed, its hypothenar muscular attachments must be moved over to the remaining little finger. Aberrant tendon attachments may restrict motion, or cause rotation of the digit by a constant unforgiving pull in a growing digit.

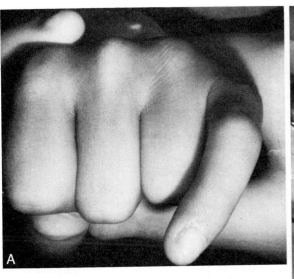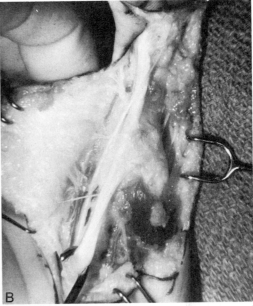

Figure 30–37. A, An accessory tendon with its abnormal pull caused malrotation of the fifth digit and a restriciton of flexion; *B,* at surgery, the abnormal tendon is shown inserting into the remains of an extra digit.

Ulnar Dimelia (Mirror Hand)

The mirror hand has many major inherent problems.[26] I will just briefly mention a few. Some of these abnormalities are shown in the preoperative photos of a child with eight digits (Fig. 30–38).

The elbow will almost always have limited motion in all directions regardless of the surgical technique, because the medial articular end of each ulna has turned around on its axis so as to make its olecranon fossa face the corresponding notch of its mate. The distal articular end of the humerus lacks a capitellum, and is composed of two ill-defined trochleas.

The wrist tends to remain flexed and ulnarly deviated, often making a wrist arthrodesis necessary because of the absence of wrist extensors, which occurs with the absence of the radial half of the forearm.

Most fingers maintain a flexed position because the extensor muscles are often absent or hypoplas-

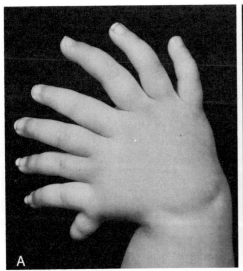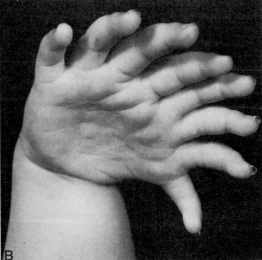

Figure 30–38. A, B, Preoperative photographs of a typical mirror hand with the findings of a flexed wrist radially deviated, and eight digits. (Courtesy of J. Dobyns. From Wood, V. E.: Congenital anomalies. *In* Green, D. P. (ed.): Operative Hand Surgery, New York, Churchill Livingstone, 1982.)

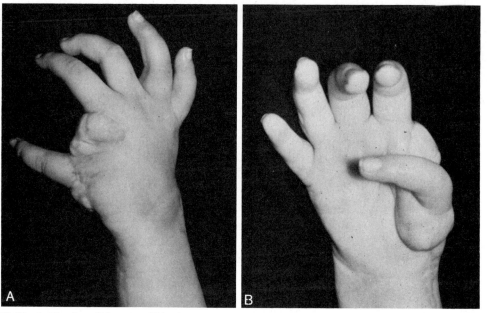

Figure 30–39. *A,* The first digit was pollicized to make a thumb, the second and third digits were filleted to make a thumb web, and the eighth ulnar digit was deleted. *B,* The amount of opposition present. These hands are never normal. (Courtesy of J. Dobyns. From Wood, V. E.: Congential anomalies. *In* Green D. P. (ed.): Operative Hand Surgery, New York, Churchill Livingstone, 1982.)

tic. If the digits cannot extend, surplus tendons may be used for transfer from amputated digits into the weak digits. The flexor carpi ulnaris may be transferred to the common extensors to improve extension.

Finally, a normal thumb can never be created because the intrinsic muscle function is weak. One must pollicize a finger, create a large thumb web out of an amputated digit, and even rotate the pollicized finger further with an osteotomy to aid the extremely weak opposition. In an attempt to gain even stronger opposition, one can transfer the strongest extensor tendon of one of the amputated digits to the pollicized finger. Even after performing all these multiple skilled maneuvers, however, one is almost always disappointed in the final result (Fig. 30–39).

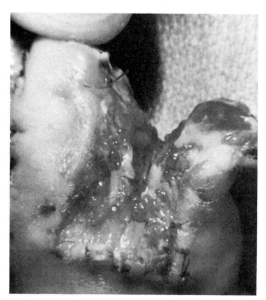

Figure 30–40. This child with a complicated acrosyndactyly developed an infection and lost the skin graft, the web for the commissure, and the normal skin on the digit.

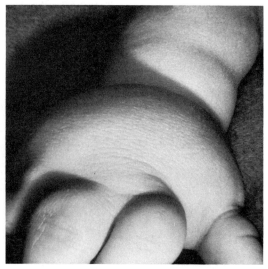

Figure 30–41. This constriction band in the forearm caused the entire hand to be edematous, swollen, firm, and functionally useless.

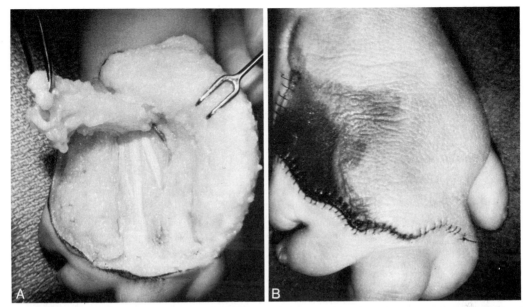

Figure 30–42. The firm fatty tissue is removed surgically *(A)*, but, because the tissue is not normal, the outer margin of the flap became dusky and necrotic *(B)*. One must be careful not to get too vigorous with the delicate skin.

CONGENITAL CONSTRICTION BAND SYNDROME

The most common form of constriction band syndrome seen has been labeled acrosyndactyly, which in most of the literature has been classified as a complex syndactyly. In a complex syndactyly such as acrosyndactyly, it is difficult to obtain good results. This is due to the fact that sinus tracts cause difficulty in designing local flaps, because neither the sinus nor the cleft is ever large enough for a normal web space. The epithelial tracts or tunnels should be carefully dissected out at surgery, and should never be buried beneath a skin graft. An epithelial sinus continues to secrete fluid if not opened and incorporated into the flaps.

In the literature, the results of most operated cases are poor because of flexed, crooked, or stiff fingers, or missing digit tips.[46] All the complications of syndactyly are possible in the treatment of acrosyndactyly (Fig. 30–40). Inherent in this anomaly are hypoplasia, brachydactyly, symphalangism, symbrachydactyly, camptodactyly, and congenital amputations.

Neurologic and vascular deprivation distal to the constriction ring is common, and the edematous tissues are firm and thickened rather than swollen and filled with fluid (Fig. 30–41). Because of decreased blood supply, many surgeons formerly recommended staged Z-plasty to remove the constriction band. More recently, though, some surgeons recommend releasing the entire band at one operation, but extreme care must be exercised to prevent necrosis at the tips of already shortened digits.

One other complication that occurs is necrosis of skin from a defatted limb (Fig. 30–42). One must never become too vigorous in attempts to do a procedure too rapidly. The skin is not normal in the way it reacts to trauma because of its decreased vascular and neurologic status.

References

1. Barsky, A. J.: Congenital anomalies of the thumb. Clin. Orthop., 15:96, 1959.
2. Barsky, A. J.: Cleft hand: Classification, incidence and treatment. J. Bone Joint Surg., 46A:1707, 1964.
3. Beasley, R. W.: Reconstructive surgery and the management of congenital anomalies of the upper extremity. *In* Swinyard, C. A. (ed.): Limb Development and Deformity Problems of Evaluation and Rehabilitation, Springfield, Il, Charles C Thomas, 1969, pp. 782–784.
4. Berger, A., and Millesi, H.: Spätergebnisee der operativen behandlung der Kamptodaktylie. Handchirurgie, 7:75, 1975.
5. Broadbent, T. R., and Woolf, R. M.: Flexion-adduction deformity of the thumb—congenital clasped thumb. Plast. Reconstr. Surg., 34:612, 1964.
6. Broudy, A. S., and Smith, R. J.: Deformities of the hand and wrist with ulnar deficiency. J. Hand Surg., 4:304, 1979.
7. Carroll, R. E., and Bowers, W. H.: Congenital deficiency of the ulna. J. Hand Surg., 2:169, 1977.
8. Carstam, N., and Theander, G.: Surgical treatment of clinodactyly caused by longitudinally bracketed diaphysis (Delta Phalanx). Scand. J. Plast. Reconstr. Surg., 9:199, 1975.
9. Crawford, H. H., Horton, C., and Adamson, J.: Congenital aplasia or hypoplasia of thumb and finger extensor tendons. J. Bone Joint Surg., 48A:82, 1966.
10. Currarino, G., and Waldman, I.: Camptodactyly. Am. J. Roentgenol., 92:1312, 1964.
11. Dell'Oro, B.: Hirperfalangia del indice y del medio. Día Médico (Buenos Aires), 7:1071, 1935.
12. Durham, J. M., and Meggitt, B. F.: Trigger thumbs in children. J. Bone Joint Surg., 56B:153, 1974.
13. Elkin, D. C.: Hereditary ankylosis of the proximal phalangeal joints. J.A.M.A., 84:509, 1925.
14. Engber, W. M., and Flatt, A. E.: Camptodactyly: An analysis of sixty-six patients and twenty-four operations. J. Hand Surg., 2:216, 1977.

15. Flatt, A. E.: Prosthetic replacement of finger joints. *In* Proceedings of the Third International Congress of Plastic Surgery, Washington, DC, Excerpta Medica, International Congress Series No. 66, 1963, pp. 945–953.

16. Flatt, A. E.: Presented at the Dixieme Congres International de Chirurgie, Orthopedie, et de Traumatologie, Paris, 1966.

17. Flatt, A. E.: Problems in polydactyly. *In* Cramer, L. M., and Chase, R. A. (eds.): Symposium on the Hand, Vol. 3, St. Louis, C. V. Mosby, 1971, pp. 150–167.

18. Flatt, A. E.: The considered use of digital joint prostheses. *In* Transactions of the Fifth International Congress of Plastic and Reconstructive Surgery, Melbourne, Butterworth, 1971, pp. 638–648.

19. Flatt, A. E.: Practical factors in the treatment of syndactyly. *In*: Symposium on Reconstructive Hand Surgery, Vol. 9, St. Louis, C. V. Mosby, 1974, pp. 144–156.

20. Flatt, A. E.: The Care of Congenital Hand Anomalies. St. Louis, C. V. Mosby, 1977, pp. 60–825.

21. Flatt, A. E., and Wood, V. W.: Rigid digits or symphalangism. Hand, 7:197, 1975.

22. Fort, A. J. A.: Des Difformites Congenitales et Acquises des Doigts, et des Moyens d'y Remedier, Paris, Adrien Delahaye, 1869.

23. Hefner, R. A.: Inherited abnormalities of the fingers. J. Hered., 15:323, 1924.

24. Jaeger, M., and Refior, H. J.: The congenital triangular deformity of the tubular bones of the hand and foot. Clin. Orthop., 81:139, 1971.

25. Jones, G. B.: Delta phalanx. J. Bone Joint Surg., 46B:226, 1964.

26. Kelikian, H.: Congenital Deformities of the Hand and Forearm, Philadelphia, W. B. Saunders, 1974, pp. 457–466.

27. Kettlekamp, D. B., and Flatt, A. E.: An evaluation of syndactylia repair. Surg. Gynecol. Obstet., 113:471, 1961.

28. Kleinert, H. E., and Greenberg, A. B.: Treatment of the reduplicated thumb. J. Bone Joint Surg., 55A:874, 1973.

29. Lankford, L. L.: Correspondence club letter, No. 1975–1. (3600 Gaston Ave., Dallas, TX, 75246, May, 1975.)

30. Mark, T. W., and Bayne, L. G.: Polydactyl of the thumb: Abnormal anatomy and treatment. J. Hand Surg., 3:107, 1978.

31. Milch, H.: Triphalangeal thumb. J. Bone Joint Surg., 33A:692, 1951.

32. Millesi, H.: Deformities of the fingers following operations for polydactylia. Klin. Med. (Vienna), 22:266, 1967.

33. Millesi, H.: Camptodactyly. *In* Littler, J. W., Cramer, L. M., and Smith, J. W., (eds.): Symposium on Reconstructive Hand Surgery, St. Louis, C. V. Mosby, 1974, pp. 175–177.

34. Miura, T.: An appropriate treatment for postoperative Z-formed deformity of the duplicated thumb. J. Hand Surg., 2:380, 1977.

35. Miura, T., and Komada, T.: Simple method for reconstruction of the cleft hand with an adducted thumb. Plast. Reconstr. Surg., 64:65, 1979.

36. Nutt, J. N., and Flatt, A. E.: Congenital central hand deficit. J. Hand Surg., 6:48, 1981.

37. Ogden, J. A., Watson, H. K., and Bohne, W.: Ulnar dysmelia. J. Bone Joint Surg., 58A:467, 1976.

38. Palmieri, T. J.: The use of silicone rubber implant arthroplasty in treatment of true symphalangism. J. Hand Surg., 5:242, 1980.

39. Reid, D. A. C.: Reconstruction of the thumb. JBJS, 42B:444–465, 1960.

40. Schramm, G.: Über die angeborene Flughautbildung (Muskulo-dysplasia patagiata congenita). Z. Orthop., 70:189, 1939.

41. Shoul, M. E., and Ritvo, M.: Roentgenologic and clinical aspects of hyperphalangism (polyphalangism) and brachydactylism: Hereditary abnormal segmentation of the hand. N. Engl. J. Med., 248:274, 1953.

42. Smith, R. J., and Kaplan, E. B.: Camptodactyly and similar atraumatic flexion deformities of the proximal interphalangeal joints of the fingers. J. Bone Joint Surg., 50A:1187, 1968.

43. Snow, J. W., and Littler, J. W.: Surgical treatment of cleft hand. *In*: Transactions of the International Society of Plastic and Reconstructive Surgery, Fourth Congress, Rome, Excerpta Medica Foundation, 1967, pp. 888–893.

44. Swanson, A. B.: A classification for congenital limb malformation. J. Hand Surg., 1:8, 1976.

45. Tuch, B. A., et al.: A review of supernumerary thumb and its surgical management. Clin. Orthop., 125:159, 1977.

46. Walsh, R. J.: Acrosyndactyly—a study of twenty-seven patients. Clin. Orthop., 71:99, 1970.

47. Wassel, D. H.: The results of surgery for polydactyly of the thumb. Clin. Orthop., 64:175, 1969.

48. White, J. W., and Jensen, W. E.: The infant's persistent thumb-clutched hand. J. Bone Joint Surg., 34A:680, 1952.

49. Wood, V. E.: Duplication of the index finger. J. Bone Joint Surg., 52A:569, 1970.

50. Wood, V. E.: Treatment of central polydactyly. Clin. Orthop., 74:196, 1971.

51. Wood, V. E.: Treatment of triphalangeal thumb. Clin. Orthop., 120:188, 1976.

52. Wood, V. E.: Hyperphalangism, report of a case. J. Hand Surg., 1:79, 1977.

53. Wood, V. E.: Polydactyly and the triphalangeal thumb. J. Hand Surg., 3:436, 1978.

54. Wood, V. E., and Flatt, A. E.: Congenital triangular bones in the hand. J. Hand Surg., 2:179, 1977.

55. Woolf, R. M., and Broadbent, T. R.: The four flap Z-plasty. Plast. Reconstr. Surg., 49:48, 1972.

31

MACRODACTYLY

Kenya Tsuge

Macrodactyly, also known as megalodactyly, is a fairly uncommon deformity that consists of an abnormal overgrowth of one or two digits, including the nail. It presents not only grotesque appearance, but there is also impairment in flexion of the digits as a result of the excessive fatty tissue on the volar aspect. It usually poses various cosmetic and functional problems.

CLINICAL FINDINGS

I have seen 23 cases of macrodactyly during the past 25 years. Of the 23 cases, 11 were males and 12 were females, with 5 involving the thumb, 13 the index finger, 9 the middle finger, 7 the ring finger, and 6 the little finger, with 14 on the right hand and 9 on the left. No genetic relationship could be noted in any of these cases. Macrodactyly also develops in the toe, and 22 cases were seen during the same period of time, with the second toe being most frequently affected.

In many cases, macrodactyly was noted at the time of birth. In some cases, the parents became aware of it when the child was 2 or 3 years old, while in others it was even later. It tended to develop more slowly in those cases noted later, but there was no essential difference between the two.

The degree of hypertrophy varies, and the growth of the affected fingers is not necessarily uniform. If there is a difference in the rate of growth on the two sides, the finger tends to deviate toward the radial or ulnar direction. In many cases marked hypertrophy of the soft tissues on the palmar side frequently causes a hyperextended position of the interphalangeal joint obstruction flexion of the finger. Generally the involvement is greatest distally, and it is not rare to find that the width and length of the nail are increased two to three times those of normal size.

Macrodactyly is not limited to the fingers, but also involves the palmar side of the hand. On palpation it presents findings of a soft mass. In some cases, the hypertrophy extends as far as the forearm, and presents such findings as hypertrophy of the median nerve. There is usually no pain nor paresthesia in the fingers, but in some cases slight paresthesia is recognized in the markedly hypertrophied fingers, especially when the hypertrophic median nerve is compressed in the carpal tunnel.

Radiographs reveal hypertrophy of the bone, and the phalanges are longer and wider, particularly in the distal end. When there is a deviation of the finger, asymmetric bone growth of both sides of the phalanges can be seen.

The cause of this entity is yet unknown but, as has been pointed out by many workers, some close relationship exists between the abnormal growth of the finger and the peripheral nerve abnormality (Fig. 31–1).[3, 5, 7, 8] In all cases, except one treated surgically, I observed that the digital nerves and their branches were enlarged to two to three times those of normal, and showed marked tortuosity. A noteworthy finding was that there was complete agreement in the sites of peripheral nerve abnormality and hypertrophy of the finger. When hypertrophy extended to the palmar area, nerve abnormality extended from the digital nerve to the common nerve. That is, the clinical area of hypertrophy and nerve abnormality coincided very well. In this sense, a new term, "nerve territory-oriented macrodactyly," (NTOM) is currently used.

Grossly, the hypertrophic nerve shows that the epineurium is thickened, lacks its normal luster, and adheres so closely to the surrounding proliferated adipose tissue that detachment is extremely difficult. The same state exists in the branches, the lobules of fat are larger than normal, and the fibrosis is noted between granules. Histologic findings show thickening of the epineurium, marked proliferation of the connective and adipose tissues, and fibrosis.

As stated above, it is obvious that a close relationship exists between overgrowth of the fingers and the peripheral nerve abnormality, but there are

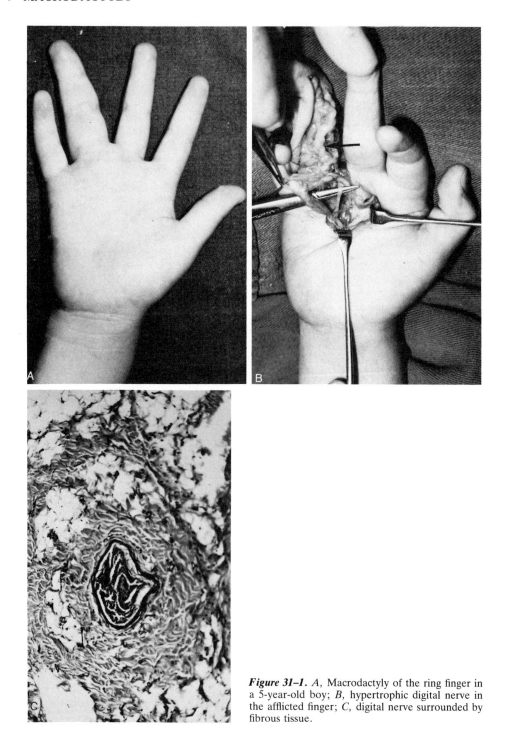

Figure 31–1. A, Macrodactyly of the ring finger in a 5-year-old boy; *B,* hypertrophic digital nerve in the afflicted finger; *C,* digital nerve surrounded by fibrous tissue.

still many unknown aspects about the development of this abnormality—for example, the mechanism involved in the cause of the hypertrophy of bone and nail. In some cases, angiography shows some hypertrophy and tortuousity of the vessels, but it is felt that they should be considered as secondary changes and not as the primary cause of this abnormality. It might be more correct to consider macro-

dactyly as a tumorous condition rather than as a congenital deformity.

TREATMENT

Treatment for macrodactyly must be individualized for each patient, but the following two prob-

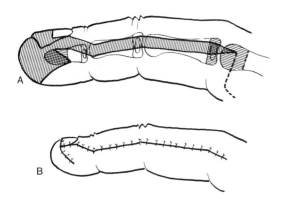

Figure 31–2. Shortening and reduction of macrodactyly. *A,* Tip and side skin are excised, and distal part of the distal phalanx and metacarpophalangeal joint are also excised; *B,* shortening and reduction have been completed.

lems should be taken into consideration. When enlargement of the finger is not too marked in an infant, further growth of the finger should be inhibited, and an attempt should be made to gain proportionality with the normal fingers by waiting for them to grow. After marked macrodactyly has developed in older children and adults, it is necessary to shorten and reduce the size from the cosmetic point of view. However, such prevention, shortening, and reduction constitute difficult problems.

Infants and Children

In the case of infants and children, treatment should be started as early as possible. First, the nail is cut and the hatched area of the fingertip is excised as shown in Figure 31–2. Then, a lateral incision is made on the convex side of the finger, the hypertrophic nerve is drawn out and isolated, and the surrounding adipose tissue is excised to the extent that it does not cause disruption of blood flow to the skin. Next, either the hypertrophic nerve or the branches are excised, after which the edges of the

skin are trimmed as necessary, and the size of the finger is reduced (Figs. 31–2 and 31–3). This procedure is usually done on one side at a time so as not to disturb the circulation. On the opposite side, the same procedure is performed after an interval of 2 to 3 months.

When the hypertrophy of the nerve is marked, and the afflicted nerve is less important in stereognosis, it should be excised. In some cases, nerve grafting may be considered thereafter.

If there is deviation of the finger, it is corrected by osteotomy and the finger is immobilized by Kirschner wires. To control the longitudinal growth of the finger, epiphyseal arrest at the proximal end of each phalanx might be considered. If the mobility of the distal interphalangeal joint is impaired, excision of the epiphyseal plate of the distal phalanx is performed and the joint is fused. The epiphyseal plate of the proximal phalanx is also excised, but that of the middle phalanx should not be excised.

Longitudinal excisional osteotomy of the phalanx will become necessary in some cases, especially for the thumb, but greater care must be taken so as not to injure the joint surface of the phalanges (Fig. 31–4).

Older Children and Adults

In the case of older children and adults, it will be necessary to shorten and reduce the size of the affected finger. In such cases, fingers are shortened according to Barsky's method, in which the distal interphalangeal joint and skin on the dorsal side are excised.[1, 7] The bulging of soft tissue that occurs on the palmar aspect of the finger is resected, together with the skin on the lateral side and fatty tissue as a secondary procedure 5 or 6 weeks after the first operation. The hypertrophic nerve branches must also be excised, and the nail reduced in size. These procedures are done on one side only, and the opposite side is subjected to the same procedures 3 months later as a third operation.

I have been using an approach that may be

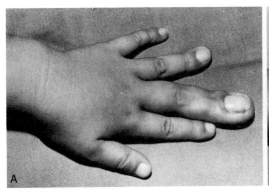
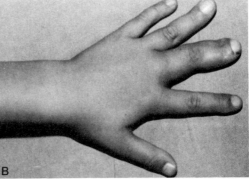

Figure 31–3. A, Macrodactyly of the middle finger in a 3-year-old boy; *B,* findings 4 years after shortening and reduction.

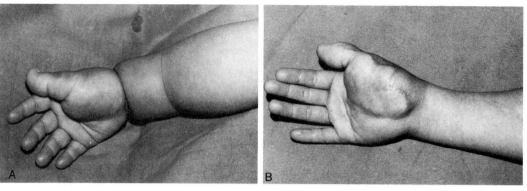

Figure 31–4. A, Macrodactyly of the thumb with hypertrophy of the forearm in a 2-year-old girl; B, findings 17 years after surgery.

considered to be the opposite to Barsky's method.[7] That is, whereas Barsky's method produces a bulge on the palmar side, my method involves a shortening procedure whereby the bulge is created on the dorsal side, which makes it particularly convenient to perform plastic procedures for the fingertip and nail (Fig. 31–5). The method involves making incisions along both midlateral sides of the finger and creating a dorsal skin flap, with the distal end attached to the nail and the dorsal third of the distal phalanx. This is retracted a suitable distance and the dorsal third of the middle phalanx is excised at an appropriate site, to which the portion of the distal phalanx is fixed. The excess portion of the

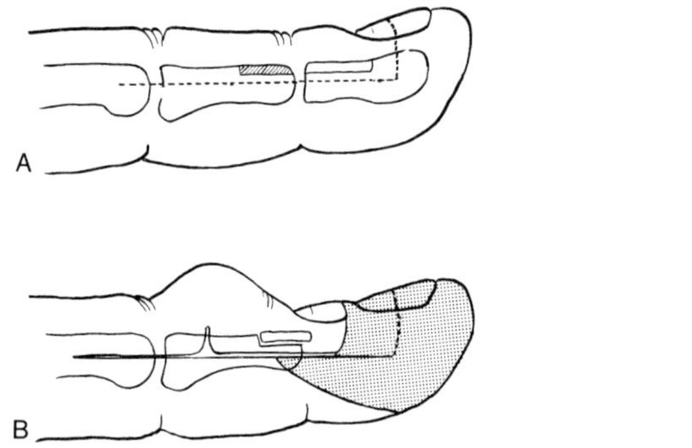

Figure 31–5. Shortening of macrodactyly. A, Incision; B, dorsal flap is retracted in wormlike fashion; C, tip of finger is excised, and partial excision of the nail is done; D, secondary surgery is performed to remove excess skin.

fingertip is excised and the nail is shortened in one procedure. A puckering of skin will be produced on the dorsal side of the finger, and the subsequent excision of the bulge and correction of size are carried out similar to the method described above.

Procedures for shortening and reduction of fingers has been discussed. However, when hypertrophy of the fingers is marked, there is probably no alternative but amputation (Fig. 31–6).

FIBROFATTY NERVE PROLIFERATION

There is an entity in which the median or ulnar nerve from the forearm to the palm becomes abnormally hypertrophic. This is found as a complication of macrodactyly or as an isolated condition, and has been given various names such as fibrofatty proliferation, fatty infiltration, lipofibroma, and lipomatous hamartoma, but in summary it is a condition whereby the nerve becomes markedly hypertrophic, reaching two to three times that of normal size or even larger.[2, 4, 6] It is caused by proliferation of fibrosis and fatty tissue in the connective tissue surrounding the nerve sheath and nerve bundles. These are considered to be the same as those seen in macrodactyly. I have seen seven cases that correspond to median or ulnar nerve abnormality and, with the exception of two cases, these occurred with macrodactyly.[8]

The symptoms are a soft mass unaccompanied by pain or tenderness, which extends from the forearm to the palm. It is often found to be present together with macrodactyly. The hypertrophic median nerve is frequently compressed at the carpal canal, causing sensory disturbance in the median nerve area.

Treatment consists of excising the hypertrophic fibrotic tissue and fatty tissue surrounding the nerve but great care must be exercised, because the separation is extremely difficult and harm may be inflicted on the nerve fibers. If compression of the median nerve is causing symptoms, decompression should be performed. If there is swelling only,

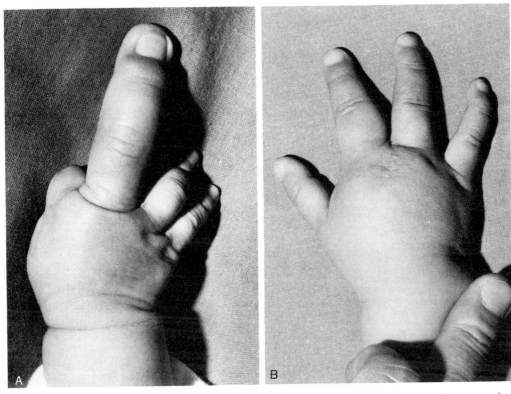

Figure 31–6. *A,* Six-month-old boy with macrodactyly of the middle finger; *B,* findings 2 years after amputation. The defect was closed using procedures for cleft hand.

without any other disturbance, it may be left as it is.

This concludes my discussion of the surgical treatment of macrodactyly and related conditions. It is extremely difficult to reduce the size of the digit, and at the same time have a digit with good cosmetic appearance and function. Furthermore, there is no effective means of checking the growth of such digits. As complications, I have often found distal interphalangeal or proximal interphalangeal joint stiffness, or both, and it is not rare for malalignment of the bone to develop. The condition is usually accompanied by deformity of the fingertip and nail. If treatment is administered to the digital nerves, sensory disturbance will naturally occur. There are no problems in the treatment of the surgical wound, but if size reduction efforts are excessive, circulatory disturbance is likely to develop, which may lead to necrosis.

Therefore, rather than attempting difficult multiple excision, if only one digit is involved it would probably be better to consider amputating the digit and performing metacarpal transfer of the adjoining digit.

References

1. Barsky, A. J.: Macrodactyly. J. Bone Joint Surg., 49A:1255, 1967.
2. Callison, J. R., Thoms, O. J., and White, W. L.: Fibro-fatty proliferation of the median nerve. Plast. Reconstr. Surg., 42:403, 1963.
3. Edgerton, M. T., and Tuerk, D. B.: Macrodactyly (digital gigantism): Its nature and treatment. *In* Littler, J. W., Cramer, L. M., and Smith, J. W. (eds.): Symposium on Reconstructive Hand Surgery, Vol. 9, St. Louis, C. V. Mosby, 1974, pp. 157–172.
4. Emmett, A. J. J.: Lipomatous hamartoma of the median nerve in the palm. Br. J. Plast. Surg., 18:208, 1965.
5. Rechnagel, K.: Megalodactylism. Report of seven cases. Acta Orthop. Scand., 38:57, 1967.
6. Rowland, S. A.: Lipofibroma of the median nerve in the palm. J. Bone Joint Surg., 49A:1309, 1967.
7. Tsuge, K.: Treatment of macrodactyly. Plast. Reconstr. Surg., 39:590, 1967.
8. Tsuge, K., and Ikuta, Y.: Macrodactyly and fibro-fatty proliferation of the median nerve. Hiroshima J. Med Sci., 22:83, 1973.

32

RADIAL AGENESIS

Douglas W. Lamb

Failure of development of the radius is a complex problem associated not only with complete or partial absence of the bone but also with failures of development or abnormalities of the associated muscles, joints, nerves, and vessels. The muscles that are usually deficient are those arising from the lateral condyle of the humerus (common extensor origin) and those normally arising from the radius. This usually means that the radial carpal extensors and the brachioradialis are absent, accounting for the weakness in dorsiflexion of the wrist and the tendency to a volar wrist deformity (see Fig. 32–8). Because the thumb is usually absent, the failure of development of the flexors, extensors, and abductors of the thumb is not of functional significance, and the main defect resulting from the failure of development of muscles of the radius is that of the index profundus. This may be of significance in regard to function following pollicization of an index finger (see below).

The structure of the joints is commonly affected. This is seen predominantly in the elbow and in the metacarpophalangeal and proximal interphalangeal joints of the fingers. In the most severe degrees of radial agenesis, however—for example, in some of those cases seen in association with thalidomide—there may be a defect in the development of the upper end of the humerus and poor glenohumeral movement. The principal abnormality of the elbow is a tendency for it to be held in extension. There is seldom any radiologic abnormality to be seen in the early years, but subsequently there may be deformities in the bony configuration of the lower humerus and upper ulna. Although this may affect flexion of the elbow, an additional factor is that the elbow flexors are usually more poorly developed than the triceps. The importance of this stiffness of the elbow in management will be discussed later in this chapter.

Stiffness of the small joints of the hand tends to be much more severe in the index and long fingers than in the ulnar two fingers. Flexion of the metacarpophalangeal joints is restricted and there is

often an abnormality of the extensor hood, which seems to be the main cause of the limited flexion rather than any abnormality in the joint itself. The proximal interphalangeal joint may be completely stiff and there is a tendency to flexion contractures with skin webbing and with abnormal development of the joint, particularly of the head of the proximal phalanx. The range of joint movement and the overall function of the hand needs careful assessment before any operative correction of the wrist deformity, because an extensive operation may not be justifiable if there is no useful function in a stiff hand.

The abnormal development of the radial side of the carpus and hand leads to the characteristic deformity known as "radial club hand" (Fig. 32–1). This deformity is often passively correctable, either completely or partially at birth. If the deformity is left uncontrolled during growth, the soft tissue structures will become contracted on the radial side so that the deformity will increase in severity.

PRINCIPLES OF MANAGEMENT

It is not surprising, therefore, that surgical attempts to correct the deformity are difficult and liable to complications and recurrence of deformity. It is important to be sure of the aims of operation and of the potential gains before embarking on any surgery. Although this is an ugly deformity, the rules relating to the surgical correction of congenital anomalies of the upper limb must be observed. Improvement of appearance is by itself seldom, if ever, justified, and the aim is to improve function. If this is always a guiding rule, disappointment to patient and surgeon and the development of complications will be less common.

It is recommended that the deformity should be corrected and controlled by splintage at night while waiting to decide if surgery is indicated. Some authorities feel that continuous splinting is advisable, but I have found that intermittent splintage at

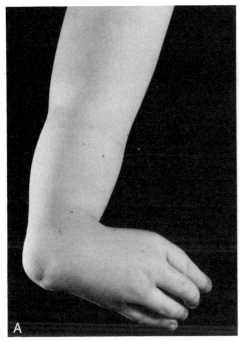 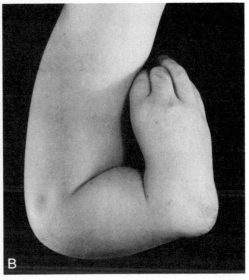

Figure 32–1. *A*, Typical deformity at the wrist in an untreated case of radial agenesis. This fixed deformity is passively incorrectable. Note the prominence of the lower ulnar head and the shortness of the forearm in this 10-year-old boy. *B*, The excellent range of active flexion at the elbow is unusually good for this condition.

night only is quite adequate in preventing fixed contractures. I use splintage also during the day to see if the overall function of the hand is as good with the wrist straight as in the deformed position, so as to help assessment regarding the advisability of straightening the wrist by operation. A careful assessment of the overall function and the ability to carry out self-care activities is necessary. The structure and range of movement of the elbow and finger joints are all-important in deciding if surgical correction is indicated. The elbow joint is often stiff in extension, and efforts should be made to mobilize the elbow. In some patients the range of elbow movement is good, but it would be wise not to correct the wrist deformity unless there is at least 90° of active elbow flexion; otherwise, the child may be unable to reach the mouth and face with the hand (Fig. 32–1*B*). In addition, it would be of little functional benefit to a child to have a wrist corrected when the hand function is severely impaired by stiffness of the joints, which is often associated with flexion contractures (Fig. 32–2).

The forearm lacks normal pronation and supination movement, and the abnormal mobility available at the deformed wrist will compensate for this. It must be appreciated, therefore, that if the wrist is straightened there will be some loss of that compensating movement. However, I have found that this is more than compensated for by increased stability at the wrist and by the improved range of movement and strength in the fingers because of

the improved mechanical advantage of the tendons. If preoperative assessment suggests that improvement in function can be obtained, then the appearance is also greatly improved and the apparent length of the forearm is enhanced.

SURGICAL PROCEDURES

A large variety of different operative procedures have been described over the last 100 years for the correction of this deformity. They may be divided into three main types.

Corrective Osteotomy of the Ulna. There are various methods. These are nearly always followed by a fairly rapid recurrence of the deformity.

Attempts to Replace the Missing Radius. These have failed, because the replaced bone has usually failed to grow. Transplant of the upper fibula with its growing epiphysis was initially promising, but the epiphysis usually closed soon after transfer. New methods of bone transfer on a vascular pedicle with microvascular anastomosis have been described, but long-term results are unknown.

Straightening the Carpus Over the End of the Ulna. The most definitive of these procedures is arthrodesis between the carpus and the lower ulna. This would affect growth, and is not advisable until the epiphysis has closed. It also has the disadvantage of leaving a stiff wrist, and the lack of movement may be of functional significance.

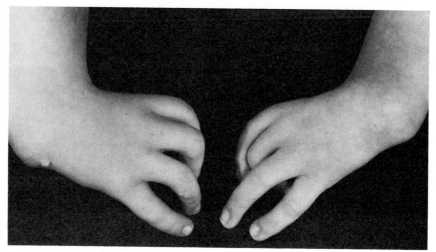

Figure 32–2. Bilateral radial agenesis in a 7-year-old boy. When referred at this stage there had been no splinting nor other treatment. Note the degree of radial deviation at the wrist, particularly the flexion contractures at the proximal interphalangeal joints of the radial two digits. The elbows were completely stiff in extension, with no active or passive flexion.

In more recent years, the most successful procedure for correcting the deformity that still retains a small amount of movement has been the operation of centralization of the carpus over the ulna. This will be described, together with complications that may arise.

Centralization of the Carpus

Any severe soft tissue contracture may have to be corrected before the definitive operation. Sometimes this is not possible by splintage, and may require Z-plasty lengthening of the skin and division of right soft tissue bands. Splintage of the wrist at night from birth will make this unnecessary.

An incision is required to provide adequate exposure of the lower end of the ulna, the carpus on the radial side of the lower ulna, and the volar aspect of the forearm to display and protect the median nerve and to expose the flexor muscles, which may require transposition or lengthening. I begin a suitable incision over the dorsoradial aspect of the hand, run obliquely to the head of the ulna, and then curve radially across the dorsal carpal crease, around the radial side of the wrist and extending up the volar aspect of the forearm (Fig. 32–3). This is a long but necessary exposure. The deep fascia is divided in the line of the incision with care for the median nerve, which will be found lying superficially on the radial aspect and must be protected. It may have divided into two main components in the lower forearm, and the radial vessels and superficial radial nerve are usually absent. Once the median nerve has been protected the carpus can be exposed on the radial aspect of the lower ulna. In the small child it will be largely cartilaginous, but the bones can usually be identified. A notch is created in the carpus wide enough to receive the

lower end of the ulna, which should be inserted to a depth equal to its transverse diameter (Fig. 32–4). This usually means removal of the lunate and capitate and sometimes some of the adjacent scaphoid

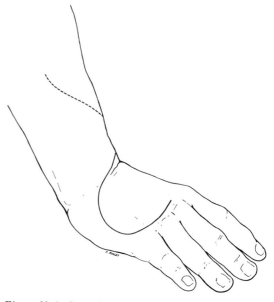

Figure 32–3. Operative approach. Most patients referred to me for operation have had no splintage nor other attempt to prevent the development of fixed contractures. In such circumstances a wide exposure has been found to be advantageous to release contractures, avoid damage to the median nerve, expose the carpus and lower ulna, and facilitate lengthening or transfer of tendons, as required. When operation is carried out early and there are no fixed contractures a less extensive procedure, particularly on the volar forearm, is satisfactory.

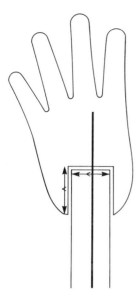

Figure 32–4. Centralization of the carpus, showing the ulna inserted into the notch created by excision of appropriate portions of carpus to a depth equal to its transverse diameter. This provides good stability, which can be maintained in the early postoperative phase by inserting a Kirschner wire along the third or fourth metacarpal, across the center of the lower ulnar epiphysis, and up the medullary cavity of the ulna. This period of fixation will allow a new capsule to form around the carpus and the lower ulna to provide stability once the wire has been removed.

or triquetrum—whatever is required to insert the ulna snugly while still retaining stability.

The lower end of ulna is identified and dissected extraperiosteally so as to avoid damage to the lower ulnar epiphysis. The carpus can now be placed over the end of the ulna and a stable situation achieved. This will leave some redundant soft tissue, including skin over the ulnar aspect, which some surgeons remove; however, it will resolve spontaneously if left. Once the wrist has been straightened the flexor tendons, in particular the superficialis, may become tight. If the fingers cannot be straightened passively, the superficialis should be lengthened at the musculotendinous junction.

The flexor carpi radialis is often a deforming factor. If this is the case, the tendon insertion should be transferred to the dorsum of the wrist.

Wrist stability is maintained by a Kirschner wire passed through the carpal notch along the fourth metacarpal shaft and out of the metacarpal head. After placing the carpus over the ulna, the Kirschner wire is passed up the ulnar medullary cavity to cross the center of the epiphysis (Fig. 32–5).

Curvature of the ulna is frequently present. This should be corrected by osteotomy at one or more sites at the same time as the centralization, using the Kirschner wire for stability.

Following release of the tourniquet, hemostasis is obtained and a compression bandage is applied. Considerable postoperative edema is common, partially due to the poor finger movements, and it is advisable to elevate the arm and hand until the

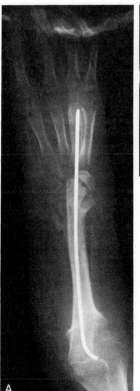

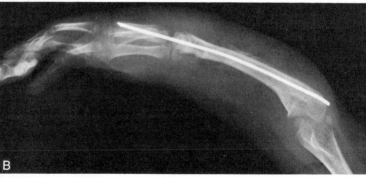

Figure 32–5. *A, B,* Postoperative fixation following centralization. The upper end of the wire has been bent in attempt to prevent extrusion of the wire.

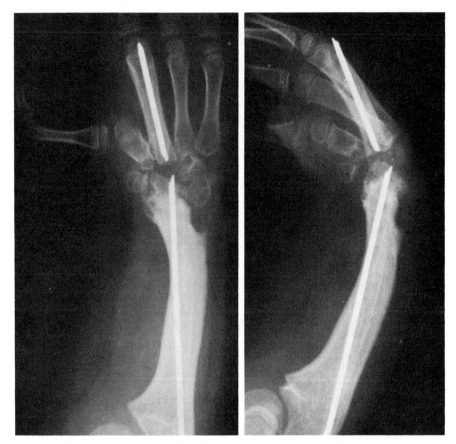

Figure 32–6. The Kirschner wire used to stabilize this wrist following centralization 2 years previously has broken, allowing some recurrence of the wrist deformity.

swelling has been reduced before applying an external plaster support.

Postoperative splintage with the Kirschner wire for 6 months is advisable. Sometimes the wire slips out and, when it does, it should either be reinserted or an external plaster support maintained until 6 months from operation.

Complications

These may be early or late.

Early Problems. Complications during or soon after surgery are unusual. Infection is very rare, and antibiotics are not used routinely. Postoperative edema and swelling are common, but these usually resolve in 3 or 4 days, and have not been a factor leading to any delay in skin healing. There have been no problems from ischemia.

Late Problems. Complications during the first 6 months after operation and while immobilization is being continued are rare. All wounds heal primarily and are usually inconspicuous, although occasionally a keloid scar is seen. There has been no example of nonunion of osteotomy of the ulna.

Fracture of the Kirschner wire at wrist level has been seen rarely; this becomes obvious with recur-

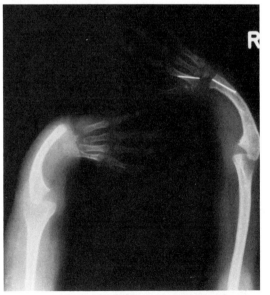

Figure 32–7. The ulnar bowing has been inadequately corrected here, allowing some recurrence of deformity even though there has been satisfactory correction of the right wrist by centralization. Corrective osteotomy of the ulna is indicated. The left wrist is untreated.

rence of deformity, and is confirmed by x-ray (Fig. 32–6). The wire should be removed and replaced.

Careful monitoring of hand function and the ability to carry out self-care activities is carried out, and pre- and postoperative functions are compared. In no case in my series has there been a loss of function following centralization.

The two main complications after centralization are recurrence of the wrist deformity and premature fusion of the lower ulnar epiphysis.

Recurrence of Deformity. Some recurrence of radial deviation is not uncommon during growth, but it is seldom severe enough to require further operation, although inadequate correction of ulnar bowing may require further osteotomy (Fig. 32–7).

A more frequent deformity is one of volar flexion due to the flexor muscles being stronger than the extensors (Fig. 32–8). The flexor carpi radialis often appears to be the main deforming muscle and, if it has not been transferred at the original operation, this should be done to try and balance the wrist.

To prevent recurrence of deformity, some form of protective corrective splintage should be used at night during growth.

Premature Fusion of the Lower Ulnar Epiphysis. In radial agenesis ulnar growth is always restricted, because the lower epiphysis closes at about the age of 12 years and the forearm is only half to two thirds of the normal length.

No operative treatment should cause premature fusion of this lower epiphysis and, provided an extraperiosteal dissection of the lower ulna is carried

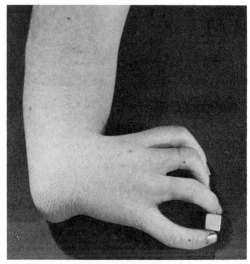

Figure 32–9. Usual pattern of prehension associated with radial agenesis in the radially deviated wrist. When it is a pure deviation, the grip between the ulnar two digits is often quite good, and of course the ulnar two digits are usually of much better structure and function than the radial two digits. When there is also a volar displacement, the ulnar prehension has to be from the dorsal aspect of the fingers, and is a much poorer grip. In my experience when the wrist is straightened by centralization, the function becomes oriented to the radial fingers but does not suffer by the correction of the wrist. In fact, the power of grip appears to be greater, presumably because of the straighter line of pull of the flexor tendons.

out and the Kirschner wire is passed across the center of the epiphysis, there is seldom any evidence of premature epiphyseal fusion. If the ulna is handled roughly or stripped subperiosteally, the Kirschner wire inserted without care, or an osteotomy carried out near the epiphysis, a very stunted ulna may result.

Prior to centralization, the characteristic prehension is with the ulnar two digits (Fig. 32–9). This is partly due to the ulnar fingers being of better structure and function than the radial digits, but also results because the ulnar border of the hand in the deformed position is the first to reach objects.

Pollicization

Following correction of the wrist the orientation for prehension is to the radial side, where the thumb is either absent or grossly deficient in the form of a "dangle" thumb (Fig. 32–10). It is useless to try and reconstruct the thumb by bone grafting and tendon transfer. To improve prehension, consideration should be given to pollicization of the index digit. The best results will be obtained in cases in which the structure and function of the index finger are normal, but this is seldom found in radial agenesis. The proximal interphalangeal joint usually has a flexion contracture and is stiff, and the index profundus is often weak or absent. Despite this, a

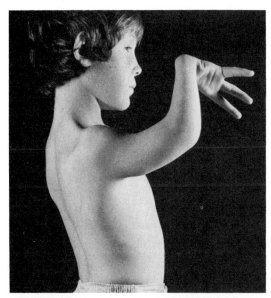

Figure 32–8. This boy has an untreated deformity of the right upper limb. There is shortness of the upper arm, limitation of shoulder elevation due to poor development of the upper humerus, and restricted active flexion of the elbow. The wrist deformity is seen to consist more of a volar deformity rather than of the characteristic radial deformity.

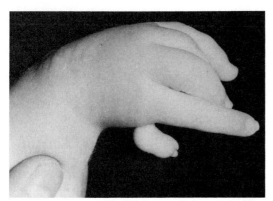

Figure 32–10. Typical "dangle" thumb (floating thumb, *pounce flottant*). It is small, has a ring constriction at its base, and is situated much more distally than the normal thumb. The thumb has no tendons and is functionless, and attempts to reconstruct this thumb by bone or tendon grafting are not justifiable—the growth potential is nil.

reasonable thumb can be provided that will improve function.

Other indications for pollicization would be the "dangle" thumb in the absence of radial aplasia, the four-fingered hand, and the five-fingered hand. In most of these circumstances the radial index finger is the most suitable digit for pollicization.

Most complications result from a lack of appreciation of the finer points and difficulties of the procedure. The incision used is that described by Barsky, with a racquet incision centered on the metacarpophalangeal joint and continuing on the radial side of the hand in a sinuous manner to form the flap for the new thumb web. To facilitate the reattachment of the intrinsic muscles to the extensor mechanism, the incision is extended along the dorsoradial aspect of the proximal phalanx of the index finger, as advocated by Buck-Grampcko (Fig. 32–11).[1] The incision is developed on the volar aspect to expose the neurovascular bundles. In radial agenesis the radial neurovascular bundle may be absent, and it is important to dissect the ulnar neurovascular bundle with great care. The metacarpal nerve to the interspace between the index and long fingers is separated into its two components proximally to the base of the palm, and the associ-

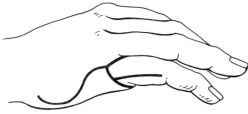

Figure 32–11. Incision for pollicization. (From Lamb, D. W.: Congenital abnormalities. *In* Lamb, D. W., and Kuczynski, K. (eds.): The Practice of Hand Surgery, Oxford, Blackwell Scientific Publications, 1981.)

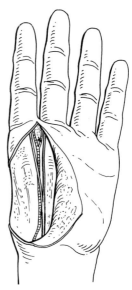

Figure 32–12. Technique of pollicization, showing the neurovascular bundle to the interspace between the index and middle fingers. The flap has been elevated to expose the nerve and vessels on the volar aspect. The artery to the middle finger has been divided, and the nerve is being separated into two components. (From Lamb, D. W.: Congenital abnormalities. *In* Lamb, D. W., and Kuczynski, K. (eds.): The Practice of Hand Surgery, Oxford, Blackwell Scientific Publications, 1981.)

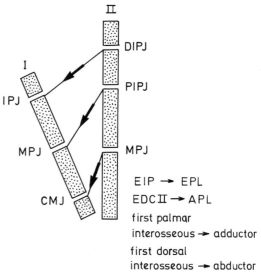

Figure 32–13. Diagram showing how the components of the index digit are transposed into the thumb. The head of the second metacarpal becomes the new trapezium. The interossei are inserted into the extensor at the level of the old proximal interphalangeal joint and what is now the metacarpophalangeal joint of the new thumb. (From Lamb, D. W.: Congenital abnormalities. *In* Lamb, D. W., and Kuczynski, K. (eds.): The Practice of Hand Surgery, Oxford, Blackwell Scientific Publications, 1981.)

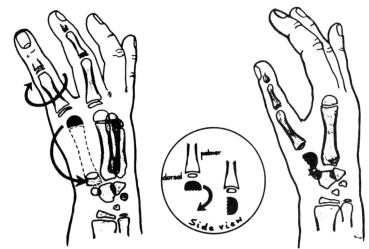

Figure 32–14. Diagram showing rotation of metacarpal head to prevent hyperextension deformity at the base of the thumb. The metacarpal head is rotated so that the palmar surface becomes proximal, and the volar plate and capsule are tightened. (From Buck-Grampcko, D.: Pollicization of the index finger. J. Bone Joint Surg., 53:1605, 1971.)

ated metacarpal artery is displayed to its division at the web, which is always much more distal than the nerve (Fig. 32–12). The neurovascular bundle should always be identified and dissected before operation proceeds, because there may be an anomaly of the nerve that prevents its separation into its two components to the index and middle fingers.

The incision is then deepened from the dorsum to expose the second interspace, and the deep transverse metacarpal ligament is divided to expose the neurovascular bundle. The first dorsal and volar interosseous muscles are now dissected subperiosteally off the second metacarpal. This is thus exposed in its length and removed to leave only the head, which is separated through the epiphyseal line. This will produce an index segment, which is now the appropriate length for a new thumb that reaches to the level of the proximal interphalangeal joint of the middle finger. The space left by the removal of the metacarpal will receive the metacarpal head to become the new trapezium. The metacarpophalangeal joint of the index finger will now become the carpometacarpal joint, and the distal joint will become the interphalangeal joint of the new thumb (Fig. 32–13). The index metacarpophalangeal joint is frequently hyperextensible due to volar plate laxity. To prevent this deformity developing at the new carpometacarpal joint (one of the ugly and frequent complications following pollicization), the metacarpal head should be rotated to tighten the volar structures (Fig. 32–14).[1] The index ray is rotated on its longitudinal axis through 150°, and the rotated head is maintained in its new position by soft tissue sutures. Before the thumb is fixed in its new position, it is important to ensure that there is no kinking of the vessel and that the nerve has been freed proximally enough to prevent it's being stretched. The tourniquet is then released and hemostasis is obtained.

The interosseous tendons are attached, one on the radial and the other on the ulnar side of the extensor tendon, to the lateral bands at the new metacarpophalangeal joint level. This will give a

boost to extension and, in particular, will provide some control of the new thumb by simulating the normal abductor-adductor function. Also, it gives considerable stability to the thumb as well as a more normal appearance (Fig. 32–15).

Complications

These may be early or late.

Early Problems. *Ischemia.* The most serious complication is ischemia of the transposed digit. This is always a possibility, especially when there is no radial vessel on the index finger. When care is taken with dissection of the ulnar neurovascular bundle and with division of the arterial branch to the middle finger well away from its bifurcation, the complication is rare. Avoid kinking of the vessel when the index finger is rotated. Arterial insufficiency will usually become evident when the tourniquet is released, and steps are taken to ensure that the vessel is not under tension nor twisted. It could develop also in the early postoperative period as a result of thrombosis, and could require re-exploration.

Arterial damage at the time of operation should be repaired, or a vein graft inserted. It is much more common for the circulation to give concern a few hours after operation due to venous insufficiency. To prevent this, it is important to preserve dorsal veins during dissection of the digit. The digit may become dusky a few hours after transposition, but circulation usually improves quickly. Persistence of signs of poor circulation generally indicates that the bandages are too tight and should be released. If there is no improvement the most likely cause is tight constriction of the new thumb web flap around the base of the transposed index finger. This should be checked and, if tight, should be released by removal of stitches.

Numbness in the Transferred Digit. This may develop due to kinking or stretching of the digital nerve, but it is unlikely if the nerve has been separated into its two components proximally into

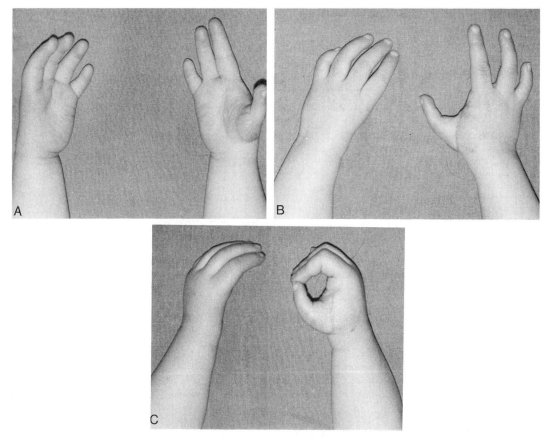

Figure 32–15. The appearance of a "thumb" that has been made from the index finger, which has been placed in good cosmetic *(A)* and functional *(B, C)* position. Note the appearance of the "thenar" area produced by the rearrangement of the first dorsal interosseous muscle and tendon. The operation was done on a 1-year-old girl with bilateral four-fingered hands. The left hand was similarly operated on at 21 months.

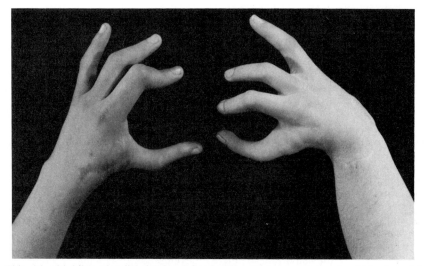

Figure 32–16. This girl, with bilateral radial club hand, has had the wrists corrected and pollicization of the index finger on each side. Note that the thumbs are proportionately too long, particularly on the left side.

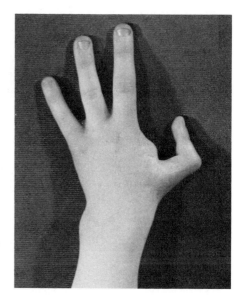

Figure 32–17. This boy has had pollicization of his index finger. As a result of not rotating the head of the metacarpal, hyperextension deformity has developed at the base of the thumb, with a compensatory flexion deformity at the metacarpophalangeal joint. This was, of course, the original proximal interphalangeal joint that already had a flexion contracture prior to transfer; it was made worse as the result of the hyperextended basal joint.

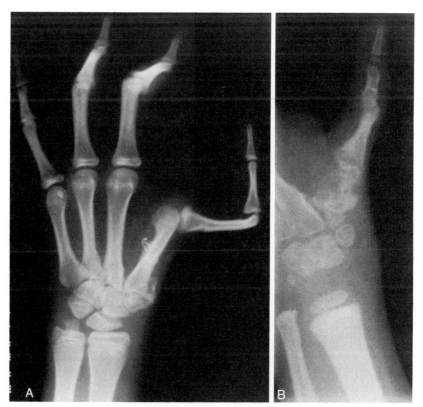

Figure 32–18. *A,* Too much of the second metacarpal has been retained and, as a result, the thumb is too long. A hyperextension deformity has occurred at the old metacarpophalangeal joint. Preserving too much of the metacarpal shaft prevents the rotation of the metacarpal head needed to correct the hyperextensibility. The preoperative flexion contracture of the proximal interphalangeal joint has increased because of the hyperextensibility at the metacarpophalangeal joint. *B,* Ideal length of thumb after resection of all the second metacarpal except for the head, which has now developed into a new trapezium. The proximal phalanx is broadening and forming a first metacarpal.

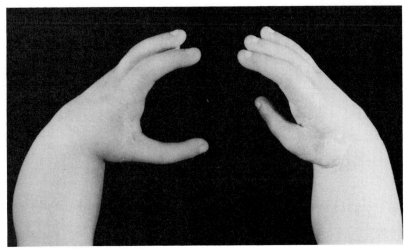

Figure 32–19. This boy had bilateral agenesis of the radius. Pollicization of the index finger was carried out on both sides. On the left side the thumb has been rotated through 140° on the long axis to lie in a good functional position, whereas on the right side inadequate rotation and abduction has resulted in a web contracture, and the thumb is now in a poor functional position.

the base of the palm. It is usually a temporary impairment of sensation and improves spontaneously.

Failure of Healing. This is most unusual but, if the new thumb web flap has been closed too tightly, there may be some superficial necrosis. To avoid this complication it is much better to close loosely or with a skin graft. Even if small areas are left open these will heal very readily in the small child.

Late Problems. *Failure of Growth.* This is only likely to occur in a transposed digit if the phalangeal epiphyses are abnormal. It has been mentioned as a complication in the past, but this was usually in cases in which attempts were made to build up a thumb that was structurally abnormal. A thumb made out of an index finger, with normal phalangeal epiphyses, shows no sign of impairment of normal growth.

Due to a fear that growth may not occur normally, there has been a tendency for many surgeons to make the thumb longer than necessary, which may lead to problems initially in healing (Fig. 32–16). It is, of course, a much less severe problem to have a thumb that is too long than one that is too short. If, in a teen-ager, the thumb appears too long, it can easily be shortened. Since I have used the technique this has not been a problem, and shortening has not been required.

Hyperextension Deformity at the Base of the Thumb. This ugly deformity has already been mentioned, and its mode of prevention described. The development of this deformity undoubtedly is detrimental to a good cosmetic result and justifies further operation to correct it (Fig. 32–17). The

metacarpal head, or new trapezium as it has become, requires freeing and rotating (as described) to correct the hyperextension (Fig. 32–18).

Inadequate Rotation of the Index Finger on Its Longitudinal Axis. This will prevent good pulp-to-pulp opposition, and may result in an adduction contracture of the new thumb web (Fig. 32–19).

It is only by release and reattachment of the first dorsal and first volar interosseous that a satisfactory looking thumb is produced (see Fig. 32–15). Failure to do this will make the thumb look like an index finger lying in a new position. The reattachment of the intrinsics is a significant factor in producing good appearance and function. The poorer the original structure and function of the index finger, the poorer the function of the new thumb will be. In radial agenesis the index profundus is often absent, meaning that the thumb will have poor interphalangeal flexion. If the index extensor tendons are poorly developed, the power of extension of the thumb will be poor. The function of the hand as a whole may be better but the performance of the new thumb will definitely be less than optimal if tendon defects are present, or if there has been impaired movement or flexion contracture in the interphalangeal joints.

Reference

1. Buck-Gramcko, D.: Pollicization of the index finger. Method and results in aplasia and hypoplasia of the thumb. J. Bone Joint Surg., 53:1605, 1971.

33

CEREBRAL PALSY

Alfred B. Swanson and
Genevieve de Groot Swanson

Reconstructive surgery for the cerebral palsied hand is rarely indicated. In certain selected cases it may be of considerable benefit to the patient. To avoid the pitfalls of inadequate results following surgery on these patients requires a consideration not only of the failures of surgical technique but also of failures in diagnosis, the evaluation of deformities, and the identification of appropriate and rewarding methods of surgical treatment and rehabilitation.

It is a great challenge to attempt to correct disturbed functional adaptations in the cerebral palsied upper extremity. It is necessary for the surgeon, therefore, to have the benefit of a sophisticated team of professionals to help in operative decision making or to ensure that the necessary decision components are carefully observed. Complications of wound breakdown, infection, inadequate dressings, and casts will not be considered here.

DEFINITION, INCIDENCE, AND CLASSIFICATION OF CEREBRAL PALSY

Cerebral palsy is a "condition characterized by paralysis, weakness, incoordination, or any aberration of motor control centers of the brain."[21] It is a challenging problem for those who would treat it.

There are an estimated 600,000 cases of cerebral palsy patients in the United States. Some form of brain damage manifested by cerebral palsy occurs in one to five newborns per every 1000 births in the United States.[6, 11] Of every seven cases, one dies, two will require custodial care for severe mental handicaps, one will require custodial care for severe physical handicaps, two will require moderate treatment, and one will require mild treatment. The improvement of prenatal care and obstetric methods

are the main factors contributing to the decreased incidence of this disorder.

The classification of cerebral palsy has been the subject of many debates. The most logical classification seems to be reference to the type of manifestation of the central motor disorder and to the distribution of the peripheral involvement.[33, 37]

The types of cerebral palsy may be classified as follows:

Type	Incidence (%)
Spastic	70
Athetoid	20
Ataxia, tremor, rigidity, other	10

Few patients have a single diagnostic involvement. Most have a mixed involvement with one type predominating. Approximately 25% of these patients have a severe loss of sensibility that will prevent usage of their hand even though their motor ability is adequate.[34]

Peripheral involvement in cerebral palsy may be classified as follows:

Involvement	Incidence (%)
Quadriplegia	50
Hemiplegia	40
Para-, mono-, triplegia	10

A comparison of the intelligence quotient (IQ) between the general population and cerebral palsied patients shows the following values:

IQ in "Normal"	IQ in CP
>90 = 75%	>90 = 25%
<70 = 3%	<70 = 50%

Associated problems presented by the cerebral palsied patient further handicap this unfortunate child, and increase the difficulties of the rehabilitation program. Speech defects are present in 75% of these patients, visual defects in 50%, hearing defects in 10%, some convulsive disorders in 30%, and laterality in 40%. A certain number of these patients also have nutritional problems, marked distractibility, incontinence, and drooling. Their psychological development and adjustment can be poor and is further complicated by parental attitudes of guilt, intolerance, or rejection.

DISTURBED MUSCLE PHYSIOLOGY AND PRINCIPLES OF TREATMENT

Separate muscle units can be affected differently in cerebral palsy. They may be spastic, flaccid, normal, weak, or contracted. Long-standing flexion deformities commonly result in myostatic contractures, which are often coupled with disturbances in the stretch reflex mechanism. There is a direct relationship between the length to which a muscle is stretched and the amount of tension developed. As the tension increases, the stretch reflex or contractile response of the muscle increases.[1] This reflex is present in all normal skeletal muscles but is overactive in spastic muscles.

Spasticity of muscles, especially of the flexors of the wrist and fingers, is common in the cerebral palsy patient. Myostatic contractures can be prevented to some degree by stretching with casts or braces. Hyperactive stretch reflexes can be abolished by destroying any portion of their arc. Selective neurectomy has been used in the past, but became contraindicated because it resulted in excessive muscle weakness. Hyperactivity of the gamma motor neurons to the muscle spindle is the main cause of spasticity.[23] Infiltration of the muscle or peripheral nerve with 1% procaine can produce temporary abatement of the spasticity. This apparently reduces the activity of the gamma system without decreasing the motor control completely. It has been suggested that dilute chemolytic agents injected directly into a peripheral nerve may selectively destroy the gamma motor fibers to decrease spasticity without seriously affecting larger motor or sensory pathways.[2, 19] Phenol 2 to 5% has been used for direct infiltration of motor branches of the ulnar and median nerves in the forearm after surgical exposure, but it should not be injected into sensory nor mixed nerves. Most cases have demonstrated only a short-term relief. A long-term appraisal of these agents will be necessary before they can be included in the treatment of cerebral palsied extremities.

Overactive reflexes and spasticity can be relieved in part by judicious shortening of the muscle to prevent its overstretching. This can be achieved either by tendon lengthening distally, or by proximal muscle origin release with distal advancement (see below). The ideal treatment for relieving spasticity, when finally discovered, will be a pharmacologic agent or surgical procedure that will decrease spasticity at the motor end-plate differentially without affecting voluntary movements.

Any physician responsible for the rehabilitation program of a cerebral palsied individual must be aware of the problems summarized above to evaluate the potential of each patient properly, select candidates for surgical improvement properly, and apply proper treatment.

Preoperative Evaluation

Definitive plans for rehabilitation of a cerebral palsy patient cannot be formulated after a single consultation. The patient must be evaluated carefully several times by the physician and by team members, including the physical and occupational therapists, before a treatment plan can be established.

The functional evaluation is done by questioning the parents, the patient when possible, and by observing patterns of hand activities while handling test objects. This functional evaluation must include observation of speed, skill, coordination, and strength in the use of the hand, hand adaptation patterns, hand-eye coordination, reach, hand placement, handedness, bilaterality, and the ability to handle test objects. Questions and observations must also be directed toward defining the patient's intelligence and capacity to perform activities of daily living.

The physical examination must include observation of the patient's voluntary control and grasp and release patterns. A grasp and release pattern must be present in a cerebral palsy patient if improvement is to be expected from a surgical procedure. Spasm, accessory movements, and muscle imbalances must be noted. The muscle tone may be flaccid, normal, or spastic in various muscle groups of the same extremity. The presence and degree of joint instability and its repercussions on hand function should be recorded. The presence of resistant deformities and the sensory status must be determined. A simple sensory test would be the blind differentiation between a marble and a cube.

The results of tenodesis procedures can be predicted by taping small aluminum splints onto the digits to stimulate the postoperative condition. Although rarely indicated, should a wrist arthrodesis be considered, the application of a plaster cast or brace can demonstrate the patient's postoperative functional potential or the preferred position for wrist fusion. Because spastic patients are especially dependent on reciprocal flexion of the wrist to obtain finger extension, a wrist fusion can be disastrous.

Deformities and Impairments

Common deformities in the cerebral palsied upper extremity include internal rotation of the arm, flexion of the elbow, pronation of the forearm, flexion of the wrist and digits, extension of the digits with swan-neck deformities, thumb-in-palm deformity, adduction of the first metacarpal, unstable joints, motor deficiencies, and sensibility defects.

Pronation deformity is common in cerebral palsy. The pronation position is functional for many hand activities, and therefore no surgical treatment may be indicated. This deformity cannot be well treated by conservative methods of stretching or exercises. Release of the insertion of the pronator teres, pronator quadratus, or both may be of some benefit in certain cases. Release of the pronator teres origin as performed by the flexor-pronator origin release procedure and by the Green procedure can also improve the problem. Occasionally, this deformity may be associated with posterior dislocation of the head of the radius or with an altered relationship of the shaft of the radius to the ulna. A long oblique osteotomy of the shaft of the radius may be necessary to bring the hand to the neutral position. In general, if supination to 0° is possible, no other treatment should be indicated. Specific surgical treatment for this deformity alone is uncommon and the results are frequently unrewarding.

The major handicap of the hand in cerebral palsy is the patient's inability to open the hand for grasp. Often the hand has good strength for closing but does not have efficient extension nor the necessary speed of extension for normal function. Instability of the fingers often precludes strong pinch and grasp. This is especially true in hyperextension deformities of the fingers. The collapse of the normal flexion arc of the digit, associated with hyperextension of the proximal interphalangeal joint and flexion of the distal interphalangeal joint, known as the swan-neck deformity, is functionally disabling and also cosmetically unattractive. These deformities are particularly severe in individuals with inherently lax ligamentous structures. The loss of the normal flexion arc of the interphalangeal joints also contributes to the inability to extend the metacarpophalangeal joint properly. Extension of the metacarpophalangeal joint is facilitated by proximal interphalangeal joint flexion.[35]

The normal functions of the contiguous articulations in the fingers and hand are interdependent. Any disturbance in one joint will affect other related joints. In cerebral palsy, these interrelated functions are profoundly affected and it may be difficult to determine whether a deformity is primary or secondary to other imbalances.

Indications for Surgery

Most patients with cerebral palsy involvement of the upper extremity are not candidates for surgical reconstructive procedures. In 10 to 20% of cases, certain selective operative procedures may assist in the patient's rehabilitation.[8, 15, 22, 25, 27, 28, 33, 37] We have developed a group of operations over a period of years in our clinic that appear to be useful. It is our impression that this type of surgery can best be

carried out in a clinic situation in which a team approach to rehabilitation is available. The need for careful preoperative evaluation of the patient's functional potential is obvious (see above).

The indications for surgery in the cerebral palsied hand include a rehabilitation potential for disabilities that are correctable by surgery in the presence of a good potential for functional and cosmetic improvement. Approximately 50% of these cerebral palsy patients are seeking cosmetic improvement. Patients with severe athetoid manifestations usually present incoordinations that will probably not benefit from any surgical procedure.

The ideal surgical candidate is one with sufficient intelligence, emotional stability, and a cooperative disposition. The patient is usually a spastic hemiplegic with good voluntary grasp and release patterns, adequate sensation in the hand, and a good functional and cosmetic potential. The defects usually presented are pronation deformity of the forearm, flexor muscle overactivity with contracture, and spasticity of the wrist and finger muscles, thumb-in-palm attitude, and hyperextension or swan-neck deformities of the proximal interphalangeal joints.

SURGICAL TREATMENT

Surgical procedures have been designed to improve the following: flexion deformity of the wrist; inability to open the hand; thumb-in-palm deformity; and swan-neck deformities.

Flexion Deformity of the Wrist

Treatment of this deformity includes the following methods:
1. Conservative stretching with bracing or casting
2. Selective lengthening of flexor tendons
3. Transfer of flexor carpi ulnaris
4. Flexor muscle origin release procedures
5. Combination of the above
6. Postoperative bracing
7. Wrist arthrodesis

Conservative attempts to correct the wrist flexion deformity by bracing or casting should precede any surgical procedure. The flexor carpi ulnaris transfer, as described by Green and Banks, is our procedure of choice for patients who present a flexion-pronation deformity of the wrist with weakness of the wrist extensors.[10] This procedure is occasionally done in association with a flexor muscle origin release procedure for finger-flexion deformity. In this situation, the proximal origin of the flexor carpi ulnaris is left intact. Bracing must always be applied postoperatively, usually for a prolonged period of time.

Arthrodesis of the wrist is performed rarely in our clinic because of the particular dependency of the cerebral palsied patient on wrist flexion to achieve finger extension. It is most important to evaluate the potential for finger extension preoperatively, because the wrist is maintained in the desired position of fusion with a plaster cast or brace. This procedure has been occasionally done in an attempt to obtain cosmetic improvement in athetoid patients.

Flexor Carpi Ulnaris Transfer

Careful assessment of the degree of deformity present before surgery and measure of the tendon balance at the wrist are important to anticipate the muscle power balance after flexor carpi ulnaris tendon transfer. It is critical to determine whether an increase in extensor power or a decrease in flexor power should be obtained to adjust the tightness of the tendon transfer correctly. The degree of wrist flexion needed to enable the patient to extend the fingers is noted. Increased extension of the wrist is provided at surgery when good finger extension is available preoperatively. If reasonable finger extension is absent, the tendon transfer should not be pulled so tight as to prevent some wrist flexion. The power of the wrist extensor muscles can be evaluated more accurately by temporarily blocking the flexors with a local anesthetic.[28]

Procedure. The basic steps of the Green procedure are the following (Fig. 33–1). A longitudinal incision is carried out from the area of insertion of the flexor carpi ulnaris distally, along the ulna over the muscle belly proximally. The flexor carpi ulnaris tendon is identified and dissected far enough distally to section the tendon at its attachment on the pisiform bone. The muscle is then carefully dissected from the ulna proximally to its origin, taking care to preserve its neurovascular supply. An oblique subcutaneous tunnel is made from the origin of the muscle, along the forearm, and around the dorsum of the wrist to the level of the extensor carpi radialis brevis tendon distally. This tendon is the favored recipient for the transfer because it is a neutral extensor of the wrist. The flexor carpi ulnaris tendon is then rerouted through this tunnel and securely woven through the extensor carpi radialis brevis tendon, about 2 to 4 cm proximal to the wrist. The tension of the transfer is carefully adjusted, and the tendon is firmly fixed with multiple interrupted 3-0 nonabsorbable sutures (Dacron). The extremity is immobilized in a long arm cast with the wrist in moderate dorsiflexion and the forearm in

supination. The cast is worn for approximately 6 weeks.

Complications. The following technical considerations are important to avoid complications in performing a flexor carpi ulnaris transfer. The flexor carpi ulnaris must be dissected far enough distally and sectioned off its attachment on the pisiform to obtain sufficient length. The muscle tendon unit must be carefully dissected, taking care to avoid the ulnar artery and the ulnar nerve and its branches. The motor branches must be protected on dissecting the unit proximally. The tendon should be directed as longitudinally as possible to its new insertion into the neutral wrist extensor, the extensor carpi radialis brevis. The second extensor retinacular compartment should be incised approximately 4 cm to allow proper interweaving of the flexor carpi ulnaris tendon into the extensor carpi radialis brevis tendon; this insertion must be securely sutured with multiple 3-0 nonabsorbable sutures (Dacron).

Cerebral palsied patients are more likely to tear out tendon suture lines, and therefore careful suturing technique and postoperative immobilization are important. The wrist should be kept extended, with the forearm at neutral or slight supination in a long arm cast for 8 weeks. Stress should be avoided for another 4 to 6 weeks in the rehabilitation program.

Extension deformity of the wrists can occur early or late. It is usually due to making the transfer too tight. The wrist should be able to be flexed to 30° with the forearm in supination. If there are inadequate wrist flexors to balance wrist extension after the flexor carpi ulnaris has been moved, late contracture can occur. Treatment of wrist contracture can include lengthening of the tendon and release of restricting scar in the tunnel of the transferred muscle.

Flexion Deformity of the Fingers

Flexion deformity of the fingers is the result of severe spasticity and myostatic contracture of the flexor muscles, and is usually associated with flexion and pronation of the wrist. Treatment of this deformity includes the following methods:

1. Attempts at conservative stretching of the muscle contracture with bracing; should always precede any surgical procedure

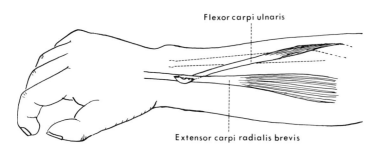

Flexor carpi ulnaris

Extensor carpi radialis brevis

Figure 33–1. The Green procedure for transfer of the flexor carpi ulnaris subcutaneously to the extensor carpi radialis brevis is the preferred method of treatment of flexion deformity of the wrist in cerebral palsy. (From Swanson, A. B.: Surgery of the hand in cerebral palsy and muscle release procedures. Surg. Clin. North Am., 48:1129, 1968.)

2. Release of the flexor muscle's origin[29]
3. Lengthening of individual tendons participating in the deformity
4. Lengthening of multiple tendons
5. Continued bracing after the surgical procedure

Flexor Muscle Origin Release

The flexor muscle origin release, which we first performed in cerebral palsied patients in 1963, allows the flexor muscles to reattach distally without interrupting their main neurovascular supply.[29] The purpose of this procedure is to obtain a new shorter resting or postural length, thereby decreasing the tension developed and the stretch reflex or contractile response of the muscle. This decreases strength as well as spasticity and contracture. The flexor origin release procedure is most useful to rebalance the extensor-flexor forces and to improve hand function.[5, 9, 12, 20, 24, 29, 32, 33, 36]

Procedure. The flexor origin procedure is specifically indicated for patients who have a voluntary grasp and release pattern, and who present flexor muscle contractures that make wrist flexion necessary to obtain finger extension. This procedure is indicated when complete finger extension cannot be achieved with the wrist in more than 30° of flexion, or when there is obvious contracture on passive extension of the fingers with the wrist in from 30 to 70° of flexion. Injection of a dilute solution of procaine into the flexor mass can also help to determine the degree of spasticity and myostatic contracture. Additional release of the pronator teres can improve the frequently associated pronation deformity. Occasionally, the lacertus fibrosus may be incised, especially if flexion contracture of the elbow is present.

The flexor release procedure is carried out through an incision starting approximately 3 cm proximal to the medial epicondyle and carried down over the ulnar proximal two thirds of the forearm (Fig. 33–2). The pronator-flexor mass is sectioned from the capsular structures over the medial epicondyle and advanced distally. The median nerve is identified and protected. The dissection is carried along the ulna, avoiding the proximal motor branches of the ulnar nerve and sectioning all the muscular attachments from the proximal ulna and interosseous membrane distally. Infrequently, if the flexor pollicis longus is to be recessed, an additional incision over the radial aspect of the forearm is made to expose the radius. The released pronator-flexor muscle mass can then be demonstrated to move 3 to 5 cm distally by hyperextending the fingers and wrist. The pronator teres, flexor digitorum sublimis and profundus, flexor carpi radialis, flexor carpi ulnaris, and palmaris longus have a new shorter resting length position. The muscle mass, especially the pronator teres, may be sutured to the underlying structures at the desired level for reattachment. If the motor branches of the ulnar nerve appear to be under tension, the ulnar nerve can be rerouted anteriorly.

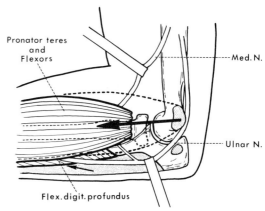

Figure 33–2. Release of the origin of the flexor-pronator muscles in the forearm. The proximal attachments are released and allowed to move 3 to 5 cm distally. The neurovascular supply is left intact. The muscle mass, especially the pronator teres, may be sutured to the underlying structures at the desired level. Because the length of the muscles is decreased, the stretch reflex is decreased and, consequently, the flexion deformity of the fingers and wrist are relieved. (From Swanson, A. B.: Surgery of the hand in cerebral palsy and muscle release procedures. Surg. Clin. North Am., 48:1129, 1968.)

Multiple drains are placed in the wound or a negative pressure drainage apparatus is used for 2 days to prevent postoperative hematoma. The fingers and wrist are held in hyperextension to maintain the distal positioning of the muscle origins in the operative dressing. The proximal interphalangeal joints are flexed to 30°. A voluminous conforming dressing and a plaster cast are applied with the elbow at 90° of flexion, the wrist and metacarpophalangeal joints in 0° of extension, and the forearm in supination. This cast is worn for approximately 3 weeks. A physical and occupational therapy program is then started. The patient is instructed to wear a modified pancake brace between treatments for 3 to 6 weeks. The brace is worn at night for an additional 3 months or longer, as necessary.

The flexor carpi ulnaris origin and its tendon can be left intact for a Green transfer in patients who present excessively weak wrist extensors preoperatively or in some patients who desire, for cosmetic reasons, the assurance that their wrist will no longer present a flexion deformity. White has performed a wrist arthrodesis in association with the flexor origin release procedure; however, this is believed to be unnecessary.[36]

Complications From Muscle Origin and Tendon Release Procedures. Complications from muscle origin and tendon release procedures can stem from injury to associated important anatomic structures during surgery. Avoiding injury to nerves and vessels requires an awareness of their location and careful tissue handling. Muscle ischemia can be prevented by incision of overlying fascia. Hematoma formation is prevented by control of all bleeders after the tourniquet has been released. The wounds are drained with standard tissue drains. Postoperative swelling should be controlled with a bulky conforming dressing and nonconstrictive splintage and elevation.

Individual Tendon Lengthening

In patients presenting contracture of selective flexor tendons of the wrist or digits, Z step-cut lengthening of individual tendons at their musculotendinous junction in the forearm can provide adequate release. This may be especially important for the flexor pollicis longus or flexor sublimis tendons.

Multiple Tendon Lengthening

Patients presenting severe clasping of the fingers into the palm with inability to extend the fingers until wrist flexion is greater than 70° may be candidates for multiple tendon releases in the forearm. These patients usually have poor functional potential and inadequate sensibility, and do not demonstrate voluntary grasp and release patterns. This type of release is appropriate for severe cases of flexion contracture of the digits and wrist to allow the patients to get the fingers permanently out of the palm for cosmetic and hygienic reasons. The surgery consists of step-cut lengthening of the tendons or, as we prefer, a transfer of the cut ends of the sublimis to the profundus tendons.[4]

The surgical procedure is carried out at the distal forearm; the sublimis tendons are cut distally and the profundus tendons are cut proximally. The proximal ends of the sectioned sublimis tendons are transferred to the distal ends of the sectioned profundi tendons with proper tension, because the fingers and wrist are in neutral position. The fingers and wrist are immobilized in extension in a long arm cast for approximately 6 weeks.

The rehabilitation program should include physical and occupational therapy in an attempt to obtain useful functional adaptations for using the hand as an assistive hand. Nighttime splinting to maintain extension should be continued for many months until the balance of extensors and flexors has been stabilized.

Intrinsic muscle tightness may become more obvious when the long finger flexors are released. Swan-neck deformities may become severe. We have done a sublimis tenodesis procedure at the proximal interphalangeal joint (see below) to correct this problem. Intrinsic muscle release procedures could be appropriate if a severe intrinsic-plus deformity occurs. This has been unnecessary in our cases. Selective preoperative local anesthetic blocks of the median nerve at the elbow can assist in predicting the postoperative condition, and should be used.

Thumb-in-Palm Deformity

The thumb-in-palm deformity in cerebral palsy can be most disabling by interfering further with already handicapped pinch and grasp patterns. This deformity has several components, and treatment must consider each factor contributing to the disability. As the fingers are flexed, the thumb may be drawn across the palm in an adducted position, or the metacarpal may be adducted and contracted with a tendency for hyperextension deformity of the metacarpophalangeal joint. The goal of treatment is to achieve adequate active abduction of the thumb. Pulp pinch can seldom be obtained in reconstruction of these thumbs; however, lateral or key pinch can be adequately restored, and is probably more useful in such cases.

The first step in the treatment of this deformity, as in any other cerebral palsy deformity, should be the application of conservative methods and bracing. When the patient presents a contracture or moderate spasticity of the intrinsic muscles, the origin of the adductor pollicis is released from the third metacarpal and the flexor pollicis is released from the volar carpal ligament.[13, 17, 29, 33] If active abduction of the thumb is weak it can be reinforced with a tendon transfer, using the brachioradialis or the flexor carpi radialis. If there is an extension deformity or instability of the metacarpophalangeal joint of the thumb, a capsulorrhaphy of this joint is done in children or an arthrodesis is done in later age groups. A flexion deformity of the distal phalanx of the thumb can be corrected by lengthening the flexor pollicis longus at its myotendinous junction or by reinforcing the extensor pollicis brevis. The intermetacarpal bone block procedure has been avoided for the treatment of the thumb-in-palm deformity in our clinic because the fixed post cannot provide accurate pinch to the fingers of an uncoordinated cerebral palsy hand. Among other drawbacks, it can also be a problem for a patient who requires crutches for walking.

Thumb Intrinsic Muscles Origin Release

Release of the thumb intrinsic muscles origins is performed through a palmar incision paralleling the thenar crease (Fig. 33–3). The arteries and nerves in the area are identified and carefully retracted. The transverse and oblique heads of the adductor pollicis are identified, and their origin is released from the third metacarpal by blunt dissection. The deep ulnar motor branch to the interosseous muscles is preserved. The motor branch of the median nerve to the thenar muscles is identified and carefully avoided. Both heads of the flexor pollicis brevis, opponens pollicis, and the distal two thirds of the abductor pollicis brevis muscles may also be sectioned at their origins to the volar carpal ligament and recessed distally; however, this is usually unnecessary. The attachment of the first dorsal interosseous to the first metacarpal may also be released in the depths of the wound after adequate retraction of the released muscles; however, this has usually not been found to be necessary. Care is taken to avoid the perforating branch of the radial artery. The wound is closed and subcutaneous drains are inserted. A bulky conforming dressing and plaster

Figure 33–3. Release of the origin of the intrinsic muscles of the thumb for thumb-in-palm deformities involving spastic adduction of the metacarpal. The transverse head and a portion of the oblique head of the adductor pollicis are released at their origin. The flexor pollicis brevis and two thirds of the abductor pollicis may occasionally be released from the transverse carpal ligament. The attachment of the first dorsal interosseous to the first metacarpal may also be released, if necessary. The motor branches of the ulnar and median nerve may be preserved. (From Swanson, A. B.: Surgery of the hand in cerebral palsy and muscle release procedures. Surg. Clin. North Am., 48:1129, 1968.)

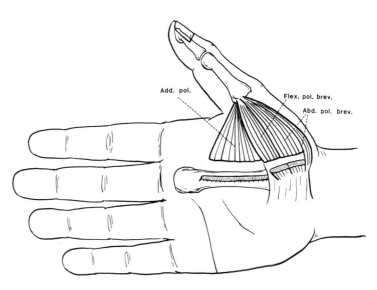

cast are applied, with the first metacarpal widely abducted. It is important to ensure that the metacarpal and not the phalanges of the thumb are abducted. A Kirschner wire may be passed between the first and second metacarpals for temporary fixation in severe cases.

Capsulorrhaphy of the Metacarpophalangeal Joint

Capsulorrhaphy of the metacarpophalangeal joint of the thumb can be done successfully in children who have hyperextension deformity of this joint. The palmar aspect of the joint is approached through a lateral incision. The proximal membranous insertions of the palmar plate are incised. The sesamoid bones and their tendinous attachments are left intact. The periosteum is stripped from the volar aspect of the neck of the metacarpal, and two small drill holes made through the bone in a vertical direction are connected with a curet to form a cavity on the volar side. The dorsal aspect of the palmar plate is roughened and fixed into the bony depression with a pull-out wire suture exiting dorsally over a button. The suture is placed through the palmar plate flap to obtain 10 to 15° of flexion of the metacarpophalangeal joint, and a Kirschner wire is placed obliquely across the joint to hold the desired degree of flexion. The pull-out suture is removed in 3 weeks and the Kirschner wire is removed in 6 weeks. This procedure has worked very well to correct hyperextension deformity if attention is paid to obtain bony union of the palmar plate to the metacarpal.

Tenodesis or capsulodesis procedures can successfully and permanently restrict joint movement if the attachment of the restraining soft tissue has good bony ingrowth. The tissue should be pulled into a bony defect that exposes cancellous bone, and should be securely immobilized until Sharpey's bone fibers grow into it. This requires about 6 weeks of absolute fixation and another 6 weeks of protec-

tion against stretching. Once bony healing into the soft tissue occurs, there should be no stretching out of the attachment as one would see with only soft tissue healing.

Fusion of the Metacarpophalangeal Joint

The metacarpophalangeal joint is fused in 10° of flexion, 5° of abduction, and slight pronation. A longitudinal wire is placed in a retrograde fashion across both the interphalangeal and the metacarpophalangeal joints, and is left extruding 5 to 10 mm from the tip of the thumb. A second wire is inserted obliquely across the metacarpophalangeal joint to maintain the position desired. The fusion area is firmly compressed to ensure good contact of the raw bone surfaces. The longitudinal wire is removed in 6 weeks, and the oblique wire may be left in place.

Tendon Transfers for the Thumb

In patients presenting weak abduction and extension of the thumb, the abductor power can be reinforced with a tendon transfer. Common tendon transfers used for the thumb in cerebral palsy include that of the flexor carpi radialis or brachioradialis to the abductor pollicis longus, extensor pollicis brevis, or extensor pollicis longus. We prefer using the brachioradialis for this transfer because it has good strength and, if well dissected proximally, it offers adequate amplitude of 3 to 4 cm.

Transfer of the brachioradialis muscle is performed using a dorsoradial incision starting at the elbow and exposing the full length of the musculotendinous unit (Fig. 33–4). The brachioradialis tendon is cut distally, and the dissection is carried proximally to the origin of the muscle. Care must be taken to preserve the radial neurovascular unit and its branches to the brachioradialis muscle. A good release will allow a greater contractural excursion of the short belly muscle. The appropriate

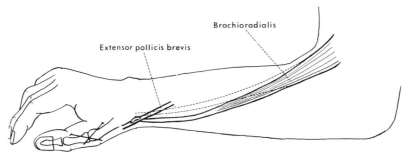

Figure 33–4. Transfer of the brachioradialis to the extensor pollicis brevis or longus or to the abductor pollicis longus. Stabilization of the metacarpophalangeal joint of the thumb either by fusion or by capsulorrhaphy is necessary to prevent hyperextension tendencies. (From Swanson, A. B.: Surgery of the hand in cerebral palsy and muscle release procedures. Surg. Clin. North Am., 48:1129, 1968.)

extensor compartment is incised longitudinally to allow either the extensor pollicis longus or brevis or the abductor pollicis to be rerouted in the line of pull of the abductors. The tendon of the brachioradialis is interwoven through the selected recipient tendons for the transfer, the tension is carefully adjusted, and the transfer is firmly secured with multiple nonabsorbable sutures. Transfer to the extensor pollicis longus is usually preferred. The metacarphalanageal joint must be stabilized either by fusion or capsulorrhaphy to prevent hyperextension tendencies. The wound is closed in layers, and drains are placed subcutaneously. A voluminous conforming dressing and a full arm plaster cast are applied with the elbow at 90° of flexion, the wrist in neutral position, and the thumb widely abducted. After 6 weeks of immobilization, acitve use of the hand is resumed with special attention to abduction exercises and long-term splinting.

Swan-Neck Deformity of the Fingers

Swan-neck deformity is common in the cerebral palsied hand, and has been studied using local anesthetic nerve blocks to determine the muscle group that is primarily causing the deformity.[27-33] It has been stated in the literature that the swan-neck deformity is due to overactive intrinsics. In some cases it was noted that, when the intrinsics were paralyzed through a distal medial and ulnar block, the deformity disappeared. In other cases, anesthetizing the interosseous branch of the radial nerve was necessary to block the long extensor muscle action before the swan-neck deformity disappeared. It was felt that both extrinsic and intrinsic muscles contributed to the deformity.

However, it appears that the main cause of the swan-neck deformity in the cerebral palsied hand is the result of a muscle imbalance caused by a chronic flexion of the wrist and metacarpophalangeal joints, and by secondary ligamentous and capsular relaxation at the proximal interphalangeal joints (Fig. 33–5).[14, 16, 26, 27, 29-31, 34, 35] The deformity is produced, basically, by the relative shortness of the central tendon as compared to the lateral tendons. It is caused by chronic tension from the long extensor and intrinsic muscles to the central tendon. Stretching of the volar capsule and ligaments allows hyperextension of the proximal interphalangeal joint to occur. The distal interphalangeal and metacarpophalangeal joints become flexed. The fingers frequently lock in extension, and the force of pinch and grasp is lost. Extension of the metacarpophalangeal joint is affected because of the loss of prox-

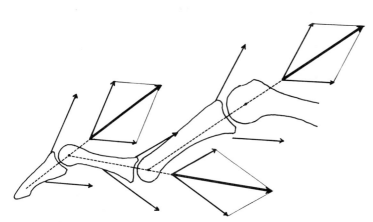

Figure 33–5. Diagram of deforming forces that contribute to swan-neck deformity. Both extrinsic and intrinsic muscles contribute to the collapse deformity; however, the main cause of deformity in cerebral palsy is chronic flexion of the wrist and metacarpophalangeal joints, with secondary ligamentous and capsular relaxation of the proximal interphalangeal joints.

imal interphalangeal joint flexion, and patients are frequently concerned about the appearance of their hand. When swan-neck collapse deformity is present, surgical treatment is indicated.[27, 29–33]

If the deformity is not too severe, surgical treatment can be directed toward relief of the overloading forces on the extension side of the proximal interphalangeal joint, either by lengthening the extensor communis tendon or by blocking its extension by tenodesis at the proximal phalanx. Relocating the dorsally displaced lateral tendons palmarward toward the center of axis of rotation of the joint will improve the balance of the retinacular ligament system, and maintaining the lateral tendons in this position may be important. Resection of the spiral or oblique fibers of the extensor expansion from the intrinsics to the central tendon may relieve some of the overloading of the central tendon attachment. If the hyperextensibility of the proximal interphalangeal joint is too great, the deformity will recur. In these cases it is necessary to prevent hyperextension if the normal flexion arc of the finger is to be restored. The simplest and most effective procedure in the flexible swan-neck deformity is to place the proximal interphalangeal joint in some initial flexion by palmar capsulorrhaphy of the proximal interphalangeal joint or, preferably, by sublimis tenodesis. The flexor sublimis tenodesis procedure, such as we have originally described, is a most useful technique to correct the swan-neck deformity of cerebral palsied hands satisfactorily.

Flexor Sublimis Tenodesis

Tenodesis of the sublimis tendon to the neck of the proximal phalanx creates a checkrein to hyperextension. Placing the proximal interphalangeal joint in 20 to 40° of flexion, as necessary to establish a functional flexor arc, re-establishes the position of the lateral tendons and the retinacular ligament and also allows the flexors to produce proximal interphalangeal joint flexion without further locking the joint in hyperextension. Correction of the hyperextension of the proximal interphalangeal joint secondarily improves initial extension at the metacarpophalangeal joint and extension of the distal interphalangeal joint. This procedure, such as used in our clinic, has successfully corrected the deformity and markedly improved the function of these hands for the past 28 years. Full flexion of the joint is possible, and this procedure therefore has definite advantages over arthrodesis.

The flexor sheath is exposed through a midlateral incision, at the proximal interphalangeal joint and incised longitudinally to expose the flexor tendons (Fig. 33–6). The palmar plate is partially resected at its proximal portion so that it will not interfere with the tenodesis. It should be noted that tenodesis of the flexor digitorum sublimis at this level will not interfere with the action of the flexor digitorum profundus. In this procedure, it is important to obtain good healing between the tendon and the bone to avoid recurrences of the deformity. Two

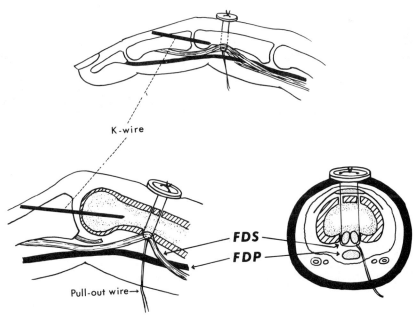

Figure 33–6. Sublimis tenodesis procedure to correct swan-neck deformities of the fingers. After placing two small drill holes through the neck of the proximal phalanx, a bed of raw bone is prepared for firm attachment of the tendon. The sublimis is pulled up well into the bone with a pull-out type suture left in place for 4 to 5 weeks. The proximal interphalangeal joint is immobilized in 20° to 40° of flexion with a Kirschner wire for a period of 6 to 8 weeks, or longer if necessary. *FDS,* flexor digitorum sublimis; *FDP,* flexor digitorum profundus. (From Swanson, A. B.: Surgery of the hand in cerebral palsy and muscle release procedures. Surg. Clin. North Am., 48:1129, 1968.)

small drill holes are placed approximately 0.25 inch apart through the palmar aspect of the neck of the proximal phalanx and connected with a curet. This will prepare a broad bony bed for attachment of the sublimis tendon. The end of the sublimis tendon is scarified and drawn up into the bone with a Bunnell-type pull-out suture.[3] The tension of the tenodesis should be adjusted to allow 20 to 40° of extension lag at the proximal interphalangeal joint. A small Kirschner wire is inserted across the proximal interphalangeal joint to maintain the desired degree of flexion throughout the healing period. The end of the wire is cut immediately under the skin, or cut so that 1 cm of wire extrudes from the skin. The cut end of the wire is capped with a plastic end.

The deep structures, including the retinacular ligament, are resutured with absorbable material. The skin is sutured, and a small drain is inserted subcutaneously. A voluminous conforming dressing is applied. If a plaster cast is used, it should include the elbow to prevent its distal migration, which could produce a straightening effect at the proximal interphalangeal joints.

The pull-out wire is removed in 4 to 5 weeks and the Kirschner wire is taken out in 6 to 8 weeks. Small aluminum splints may be taped onto the fingers to hold the proximal interphalangeal joint in flexion if the Kirschner wire needs to be removed prematurely, or if further immobilization is desired. It should be explained to the patient that the goal of the procedure is to obtain some degree of flexion contracture to prevent efforts to mobilize the fingers in extension.

This procedure can be performed in conjunction with other reconstructive procedures in the cerebral palsied hand. It has been used in our clinic to control disabling hyperextension deformities of the proximal interphalangeal joint from residuals of cerebral palsy, poliomyelitis, and rheumatoid arthritis. Postoperative recurrence of the deformity may be due to inadequate fixation of the tendon to the bone and to inadequate postoperative fixation of the joint. Proper application of the sublimis tenodesis procedure, as described above, should obviate these problems.

Wrist Arthrodesis Complications

Wrist arthrodesis complications include failure to fuse, injury of the distal epiphysis of the radius or ulna, poor position of the hand for function because of inadequate finger extension, and inability to place the hand in functional positions. The wrist should always be placed in the desired position in a cast preoperatively to evaluate the patient's functional adaptations, especially for extension of the fingers. If the patient cannot extend the digits with the wrist in extension, the fusion should not be done. Fusion should not be done across open epiphyses. Bone grafts can be taken from the ilium to facilitate healing. Internal fixation with Kirschner wires and staples is useful. Placing a portion of the extensor

retinaculum over the graft area and under the tendons will help to prevent adhesions of these structures.

BRACING OF THE SPASTIC HAND

Flexor muscles should not be stretched by extending the finger joints, because this may be a major cause of hyperextension deformities of the proximal interphalangeal joints. The normal arches of the palm and fingers should be respected and maintained. Myostatic contractures of the finger and wrist flexor muscles are best stretched by extending the wrist, not the fingers. The muscles should never be stretched at the expense of the joints.

A recommended night splint for a spastic hand is a modified pancake splint shaped of aluminum and covered with leather.[29, 32, 33] It is built up under the palmar arch and the proximal interphalangeal joints. The thumb is held abducted and extended to stretch the intrinsic muscles and the long thumb flexor. Finger and wrist flexors are then stretched by dorsiflexing the wrist portion of the splint.

CLASSIFICATION OF RESULTS AND EXPECTATIONS

The results of operative procedures for cerebral palsy in the upper extremity are difficult to predict and reproduce. Careful preoperative and postoperative evaluations are especially important in these patients. A useful classification of results for the hand as devised by the senior author is shown in Table 33–1.

We have described in this chapter selected deformities in the upper extremity related to muscle imbalance, spasticity, contracture, and joint instability associated with cerebral palsy that may be helped by certain surgical procedures. In the planning of the rehabilitation program, it is most important to repeat carefully the preoperative evaluation, record the functional and anatomic disabilities, and define the functional and cosmetic potentials, considering first the patient, then the extremity, and then the hand, in that order. Existing functional adaptations must never be sacrificed. A continued rehabilitation program must be planned. The postoperative progress and results must be evaluated objectively. In spite of all these considerations, one cannot expect to gain a normal hand.

Avoiding complications in the surgical treatment of the cerebral palsied hand depends on an understanding of the variety of types and severity of neurologic involvement. A very careful evaluation of the hand, as well as its relationship to the patient as a whole and proper selection of operative procedures that are carefully designed and performed, are essential to avoid disastrous complications. A postoperative rehabilitation program that considers the special needs of the cerebral palsy child is also of great importance. Proper application of these

Table 33–1. CLASSIFICATION OF RESULTS OF OPERATIVE PROCEDURES FOR CEREBRAL PALSY OF THE UPPER EXTREMITY

Characteristics	Excellent	Good	Fair	Poor
Grasp and release	Good	Good	Fair	Poor
Pinch	Tip, lateral, pulp	Lateral and pulp	Lateral	Poor
Hand placement	Good	Good	Fair	Poor
Control	Good	Good	Fair	Poor
Extension of fingers with wrist	To + 30°	From 0 to + 30°	From − 30 to 0°	At − 30°
Supination	> 45°	0 to 45°	To 0°	Not active
Joints	Stable	Stable	Unstable	Unstable
Sensibility	Good	Good	Fair	Poor
Activities of daily living	Good	Fair	Poor	None
Other	Integrated digit function		Helping hand	Hand—passive

concepts can result in improved function in selected cerebral palsy cases.

References

1. Bechtol, C. O.: Muscle physiology. *In* American Academy of Orthopaedic Surgeons: Instructional Course Lectures. Vol. 5, Ann Arbor, J. W. Edwards, 1948, pp. 181–189.
2. Boyd, I. A., et al.: The Role of the Gamma System in Movement and Posture, Association for the Aid of Crippled Children, St. Louis, The C. V. Mosby Co., 1964.
3. Boyes, J. H.: Bunnell's Surgery of the Hand, 4th ed., Philadelphia, J. B. Lippincott, 1964.
4. Braun, R. M., Guy, T. V., and Roper, B.: Preliminary experience with superficialis-to-profundus tendon transfer in the hemiplegic upper extremity. J. Bone Joint Surg. [Am.], 52:466, 1974.
5. Braun, R. M., Mooney, V., and Nickel, V. L.: Flexor-origin release for pronation-flexion deformity of the forearm and hand in stroke patients. An evaluation of the early results in eighteen patients. J. Bone Joint Surg., 52A:907, 1970.
6. Denhoff, E., and Robinault, I. P.: Cerebral Palsy and Related Disorders—A Developmental Approach to Dysfunction, New York, McGraw-Hill, 1960.
7. DeVries, J. S.: Encephalopathia Infantilis. A Study Based on Patients and Orthopaedic Procedures, Asten, N. Br., The Netherlands, Schrik's Drukkerij, 1967.
8. Goldner, J. L.: Reconstructive surgery of the hand in cerebral palsy and spastic paralysis resulting from injury to the spinal cord. J. Bone Joint Surg., 37A:1141, 1955.
9. Gorynski, T., and Jedrzejewska, H.: Chirurgiczne leczenie zniekształcen i zabursen czynnosciowych nadgarstka i palcow w porazeniah mozgowych. Chir. Narzadow Ruchu Ortop. Pol. 25:621, 1960.
10. Green, W. T., and Banks, H. H.: Flexor carpi ulnaris transplant and its use in cerebral palsy. J. Bone Joint Surg., 44A:1343, 1962.
11. Illingworth, R. S.: Recent Advances in Cerebral Palsy. Boston, Little, Brown & Company, 1958.
12. Inglis, A. E., and Cooper, W.: Release of the flexor-pronator origin. J. Bone Joint Surg., 48A:847, 1966.
13. Inglis, A. E., Cooper, W., and Bruton, W.: Surgical correction of thumb deformities in spastic paralysis. J. Bone Joint Surg., 52A:253, 1970.
14. Kaplan, E. B.: Functional and Surgical Anatomy of the Hand, 2nd ed., Philadelphia, J. B. Lippincott, 1965.
15. Keats, S.: Operative Orthopaedics in Cerebral Palsy, Springfield, IL, Charles C Thomas, 1970.
16. Landsmeer, J. M. F.: The anatomy of the dorsal aponeurosis of the human finger and its functional significance. Anat. Rec., 104:31, 1949.

17. Matev, I.: Surgical treatment of spastic "thumb-in-palm" deformity. J. Bone Joint Surg., 45B:703, 1963.
18. Moberg, E.: Objective methods for determining the functional value of sensibility in the hand. J. Bone Joint Surg., 40B:454, 1958.
19. Mooney, V., Frykham, G., and McLamb, J.: Current status of intraneural phenol injections, Clin. Orthop., 63:122, 1969.
20. Page, C. M.: An operation for the relief of flexion-contracture in the forearm. J. Bone Joint Surg., 5:233, 1923.
21. Perlstein, M. A.: Infantile cerebral palsy. Classification and clinical correlations. J.A.M.A., 149:30, 1952.
22. Phelps, W. M.: Long-term results of orthopaedic surgery in cerebral palsy. J. Bone Joint Surg., 39A:53, 1957.
23. Samilson, R. L., and Morris, J. M.: Surgical improvement of the cerebral palsied upper limb. J. Bone Joint Surg., 46A:1203, 1964.
24. Scaglietti, O.: Sindromi cliniche immediate e tardive da lesioni vascolari nelle frature degli arti, Vol. 8, Archivio Putti, di Chirurgia Degli Organi di Movimento, 1957.
25. Steindler, A.: Pathokinetics of cerebral palsy. *In* American Academy of Orthopaedic Surgeons: Instructional Course Lectures, Vol. 9, Ann Arbor, J. W. Edwards, 1952, pp. 118–129.
26. Sunderland, S.: The actions of the extensor digitorum communis, interosseous and lumbrical muscles. Am. J. Anat., 77:189, 1945.
27. Swanson, A. B.: Surgery of the hand in cerebral palsy and the swan-neck deformity. J. Bone Joint Surg., 42A:951, 1960.
28. Swanson, A. B.: Considerations for surgery of the hand in cerebral palsy. Bull. N.Y. Acad. Med., 10:170, 1964.
29. Swanson, A. B.: Surgery of the hand in cerebral palsy. Surg. Clin. North Am., 44:1061, 1964.
30. Swanson, A. B.: Pathomechanics of the swan-neck deformity. J. Bone Joint Surg., 47A:636, 1965.
31. Swanson, A. B.: Treatment of the swan-neck deformity in the cerebral palsied hand. Clin. Orthop., 48:167, 1966.
32. Swanson, A. B.: Surgery of the hand in cerebral palsy and muscle release procedures. Surg. Clin. North Am., 48:1129, 1968.
33. Swanson, A. B.: Surgery of the hand in cerebral palsy. *In* Flynn, J. E. (ed.): Hand Surgery, 3rd ed., Baltimore, Williams & Wilkins, 1982, pp. 476–488.
34. Tachdjian, M. O., and Minear, W. L.: Sensory disturbances in the hands of children with cerebral palsy. J. Bone Joint Surg., 40A:85, 1958.
35. Tubiana, R., and Valentin, P.: The physiology of the extension of the fingers. Surg. Clin. North Am., 44:907, 1964.
36. White, W. F.: Flexor-muscle slide in the spastic hand. J. Bone Joint Surg., 54B:453, 1972.
37. Zancolli, E. A., Goldner, L. J., and Swanson, A. B.: Surgery of the spastic hand in cerebral palsy: Report of the Committee on Spastic Hand Evaluation. J. Hand Surg., 8 (Part 2):766, 1983.

INDEX

Superficial palmar arch (*Continued*)
variations in anatomy of, *3*, 3–4
Supernumerary digits, 338–344
Suture(s), placement of, in repair of
flexor tendon injuries, 31, *32*
Swan-neck deformity, 27, *27*
as complication of tendon transfer,
for ulnar nerve paralysis, 62–64, *63*
improper flexor tendon repair and, 36
in cerebral palsy, 370, *370*
treatment of, *371*, 371–372
in rheumatoid arthritis, 245, *245*
in children, 266, *266*
of thumb, in rheumatoid arthritis,
246, *246*
Sympathectomy, for pain of reflex sympathetic dystrophy, 91, 172
Sympathetic dystrophy, reflex. See *Reflex sympathetic dystrophy.*
Sympathetic nerve block, for pain in reflex dystrophy, *88–90*, 89, 91
after surgery for Dupuytren's disease, 298
Symphalangism, *328*
adaptation to, 328–329
treatment of, *329*, 329–330
Syndactyly, 330
central polydactyly with, 340–342
in Apert's syndrome, 332, *333*
treatment of, 330–331
complications of, 330–332, *330–332*
Synovitis, in reaction to rod, in staged
flexor tendon grafting, 36–37, *37*
in rheumatoid arthritis, involving
shoulder, 240–241
involving wrist, 241, *244*
Systemic response pain, in reflex sympathetic dystrophy, 91–92
treatment of, 92

Tactile gnosis, 307
Teeth wounds, of hand, 43, 235, *315*,
316, *316*
Temperature, digital, as index of blood
flow status, 7, *7–8*, 9
Tendon(s). See also specific structures,
e.g., *Flexor tendons.*
adhesions of, at site of fracture of
phalanx, 139–142, *140, 141*
in reconstructed hand, 323
injuries of, crushing, 217(t), 223–224
fracture of distal radius and, 169–
170
fracture of phalanx and, 139, *140*
rupture of, missed diagnosis of, 319,
319
severance of, 317, *317*, *318*, *320*
thumb, rupture of, in rheumatoid arthritis, 246
Tendon flap, retrograde, for boutonnière deformity, 42, *42*
Tendon graft, restoration of extensor
function with, 45–46
limiting of, to metacarpophalangeal
joint, *45*, 46
Tendon transfer, for extensor tendon
injuries on dorsum of hand, 45, *45*

Tendon transfer (*Continued*)
for paralysis of hand, 50–68. See also
under nerve sites of paralysis.
complications of, 50–68
for thumb-in-palm deformity, in cerebral palsy, 369–370, *370*
Tenodesis, slackening of, as complication, of hand and elbow procedures, in upper extremity surgery
for tetraplegia, 126
Tenolysis, for extensor tendon adhesions, 46–47
in treatment of boutonnière deformity, 43, *43*
for tendon adhesions, at site of fracture of phalanx, *141*, 142
Tenosynovitis, infection and, 233
complications of, 234–235
treatment of, 233–234, *234*
stenosing, of thumb, in rheumatoid
arthritis, 246
Tetraplegia, loss of upper extremity
function in, 123(t)
surgery for, complications of, 124–
126
construction of hand grip in, 123–
124, *124*
complications of, 125–126
goals of, 127
rehabilitation after, 125–126
restoration of elbow extension in,
123, *124*
complications of, 125–126
Thenar compartment of hand, 5
Thenar space, 232
abscess of, 233, *233*
incisions for drainage of, 233
Thermal injuries. See *Burn(s).*
Thermography, blood flow studies with,
7
Thrombosis, risk of, in upper extremity
trauma, 225, 226
Thumb, abduction of, loss of, radial
nerve injury and, 94, *95*
amputation of, cold intolerance in
stump as complication of, 203
replantation after, and loss of motion, 209
retention vs. resection of stump in,
200, *202*
bite injury of, *316*
boutonnière deformity of, in rheumatoid arthritis, 245, *246*
contracture of, improper immobilization and, *324*
contracture of soft tissue of, as congenital anomaly, 333–334
dangle (floating), in radial agenesis,
357, *358*
extension of, loss of, radial nerve injury and, 94, *95*
flexor tendon injuries of, zone classification of, 22(t)
growth of, excessive, *350*
hypoplastic, stretching of, 326, *326*
interphalangeal joint of, flexion of, in
ulnar nerve injury, 97, *97*
intrinsic muscles of, release of origin
of, for thumb-in-palm deformity, in
cerebral palsy, 368–369, *369*